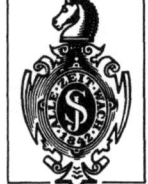

R.P. Sengupta · V.L. McAllister

Subarachnoid Haemorrhage

Foreword by Sir John Walton

With 243 Figures and 130 Tables

Springer-Verlag
Berlin Heidelberg NewYork Tokyo

R.P. Sengupta, MSc, FRCS, FRCS (Ed)
Consultant Neurosurgeon
Newcastle General Hospital
Westgate Road
Newcastle upon Tyne NE4 6BE

V.L. McAllister, DMRD, FRCR
Consultant Neuroradiologist
Regional Neurological Centre
Newcastle General Hospital
Westgate Road
Newcastle upon Tyne NE4 6BE

ISBN-13:978-1-4471-1385-0   e-ISBN-13:978-1-4471-1383-6
DOI: 10.1007/978-1-4471-1383-6

Library of Congress Cataloging-in-Publication Data
Sengupta, R.P. (Ram Prasad), 1937–   . Subarachnoid haemorrhage.
Includes bibliographies and index. 1. Subarachnoid hemorrhage. 2. Intracranial aneurysms. I. McAllister, V. (Victor), 1941–   . [DNLM: 1. Cerebral Aneurysm. 2. Subarachnoid Hemorrhage-diagnosis. 3. Subarachnoid Hemorrhage-therapy. WL 200 S476s] RC394.H37S46 1985 616.8'1 85-12669
ISBN-13:978-1-4471-1385-0 (U.S.)

Filmset by Polyglot Pte Ltd. Singapore.

2128/3916 543210

Foreword

Ever since I began my training in internal medicine and subsequently in neurology, I have been interested in subarachnoid haemorrhage and indeed chose this topic as a subject of study for my Doctorate in Medicine. It was because the information derived from a retrospective study of 312 patients proved to be so interesting that I published a monograph on the subject 30 years ago. My first reaction on reading this splendid book by my former colleagues in Newcastle, Mr. Sengupta and Dr. McAllister, was one of realisation of the extent to which knowledge about the condition and principles of management have been transformed. This splendidly comprehensive volume carefully reviews the earlier literature, analyses the anatomical, pathophysiological and clinical features of the condition in consummate detail and goes on to consider in depth all of those issues relating to investigation and medical and surgical management which continue to present challenges to neurologists and neuro-surgeons alike.

When I began my personal study, angiography had still to be introduced as a routine method of radiological diagnosis in many centres in the U.K. and we were largely dependent upon clinical methods of diagnosis and assessment. How interesting it is to see that now, very properly, computerised tomography (CT scanning) takes precedence as an initial diagnostic instrument over angiography, and that lumbar puncture, once thought to be obligatory for diagnosis, is being used less and less since its dangers were fully appreciated.

As one scans through the pages of this volume, one cannot fail to be impressed by the comprehensive coverage of the subject which the authors have achieved. Each time I considered whether they might conceivably have overlooked some minor point of interest of which I had become aware over the years, I looked for it and it was there. Superbly illustrated, clearly written and thoroughly referenced, this volume will, I am sure, be very successful. All of those with an interest in the subject, whether they be physicians in internal medicine, pathologists, anaesthetists or radiologists, and of course neurologists and neurosurgeons in particular, would profit from possessing this book to which I have no doubt they would wish to turn regularly for information and advice about the condition and its management. Mr. Sengupta and Dr. McAllister have done a thorough workmanlike job and deserve our thanks and congratulations.

Green College, Oxford   Sir John Walton, TD, MA, MD, DSc, FRCP

Preface

It is nearly 30 years since Sir John Walton published his classic book on subarachnoid haemorrhage from Newcastle. Since then, there have been revolutionary advances in the diagnosis and the medical and surgical management of this clinical syndrome. The authors believe, therefore, that there is a need for an up-to-date monograph on subarachnoid haemorrhage.

A ruptured intracranial aneurysm is by far the commonest cause of subarachnoid haemorrhage. The fate of those harbouring a ruptured aneurysm is grim indeed. It has been estimated that three out of every five of these patients will die at the end of the first year, one will be disabled and only one will lead a normal life. Therefore, the neurosurgeon's task is to treat it in time before another haemorrhage occurs. This is reflected in the larger proportion of the book dealing with the diagnosis and management of cerebral aneurysms. However, less common causes of subarachnoid haemorrhage are also included. The development in anaesthesiology and microsurgical techniques has resulted in improved outcome following surgery for intracranial aneurysms and arteriovenous malformations.

The clinical picture of a major subarachnoid haemorrhage is well known, but it is not widely recognised that a large proportion of aneurysms produce a warning leak before a major haemorrhage. Since the result of surgery at this stage is ideal, recognition of a minor subarachnoid haemorrhage is of paramount importance. The best chance of survival following subarachnoid haemorrhage depends not only on its early recognition and prompt referral to a neurological centre, but also on appropriate medical management by the first attending physician. For this purpose, early management of subarachnoid haemorrhage at the primary hospital has been clearly defined.

The introduction of the CT scanner has opened up new vistas in our understanding of the natural history and living pathology of subarachnoid haemorrhage, and has proved invaluable in the management of patients with subarachnoid haemorrhage.

In writing this book, personal experience of 1000 patients with subarachnoid haemorrhage of varied aetiology, drawn from a geographically defined population of two and a half million, during a 10-year period, has been taken into account. The first 500 cases of intracranial aneurysms operated upon by one of the authors (RPS), between 1969 and 1980, have been analysed in detail. To identify the source of haemorrhage, patients with proved subarachnoid haemorrhage admitted between January 1980 and March 1983 have been critically evaluated. To assess the role of CT scan in the management of subarachnoid haemorrhage, a consecutive series of 500 patients has been studied. Since the incidence of subarachnoid haemorrhage in children is rare, we reviewed the records of all the children admitted with proven subarachnoid haemorrhage to the Regional Neurological Centre since 1960.

The improvements in anaesthetic techniques have contributed much to the success of surgical management, and this is reflected by devoting a chapter entirely to them. This is written by Dr. J. D. Whitby, who took an active part in the management of patients with aneurysmal subarachnoid haemorrhage since 1950.

This book, although reflecting a personal viewpoint, nevertheless will outline the mainstream of thought on the subject of subarachnoid haemorrhage, and will be a comprehensive reference work for those engaged in the field of subarachnoid haemorrhage.

Acknowledgements

We are especially indebted to Dr. V. R. Sastry Kolluri and Dr. Peter Gates for their invaluable assistance in preparing this book. We are very grateful to our colleagues who have entrusted their patients to our care, the experience of which provided the basis for this book. We are also grateful to Dr. David Bates, Professor John Hankinson and Dr. Ian Wagstaff for their constructive criticism and advice. We are indebted to Professor B. Worthington for the section on MRI in Chapter 17. Our deepest appreciation is extended to Dr. Robert Perry and Dr. D. P. Purohit for providing pathological illustrations, to Mr. Angus McNay for statistical analysis and to Mr. D. Hammersley for drawings. Grateful thanks are due to our junior colleagues, particularly Dr. Goran Algers, Dr. Y. T. Kan and Dr. Subba Rao for helping in analysing patient's data. We wish to acknowledge the radiographers, physiotherapists, theatre technicians and the nursing staff in the Regional Neurological Centre, particularly Sisters E. Murphy and M. Walls, whose alert care is essential in the successful treatment of our patients. We extend our grateful thanks to Miss A. Phillips for her diligent painstaking and superb secretarial assistance, and to Miss A. Kellett for her expertise in producing the illustrations.

We are happy to acknowledge permission to reproduce certain illustrations, and these are mentioned in the legends to the figures concerned.

Finally, we are greatly indebted to Mr. Michael Jackson of Springer-Verlag for the patience with which he has awaited the manuscript, and for his sympathetic understanding of the reasons for delay.

Newcastle 1986   R. P. Sengupta
                                                                                   V. L. McAllister

Contents

1 Historical Review

Subarachnoid haemorrhage (SAH) may have been recognised in ancient and biblical times, and the literature pertaining to this can be found in Walton's monograph entitled "Subarachnoid Haemorrhage" (Walton 1956). However, SAH as a definite clinical entity has only been recognised for less than 200 years. The major cause of SAH is a ruptured aneurysm, and this historical review will concentrate on milestones in the understanding and management of aneurysmal SAH. There are also less common causes, and historical aspects of these will be discussed in subsequent chapters.

Although Morgagni (1761), Professor of Anatomy at Padua, is often quoted as being the first to describe an intracranial aneurysm, he simply implied that the existence of such an entity was probable. Biumi of Milan in 1765 gave a clear-cut description of an unruptured cavernous sinus aneurysm seen at post mortem in a 52-year-old female. Thirty years elapsed before the description of a second case, a female who died in 1792 at the age of 69. At autopsy an aneurysm was seen arising from the internal carotid artery on each side of the sella turcica (Bull 1962).

In 1813 Blackhall (Fig. 1.1) observed clinically an SAH in a 20-year-old female, who subsequently died, and at post mortem a ruptured basilar artery aneurysm was found with blood in the ventricular system and subarachnoid space. This probably represents the first account of a ruptured intracranial aneurysm.

Further isolated case reports appeared, but the credit for the first systematic analysis of the symptoms due to ruptured intracranial aneurysm should go to Brinton (1850–51). He analysed 52 cases collected from the literature, and came to the following conclusions: the average age of presentation was 40 years, the range being from birth to old age. The sex incidence was 2 to 1 in favour of males; one-third of the aneurysms were located on the basilar artery, while equal numbers occurred on the anterior cerebral, the middle cerebral and the internal carotid arteries. He

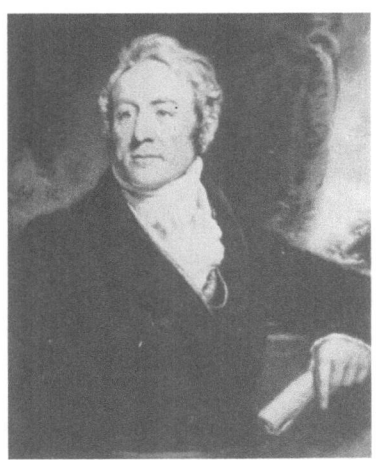

Fig. 1.1. J. Blackhall.

classified the aneurysms, depending on their size, into filbert (a cultivated hazel), pea and walnut. Half of the aneurysms were the size of a filbert, one-quarter the size of a pea, and the other quarter the size of a walnut. Where the outcome was fatal, 50% died of rupture; epileptiform attacks, coincidental disorders, e.g. an accident, inflammatory conditions of the brain, and local pressure from the space-occupying effect of haematoma each accounted for 12.5% of deaths. In 1859, Gull added 11 more cases to those reported by Brinton (1850–51) and stressed the importance of headache as a symptom, when he stated:

> As with all tumours, so with an intracranial aneurysm, headache, though difficult to estimate strictly, is one of the most important symptoms. The character of it, which should most arrest our attention, is its constant recurrence and its often distressing severity with concomitant disturbance of cerebral function. All care, however, will often fail to enable us to form a correct opinion, even should we, as some have suggested, auscultate the cranium for an aneurysmal murmur.

He also added:

> Intracranial aneurysms often serve to illustrate to us how much the whole nutrition of the brain may be affected by the operation of a strictly local lesion.

In 1860, Holmes described the clinical features and post-mortem appearances of an aneurysm of the internal carotid artery in the cavernous sinus of a 16-year-old boy. In 1868 Charcot and Bouchard described the microaneurysms which bear their names. A few years later Bramwell (1886) published an excellent clinicopathological correlation of two cases of SAH.

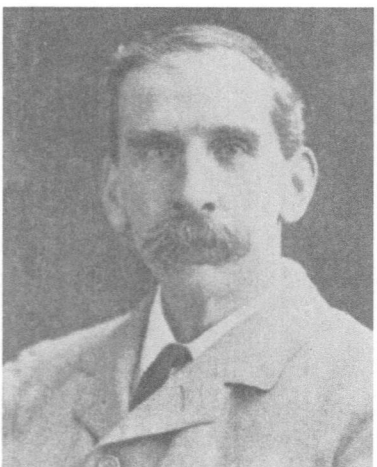

Fig. 1.2. Sir Victor Horsley.

The earliest attempt at surgical treatment of a ruptured cerebral aneurysm was by Sir Victor Horsley in 1885 (Fig. 1.2), quoted by Keen (1890). He diagnosed an aneurysm at the base of the brain pressing upon the chiasm, for which he successfully ligated both the carotid arteries in the neck. He later confirmed the diagnosis of an aneurysm at craniotomy. Eppinger (1887) suggested that these aneurysms, in the absence of any signs of inflammation, were of congenital origin and due to an inborn defect of the elastic properties of the arterial wall. In 1907 Beadles analysed 555 cases collected from the literature and classified the aneurysms into four groups:

1. Those that presented with an apoplectic attack
2. Those that had symptoms suggestive of a cerebral tumour prior to fatal apoplexy
3. Those that had symptoms of cerebral tumour without apoplexy
4. Those that were an incidental finding at post-mortem examination

The first attempt to classify cerebral aneurysms on a pathological basis, into infective, congenital and degenerative, was that of Turnbull (1918). In 1891 Quincke (of Kiel) introduced the technique of lumbar puncture and it soon became a practical aid in the differential diagnosis of apoplexy. Froin (1904) and Matas (1938) described the changes that occur in the cerebrospinal fluid following SAH. In 1923, Symonds described in detail the clinical picture of SAH and divided the signs into three groups: neighbourhood signs due to the local compression by the aneurysm, those of the disease causing the aneurysm, and signs of leakage from the aneurysmal sac. He was also one of the first to describe the early recurrence of bleeding from ruptured aneurysms.

The most significant milestone in the evolution of our understanding and practical management of patients with SAH was the introduction of the technique of cerebral angiography in 1927, by Moniz (Fig. 1.3). The first aneurysm was demonstrated angiographically in 1931 (Dott 1933; Moniz 1933). In 1931 Collier emphasised the importance of entertaining SAH as a differential diagnosis when dealing with a clinical picture similar to that of encephalitis, and discussed the different modes of presentation of SAH.

In 1926 Grey Turner (quoted by Nattrass 1928) ligated the internal carotid artery in a patient suspected to be suffering from a right internal carotid artery aneurysm which had produced first, second, third, fifth and sixth cranial nerve palsies

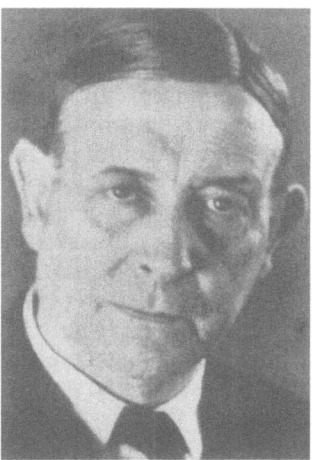

Fig. 1.3. Egaz Moniz.

as well as frontal lobe signs. One year after the ligation there was some improvement in the external ocular movements and no trace of anosmia. The left hemiparesis had resolved and the frontal lobe function had improved (Nattrass 1928).

The modern era of treating SAH patients by directly attacking the source of the haemorrhage started when Dott (1933; Fig. 1.4) wrapped a carotid bifurcation aneurysm (which had been demonstrated at angiography) with muscle, on 22 April 1931. McConnell (1937) opened an intracranial aneurysm and packed the sac with muscle, with an improvement in the symptoms to such an extent that the patient was considered to be cured.

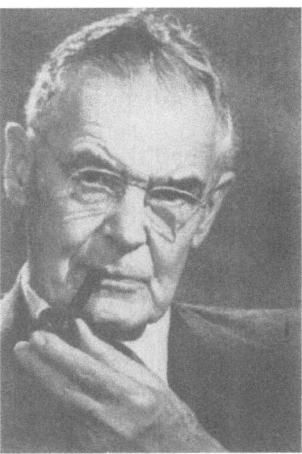

Fig. 1.4. Norman M. Dott.

The first successful clipping of the neck of an aneurysm in a 43-year-old male, who presented with ptosis of the right eye, was performed in 1938 by Dandy, and was a turning point in the ultimate goal of excluding the aneurysmal sac without interfering with the circulation in the vessel of origin. Fincher (1939) trapped an aneurysm of the internal carotid artery between an intracranial clip and a ligature in the neck. In 1939, Russell reported a 12-year-old boy in whom an anterior cerebral artery aneurysm, arising at the junction of the anterior communicating artery and circle of Willis, was successfully excised (by Dr Cone). Dandy (1944), in his excellent monograph *Intracranial Arterial Aneurysms*, reported four cases in which the neck of the aneurysm was clipped successfully. He also mentioned ligating the vertebral artery in the management of basilar artery aneurysm. However, in one case in which he attempted to ligate both the vertebral arteries at an interval, the patient died immediately after the application of the artery forceps to the second side.

While surgeons were attacking the source of origin of the subarachnoid haemorrhage directly, simultaneous developments in anaesthesia (see Chap. 9), operative technique and surgical instruments were taking place. In 1953 White and Sweet utilised the technique of hypothermia to enable them to occlude the cerebral blood flow transiently while they were operating upon patients with arteriovenous malformations (Lougheed and Marshall 1969a). Botterell et al. (1958) claimed improved results with hypothermia and they argued that it provided protection against anoxia during temporary cervical occlusion of the carotid or vertebral arterises. There was also a marked reduction in the brain volume which they argued helped for easier dissection. Uihlein et al. (1962) reported their experience of deep hypothermia associated with circulatory arrest (the hypothermia, as low as 11°C, was produced by whole body perfusion). They obtained a successful result in 11 out of 14 patients with an intracranial aneurysm which had been operated upon using such a technique. This initial enthusiasm, however, was not sustained, and in 1964 Drake et al. felt that although superb exposure of the aneurysm and its relation to other vessels was provided with circulatory arrest, it did not decrease the hazards of vasospasm and associated ischaemic complications, and, furthermore, that additional hazards were created by deep hypothermia. A similar view was expressed by MacCarty et al. (1964) only 3 years after they themselves had suggested the use of profound hypothermia in the surgical management of intra-cranial aneurysm. Hamby (1963), in a comparative study of 94 cases, was unable to find any improvement in the survival rate of patients operated upon under moderate hypothermia.

As the earlier results of direct clipping of some aneurysms were not always satisfactory (owing to their peculiar anatomical situation or the presence of a broad neck), surgeons, in an attempt to prevent rebleeding from the aneurysm, introduced the technique of reinforcement of the sac. Hunter et al. (1956), in animal experiments, found methyl methacrylate with acetone to be the least irritating agent, and Dutton (1956) used this substance to wrap aneurysms in three patients. In 1962, Selverstone et al. laid down the criteria for the ideal coating material. It had to be non-toxic and non-irritant, should adhere to the vessel wall intimately without leaving a dead space, be insoluble in body fluids, flexible, stable dimensionally, and provide immediate reinforcement. They used polyvinyl, polyvinylidene chloride copolymer (Selverstone and Ronis 1958; Selverstone 1962). Todd et al. (1962) used a silicone preparation for wrapping the aneurysm in three patients. Messer et al. (1963) used methyl-2-cynoacrylate (a watery substance which polymerises in the presence of moisture and pressure, forming an adherent film) successfully in a 34-year-old Negro woman to encourage thick fibrosis around the sac of a left middle cerebral artery aneurysm. Wrapping the whole sac in sterile muslin gauze and a layer of temporal fascia was advocated by Gillingham (1958).

Coating the aneurysm is not always possible, and is sometimes unnecessary, for example giant aneurysms which have a very thick sac do not usually rupture, and, furthermore, are technically difficult to clip by direct surgery because of their anatomical situation. Although the principle of proximal ligation of the feeding vessel has been practised since the days of Hunter, it soon became apparent that ligation of the carotid artery in the treatment of intracranial aneurysms led, on occasions, to cerebral ischaemia. To encourage the opening of collaterals, Selverstone and White (1951) described the technique of gradually occluding the internal carotid artery in the neck by means of a stainless steel clamp. The advantage of this clamp was that the blood flow could be increased at any time, should partial occlusion not be tolerated by the patient. Crutchfield (1959), on the same principle, developed another clamp which was smaller and less complicated to use. Recently the technique of external carotid to internal carotid anastomosis as described by Yasargil (1967) has been used to reduce the risk of cerebral ischaemia following internal carotid ligation (Sengupta 1982).

Olivecrona developed a long silver clip which was an improvement over the conventional silver clips of ordinary length in that it could be removed after application if necessary (Tovi 1955; Gillingham 1958). This clamp was larger and flatter and was corrugated on its inner aspect. As aneurysms almost invariably bleed from the fundus, Tovi (1955) felt that it was this portion of the aneurysm which should be isolated from the circulation. For this purpose, he constructed a triangular silver clip with blades which had a wide base. Scoville (1966) developed the torsion bar spring clip, the loop of which is no larger than the width of the jaws. These clips were lightweight and could also be applied temporarily or permanently. Numerous improvements in the design of the aneurysmal clip have occurred in recent years to suit the need for any individual aneurysm.

Greenwood (1940) developed forceps with two blades, insulated from each other (the bipolar diathermy), in which the current passes from one tip to the other, coagulating only the tissues in between. This is of great advantage while working in depths and where other vital structures are involved. Drew (1955) used an insulating plastic coat for neurosurgical instruments, and such instruments can be autoclaved and are resistant to ordinary wear and tear. The plastic was a polymer of biflurochloroethylene.

Another important development was the introduction of the operating microscope. Nylen was probably the first to use a monocular microscope for otological surgery in 1921 (Nylen 1954), and Holmgren (1923) developed the binocular instrument, also for use in otological surgery. Jacobson et al. (1962) used the binocular microscope for endarterectomy of the middle cerebral artery, and Adams and Witt (1964) probably were the first to apply the microscope to intracranial aneurysm surgery.

Pool and Colton (1966) described their experience in operating on 13 intracranial aneurysms and 3 arteriovenous malformations with the help of the operating microscope, and stressed the advantage of good illumination and magnification of the anatomical details during aneurysmal surgery. In 1965 Lougheed and Marshall (1969b) introduced the diploscope and with it, for the first time, both the surgeon and his assistant had good binocular vision with magnification of the operation field. However, it was Yasargil (Fig. 1.5) who emphasised the enormous value of the oper-

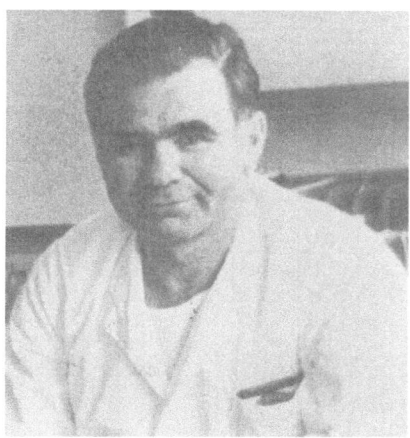

Fig. 1.5. M.G. Yasargil.

ating microscope in the surgical treatment of intracranial aneurysms.

Simultaneously with the advances in the technique of excluding aneurysms from the circulation by direct surgery, other avenues of operative treatment were being explored in order to reduce the serious complications and mortality associated with major intracranial surgery. Many of these have not survived the test of time.

Logue (1956) developed the technique of proximal clipping of the anterior cerebral artery supplying the sac. He used a lateral approach along the Sylvian fissure without any exposure or disturbance of the aneurysmal sac. The occlusion was designed to reduce the pulse pressure on the aneurysm.

Werner et al. (1941) used wiring and electrothermic coagulation in a 16-year-old schoolgirl who had a giant aneurysm of the right internal carotid artery. This was increasing in size despite ligation of both common carotid arteries in stages. They introduced 30 ft (9 m) of 34-gauge coiled silver wire into the sac using a special needle; the wire was heated to 80°C for 40 s, using the principle developed by Blakemore and King (1938) in the treatment of aneurysms of the aorta. Gallagher (1963, 1964), in order to obliterate the aneurysm by encouraging intraluminal thrombosis, inserted hog hair into the sac of the aneurysm with a special gun, so that the root of the hair emerged first. With this technique of piloejection, the normal negative charge of the intima was thought to be reversed due to damage and the negatively charged circulating elements migrated to the intima, thus producing a thrombus. Each shaft of hair was capable of causing a limited amount of thrombosis and thus multiple hairs needed to be injected.

Mullan et al. (1964), following the lead given by Sawyer and Pate (1953), suggested the use of intraluminal electrodes based on the bioelectric phenomenon of intravascular thrombosis. They also suggested that to prevent clot lysis, an antifibrinolytic agent, such as epsilon aminocaproic acid, should be used in the immediate posthaemorrhage stage. Luessenhop and Velesquez (1964) produced thrombosis of the sac of an aneurysm by temporary occlusion of the orifice with a Silastic sphere. This sphere, with 4–0 silk attached to it, was floated up via the carotid artery to the neck of the aneurysm, and subsequent angiography showed non-filling of the aneurysm. Autopsy later showed adherent clot in the neck of the aneurysm, but thrombosis had not obliterated the entire lumen. There was no obstruction to the flow through the carotid artery. Drake and Vanderlinden (1967) warned of the danger of incomplete obliteration of an aneurysm as it had the capacity to enlarge and cause fatal rebleeding at a later stage. They advised plastic coating of the residual portions of the aneurysm and then wrapping with muscle. They also advocated postoperative angiography to confirm the complete obliteration of the aneurysm. Rothenberg et al. (1962) developed angiotactic surgery and in a preliminary report they showed that in experimental animals (canines) an intravascular implant could be placed at a distance from the arteriotomy and that intimal growth encased it permanently. With this technique the aneurysmal opening into the parent artery could be occluded. Riechert and Mundinger (1964) described two cases in which combined stereotactic operation and craniotomy in two stages were used to reduce the vascular supply to angiomas and aneurysms. In 1974 Mullan published his experience with surgical thrombosis of intracranial berry aneurysms and caroticocavernous fistulae. In giant aneurysms he introduced fine copper wire (which was thrombogenic) and beryllium–copper alloy wire (which was not thrombogenic but served as a packing material) into the aneurysm through fine needles. Of the 15 patients treated in this way, in 12 there was satisfactory thrombosis. There were two operative deaths and two late deaths; in one patient the aneurysm continued to enlarge and death occurred 1 year later. Mullan also produced thrombosis electrically, by inserting copper-plated steel wire across the neck (stereotactically) at 1-mm intervals and passing 0.5–1 mA of direct current through each needle for 5 min. Mild thrombosis was initiated and permanent fibrosis resulted. Of 61 patients subjected to this procedure, there were 4 operative deaths; in 8 the occlusion was incomplete, and the patients died 1–66 days later due to rebleeds. New eddies and stresses within the aneurysmal sac set up by the partial thrombus probably contributed to the rebleed, and Mullan concluded that partial thrombosis was worse than none at all. In his opinion, this technique was not applicable for large aneurysms and in patients who were in a poor clinical condition. However, he found wire thrombosis suitable for the majority of these large aneurysms, but not in those where distal branches originate from the sac of the aneurysm. He also warned that if the aneurysm was already partially thrombosed, then the insertion of wire carried the risk of distal embolisation from the sac.

Cahan and Rand (1973) also used a stereotactic method to treat a paraventricular arteriovenous malformation (AVM). Kandel and Peresedov (1977) developed a stereotactic technique to clip inaccessible aneurysms and to occlude the feeding vessel supply in deep-seated AVMs. There was no mortality in the eight cases they initially described.

A new method for intravascular thrombosis by injecting iron and holding it in place by a stereotactically placed magnet was developed by Alksne et al. (1966), and early results were quite encouraging in good-risk patients (Alksne 1971; Rand and Mosso 1973). Debrun et al. (1978) used a detachable balloon in the management of aneurysms.

For many years aneurysms of the posterior circulation were considered to be inoperable. However, Drake (Fig. 1.6) has shown that these aneurysms can also be surgically treated with acceptable risk.

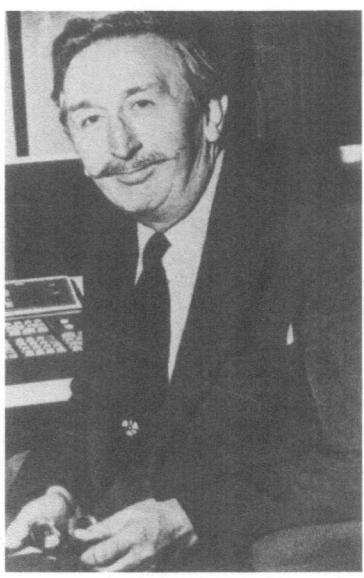

Fig. 1.7. Sir Geoffrey Hounsfield.

An understanding of the relationship of the neurological condition of the patient on admission and at the time of operation to the final outcome has led to the establishment of different modes of classifying severity (Botterell et al. 1956; Nishioka 1966; Hunt and Hess 1968; Nibbelink et al. 1977), and has to a great extent rationalised the management in a given patient population.

One of the unresolved problems of aneurysmal SAH is the onset of cerebral vasospasm. Robertson (1949) observed that cerebral infarct following SAH was due to ischaemia from vasospasm. Ecker and Riemenschneider (1951) demonstrated angiographic vasospasm in patients with SAH. The mechanism of vasospasm and its treatment still remain speculative and are discussed in greater detail in Chap. 12.

The first monograph dealing with SAH was published less than 30 years ago when Walton (1956) reviewed 312 cases in detail.

The co-operative study (Sahs et al. 1966) provided a detailed examination of over 6000 patients with SAH, and today it still represents the largest existing collection of critically analysed material on the subject.

One must finally mention CT scanning, a revolutionary milestone in the management of SAH. Hounsfield's (1973; Fig. 1.7) great discovery will not only confirm the diagnosis and the site of the bleed, but will also demonstrate the complications of SAH.

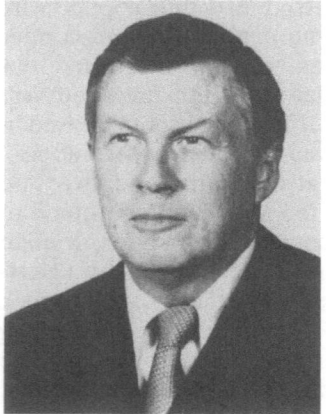

Fig. 1.6. Charles G. Drake.

References

Adams JE, Witt JA (1964) The use of the otological microscope in the surgery of aneurysms. Presented at The Seventeenth Annual Meeting of The Neurological Society of America, Litchfield Park, Arizona

Alksne JF (1971) Stereotactic thrombosis of intracranial aneurysms. N Engl J Med 284:171–174

Alksne JF, Fingerhut AG, Rand RW (1966) Magnetically controlled metallic thrombosis of intracranial aneurysms. Surgery 60:212–218

Beadles CF (1907) Aneurysms of the larger cerebral arteries. Brain 30:285–336

Biumi F (1765) Observationes anatomicae observatio V. In Sandifort: Thesaurus dissertationum. Lugd Bat S & J Lightmans 3:373–379

Blackhall L (1813) Observations on the nature and cure of dropsies. Longman, London, p. 126

Blakemore AH, King BG (1938) Electrothermic coagulation of aortic aneurysms. JAMA 111:1821

Botterell EH, Lougheed WM, Scott JW, Vanderwater SL (1956) Hypothermia and interruption of carotid or carotid and vertebral circulation in the surgical management of intracranial aneurysms. J Neurosurg 13:1–42

Botterell EH, Lougheed WM, Morley TP, Vanderwater SL (1958) Hypothermia in the surgical treatment of ruptured intracranial aneurysms. J Neurosurg 15:4–18

Bramwell B (1886) Clinical and pathological memoranda illustrated. Edinburgh Med J 32(2):97–108

Brinton W (1850–51) Report on cases of cerebral aneurysms. Trans of the Pathol Soc Lond 3:47–49

Bull J (1962) A short history of intracranial aneurysms. Lond Clin Med J 3:47–61

Cahan LD, Rand RW (1973) Stereotaxic coagulation of a paraventricular AWM. Case report. J Neurosurg 39:770–774

Charcot JM, Bouchard C (1868) Nouvelles recherches sur la pathogenie de l'hemorrhagie cerebrale achives de physiologie normale et de pathologie. Arch Physio (Paris) 1:110–127

Collier J (1931) Cerebral haemorrhage due to causes other than arteriosclerosis. Br J Med II:519–521

Crutchfield WG (1959) Instruments for use in the treatment of certain intracranial vascular lesions. J Neurosurg 16:471–474

Dandy WE (1938) Intracranial aneurysms of the internal carotid artery. Ann Surg 107:654–659

Dandy WE (1944) Intracranial arterial aneurysms. Comstock, New York

Debrun G, Lacour P, Caron JP, Hurth M, Comoy J, Keraval Y (1978) Detachable balloon and calibrated-leak balloon techniques in the treatment of cerebral vascular lesions. J Neurosurg 49:635–649

Dott NM (1933) Intracranial aneurysms. Cerebral arterioradiography: surgical treatment. Trans Med Chir Soc Edin 40:219–240

Drake CG, Vanderlinden RG (1967) The late consequences of incomplete surgical treatment of cerebral aneurysms. J Neurosurg 27:226–238

Drake CG, Barr HWK, Coles JC, Gergely NF (1964) The use of extracorporeal circulation and profound hypothermia in the treatment of ruptured intracranial aneurysms. J Neurosurg 21:575–581

Drew JH (1955) An insulating plastic coat for neurosurgical instruments. J Neurosurg 12:523–524

Dutton JEM (1956) Intracranial aneurysms. A new method of surgical treatment. Br Med J II:585–586

Ecker A, Riemenschneider PA (1951) Arteriographic demonstration of spasm of the intracranial arteries with special reference to saccular artery aneurysm. J Neurosurg 8:660–667

Eppinger H (1887) Pathogenesis (histogenesis and hemologie) der Aneurysmen einschliesslich des Aneurysm equi verminosum. Arch Klin Chir 35 (Suppl.):1–563

Fincher EF (1939) An aneurysm of the internal carotid artery treated surgically. Yale J Biol Med 11:423–424

Froin G (1904) Les hemorrhagies sous-arachnoidiennes et le mecanisme de l'hematolyse en general. Theses de Paris. Steinher, Paris

Gallagher JP (1963) Obliteration of intracranial aneurysm by pilojection. JAMA 183:231–236

Gallagher JP (1964) Pilojection for intracranial aneurysms. Report of progress. J Neurosurg 21:129–134

Gillingham FJ (1958) The management of ruptured intracranial aneurysms. Ann R Coll Surg Engl 23:89–117

Greenwood J Jr (1940) Two point coagulation. New principle and instrument for applying coagulation current in neurosurgery. Am J Surg 50:267–270

Gull W (1859) Cases of aneurysms of the cerebral vessels. Guy's Hosp Rep 3rd series 5:281–304

Hamby WB (1963) Intracranial surgery for aneurysm. Effect of hypothermia upon survival. J Neurosurg 20:41–45

Holmes T (1860–61) Aneurysm of the internal carotid artery in the cavernous sinus. Post mortem appearances. Trans Path Soc Lond 12:61–63

Holmgren G (1923) Some experiences in surgery of otosclerosis. Acta Otolaryngol Stockh 5:460–466

Hounsfield GN (1973) Computerised transverse axial scanning (tomography) Part 1: Description of system. Br J Radiol 46:1023–1047

Hunt WE, Hess RM (1968) Surgical risk as related to time of intervention in the repair of intracranial aneurysms. J Neurosurg 28:14–20

Hunter CR, Mayfield FH, McBride RH, Lattinville HE (1956) Intracranial implantation of liquid plastic in the experimental animal (Macaque). Possible clinical application in surgical management of intracranial aneurysm. Surg Forum 7:539–544

Jacobson JH, Wallman LJ, Schumacher GA, Flanagan M, Suarez FL, Donaghy RMP (1962) Microsurgery as an aid to middle cerebral artery endarterectomy. J Neurosurg 19:108–115

Kandel EL, Peresedov VV (1977) Stereotaxic clipping of arterial aneurysms and AVM. J Neurosurg 46:12–23

Keen WW (1890) Intracranial lesions. Med News, A Weekly Medical Journal, Philadelphia 57:439–450

Logue V (1956) Surgery in spontaneous subarachnoid haemorrhage. Operative treatment of aneurysm on the anterior cerebral and anterior communicating artery. Br Med J I:473–479

Lougheed WM, Marshall BM (1969a) The place of hypothermia in the treatment of intracranial aneurysms. Prog Neurol Surg 3:115–148

Lougheed WM, Marshall BM (1969b) The diploscope in intracranial aneurysms surgery—results in 40 patients. Can J Surg 12:75–82

Luessenhop AJ, Velesquez AC (1964) Observations on the tolerance of intracranial arteries to catheterisation. J Neurosurg 21:85–91

MacCarty CS, McHenfelder JD, Uihlein A (1964) Treatment of intracranical vascular disorders with aid of profound hypothermia and total circulatory arrest—3 years experience. J Neurosurg 21:372–377

Matas R (1938) Aneurysms of the circle of Willis. Ann Surg 107:660–680

McConnell AA (1937) Subchiasmal aneurysm, treatment by implantation of muscle. ZB Neurochir 2:269–274

Messer HD, Strenger L, McVee HJ (1963) Use of plastic adhesive for reinforcement of a ruptured intracranial aneurysm. J Neurosurg 20:360–362

Moniz E (1927) L'encephalographie arterielle, son importance dans la localisation des tumeurs cerebrales. Rev Neurolog 2:72–90

Moniz E (1933) Aneurisme intra-cranien de la carotid interne droit rendu visible par l'arteriographie cerebrale. Rev D'oto Neuro-Ophthal 11:746–748

Morgagni JB (1761) De sebidus et causis morborum per anatomen in sagatis venetis et topog remondiama. Book 1. Letter 4 2VXCVI:298

Mullan S (1974) Experiences with surgical thrombosis of intracranial berry aneurysms and carotid cavernous fistulae. J Neurosurg 41:657–670

Mullan S, Beckman F, Vailati G, Karasick J, Dobben G (1964) An experimental approach to the problem of cerebral aneurysms. J Neurosurg 21:838–845

Nattrass FJ (1928) Aneurysm of the carotid artery in cavernous sinus—ligature of internal carotid artery: recovery. Edin Med J 35:30–32

Nibbelink DW, Torner JC, Henderson WG (1977) Intracranical aneurysm and subarachnoid haemorrhage—a report on a randomised treatment study. II A Regulated bedrest. Stroke 8:202–218

Nishioka H (1966) Evaluation of the conservative management of ruptured intracranial aneurysm. J Neurosurg 25:574–592

Nylen CO (1954) The microscope in aural surgery, its first use and later developments. Acta Otolaryngol Stockh 116 (Suppl.):226–240

Pool JL, Colton HP (1966) The dissecting microscope for intracranial vascular surgery. J Neurosurg 25:315–318

Quincke H (1891) Die Lumbarpunction des Hydrocephalus. Berlin Klin Wochenschr 28:929–965

Rand RW, Mosso JA (1973) Treatment of cerebral aneurysm by stereotactic ferromagnetic silicone thrombosis. Hull, Los Angeles Neurol Soc 38:21–23

Riechert T, Mundinger F (1964) Combined stereotaxic operation for treatment of deep-seated angiomas and aneurysms. J Neurosurg 21:358–363

Robertson EG (1949) Cerebral lesions due to intracranial aneurysm. Brain 72:150–185

Rothenberg F, Penka EJ, Conway LW (1962) Angiotactic surgery: preliminary studies. J Neurosurg 19:877–883

Russell CK (1939) Spontaneous subarachnoid haemorrhage following rupture of congenital aneurysm of the anterior communicating artery of the circle of Willis. Trans Am Neurol Assoc 65:130–134

Sahs AL, Perett GE, Locksley HB, Nishioka H (1966) Intracranial aneurysms and S.A.H. A co-operative study. JB Lippincott, Philadelphia Toronto

Sawyer PN, Pate JW (1953) Bio-electric phenomena as aetiological agents in intravascular thrombosis. Surgery 34:491–500

Scoville WB (1966) Miniature torsion bar spring aneurysm clip. J Neurosurg 25:97

Selverstone B (1962) Aneurysms at middle cerebral trifurcation: treatment with adherent plastics. J Neurosurg 19:884–886

Selverstone B, Ronis N (1958) Coating and reinforcement of intracranial aneurysm with synthetic resin. Bull Tuffs N Engl Med Centre 4:8–12

Selverstone B, White JCS (1951) A new technique for gradual occlusion of the carotid artery. Arch Neurol Psychiat Chicago 66:246

Selverstone B, Dehghan R, Ronis N, Deterling RA, Callow AD (1962) Adherent synthetic resins in experimental arterial surgery. Arch Surg 84:80–84

Sengupta RF (1982) Special indications of external/internal bypass operation. Neurosurg Rev 5:107–112

Symonds CF (1923) Contribution to the clinical study of intracranial aneurysm. Guy's Hosp Rep 4th Series 73:139–158

Todd EM, Shelden CH, Crue BL Jr, Pudenz RH, Agnew WF (1962) Plastic jackets for certain intracranial aneurysms. JAMA 179:935–939

Tovi D (1955) New instrument to obliterate intracranial saccular aneurysm. J Neurosurg 12:525–527

Tuhy JE, Maurice GL, Niles NR (1958) Wegener's granulomatosis. Am J Med 25:638–646

Turnbull HM (1918) Intracranial aneurysms. Brain 41:50–56

Uihlein A, Terry HR, Payne WS, Kirklin JW (1962) Operation on intracranial aneurysms with induced hypothermia below 15°C and total circulatory arrest. J Neurosurg 19:237–239

Walton JN (1956) S.A.H. E. & S. Livingstone, Edinburgh London

Werner SC, Blakemore AH, King BC (1941) Aneurysm of internal carotid artery within skull, wiring and electrothermic coagulation. JAMA 116:578–582

Yasargil MG (1967) Experimental small vessel surgery in the dog including patching and grafting of cerebral vessels and the formation of functional extra-cranial shunts. In: Donaghy RMP, Yasargil MG (eds) Micro-vascular surgery. Thieme, Stuttgart, pp 87–126

2 Anatomy of the Cerebral Vessels

Introduction

The brain is unique among the organs of the body since it has no regenerative power and the highest metabolic need. The brain accounts for only 2% of the body weight, yet it receives 16.6% of the total cardiac output and consumes 20% of the oxygen used by the whole body (Bowsher 1961).

The major arteries supplying the brain are the paired internal carotid and vertebral arteries. These are joined to one another at the base of the brain in the form of an arterial circle, the circle of Willis, which was first described by the famous English physician Thomas Willis (Figs. 2.1, 2.2).

Anatomical variations in the circle of Willis are well known to neuroanatomists and are also important to the neurosurgeon, since physiological variations of the cerebral circulation through the circle of Willis may be a potential cause of poor surgical results. The increasing use of the operating microscope has created the need for an accurate understanding of the microsurgical anatomy of the cerebral vessels, in particular the small-calibre perforating vessels which may not be demonstrated at angiography.

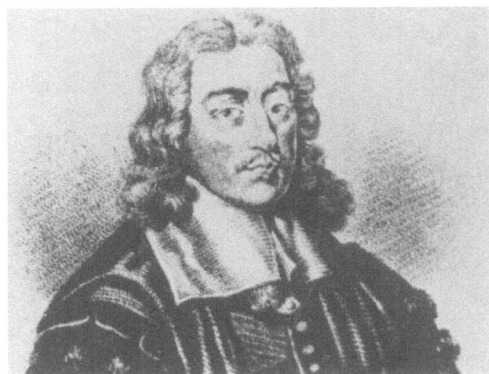

Fig. 2.1. Thomas Willis.

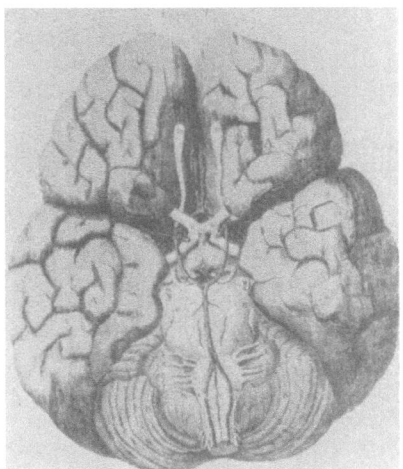

Fig. 2.2. Drawing of the circle of Willis by Christopher Wren, carried out at Willis's request.

This chapter will concentrate on specific features of vascular anatomy and anatomical variations of particular surgical importance.

Circle of Willis (Fig. 2.3)

Starting from the midline in front, the circle consists of the anterior communicating, anterior cerebral, a short segment of the internal carotid, posterior communicating and posterior cerebral arteries and the basilar bifurcation, then it continues to the starting point in reverse order. The primary purpose of the circle of Willis is to assure a good supply of blood to all areas of the brain. It also assures equal pressure in all the three major arteries. The haemodynamic virtues of the circle are apparent in two clinical situations.

1. It is not unusual to discover incidental occlusion of one or more of the major arteries in the neck without clinical deficit.
2. Surgical occlusion of major vessels to treat cerebral aneurysms relied upon this unique collateral circulation.

The classical textbook description of a symmetrically paired appearance of the vessels forming the circle of Willis is not the rule however. This entity is anatomically complete in only 52% of the normal population (Alpers et al. 1959).

To understand the variations in the circle of Willis it is necessary to look back at the development of the cerebral vascular system.

Embryology

Only in humans and a few other vertebrates do the carotid and vertebral circulations contribute in an equal manner to the cerebral circulation in early foetal life.

At 24 days of gestation the internal carotid artery appears in the foetus, which is only 3 mm in size (Padget 1944). Within 4 days, this artery separates into primitive cranial and caudal divisions. The caudal division of each side winds round the mesencephalon and the two fuse with each other to form the upper part of the basilar artery. The cranial division subdivides into the future middle cerebral and anterior cerebral arteries. At 44 days of gestation the anterior communicating artery is differentiated, and by 49

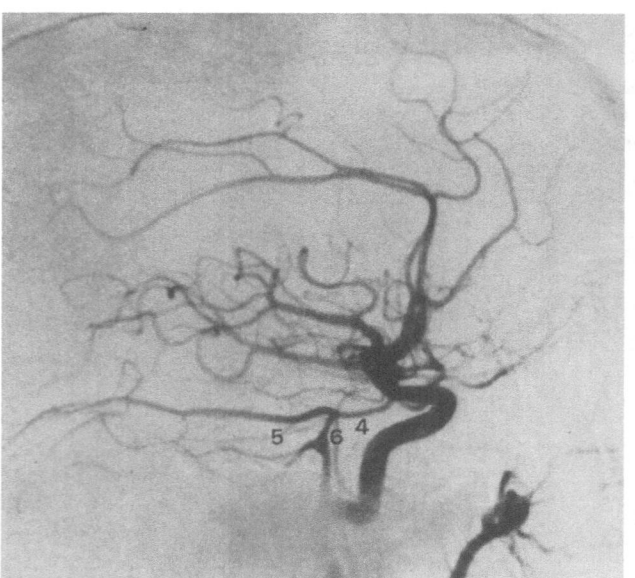
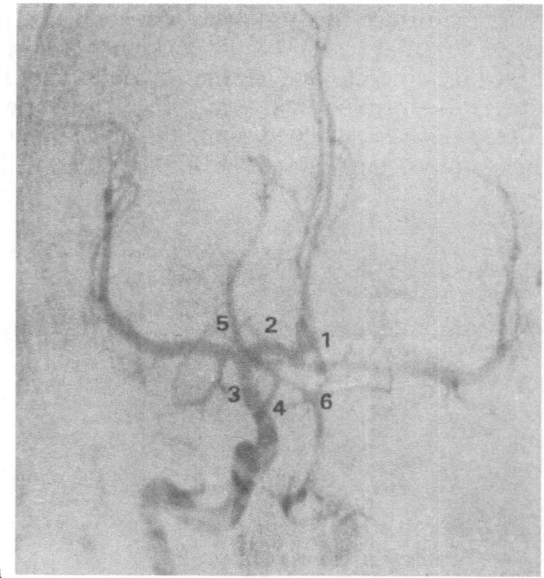

Fig. 2.3. Right carotid angiogram (**a** lateral and **b** Townes projection) which shows the circle of Willis remarkably well. *1,* anterior communicating artery; *2,* A₁ segment of the anterior cerebral artery; *3,* internal carotid artery; *4,* posterior communicating artery; *5,* posterior cerebral artery; *6,* basilar bifurcation.

days of gestation the circle of Willis is completed. At 4 months the typical symmetrical circle of Willis is present. This is then moulded by physiological factors and the calibre of each segment becomes proportional to the circulatory function of that segment. As the demand from the carotid system grows due to the rapidly developing telencephalon, the vertebral system begins to contribute and the terminal part of the foetal posterior cerebral artery now receives blood entirely from the basilar artery, while its proximal part becomes attenuated to form the slender posterior communicating artery. During this process of attenuation and enlargement several variations in the circle occur.

As a result of the persistence of embryological arteries, there are anastomotic channels between the internal cartoid artery and the basilar arteries. A persistent trigeminal artery is the most common anastomosis and occurs in about 0.2% of angiograms. It connects the cavernous segment of the internal carotid artery to the basilar artery below the superior cerebellar artery origin. The hypoglossal artery is a persistent embryonic anastomosis from the upper cervical segment of the internal carotid artery through the anterior condylar canal, joining the basilar artery close to its origin. A persistent otic artery which communicates the petrous segment of the internal carotid artery through the internal auditory canal, with the basilar artery, may occur rarely. The increased incidence of aneurysm formation in association with the carotid—basilar anastomosis—is discussed in Chap. 7 (see Fig. 7.59).

Types of Variation

The various anomalies of the circle may be classified in the following manner (Fig. 2.4).

1. Hypoplasia of communicating arteries, e.g. anterior and posterior, but this is extremely rare.
2. Hypoplasia of the divisional branch of the basilar artery, e.g. foetal posterior cerebral artery.
3. Hypoplasia of the proximal stem of the anterior cerebral artery, e.g. hypoplastic A_1 segment of the anterior cerebral artery.
4. A combination of hypoplasia of the divisional branch of the basilar artery (foetal posterior cerebral artery) and proximal stem of the anterior cerebral artery (hypoplastic A_1 segment).

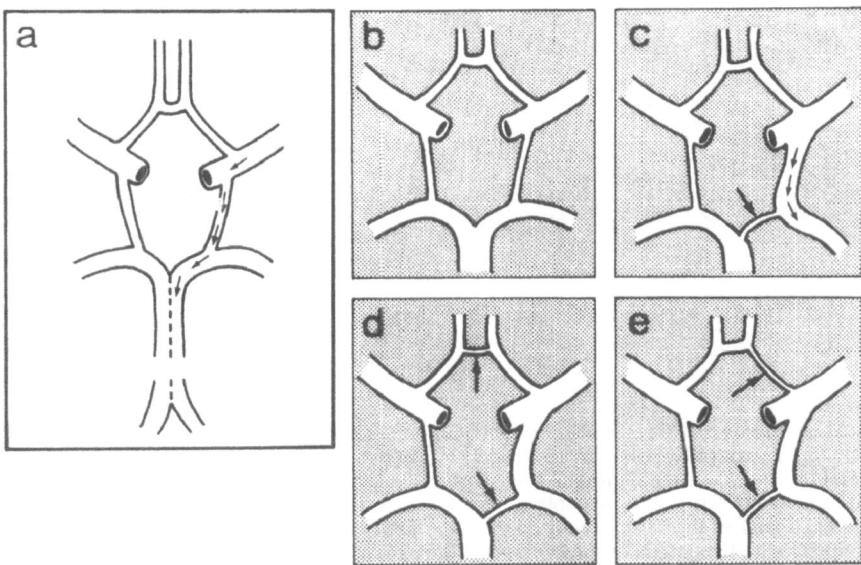

Fig. 2.4. Classification of types of variation of the circle of Willis.

Incidence of Variations

In 1953 Rigg analysed statistically the different
forms of circle of Willis observed in 1947 auto-
psies ir adults who had presented with clinical
manifestations of neural dysfunction. They were
divided into eight anatomical types which are
illustrated in Fig. 2.5. In only 18% of cases was a
classically normal circle of Willis present (type 1).
The most common type of anomaly found (type
3) was unilateral hypoplasia of an anterior cerebral artery (25% of cases). In 16% of cases there
was unilateral hypoplasia of a divisional branch of
the basilar artery which was usually associated
with partial or complete internal carotid origin of
the homolateral posterior cerebral artery (type
4). In 11% of cases there was hypoplasia of both
divisional branches of the basilar artery associated with partial or complete internal carotid
origin of both posterior cerebral arteries (type 5).
Riggs found complete absence of a component of
the circle of Willis to be very rare. Even though
one component is extremely hypoplastic, a tiny
vessel can usually be seen to bridge the area

between the two normally related arteries of the
circle.

Anomalies of the circle of Willis, by inducing
haemodynamic changes in blood flow, impose
stresses on the weak parts of arteries, namely at
the bifurcations, and result in the development of
an aneurysm. In addition, physiological alterations in blood flow through the circle of Willis
resulting from such anomalies may have an
important bearing on the potential results of
aneurysm surgery.

Internal Carotid Artery

This arises from the common carotid artery at the
cranial edge of the thyroid cartilage. It runs a
straight course in the neck without branches and
enters the carotid canal. Within the canal the
vessel runs perpendicularly upward and then
turns abruptly forward and medially towards the
front of the petrosal apex where the artery

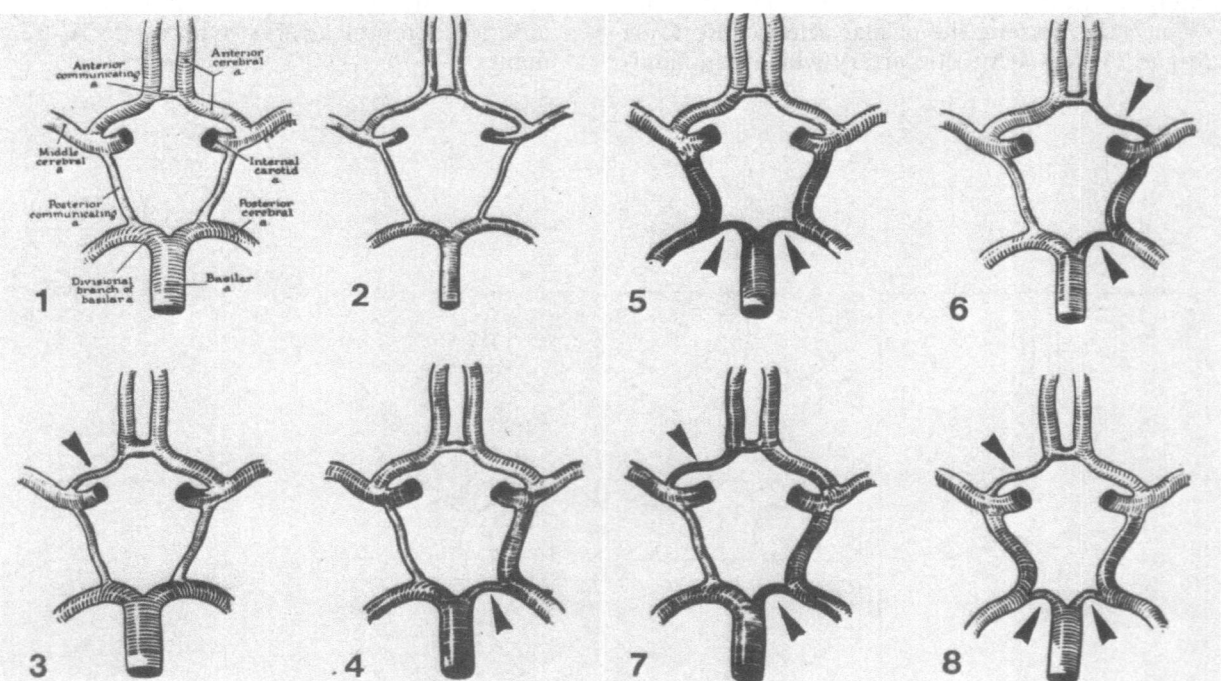

Fig. 2.5. Types of circle of Willis found at autopsy and their incidence: *type 1*, normal circle of Willis (18%); *type 2*, normally
formed circle of Willis but all the components are rather small (6%); *type 3*, hypoplasia of the proximal stem of the anterior
cerebral artery (25%); *type 4*, unilateral hypoplasia of the divisional branch of the basilar artery (16%); *type 5*, hypoplasia of
both divisional branches of the basilar artery (11%); *type 6*, hypoplasia of the proximal stem of the anterior cerebral artery
combined with hypoplasia of the divisional branch of the basilar artery on the same side (8%); *type 7*, hypoplasia of the proximal
stem of the anterior cerebral artery together with hypoplasia of the lateral divisional branch of the basilar artery (8%); and *type
8*, unilateral hypoplasia of the proximal stem of the anterior cerebral artery together with bilateral hypoplasia of the divisional
branches of the basilar artery (8%).

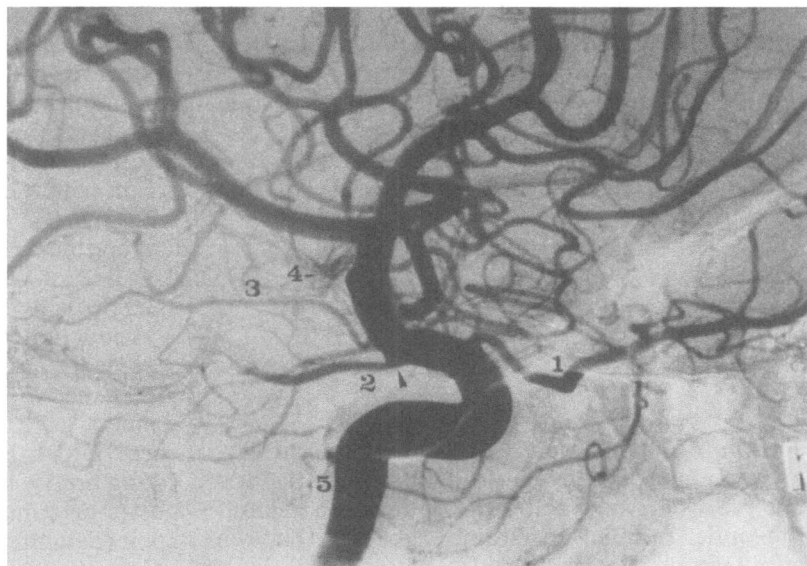

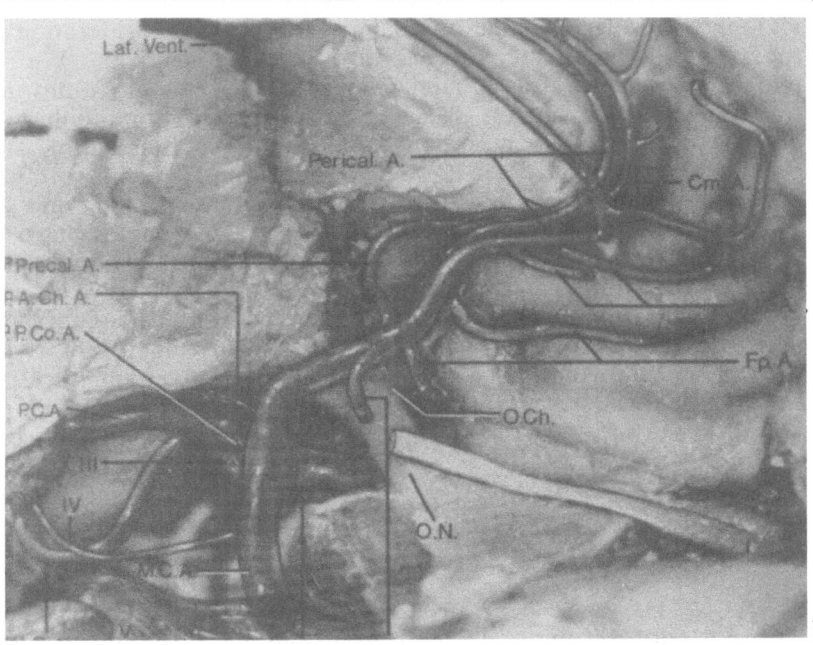

Fig. 2.6. a Carotid angiogram (magnification lateral projection) showing the three main branches of the internal carotid artery. *1*, ophthalmic artery; *2*, posterior communicating artery; *3*, anterior choroidal artery; *4*, lenticulostriate arteries; *5*, meningo-hypophyseal trunk. Notice that there is an infundibulum at the origin of the posterior communicating artery (*arrowhead*). b Anatomical dissection with one cerebral hemisphere removed to expose the midline structures and medial surface of the hemisphere. The relationship of the anterior cerebral artery (*ACA*) to the optic nerve (*O.N.*) and optic chiasma (*O.Ch.*) is shown. The posterior communicating artery (*P.Co.A.*), posterior cerebral artery (*P.C.A.*) and anterior choroidal artery (*A.Ch.A.*) pass above the oculomotor nerve (*III*). (By courtesy of Perlmutter and Rhoton 1978)

emerges from the foramen lacerum in the body of the sphenoid. It then climbs almost vertically above the foramen lacerum in a groove on the lateral side of the sphenoid sinus where it is closely associated with the frontal pole of the gasserian ganglion. It then runs an S-shaped curve, horizontally and forward in the outer wall of the cavernous sinus. The internal carotid artery then turns abruptly upwards, grooving the medial margin of the anterior clinoid process. During this vertical ascent the internal carotid artery pierces the inner layer of the dura to become an intradu-

ral structure. It then doubles back upon itself, passing below the anterior perforated substances to the medial end of the Sylvian fissure where it dividies into the anterior and middle cerebral arteries.

The internal carotid artery can therefore be divided into four segments: cervical, intrapetrosal, cavernous sinus and intradural.

The internal carotid artery gives rise to three important branches (Fig. 2.6a, b)—(a) the ophthalmic artery, (b) the posterior communicating artery, and (c) the anterior choroidal artery—

before it divides into the anterior and middle cerebral arteries. In addition, the meningohypophyseal trunk (Fig. 2.6a) arises from the internal carotid artery, where it enters the cavernous sinus and supplies the posterior lobe of the pituitary and meningeal branches to the tentorium and dura on the clivus, dorsum sellae and adjacent petrous bones.

Ophthalmic Artery

The first major branch, the ophthalmic artery, arises from the convexity of the carotid siphon and passes forward below the optic nerve to enter the optic foramen. Anatomical studies (Hayreh and Dass 1962; Renn and Rhoton 1975) have identified the origin of the ophthalmic artery as the point at which the internal carotid artery pierces the dura. The ophthalmic origin was intradural in approximately 89% of dissections, lying at the level of penetration of the dura by the internal carotid artery in 83%, or within 1 mm distal to this point in 6.5%. In the remaining 10.5% of cases the artery arises extradurally. The ophthalmic artery provides a very important landmark on the lateral carotid angiogram therefore, and an aneurysm arising from the internal carotid artery from a point more than 1 mm proximal to the origin of the ophthalmic artery can be reasonably regarded as extradural (Punt 1979).

Posterior Communicating Artery

The posterior communicating arteries join the two internal carotid arteries with the proximal parts of the posterior cerebral artery. They vary from 4 to 14 mm in length, and the calibre of the vessel is usually thinner than that of the posterior cerebral artery that extends beyond it (Fig. 2.7a). Although embryologically the posterior cerebral artery arises from the internal carotid artery, by birth it has become a terminal branch of the basilar artery. Direct origin of the posterior cerebral artery from the internal carotid artery (foetal type posterior cerebral artery) may be found (Fig. 2.7b, c) in 15%–40% of cases (Alpers et al. 1959; Kaplan and Ford 1966; Saeki and Rhoton 1977).

The neurosurgeon, in operating on posterior communicating artery aneurysms, certainly must be aware of the situation in which the posterior communicating artery constitutes the main or sole source of the posterior cerebral artery supply. Sengupta (1975) has shown that in cases of posterior communicating artery aneurysm, patients with a foetal posterior cerebral artery are more susceptible to cerebral ischaemia from vasospasm or cerebral occlusion than those with a normal artery arising from the basilar bifurcation.

A junctional dilatation or infundibulum may be seen at the origin of the posterior communicating artery (see Fig. 2.6a). An infundibulum has been defined as a triangular or rounded dilatation occurring at the origin of the posterior communicating artery, measuring less than 3 mm, with the posterior communicating artery arising from its apex (Saltzman 1959). Some authors regard it as being pre-aneurysmal, but certainly no serious consideration is usually given to its surgical removal. We have definitely documented at angiography in our department enlargement of an infundibulum to produce a definite posterior communicating artery aneurysm which has subsequently produced a subarachnoid haemorrhage (Patrick and Appleby 1983), and other such examples have been reported in the literature (Yoshimoto and Suzuki 1974; Taveras and Wood 1976; Waga and Morikawa 1979).

The term posterior communicating artery aneurysm is perhaps misleading since it is exceedingly rare for an aneurysm actually to arise from the posterior communicating artery itself (Kamiyama et al. 1979). Pia (1979), however, describes two types that do so: a fusiform type without a definable neck arising in association with an infundibulum of the posterior communicating artery, and a rarer saccular aneurysm as illustrated by Kamiyama et al. (1979). The majority of such aneurysms arise from the lateral wall of the internal carotid artery between the origin of the posterior communicating artery and that of the anterior choroidal artery. Anatomical knowledge of these vessels is therefore important, since they will have to be dissected away from the aneurysm prior to clipping. The anterior choroidal artery is not infrequently involved within the wall of aneurysm or densely fused to it, especially if the aneurysm is over 5 mm in size at its base (Kempe 1968).

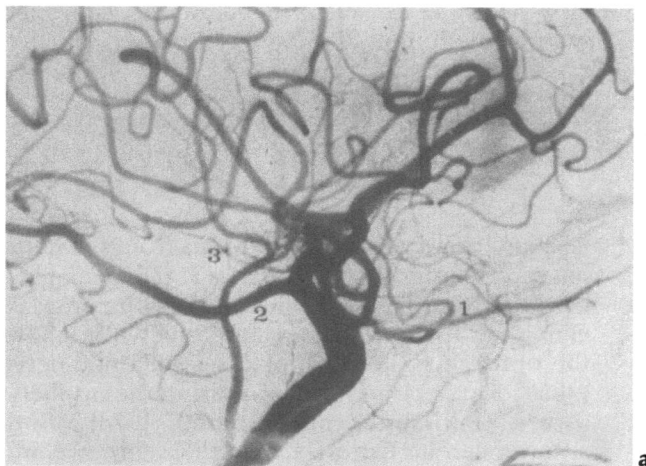

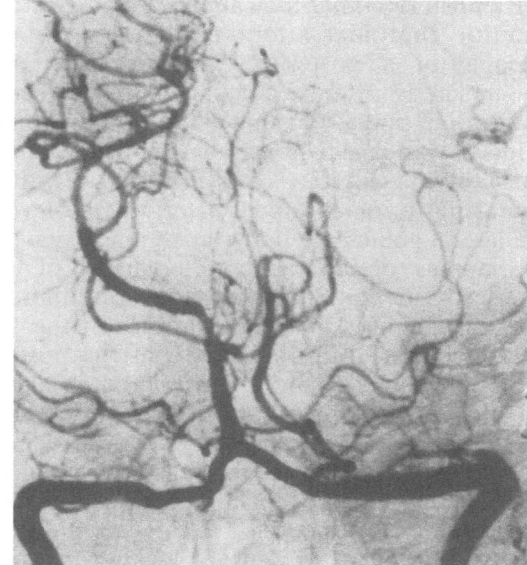

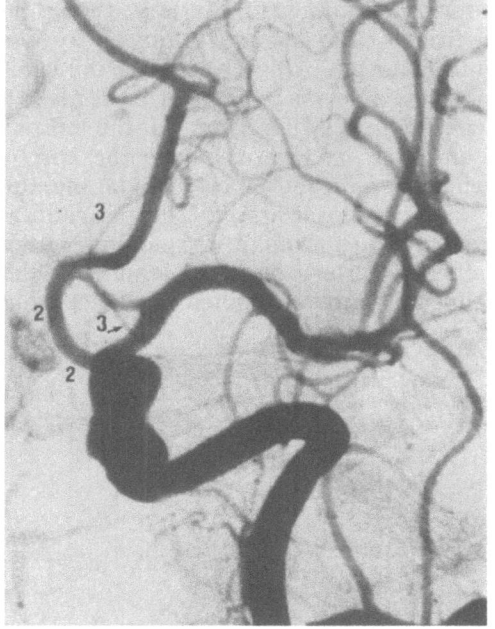

Fig. 2.7. Left carotid angiogram (**a** lateral and **b** Townes oblique projection) showing a foetal left posterior cerebral artery. *1*, ophthalmic artery; *2*, foetal posterior cerebral artery; *3*, anterior choroidal artery. **c** Vertebral angiography confirms that the left posterior cerebral artery does not fill from the basilar system.

Anterior Choroidal Artery

This artery arises from the posterolateral aspect of the internal carotid artery, about 2–3 mm above the origin of the posterior communicating artery (see Fig. 2.6a, b). The artery runs upwards and posteriorly in the ambient cistern, closely related to the posterior cerebral artery and basal vein of Rosenthal. It then passes through the choroidal fissure to enter the temporal horn of the lateral ventricle, its point of entry sometimes showing as a characteristic right-angled kink on the lateral angiogram. The artery then continues to follow the choroid plexus of the temporal horn around the atrium and terminates near the foramen of Munro. In the lateral arterial phase of the angiogram, a typical blush showing the outline of the temporal horn may be seen. The artery contributes to the vascular supply of the optic tract, cerebral peduncle, uncus, lateral geniculate body, anterior perforated substance, tip of the temporal lobe, dentate gyrus and fornix, and pulvinar of the thalamus. The effects of occlusion of the anterior choroidal artery were first described by Foix et al. (1925) and consist of a contralateral hemiplegia, hemianaesthesia and hemianopsia.

Kempe (1968) has indicated that damage to the anterior choroidal artery during, for instance, clipping of a posterior communicating artery aneurysm, is often accompanied by no serious effects. He points out that, based on anatomical studies, one can demonstrate a constant anastomosis of the anterior choroidal artery with the lateral posterior choroidal artery at the level of the lateral geniculate body, as well as a generous overlapping of the capillary territories of these arteries. Other studies have shown that there are also anastomoses between branches of the anterior choroidal artery and those of the posterior communicating, posterior cerebral, internal carotid and middle cerebral arteries. The presence of these anastomoses explains the inconsistent consequences of anterior choroidal artery occlusion.

In a study of 453 congenital or acquired arteriovenous malformations, Perret and Nishioka (1966) found that 18% were located in the intraventricular or periventricular regions, and that the anterior choroidal artery and posterior choroidal artery contributed to their supply. These vessels may also supply arteriovenous malformations located in the basal ganglia, temporal lobe, midbrain, geniculate bodies and thalamus. A detailed study of the microsurgical anatomy of the anterior choroidal artery is provided in the article by Rhoton et al. (1979) and of the choroidal arteries by Fujii et al. (1980).

Anterior Cerebral Artery

The anterior cerebral artery arises from the internal carotid artery as it bifurcates at the medial end of the sylvian fissure at the level of the anterior clinoid process. It passes anteromedially above the optic chiasma (70% of cases) or optic nerve (30% of cases) and enters the interhemispheric fissure (Perlmutter and Rhoton 1978). Both anterior cerebral arteries, near their entrance into the interhemispheric fissure, are joined together by the anterior communicating artery; they then ascend in front of the lamina terminalis to pass into the interhemispheric fissure. Above the lamina terminalis the anterior cerebral arteries make a smooth curve around the genu of the corpus callosum and pass backwards above the corpus callosum in the pericallosal cistern, taking the name of the pericallosal artery. The pericallosal artery then continues around the splenium of the corpus callosum (artery of the splenium of the corpus callosum) and terminates in the choroid

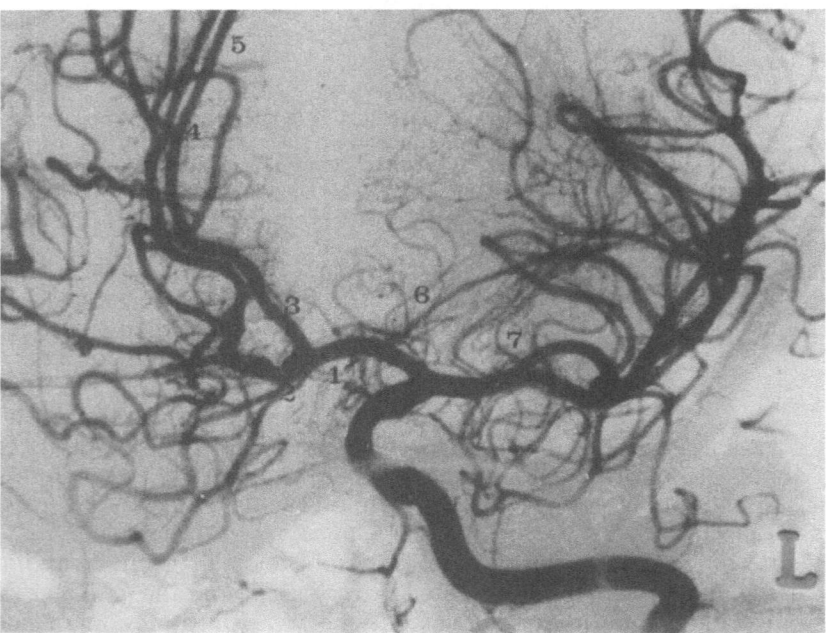

Fig. 2.8. Carotid angiogram (magnified oblique projection through the orbit) showing the three major segments of the anterior cerebral artery. *1*, A$_1$ segment; *2*, anterior communicating artery; *3*, A$_2$ segment; *4*, point of origin of the callosomarginal artery; *5*, pericallosal artery; *6*, anterior choroidal artery; *7*, lenticulostriate arteries.

plexus in the roof of the third ventricle. There is usually anastomosis between branches of the artery of the splenium of the corpus callosum and the splenial branches of the posterior cerebral artery.

From the surgical point of view, the anterior cerebral artery can be divided into three segments (Fig. 2.8).

1. The segment from the carotid bifurcation to the point of origin of the anterior communicating artery is known as the horizontal part, proximal anterior cerebral or A_1 segment.
2. The segment distal to the anterior communicating artery up to the point of origin of the callosomarginal artery is called the vertical part or A_2 segment.
3. The part distal to the origin of the callosomarginal artery is termed the pericallosal artery.

A_1 Segment of the Anterior Cerebral Artery

It is of considerable surgical importance to appreciate that this part of the anterior cerebral artery runs forward and medially from the carotid bifurcation (see Fig. 10.18). Dunker and Harris (1976) have emphasised the importance of knowing the sites of origin, course and parenchymal distribution of branches of the A_1 segment or proximal anterior cerebral artery in order to avoid manipulations which might produce severe neurological deficits.

There are branches that originate from the anterior cerebral artery just distal to the internal carotid artery bifurcation which supply the genu and the contiguous posterior limb of the internal capsule and the rostral thalamus. Branches from the proximal 4 mm supply the anterior limb of the internal capsule, the neighbouring hypothalamus, anterioventral putamen and pallidum. The remaining anterior cerebral artery, proximal to the anterior communicating artery, sends branches to the optic chiasma, the adjacent hypothalamus and the anterior commissure (Fig. 2.9).

The recurrent artery of Heubner, in a study by Perlmutter and Rhoton (1978), can be seen to arise from the A_2 segment in 78% of cases (Fig. 2.10), from the A_1 segment in 14%, and at the level of the anterior communicating artery in 8% of cases. From its origin it turns laterally, and in the majority of cases passes in very close relationship to the superolateral aspect of the proximal anterior cerebral artery or A_1 segment.

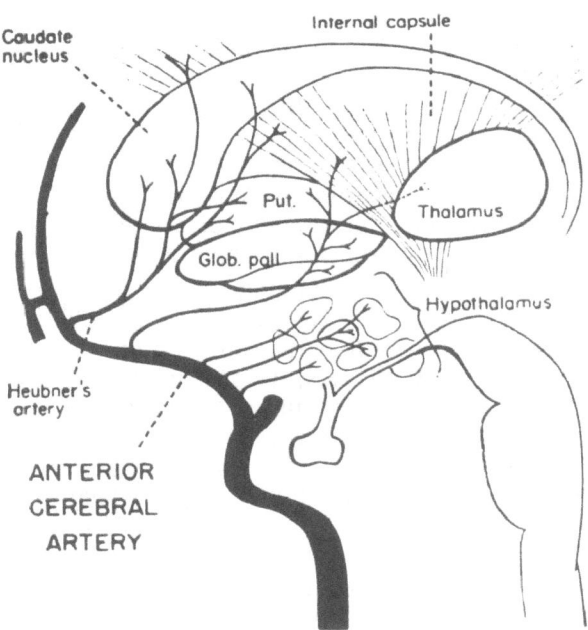

Fig. 2.9. Distribution of supply of the anterior cerebral artery. (By courtesy of Dunker and Harris 1976)

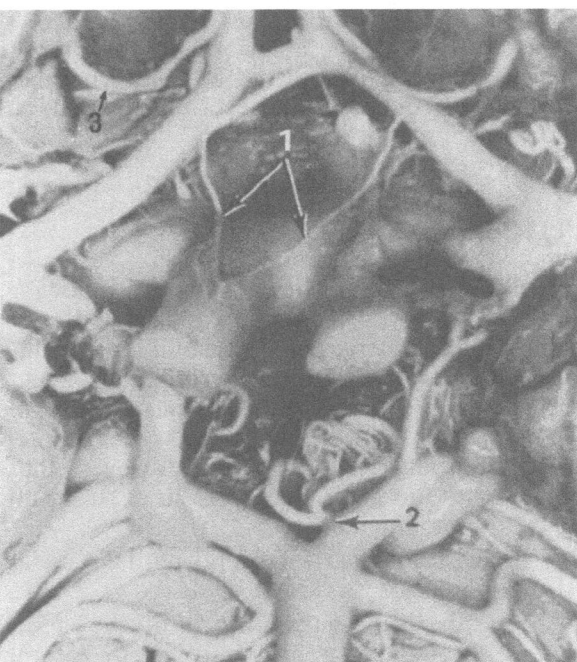

Fig. 2.10. Photograph of the base of the brain with the circle of Willis injected. There is a prominent anterior communicating artery. *1*, arteries to the optic chiasm; *2*, thalamoperforating arteries from the basilar bifurcation; *3*, artery of Heubner (By courtesy of Wollschlager 1974)

At the level of the internal carotid bifurcation it turns upwards and backwards to enter the anterior perforated substance. Heubner's artery supplies much of the striatum and the internal capsule rostral to the anterior commissure. Angiographically this vessel is best demonstrated on the AP projections, being indistinguishable on the lateral projection (see Fig. 2.13).

A₂ Segment of the Anterior Cerebral Artery

This segment gives few central branches but several cortical branches (see Fig. 2.6b). A few centimetres distal to the anterior communicating artery there arises the orbitofrontal artery, which supplies the orbital surface of the frontal lobe and the gyrus rectus. It anastomoses with orbitofrontal branches of the middle cerebral artery. The neurosurgeon may encounter this artery after a small portion of the gyrus rectus has been removed. The frontopolar artery arises in the region of the genu of the corpus callosum and runs anteriorly in the subfrontal sulcus. It supplies most of the pole of the frontal lobe, extending medially to the corpus callosum. The callosomarginal artery originates at the top of the corpus callosum and runs for a short course parallel to the main trunk of the anterior cerebral artery in the callosomarginal sulcus. It sends branches which supply the medial aspect of the frontal lobe above the corpus callosum.

Pericallosal Artery

From this artery branches arise to the following.

1. The medial surface of the frontal lobe, including the superior frontal gyrus and cingulate gyrus, some supply to the paracentral lobule through its anterior middle and posterior internal frontal artery branches. However, these branches may on occasions arise from the callosomarginal artery.
2. The paracentral artery supplying the paracentral lobule.
3. Branches to the medial aspect of the parietal lobe through its superior and inferior internal parietal artery branches.

Small branches also connect with the corpus callosum as the pericallosal artery passes along it. The reader is referred to the excellent text by Salamon and Huang (1976) for a detailed description of the course and distribution of these branches.

Anterior Communicating Artery

This artery has an average length of 4 mm and may consist of single or multiple channels. Almeida (1931) distinguished approximately 20 anatomical forms. In the past, the anterior communicating artery was described as having no branches in humans (Critchley 1930) or as inconsistently possessing a single callosal branch (Gullilan 1968; Stephens and Stilwell 1969). Dunker and Harris (1976) observed no fewer than three branches arising from the anterior communicating artery in a careful examination of 20 brain specimens from patients without neurological disease. They showed that these supplied the fornix, corpus callosum, septal region and anterior cingulum.

Several observations of surgical importance can be made:

1. The proximal anterior cerebral artery (A₁ segment), particularly its most proximal end, gives most of the vital central perforating branches (Fig. 2.11), which are not visible on angiography. These consistently supply the genu and contiguous posterior limb of the internal capsule, the rostral thalamus and much of the hypothalamus. Damage to these vessels by surgical occlusion or manipulation could readily produce a hemiparesis with brachial preponderance and significant personality changes. In this respect, this part of the artery is more important than the artery of Heubner, which supplies the most anterior striatum and anterior limb of the internal capsule, and thus the artery of Heubner is not the only vessel responsible for hemiparesis.

2. The anterior communicating artery itself contributes very little central vascular supply, and its areas of distribution have an alternative source of supply. Nevertheless, it does supply branches to prominent structures in the limbic system (e.g. fornix, septal region, corpus callosum and anterior cingulum) and this may explain the proportion of permanent personality changes which may occur in patients with ruptured anterior communicating artery aneurysm.

3. As the anterior cerebral artery runs forwards and medially from its origin, the region of the anterior communicating artery lies anterior to the bifurcation point. Surgical exploration of this

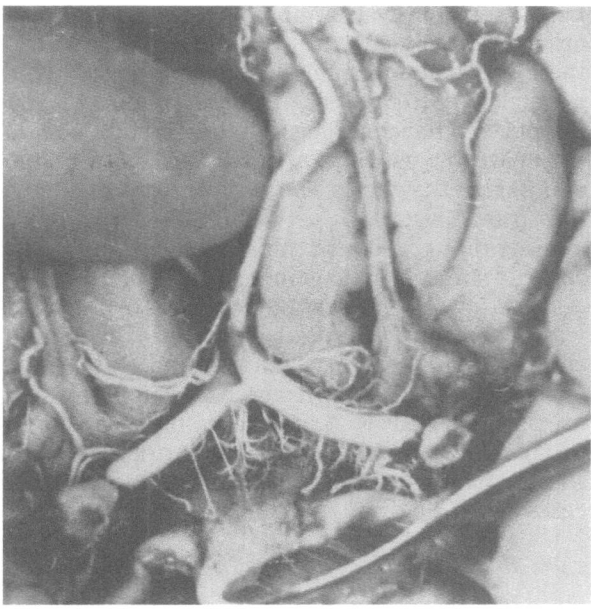

Fig. 2.11. Photograph of the base of the brain with the anterior cerebral and anterior communicating arteries injected. Multiple small perforating arteries arising from the A_1 segment of the anterior cerebral artery, and the anterior communicating artery, are demonstrated. (By courtesy of Lin and Kricheff 1974)

region is unnecessary and it may be harmful to dissect out the proximal part or A_1 segment of the anterior cerebral artery, since the anterior communicating artery can be explored with less retraction of the brain.

Anomalies of the Anterior Cerebral Artery

Anatomical variations are considerable, and in patients harbouring an aneurysm are even more pronounced. For a proper understanding of the pathological problems following subarachnoid haemorrhage and for planning surgical therapy these variations should be fully appreciated.

Normal Brains

Alpers et al. (1959) examined 350 normal adult brains, and showed anomalies of the anterior cerebral artery in 43 cases (12%) (Fig. 2.12). The abnormalities were predominantly in accessory vessels, such as a triple anterior cerebral artery in 28 cases. In six cases there was fusion of both anterior cerebral arteries to form a single vessel (azygous anterior cerebral artery) for a variable distance. A hypoplastic anterior cerebral artery was present only in eight cases (2%). There was more than one anterior communicating artery in 9% of cases.

Baptista (1963), in a review of the literature, found 23 cases of azygous anterior cerebral artery in 2153 adult brains (1%). He described three types of anomalies occurring in the distal anterior cerebral artery.

1. A true azygous artery from which all major branches are given off to both hemispheres.

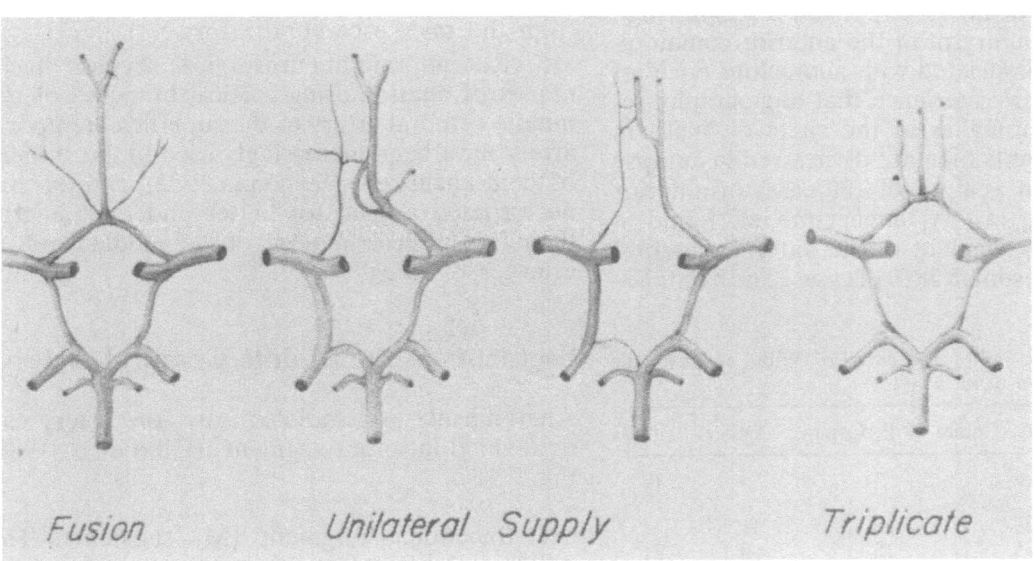

Fig. 2.12. Anterior cerebral artery variations (after Alpers)

2. A bihemispheric anterior cerebral artery where both right and left anterior cerebral arteries are present, but one is rudimentary and most of the major branches to both hemispheres arise from the other anterior cerebral artery.
3. A triple anterior cerebral artery with an accessory anterior cerebral artery arising from the anterior communicating artery. This artery is often called the anterior middle cerebral artery or the medial artery of the corpus callosum. It is only occasionally demonstrated angiographically.

In the presence of a single so-called azygous artery, there is a higher incidence of peripheral anterior cerebral arteries (see Fig. 10.19). This type of variation is different from that seen in aneurysm cases.

Variations in Brains Harbouring Saccular Aneurysms

Wilson et al. (1954) studied 114 specimens of the circle of Willis from patients with ruptured aneurysm (Table 2.1). Their figures showed a very high association between aneurysm and anomalies of the circle of Willis. In 73 cases (64%) one of the anterior cerebral arteries was hypoplastic. It is important to note from their figures that anterior communicating aneurysms are more frequently associated with a hypoplastic anterior cerebral artery and posterior communicating artery aneurysms with a foetal posterior cerebral artery. Kirgis et al. (1966) found a similar high incidence of aneurysm of the anterior communicating artery associated with anomalous circle of Willis. It is our experience that angiography reveals fewer anomalies of the circle of Willis in aneurysm patients than are discovered in autopsy material. In an analysis of 100 cases of anterior communicating artery aneurysm we found a hypoplastic A_1 segment of the anterior cerebral artery to be present in 28% of cases. The hypoplastic A_1 segment was combined with a foetal posterior cerebral artery in 8% of cases. In one case there was a hypoplastic A_1 segment together with a persistent trigeminal artery. Norlen and Barnum (1953) have emphasised the different circulatory patterns which may occur through the anterior part of the circle. The various types of circulation are illustrated in Chap. 7 (on cerebral angiography) and are more fully discussed as regards surgical management in Chap. 10.

Kwak et al. (1979), in an analysis of 296 cases with a single aneurysm of the anterior communicating artery, described fenestration or the presence of more than two anterior communicating arteries in 17 cases (5.7%) and abnormal vessels of anterior communicating artery origin, such as the median artery of the corpus callosum, in 13 cases (4.4%).

Middle Cerebral Artery

The middle cerebral artery is the largest and the most anatomically complex of the cerebral arteries. A knowledge of its anatomy is important for several reasons.

1. The middle cerebral artery is a common site for aneurysms, which usually arise near major divisions of the main trunk of the artery, most commonly a bifurcation or trifurcation.
2. The majority of intracranial arteriovenous malformations receive part of their blood supply from the middle cerebral artery.
3. Recent microneurosurgical bypass techniques of anastomosing cortical branches of the middle cerebral artery to the superficial temporal artery have been increasingly used in the surgery of giant aneurysms (Sengupta 1982), and this has necessitated a need for better understanding of the microsurgical anatomy of the middle cerebral artery.

Segments of the Middle Cerebral Artery

Anatomically and radiologically, the artery can be divided into four segments (Gibo et al. 1981; Fig. 2.13).

1. Sphenoidal segment (M_1 segment). The middle cerebral artery, from its origin from the internal carotid artery bifurcation, runs in a hori-

Table 2.1. Anomalies of the circle of Willis and saccular aneurysms (Wilson et al. 1954)

	A. Comm.	P. Comm.	Others	Total
Normal circle	2	5	3	10
Hypoplastic				
ACA	28	8	11	47
Foetal PCA	5	18	8	31
Combined	12	9	5	26

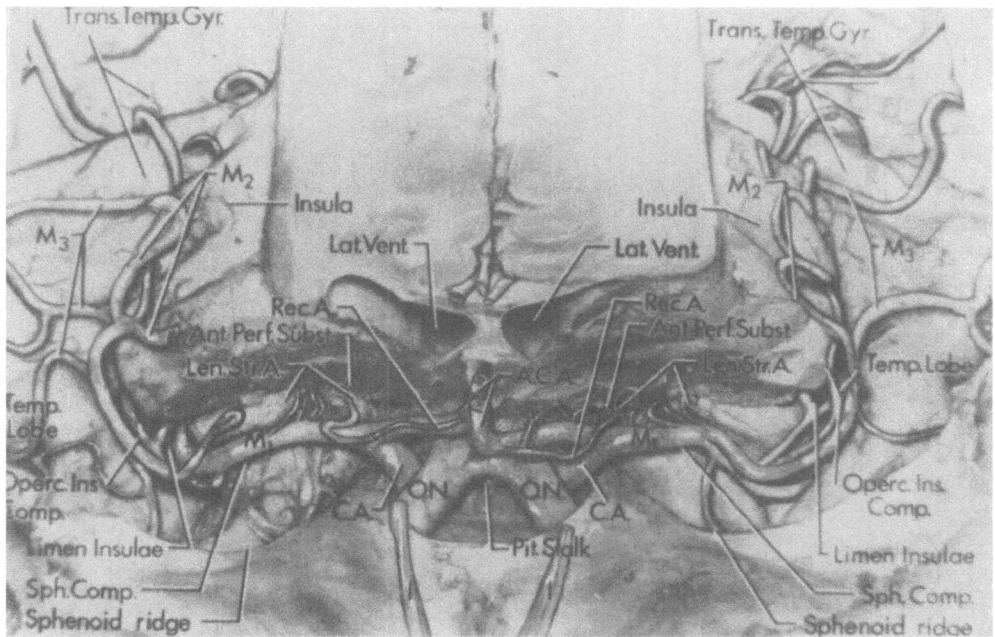

Fig. 2.13. Relationships of the M_1 segment of the temporal lobe (*Temp. Lobe*), the M_2 segment to the insular and the M_3 segment to the transverse temporal gyri (*Trans. Temp. Gyrx.*) are clearly shown. The lenticulostriate arteries (*Len. Str. A.*) arise from the M_1 segment and enter the anterior perforated substance. The course of the recurrent artery of Heubner (*Rec. A*) is clearly shown. (By courtesy of Gibo et al. 1981)

zontal lateral course parallel to the sphenoid ridge to enter the sylvian fissure. The sphenoidal segment is between the frontal lobe above and the temporal lobe below. At the level of the anterior perforated substance, it gives rise to the lenticulostriate arteries. In some cases there may be a proximal origin of the fronto-orbital artery from the middle of the sphenoidal segment.

2. Insular segment (M_2 segment). The middle cerebral artery then turns 90° and enters the depths of the sylvian fissure where it lies on the insula. It then divides into its major branches which supply the external surface of the frontal, parietal, temporal and occipital lobes.

3. Opercular segment (M_3 segment). The major branches pass out of the Sylvian fissure and course round the frontoparietal and temporal operculum to reach the external surface of the hemisphere.

4. Cortical segment (M_4 segment). The terminal branches of the middle cerebal artery have characteristic courses running either on the surface or deep within the sulci.

Variations in Branching of the Middle Cerebral Trunk

Most middle cerebral aneurysms are located at the point of division of the main trunk of the middle cerebral artery into its two or three major branches. These branches will need to be dissected free under microscopic control before the aneurysm is clipped. The pattern of major division of the middle cerebral artery trunk, however, is extremely variable with regard to both site (medial or lateral) and number of branches (single trunk, bifurcation, trifurcation or multiple middle cerebral artery trunks; Fig. 2.14). Krayenbuhl and Yasargil (1968) analysed the variations of branching of the middle cerebral artery trunk and showed that there was a trifurcation-type branching in 25% of cases, pseudobifurcation in 18.5%, lateral bifurcation in 48%, and a medial bifurcation in 2.5%. In 6% of cases there was an early origin of the fronto-orbital artery from the sphenoidal segment of the middle cerebral artery (Fig. 2.14). Gibo et al. (1981) stated

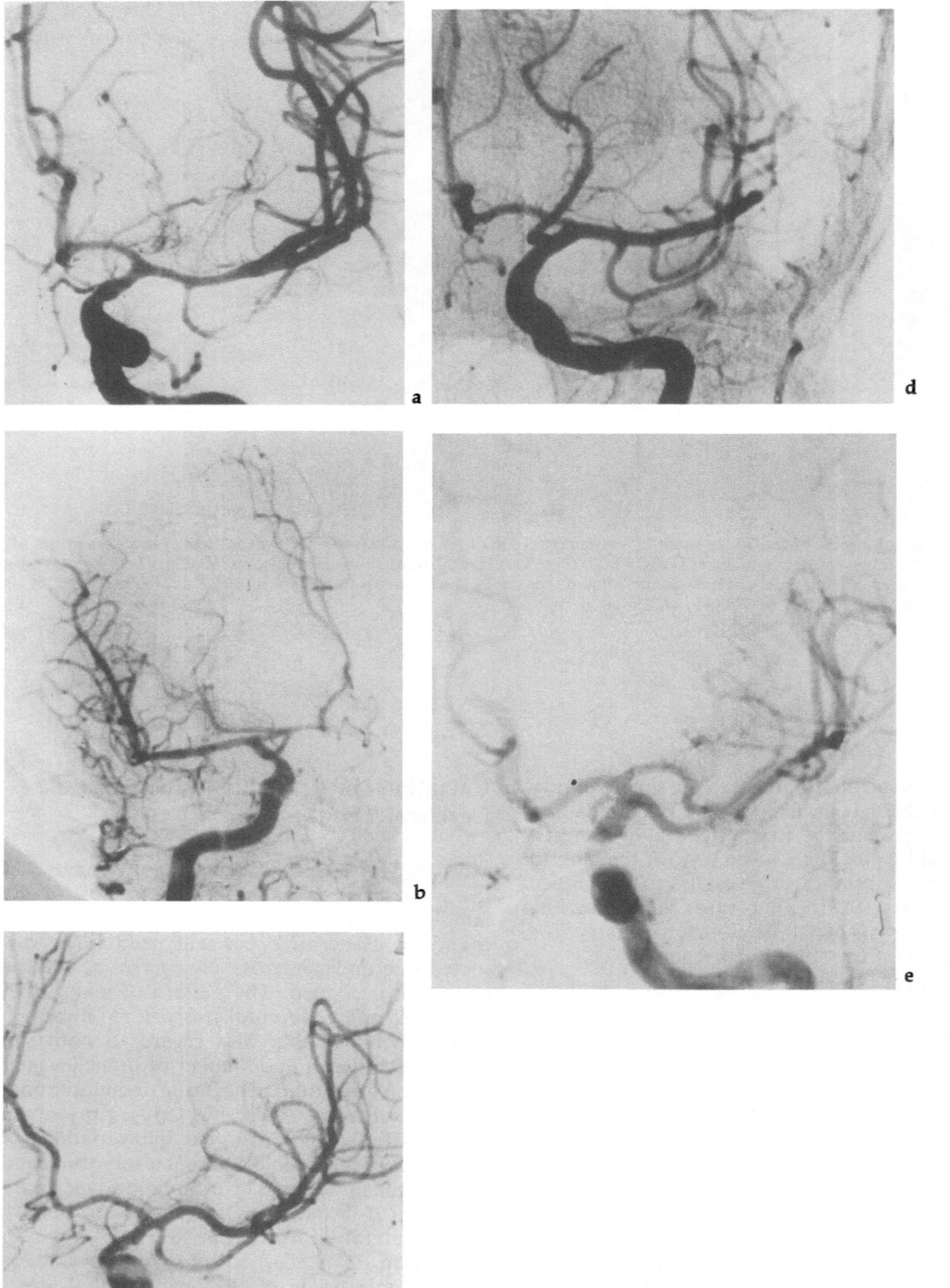

Fig. 2.14a–e. Variations in branching of the middle cerebral trunk:
a bifurcation; **b** trifurcation; **c** early bifurcation; **d** multiple trunks;
e accessory middle cerebral artery.

that the main trunk of the middle cerebral artery may divide in one of three ways: bifurcation (78% of hemispheres), trifurcation (12%), or division into multiple trunks (10%). The middle cerebral arteries that bifurcated were divided into three groups: equal bifurcation (18%), inferior trunk dominant (32%), or superior trunk dominant (28%). The surgical implications of this variable branching pattern lie in the fact that aneurysms arising from a normally situated bifurcation or trifurcation in the sylvian fissure will be away from the important perforating vessels, while those arising on the M_1 segment or from an early bifurcation will be closely related to them (see Fig. 7.10).

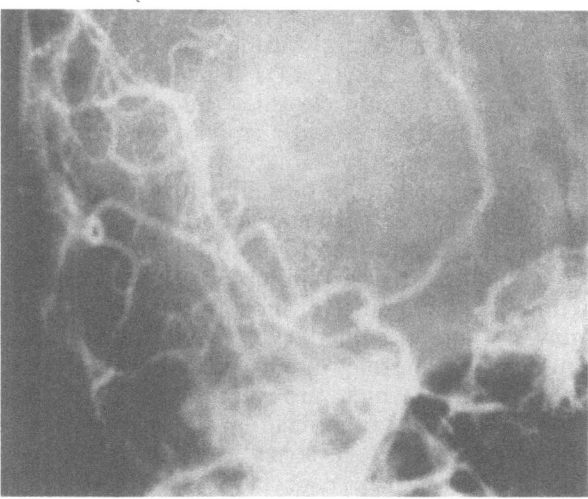

Fig. 2.15. Accessory middle cerebral artery with an aneurysm at its origin.

Middle Cerebral Artery Branches

These branches are best demonstrated on the lateral angiographic projection.

The middle cerebral artery supplies:

1. Frontal branches, e.g. orbitofrontal artery, prefrontal, precentral and central arteries
2. Parietal branches, e.g. anterior and posterior parietal arteries and the angular gyrus artery
3. Temporal branches, e.g. anterior, middle and posterior temporal arteries, the temporo-occipital artery and the temporopolar artery

(For a detailed consideration of the origin, course, distribution and variations of the middle cerebral artery branches, the reader is referred to the excellent descriptions by Salamon and Huang 1976.)

Anomalies of the Middle Cerebral Artery

These are less frequently encountered than with other cranial arteries. Two types of anomaly may be found:

1. A duplicated middle cerebral artery is a second artery that arises from the internal carotid artery.
2. An accessory middle cerebral artery is one that arises from the anterior cerebral artery, usually near the origin of the anterior communicating artery.

The accessory middle cerebral artery is distinguished from the recurrent artery of Heubner by the fact that the latter vessel enters the anterior perforated substance whereas the accessory middle cerebral artery courses lateral to this area and sends branches to the cortical areas normally supplied by the middle cerebral artery.

Crompton (1962) and Jain (1964) found the incidence of such anomalies to be about 3%. Crompton found 11 anomalies in his study of 347 hemispheres, 10 duplicate and 1 anomalous artery. Jain (1964) found 10 anomalies in 300 hemispheres, 2 duplicate and 8 anomalous arteries. Stabler (1970) reported (from our department) two cases of duplicated middle cerebral artery, including one with an aneurysm at its origin (Fig. 2.15). In his report, he used the term accessory middle cerebral artery both for branches from the internal carotid artery and from the anterior cerebral artery.

Lenticulostriate Arteries (Thalamostriate Arteries)

The lenticulostriate arteries were described by Heubner in 1872. They arise from the superior surface of the sphenoidal segment of the middle cerebral artery to penetrate the anterior substance (Fig. 2.13). They run upwards with a characteristic S-shaped curve produced by an initial slight concave curve laterally as they penetrate the anterior perforated substance, followed by a more prominent concave curve medially as they run across the lateral surface of the lentiform nucleus (Figs. 2.8, 2.14). The lenticulostriate arteries are usually classified into a larger and longer lateral group and a smaller medial group. At angiography they are best demonstrated on the AP projections, especially with magnification (See Figs. 2.8, 2.14). They can be identified in the lateral projection (see Fig 2.6) but they are usually obscured by the middle cerebral branches. Those in the medial group are very small, and may not be identified even with magnification studies. The lateral group usually consists of six to eight vessels which are typically clearly seen (Fig. 2.8, 2.14). Identification and protection of the lenticulostriate arteries at surgery is of extreme importance, especially when aneurysms arise at the junction of the middle cerebral artery and the lenticulostriate arteries.

Posterior Cerebral Artery

The posterior cerebral artery, as mentioned previously, is usually the terminal branch of the basilar artery. The part of the artery between its origin and the posterior communicating artery is usually referred to as the P_1 segment (Krayenbuhl and Yasargil 1968; Zeal and Rhoton 1978). The artery then runs from the posterior communicating artery within the penduncular and ambient cisterns and terminates at the posterior aspect of the midbrain (P_2 segment). In this part of its course the artery is separated from the superior cerebellar artery by the oculomotor nerve. The artery then continues through the quadrigeminal cistern to the region of the quadrigeminal plate, and finally ends at the anterior limit of the calcarine fissure (P_3 segment).

The posterior cerebral artery branches can be divided into three groups (Zeal and Rhoton 1978).

1. Central or brainstem branches, which are of two types.
a) Direct perforating arteries, e.g. thalamoperforating arteries arising from the P_1 segment and thalamogeniculate and peduncular perforating arteries from the P_2 segment (Fig. 2.16).
b) Circumferential arteries, e.g. the short and long circumflex arteries. These usually arise from the P_1 segment and encircle the midbrain, sup-

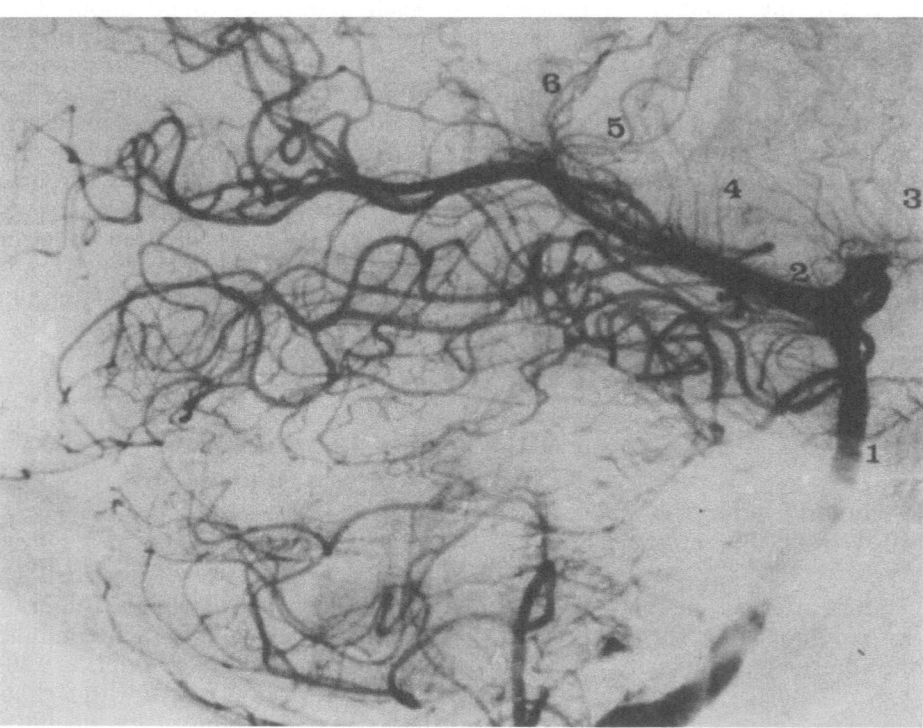

Fig. 2.16. Magnified lateral vertebral angiogram. *1*, basilar artery; *2*, posterior cerebral artery; *3*, thalamo-perforating arteries; *4*, thalamogeniculate arteries; *5*, medial posterior choroidal artery; *6*, lateral posterior choroidal artery.

plying branches as far posteriorly as the colliculi. Those arteries reaching only the geniculate bodies are called short circumflex arteries; those reaching the colliculi are called the long circumflex arteries.

2. Branches to the choroid plexus through the medial and lateral posterior choroidal arteries (Fig. 2.16). Both branches usually arise from the P_2 segment of the posterior cerebral artery, with the medial posterior choroidal artery entering the roof of the third ventricle, and the lateral posterior choroidal arteries passing over the pulvinar of the thalamus to enter the lateral ventricle. The choroidal arteries supply AVMs and tumours arising in and adjacent to the choroid plexus and ventricular system.

3. Cerebral branches of the posterior cerebral artery, which include the inferior temporal group of arteries, the parieto-occipital, calcarine and splenial (posterior pericallosal artery) branches.

Aneurysms may occasionally arise from the posterior cerebral artery itself, the most common sites of origin being at the junction of the posterior communicating artery and the P_1 segment of this vessel, and at the first major branches at the side of the midbrain (see Figs. 7.33 and 17.5).

Vertebrobasilar System

Vertebral Artery

The vertebral arteries arise from the subclavian artery. They ascend over the lateral mass C7 and then traverse the upper cervical foramen transversarium. The arteries then run posteriorly over the posterior arch of the atlas and forward and cranially to penetrate the dura at the level of the foramen magnum, becoming intracranial in location. The vertebral artery in its extracranial course gives rise to several branches which may be identified at angiography (Fig. 2.17): (a) muscular branches, (b) the anterior meningeal artery which supplies the dura in front of the foramen magnum, (c) the posterior meningeal artery which supplies the medial part of the dura of the posterior fossa and falx cerebelli, and (d) the anterior spinal and posterolateral arteries to the spinal cord.

The posterior inferior cerebellar artery represents the major branch of the intracranial portion of the vertebral artery. The vertebral arteries

are frequently asymmetric in size, and in 13% of cases may terminate as a PICA (Fig. 2.18).

Posterior Inferior Cerebellar Artery (PICA)

The anatomy of the PICA is very variable, but important to understand because aneurysm formation at the vertebral artery PICA, junction is not uncommon. In addition, aneurysms may arise on the PICA distal to its origin, (see Fig. 7.32; Hudgins et al. 1983) so that a knowledge of its complete course is necessary. The PICA arises from the vertebral artery, at the level of the olive in about 92% of cases (Salamon and Huang 1976), and this point usually lies about 10 mm above the foramen magnum (Lister et al. 1982). It may have a lower (5%; see Fig. 2.17) or higher

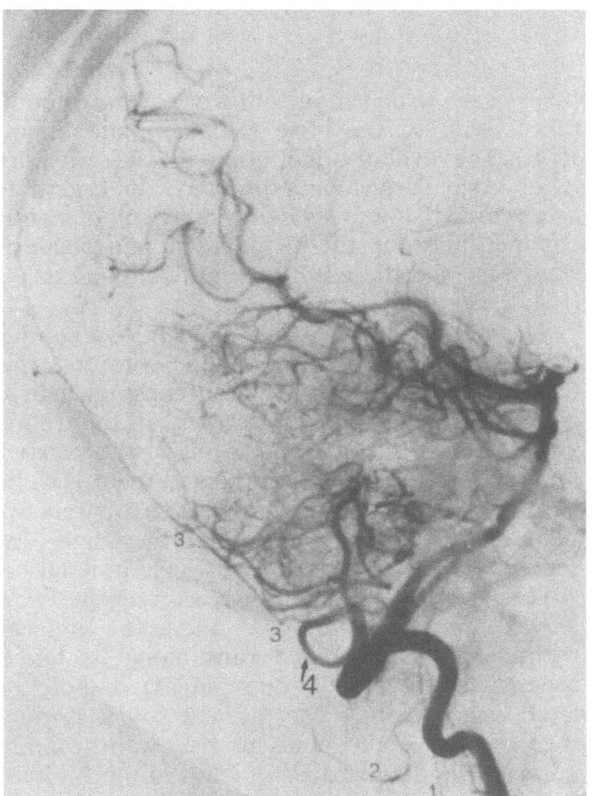

Fig. 2.17. Lateral vertebral angiogram. *1*, anterior spinal artery; *2*, muscular branches; *3*, posterior meningeal artery; *4*, posterior inferior cerebellar artery (PICA). Notice the PICA has a low origin (*arrow*) from the vertebral artery; compare with Fig. 2.21.

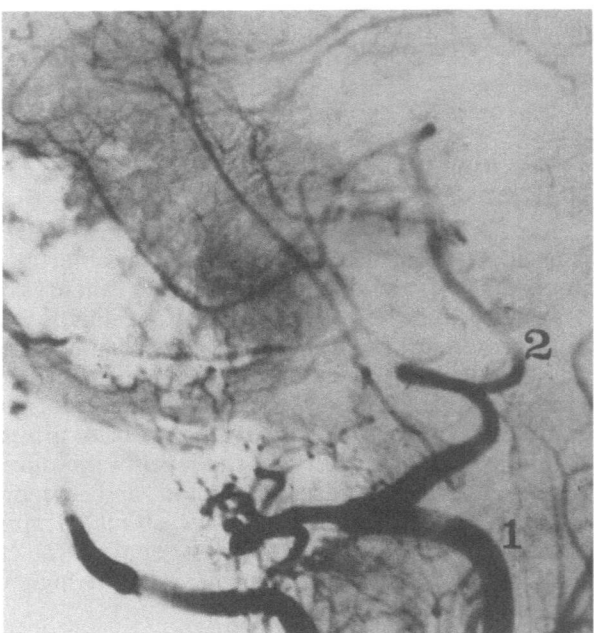

Fig. 2.18. Vertebral artery (*1*) ending as a PICA (*2*)

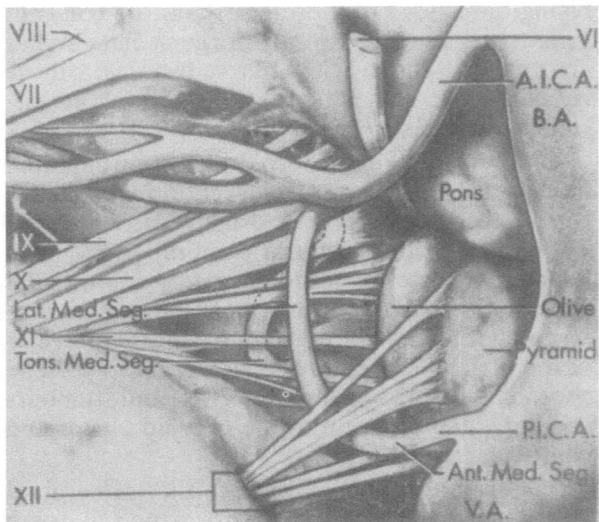

Fig. 2.19. Diagram showing the origin of the PICA from the vertebral artery and the relationship of its anterior medullary and lateral medullary segments to the olive and hypoglossal nerve (*XII*), accessory nerve (*XI*), vagus nerve (*X*) and glossopharyngeal nerve (*IX*). (By courtesy of Hudgins et al. 1983)

(3%) origin from the vertebral artery based on its relationship to the olive (Salamon and Huang 1976). The level of origin of the PICA is obviously of great surgical importance with regard to access to such aneurysms since they will be tightly confined between the medulla, the anterolateral skull base and the ninth to twelfth cranial nerves (Fig. 2.19).

The subsequent course of the PICA is complicated but understandable, if one considers that this artery has three points that it must reach in its course—(a) the choroid plexus of the fourth ventricle, (b) the inferior vermis of the cerebellum, and (c) the inferior surface of the cerebellar hemisphere—and that en route it encounters two "anatomical obstructions", first the olive, and second the cerebellar tonsil which it needs to circumvent (Fig. 2.19). From its origin the PICA leaves the front of the medulla (anterior medullary segment) and runs along its lateral aspect (lateral medullary segment), closely related to and taking a very variable course through the rootlets of the ninth to the twelfth cranial nerves. The major cause of surgical morbidity in PICA vertebral aneurysms is the inadvertent disruption of such nerve roots. The first structure it encounters is the olive, which it may circumvent, either by passing round its superior or inferior aspects or round its middle. Once the PICA has

circumvented the olive it then runs up or down on the posterior aspect of the medulla (posterior medullary segment) to reach the medial surface of the tonsil. It may then go round the tonsil in one of three ways: round its middle, its inferior pole, or its superior pole (supratonsillar segment). In its course, therefore, it presents two loops, which can be identified on the lateral vertebral angiogram (Fig. 2.20). The first loop enables it to go around the olive and reach the back of the brainstem (called the caudal loop), and the second to go around the tonsil (called the cranial loop). The peak of the cranial loop is called the choroidal point and is closely related to the floor of the fourth ventricle. The PICA always supplies branches to the choroid plexus of the fourth ventricle, usually from the area of the choroid point, as well as branches to the inferior vermis of the cerebellum (vermian branches), tonsils and cerebellar hemisphere (hemisphere branches). The PICA may be absent unilaterally in 26% of cases and bilaterally in 2% of cases. In 16% of cases it is hypoplastic (Salamon and Huang 1976). The PICA and anterior inferior cerebellar artery (AICA) show an inverse relationship in size, and if the PICA is hypoplastic, the AICA invariably will be large and supply its usual territory as well as part or all of the territory of the PICA.

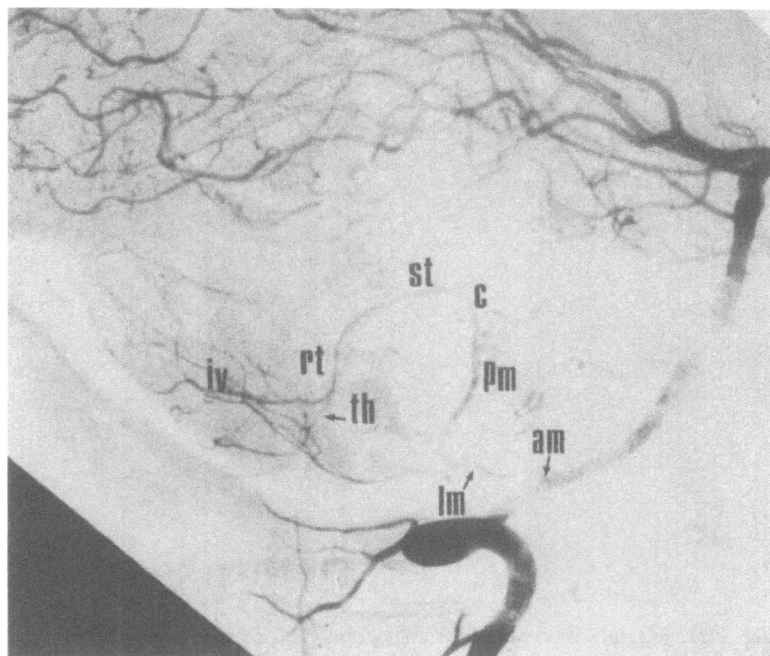

Fig. 2.20. Lateral magnified vertebral angiogram showing the course and distribution of the PICA. *am*, anterior medullary segment; *lm*, lateral medullary segment; *pm*, posterior medullary segment; *c*, choroid point; *st*, supratonsillar segment; *rt*, retrotonsillar segment; *iv*, inferior vermian segment; *th*, tonsillo-hemispheric branch; *am* + *lm* + *pm*, caudal loop (medullary loop); *pm* + *st* + *rt*, cranial loop (tonsillar loop).

Basilar Artery

The basilar artery lies between the two sixth cranial nerves at its origin from the vertebral arteries near the pontomedullary junction, then runs upwards on the belly of the pons to terminate near the pontomesencephalic junction where it is closely related to both third cranial nerves. There are, however, numerous variations in the configuration, length and degree of meandering over the midline of the basilar artery. Its course over the pons can be straight, curved or S-shaped. It frequently curves away from the side of the dominant vertebral artery. The level of termination of the basilar artery (basilar bifurcation) is also subject to considerable variation which is of importance from the surgical anatomy point of view (see Fig. 10.36). In 20% of cases it lies below and in 30% of cases above the level of the posterior clinoid process. In some cases (especialy in the elderly) the basilar tip may reach the floor of the third ventricle or bend forwards into the interpeduncular cistern (Greitz and Lofstedt 1954). The basilar bifurcation may show an area of widening, giving it a cobra-like appearance in some cases, and this should not be misinterpreted as an aneurysm.

The main branches of the basilar artery include (Fig. 2.21):

1. The superior cerebellar arteries
2. Perforating arteries to the pons
3. The anterior inferior cerebellar artery (AICA)

The posterior and lateral surfaces of the upper centimetre of the basilar artery are a rich source of perforating arteries, which are clearly demonstrated on magnification studies in the lateral projection (see Figs. 2.10, 2.16). There are usually no perforating branches arising from the anterior surface of the basilar artery. The significance of this lies in the fact that anteriorly projecting aneurysms arising from the basilar bifurcation will lie free of these important perforating arteries and would be, therefore, more amenable to surgery than a posteriorly directed basilar bifurcation aneurysm, which will be intimately related to these perforating arteries (see Fig. 7.26a).

Anterior Inferior Cerebellar Artery (AICA)

This artery arises from the lower third of the basilar artery, courses around the anterior and anterolateral surface of the pons, and runs laterally towards the flocculus, which may be local-

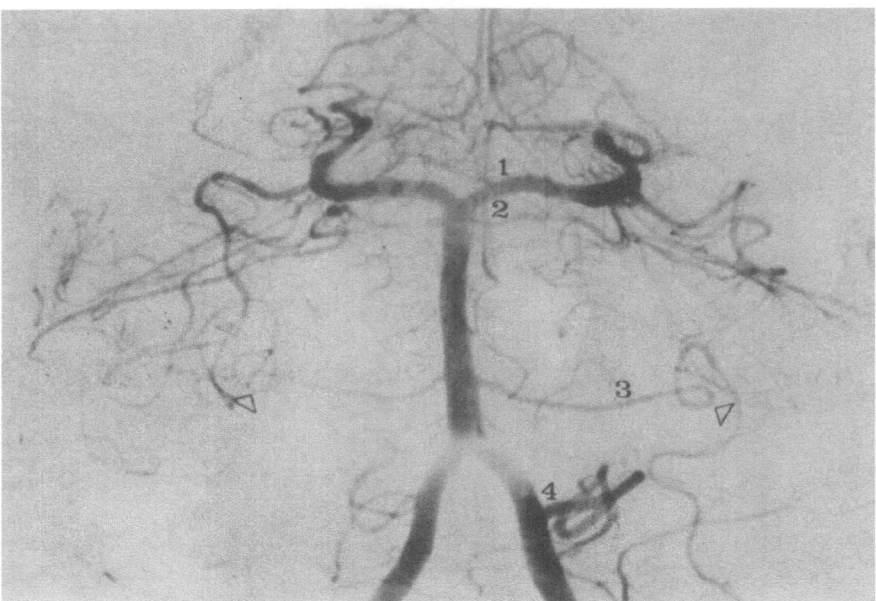

Fig. 2.21. Magnification vertebral angiogram AP projection. *1*, posterior cerebral artery; *2*, superior cerebellar artery; *3*, anterior inferior cerebellar artery (*open arrowheads* indicate floccular loop); *4*, posterior inferior cerebellar artery.

ised at angiography by a characteristic loop (Fig. 2.21). It gives branches to the internal auditory canal and supplies all the inferior surface of the cerebellar hemisphere not supplied by the PICA. It should be emphasised again that there is a considerable overlap of the territory supplied by the PICA and AICA. Anterior inferior cerebellar artery aneurysms are rare; Johnson and Kline (1978) found only 12 cases reported in the world literature.

Superior Cerebellar Artery

The superior cerebellar artery arises from the basilar trunk before its bifurcation, although in about 20% of cases it does so directly from the posterior cerebral artery. The calibre of the superior cerebellar artery is smaller than that of the posterior cerebral artery. The artery may be single, double, or occasionally triple. It runs round the cerebral peduncle of the midbrain in the ambient cistern parallel to the posterior cerebral artery and is separated from it at its origin by the third cranial nerve, the posterior cerebral artery being just above and the superior cerebellar artery just below the tentorial edge. The superior cerebellar artery then passes between the trigeminal and oculomotor nerves into the sulcus

between the mesencephalon and the cerebellum. It then divides into a midline superior vermian artery and lateral hemisphere branches.

Venous Anatomy

A knowledge of the cerebral venous anatomy is especially important in the surgical treatment of arteriovenous malformations. It is essential in the surgery of arteriovenous malformations that arterial feeders be ligated before interruption of the main venous drainage is attempted. There may, of course, be difficulties in differentiating feeding arteries from the draining veins, which may become arterialised.

The cerebral venous system essentially consists of a superficial group of veins draining via the superficial cortical veins into the superficial dural sinuses (sagittal sinus) and a deep group which drains the deep grey and white matter and the choroid plexus of the lateral ventricles into the deep dural sinuses (inferior sagittal sinus and straight sinus; Fig. 2.22).

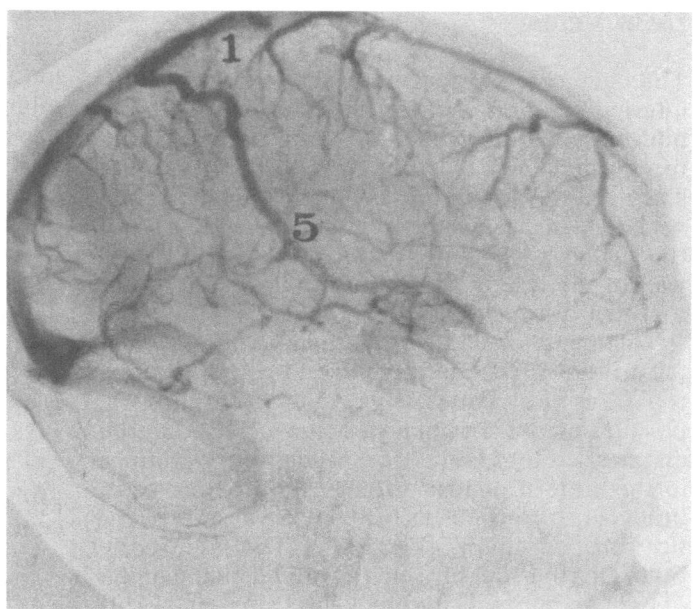

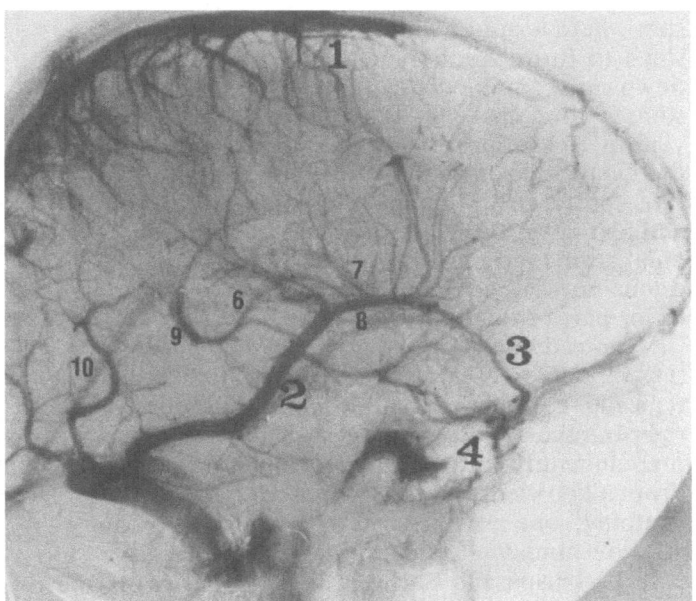

Fig. 2.22. Lateral carotid angiogram, venous phase. *Superficial veins*: *1*, sagittal sinus; *2*, vein of Labbé; *3*, superficial middle cerebral vein; *4*, cavernous sinus; *5*, vein of Trolard. *Deep veins*: *6*, internal cerebral vein; *7*, thalamostriate vein; *8*, venous angle; *9*, vein of Galen; *10*, straight sinus.

Superficial Veins

The patterns of superficial drainage of the cerebral hemispheres are extremely variable. However, the prominent veins that may be demonstrated at angiography include the following:

1. The vein of Trolard in the posterior frontal region which drains upwards into the superior sagittal sinus.

2. The vein of Labbé, which runs posteriorly in the temporal region to drain into the lateral sinus.

3. The superficial middle cerebral vein, which extends anteriorly in the outer limits of the sylvian fissure and runs over the anterior surface of the temporal lobe to drain into the cavernous sinus.

Deep Veins

The deep cerebral venous system consists of two internal cerebral veins and their tributaries. The internal cerebral veins are paired midline structures running in the roof of the third ventricle. They are formed by the confluence of the septal vein (which lies in the septum pallucidum) and the thalamostriate vein (which lies in the lateral wall of the lateral ventricle) in the region of the foramen of Munro.

The angle formed by the junction of the thalamostriate with the internal cerebral vein is referred to as the venous angle, and it outlines the position of the foramen of Munro. It should be emphasised that there are considerable variations in the pattern of formation of the internal cerebral vein. It runs posteriorly, taking a characteristic S-shaped course (Fig. 2.23). The great cerebral vein (the vein of Galen), formed by the union of the two internal cerebral veins, runs backwards and upwards to the splenium of the corpus callosum where it unites with the inferior longitudinal sinus to form the straight sinus, which extends downwards and medially to the confluence of the sinuses (torcular). The basal cerebral vein (the vein of Rosenthal) is formed by the junction of the deep anterior and middle cerebral veins, and runs posteriorly around the midbrain in the ambient cistern, together with the anterior choroidal artery and the posterior cerebral arteries. It drains into either the vein of Galen or the posterior part of the internal cerebral vein.

Venous drainage at the torcular (confluence of the venous sinuses) is extremely variable, but typically the superior sagittal sinus drains into the right transverse sinus and the straight sinus drains predominantly into the left transverse sinus. From a knowledge of the normal cerebral venous anatomy, one can predict from the site of an arteriovenous malformation its venous drainage.

In Parkinson and Bacher's (1980) series of 100 supratentorial arteriovenous malformations, drainage into the superior sagittal sinus occurred in 42% of cases, the vein of Galen in 12%, the parasellar plexus in 6% and the petrosal sinus in 3%.

Posterior Fossa Venous Anatomy

The posterior fossa venous system can be divided according to its direction of drainage into three groups (Huang and Wolf 1974).

1. Superior or Galenic drainage group. This will include veins draining from the mesencephalon, e.g. anterior pontomesencephalic vein, the internal mesencephalic vein and the posterior mesencephalic vein, and cerebellar tributaries, of which the main ones include the precentral cerebellar vein and the superior vermion vein. The precentral cerebellar vein provides an important landmark of the fourth ventricle.

2. Anterior or petrosal draining group. Venous drainage from the anterior aspect of the brainstem and cerebellum usually occurs into the petrosal vein, which lies in the cerebellopontine cistern and in turn drains into the superior petrosal sinus.

3. Posterior or tentorial drainage group. This group includes the inferior vermion vein and the superior and inferior hemispheric veins.

There are, however, frequent anastomotic communications between the three groups.

References

Almeida F de (1931) Note sur les collatérales de l'artère communicante cérébrale anterieure. Arch Anat Antrop Lisbon 13:551–556

Alpers BJ, Berry RG, Paddison RM (1959) Anatomical studies of the circle of Willis in normal brain. Arch Neurol Psychiatry 81:409–418

Baptista AG (1963) Studies on the arteries of the brain—the anterior cerebral artery, some anatomical features and their clinical implications. Neurology 13:825–835

Bowsher D (1961) Introduction to neuroanatomy. Blackwell Scientific, Oxford, pp 99–105

Critchley M (1930) The anterior cerebral artery and its syndromes. Brain 53:120–165

Crompton MR (1962) Pathology of ruptured middle cerebral aneurysm with special reference to difference between the sexes. Lancet II:421–425

Dunker RO, Harris AB (1976) Surgical anatomy of the proximal anterior cerebral artery. J Neurosurg 44:359–367

Foix DH, Chavany JA, Hillemand P (1925) Obliteration de l'artère choroidienne anterieure ramollissement cerebral hémiplégie, hémianasthesie et hémianopsie. Soc d'Ophtal (May)

Fujii K, Lenkey C, Rhoton AL (1980) Microsurgical anatomy of the choroidal arteries, lateral and third ventricles. J Neurosurg 52:165–188

Gibo H, Carver CC, Rhoton AL, Leukey C, Mitchell RJ (1981) Microsurgical anatomy of the middle cerebral artery. J Neurosurg 54:151–169

Gillilan LA (1968) The arterial and venous blood supplies to the fore-brain (including the internal capsule) of primates. Neurology 18:653–670

Greitz T, Lofstedt S (1954) The relationship between the third ventricle and the basilar artery. Acta Radiol (Stockh) 42:85–100

Hayreh SS, Dass R (1962) The ophthalmic artery—origin and intracranial and intracanalicular course. Br J Ophthalmol 46:65–98

Heubner A (1872) Zur Topographie der Ernährungsgebiete der einzelnen Hirnarterien. Zbl Med Wiss 52:817–821

Huang YP, Wolf BS (1974) Veins of the posterior fossa. In: Newton TH, Potts DB (eds) Radiology of the skull and brain, vol 2, Book 3. CV Mosby, St Louis, Miss., pp 2155–2216

Hudgins RJ, Day AL, Quisling RG, Rhoton AL, Sypert GW, Gercia-Bengochlea F (1983) Aneurysms of the posterior inferior cerebellar artery. J Neurosurg 58:381–387

Jain KK (1964) Some observations on the anatomy of the middle cerebral artery. Can J Surg 7:134–139

Johnson JH, Kline DG (1978) Anterior inferior cerebellar artery aneurysm. J Neurosurg 48:455–460

Kamiyama K, Sakarai Y, Suzuki J (1979) Aneurysm of the posterior communicating artery itself. In: Suzuki J (ed) Cerebral aneurysms. Neuron, Tokyo, pp 275–277

Kaplan HA, Ford DH (1966) The brain vascular system. Elsevier, Amsterdam New York

Kempe L (1968) Operative neurosurgery, vol 1: Cranial, cerebral and intracranial vascular diseases. Springer, Berlin Heidelberg New York

Kirgis HD, Fisher WL, Llewellyn RC, Peebles EMCC (1966) Aneurysms of the anterior communicating artery and gross anomalies of the circle of Willis. J Neurosurg 25:73–78

Krayenbuhl HA, Yasargil MG (1968) Cerebral angiography. Butterworths, London, pp 54–66

Kwak R, Niizuma H, Hatanaka M, Suzuki J (1979) Anterior communicating artery aneurysms accompanied with anomalies of the anterior communicating artery. In: Suzuki J (ed) Cerebral aneurysms. Neuron, Tokyo, pp 193–198

Lin J, Kricheff I (1974) Normal anterior cerebral artery complex. In: Newton TH, Potts DG (eds) Radiology of the skull and brain, vol. 11, Book 2. CV Mosby, St Louis, pp 1319–1410

Lister JR, Rhoton AL Jr, Matsushima T, Pearce DA (1982) Microsurgical anatomy of the posterior inferior cerebellar artery. Neurosurgery 10:170–199

Norlen G, Barnum AS (1953) Surgical treatment of aneurysm of the anterior communicating artery. J Neurosurg 10:634–650

Padget DH (1944) In: Dandy WE (ed) The circle of Willis. Its embryology and anatomy in intracranial arterial aneurysms. Cornstock, Ithaca, New York, pp 67–90

Parkinson D, Bachers G (1980) Arterio-venous malformations—summary of 100 consecutive supratentorial cases. J Neurosurg 53:286–299

Patrick D, Appleby A (1983) Familial intracranial aneurysm and infundibular widening. Neuroradiology 25:329–334

Perlmutter D, Rhoton AL (1978) Microsurgical anatomy of the distal anterior cerebral artery. J Neurosurg 49:204–228

Perret G, Nishioka E (1966) Report on the co-operative study of intracranial aneurysms and subarachnoid haemorrhage.

Section 5, arterio-venous malformations—an analysis of 545 cases of craniocerebral arterio-venous malformations and fistulae reported to the co-operative study. J Neurosurg 25:467–490

Pia HW (1900) Aneurysms of the internal carotid artery (ICA) and posterior communicating artery (PCOA) and anterior choroidal artery (ACha) region. In: Pia HW, Langmaid C, Zierski J (eds) Cerebral aneurysms. Advances in diagnosis and therapy. Springer, Berlin Heidelberg New York, pp 93–95

Punt J (1979) Some observations on aneurysms of the proximal internal carotid artery. J Neurosurg 51:151–154

Renn WH, Rhoton AL Jr (1975) Microsurgical anatomy of the sellar region. J Neurosurg 43:288–298

Rhoton AL Jr, Fujii K, Fradd B (1979) Microsurgical anatomy of the anterior choroidal artery. Surg Neurol 12:171–187

Rigg HE (1953) In: Hodes PJ, Campey F, Rigg HE, Bly P (eds) Cerebral angiography; fundamentals in anatomy and physiology. Am J Roentgenol Radium Therapy Med 70:61

Saeki N, Rhoton AL Jr (1977) Microsurgical anatomy of the upper basilar artery and the posterior circle of Willis. Neurosurg 46:563–578

Salamon G, Huang YP (1976) Radiologic anatomy of the brain. Springer, Berlin Heidelberg New York

Saltzman GF (1959) Angiographic demonstration of the posterior communicating and posterior cerebral arteries. Acta Radiol [Diagn] 54:114–122

Sengupta RP (1975) Anatomical variations in the origin of the posterior cerebral artery demonstrated by carotid angiography, and their significance in the direct surgical treatment of posterior communicating aneurysms. Neurochirurgia 18:33–42

Sengupta RP (1982) Management of large and giant aneurysms. Neurosurg Rev 5:173–178

Stabler J (1970) Two cases of accessory middle cerebral arteries, including one with an aneurysm at its origin. Br J Radiol 43:314–318

Stephens RB, Stilwell DL (1969) Arteries and veins of the human brain. Charles C Thomas, Springfield, Ill., pp 30–33

Taveras J, Wood E (1976) Diagnostic neuroradiology, vol 2. Williams & Wilkins, Baltimore, p 585

Waga S, Morikawa A (1979) Aneurysm developing on the infundibular widening of the posterior communicating artery. Surg Neurol 11:125–127

Wilson G, Riggs HE, Rupp C (1954) The pathologic anatomy of ruptured cerebral aneurysms. J Neurosurg 11:128–134

Wollschlager G, Wollshlager PB (1974) The circle of Willis. In: Newton TH, Potts DG (eds) Radiology of the skull and brain, vol 2, Book 2. CV Mosby, St Louis, pp 1171–1201

Yoshimoto T, Suzuki T (1974) Eight year demonstrated study of an aneurysm's growth at the origin of the posterior communicating artery. Neurol Surg (Tokyo) 2:571–573

Zeal AA, Rhoton AL Jr (1978) Microsurgical anatomy of the posterior cerebral arteries. J Neurosurg 48:535–559

3 Pathophysiology

The clinical management of patients with SAH is often assisted by an appreciation of the pathophysiological changes produced within the brain. The excellent descriptions of various pathological aspects by Tomlinson (1959), Crompton (1964) and others is based on autopsy studies, including those of patients who died within 24–48 h from massive SAH, and of patients with a less severe initial haemorrhage who later succumbed to complications such as hydrocephalus and cerebral infarction. Patients with massive haemorrhage can rarely be helped by any form of medical or surgical treatment. It is, therefore, more useful to know the pathological changes accompanying less severe haemorrhage since appropriate treatment in these patients may assist recovery. On the clinical side, computerised axial tomography (CAT) has given greater insight into complications which formerly often proved fatal. The pathological changes seen after SAH depend largely on the severity of the bleed, and, to a lesser extent, on the source, location and underlying cause.

The pathology—and thus the clinical relevance—of massive, major and minor degrees of SAH differ, and they will be discussed individually. The first part of this chapter deals with the pathological changes seen in relation to the severity of haemorrhage, irrespective of its aetiology. The second section deals with the aetiology of SAH and its most common cause, berry aneurysm, as well as discussing some of the unusual causes of aneurysmal SAH. Rarer causes will be dealt with in more detail in Chap. 5, "Differential Diagnosis", and the pathology of arteriovenous malformations will be discussed in Chap. 13.

Massive or Catastrophic Haemorrhage

In this category 35%–40% of patients die from the initial bleed without ever regaining consciousness. Such catastrophic haemorrhage usually occurs from rupture of an intracranial aneurysm (although obviously not all aneurysmal ruptures give rise to massive haemorrhage) and is associated with raised intracranial pressure. Following profuse bleeding from an aneurysm, the spread of blood varies according to the location and projection of the bleeding source.

Blood in the Subarachnoid Space

After a massive SAH, blood in the subarachnoid space may accumulate to such an extent that it obscures many anatomical features on the brain surface, particularly in the basal cisterns and ventral surface of the brainstem (Fig. 3.1). The source of such massive haemorrhage is usually an aneurysm arising from the circle of Willis.

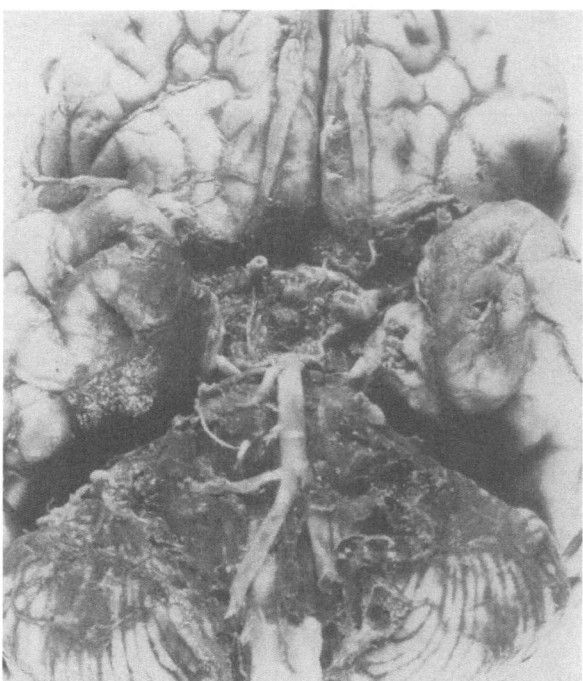

Fig. 3.1. This photograph of the ventral, basal brain surface illustrates massive subarachnoid haemorrhage in the circle of Willis region and over the ventral surface of the pons, medulla and cerebellum. Basal subarachnoid haemorrhage of this degree, especially over the ventral pons, is usually rapidly fatal. At autopsy the vertebral and basilar arteries and their branches were totally obscured by overlying blood clot. This has been partially cleared to reveal thin walled, patent vessels. In this case the source of bleeding proved to be an anterior communicating aneurysm. Blood had also extended in a retrogressive fashion into the fourth ventricle via its outlet foramina.

Subdural Haematoma

In 10%–17% of patients, subdural extension of the haemorrhage from the basal cisterns follows massive SAH (Russell 1954; Stehbens 1959). These subdural haematomas may be divided into three clinical grades, depending on their severity (Clarke and Walton 1953).

Grade 1. Haemorrhage into the subdural space as a result of extension of a massive and rapidly fatal haemorrhage.

Grade 2. A clinically significant subdural haematoma but of insufficient size to prove fatal.

Grade 3. A haematoma that is small and insignificant.

Walton (1956) maintained that subdural bleeding often occurs from aneurysms which project through the arachnoid into the subdural space.

Intracerebral Haemorrhage

Intracerebral haematomas are quite common complications in catastrophic SAH and various aspects are discussed by Fearnside (1916), Collier (1931), Richardson and Hyland (1941), Walton (1956), Freytag (1966) and Hijdra and Gijn (1982).

Aneurysms which are anatomically adjacent to or embedded in the brain frequently produce intracerebral haematomas. Thus, the location of an intracerebral haematoma depends upon the site of the aneurysm: anterior communicating artery aneurysms may cause frontal lobe haematomas (Fig. 3.2) by rupture of an aneurysm embedded in the medial frontal lobe, subcallosal gyrus. In this situation organized blood clot and fibrous tissue from previous minor haemorrhage may direct blood into the brain itself, the haematoma tracking into the grey and white matter of the anterior frontal lobe. It may also rupture into the lateral ventricle and cause intraventricular haematoma. Middle cerebral artery aneurysms may give rise to a sylvian fissure haematoma (Fig. 3.3a) or haemorrhage into the temporal lobe if they are embedded in the superior temporal gyrus (Fig. 3.3b) brain substance. Arteriovenous malformations in the cerebral hemispheres may also give rise to intracerebral haematomas if they bleed profusely.

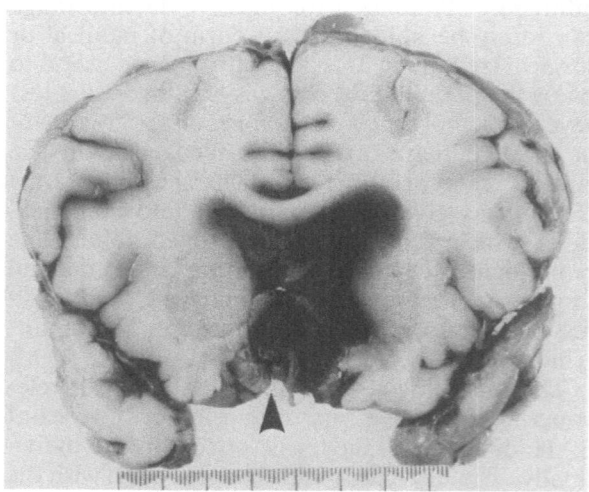

Fig. 3.2. This frontal coronal section illustrates a common mechanism by which intracerebral and intraventricular haemorrhage arises from rupture of a saccular (berry) aneurysm. In this case an anterior communicating aneurysm (*arrowhead*) was partially embedded in the gyrus rectus. Bleeding from the aneurysm occurred into this gyrus and then extended into the lateral ventricle(s).

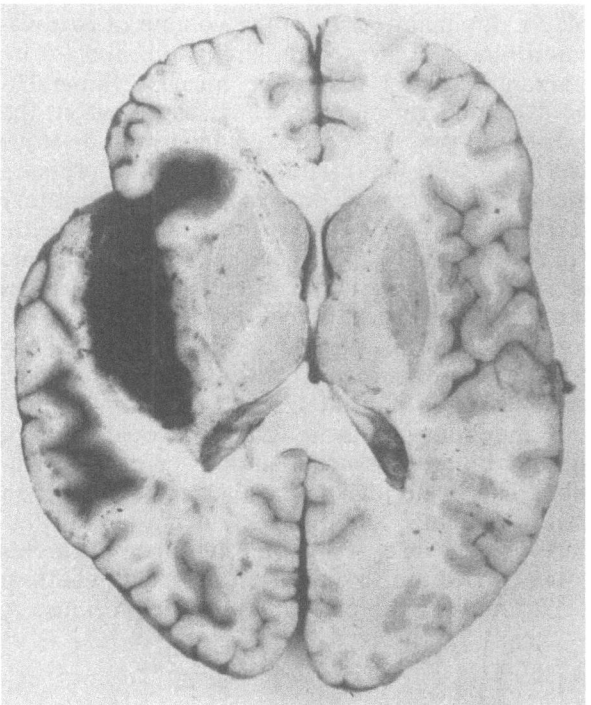

Intraventricular Haemorrhage

An intraventricular haematoma is a frequent finding in autopsy studies of SAH (Fig. 3.4). Until recently, pathologists maintained that intraventricular haemorrhage was invariably fatal. With the advent of CT, it is now realised that extension of subarachnoid blood into the ventricle can also occur in non-fatal haemorrhages, which are usually due to lesions lying in the circle of Willis, projecting towards the ventricular system, such as aneurysms of the anterior communicating artery (see above), the internal carotid bifurcation or the basilar bifurcation. When the blood spreads through the ventricular system it may block the CSF pathways (Fig. 3.5). Blood also enters the ventricles retrogressively via the fourth ventricular outlet foramina. Acute hydrocephalus resulting from a blocked ventricular system may be fatal if not recognised and treated.

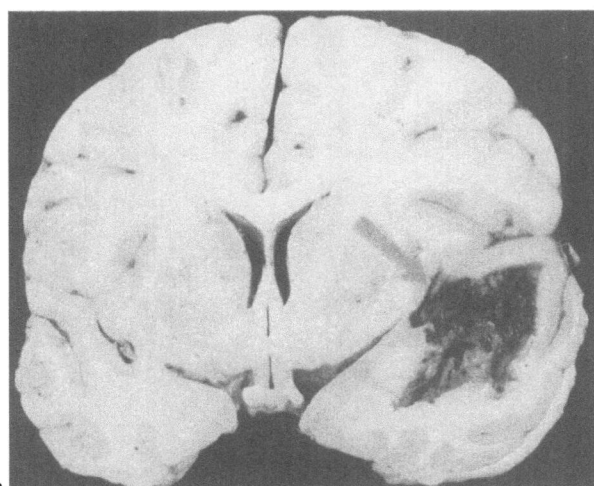

Fig. 3.3. a A hemispheric axial section illustrating massive subarachnoid haemorrhage almost entirely confined to the left sylvian fissure. The source of the bleeding proved to be a ruptured left middle cerebral aneurysm, and the space occupying effect of the sylvian fissure haematoma resulted, terminally, in tentorial herniation. **b** An intracerebral temporal lobe haematoma has followed rupture of a middle cerebral aneurysm which was embedded in temporal grey matter (*arrow*). In addition to a local space occupying effect in the temporal lobe caused by the haematoma, more generalized oedema in the left hemisphere has resulted in a slight left to right shift of hemispheric structures. This is frequently followed, or accompanied by, tentorial—midbrain—herniation.

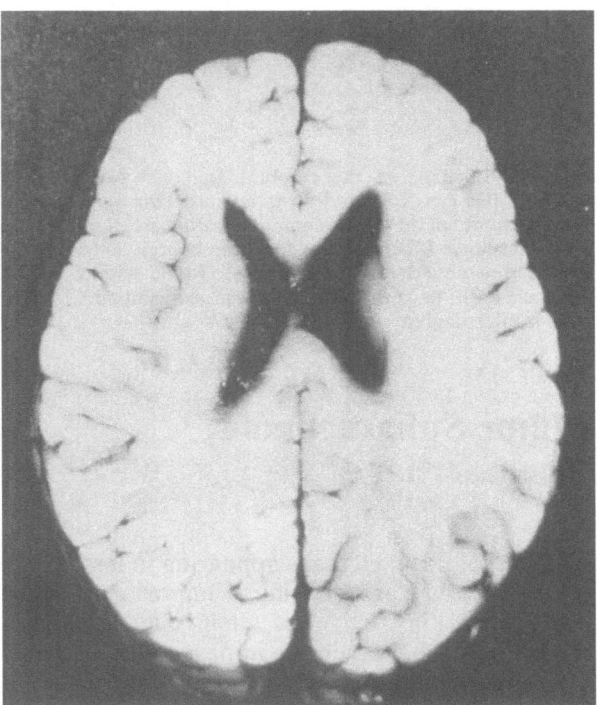

Fig. 3.4. Extensive intraventricular haematoma. The source of the haemorrhage was an internal carotid artery bifurcation aneurysm.

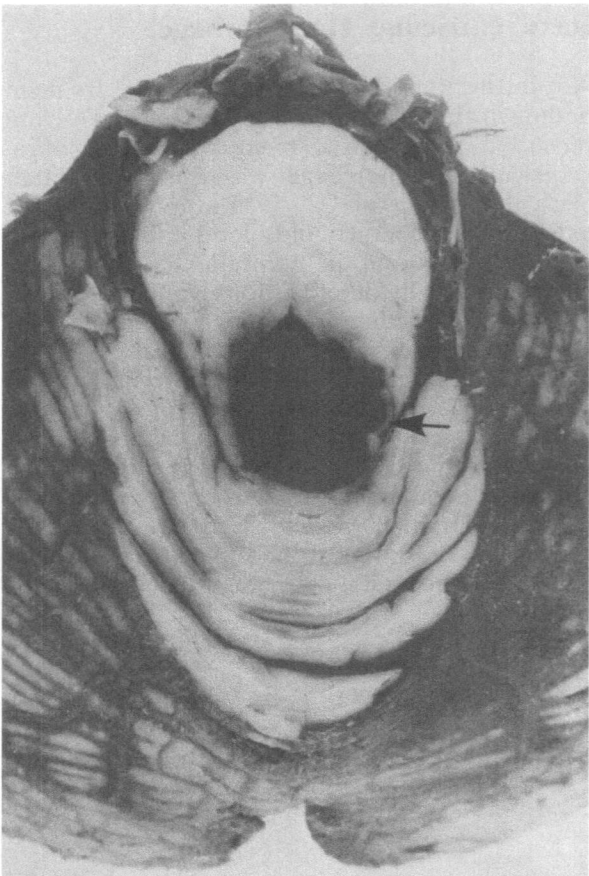

play a dominant role: (a) the volume of extravasated blood, (b) vasomotor reaction, and (c) intracranial spatial buffering capacity. Subarachnoid haemorrhage may be arrested when the extradural pressure approximates to the diastolic blood pressure, and within minutes the pressure gradually decreases due to the compensatory mechanisms. When the intracranial pressure approaches the systolic blood pressure at the time of rupture, both aneurysm leakage and cerebral blood flow will be arrested, and if the compensatory mechanisms do not result in lowered intracranial pressure, irreversible brain damage may occur. In non-fatal cases, intracranial pressure may remain elevated, but reflex elevation of systolic blood pressure maintains cerebral perfusion. This acute phase may lead to a stabilisation of the patient's condition. Reducing blood pressure (by the use of hypotensive agents) at this stage carries the risk of interfering with cerebral perfusion and therefore may be deleterious. A

Fig. 3.5. Blockage of the cerebral aqueduct (at midbrain level) in this case followed an intraventricular haemorrhage due to rupture of an anterior communicating artery aneurysm. In this instance CSF drainage from the lateral ventricles was impaired at aqueductal level (*arrow*). Blood within the 4th ventricle itself, or at its outlet foramina, may impair CSF flow to a similar degree.

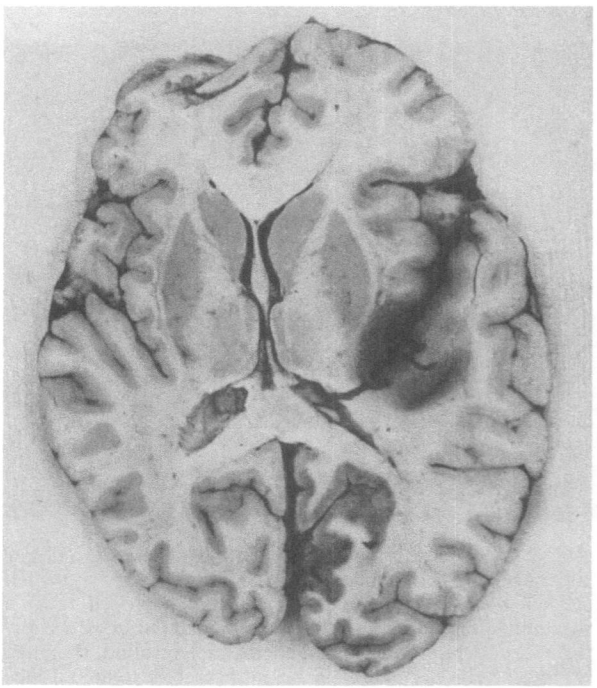

Major Subarachnoid Haemorrhage

The pathological changes appearing in less severe forms of SAH are of clinical importance, since a detailed knowledge of their effects enables measures to be taken to improve the patient's condition.

Raised Intracranial Pressure

Studies of intracranial pressure (Nornes and Magnaes 1972; Nornes 1973) aid in understanding the dynamic pathophysiology of SAH. Three factors

Fig. 3.6. Rupture of a berry aneurysm on the right middle cerebral artery has produced a moderate accumulation of blood in the right sylvian fissure. More generalised right hemisphere infarction has followed the initial bleed and a degree of right to left shift is apparent in frontal and basal ganglial regions. Tentorial herniation produced compression of the right posterior cerebral artery, with infarction of the medial occipital lobe. The latter is visible as partially haemorrhagic, oedematous grey matter.

persistent or secondary rise in intracranial pressure, in contrast, may be related to severe complications, including space-occupying haematoma, obstruction of CSF pathways, and brain swelling due to ischaemia (Fig. 3.6). These factors will further decrease cerebral blood flow and a vicious circle will ensue, unless appropriate therapeutic measures are undertaken.

Intracerebral Intraventricular Haematomas, and Those in the Basal Cisterns

These complications occur more frequently than has previously been appreciated. With the introduction of computerised axial tomography, such haematomas can be readily recognised and, if appropriate, treated by surgical evacuation. A further point of interest is that the amount of blood in the basal cisterns may determine whether or not cerebral vasospasm develops (Fisher et al. 1980; Mizukami et al. 1980).

Hydrocephalus

Bagley (1928) first reported hydrocephalus arising as a consequence of SAH, and since then it has been recognised as a more frequent complication, occurring between 2 and 12 weeks after SAH (Foltz and Ward 1956). The incidence varies between 10% and 35% (Galera and Greitz 1970; Yasargil et al. 1973; Raimondi and Torres 1973). Although varying degrees of fibrosis of the leptomeninges are a permanent feature after SAH, clinically, its amount usually reflects the extent of bleeding. If mild, no clinically significant consequences may occur, but if severe, hydrocephalus may develop. Hydrocephalus occurring in the early stages of SAH is almost invariably due to blood and cellular exudates blocking the basal cisterns and the foramen of the fourth ventricle (Kibler et al. 1961; see Figs. 3.1, 3.5). Yasargil et al. (1973) found hydrocephalus more common in patients with multiple rather than a single episode of SAH. Hydrocephalus is also more common after rupture of anterior communicating artery aneurysms than after those on the middle cerebral artery (Shulman et al. 1963). This may reflect the fact that (a) middle cerebral aneurysms lie in more intimate contact with cerebral tissue in the sylvian fissure, and hence the haemorrhage is localised to the sylvian fissure (Fig. 3.3a) and is more intracerebral than subarachnoid, and (b)

after rupture of an anterior communicating artery aneurysm the blood is often directed into the basal subarachnoid space, whereas after middle cerebral artery rupture the blood flows and accumulates in the sylvian fissure (Shulman et al. 1963). In the majority of patients who develop hydrocephalus, no active treatment is necessary and the condition resolves. Permanent CSF drainage procedures are required in only a small number of patients.

Cerebral Ischaemia and Infarction

A considerable proportion of the permanent damage inflicted upon the brain after SAH is due to ischaemic infarction. Though cerebral arterial vasospasm plays a major role in the development of such ischaemic changes, the factors which lead to ischaemia and infarction are not known with certainty and are a matter of recurrent debate. Cerebral ischaemia and infarction after SAH were first described by Richardson and Hyland in 1941. Since then, several other authors (Tomlinson 1959; Birse and Tom 1960; Smith 1963; Crompton 1964; Schneck 1964) have made important contributions to the understanding of the pathology. Cerebral infarction is usually restricted to the area of the brain in which the aneurysm is found, and often occurs within the territory of supply of the vessel on which the aneurysm arises. In patients with fatal SAH, infarction is found in at least one-third of the cortical territory of a major cerebral artery. In patients with rupture of the anterior communicating artery aneurysm, infarction frequently occurs in the hypothalamic region (Crompton 1964). Suggested aetiological factors include vascular spasm (Robertson 1949), thrombosis occurring in the arteries (Courville 1965), and circulatory interference due to pressure of the aneurysm on the artery (Meadows 1951; Courville 1965). Both vascular thrombosis and local pressure effects were largely discounted as possible factors restricting the blood supply by Tomlinson in 1959. Though there is still considerable controversy as to the degree of correlation between angiographic vascular narrowing and cerebral ischaemia, it is certain that vasospasm plays a major role in the production of cerebral ischaemia and/or infarction. The aetiology of vasospasm and its significance will be discussed in more detail in Chap. 12. Several secondary changes can occur in the brain after SAH, either as a result of the haemorrhage itself or of its associated complications. These include herniation of the midbrain through the tentorium and even compression of the lower brainstem, which frequently results in irreversible haemorrhage in the brainstem (Fig. 3.7). In a massive haemorrhage, blood rapidly occupies all the available subarachnoid space, whereas in a major haemorrhage associated with a haematoma, oedema develops around the haematoma site and increases intracranial tension. Such oedema is also seen as a result of infarction. Whatever the actual mechanism for cerebral oedema production, the end result is a space-occupying effect with a subsequent rise in intracranial pressure.

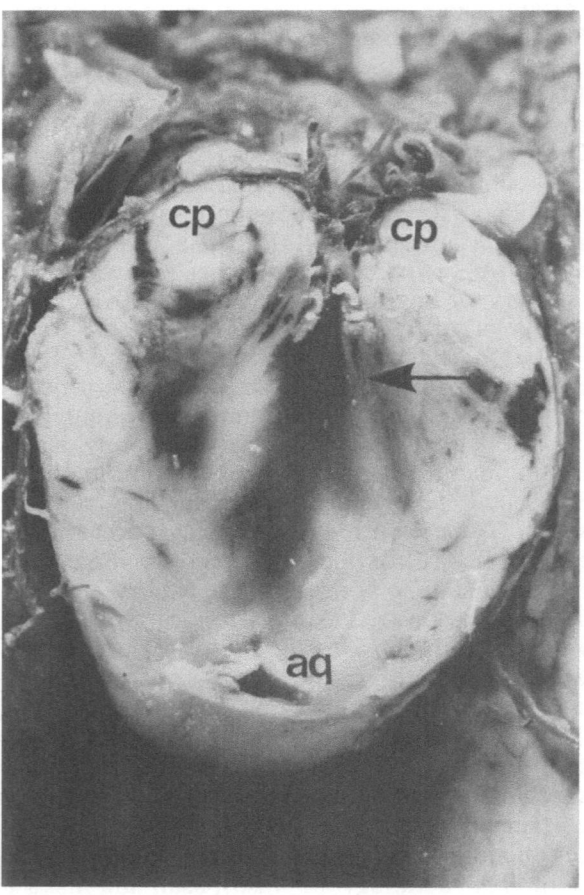

Fig. 3.7. Fatal midbrain herniation followed rupture of a middle cerebral aneurysm and cortical infarction. A central midbrain haemorrhage (*arrow*) is accompanied by smaller haemorrhages in the cerebral peduncles (*cp*). The aqueduct (*aq*) is free of blood and contrasts with the aqueduct in Fig. 3.5.

Pathological Changes Associated with Minor Haemorrhage

The pathological effects of a minor SAH are usually minimal, and there has been little interest in them in the past. Though Gillingham (1958) pointed out the significance of such haemorrhage, their importance has only recently been appreciated. In patients with fatal SAH one often finds pathological evidence of previous bleeding. Although this is most commonly associated with intracranial aneurysms, it can also occur in AVMs.

In minor haemorrhages the pathological changes are largely confined to the microscopic level (Nystrom 1963). Evidence of previous minor haemorrhage in an aneurysm wall is a common finding in pathological studies and can be due to blood extravasated from the vasa vasorum passing through fenestrations in the elastic layer (Nystrom 1963). Blood clots within the sac of a large aneurysm are also a common finding, and reflect circulatory disturbances in the aneurysm itself. Such blood clots may occasionally be demonstrated on CT scan. A sudden leak into the wall of an aneurysm may give rise to the clinical features of a diffuse SAH, but without significant blood in the cerebrospinal fluid, a point of clinical importance since it can be falsely concluded that SAH has not been responsible for the patient's headaches. Further, a clot sealing such a minor leak may dissolve, resulting in a major haemorrhage some time after the initial small leak. Aneurysms that enlarge often become loculated with irregular thickening of the wall. In areas of low haemodynamic pressure within such loculi, stasis of blood may lead to clot formation and eventual calcification within the wall. An appreciation of minor haemorrhages has an important role in the management of intracranial aneurysms; they may be seen by the clinician as "sentinel" or warning headaches. Such a case was documented by Ball (1975), who described a previously healthy woman of 22 years who experienced a sudden headache on the left side, and 5 days later complained of backache, for which all investigations proved negative. Six weeks after the initial symptoms she was admitted deeply comatose and died within 3 h. Post-mortem examination revealed massive SAH from a ruptured middle cerebral artery aneurysm. A plug of white firm material (presumably organised fibrin) filled most of the fundus of the aneurysm, and, apart from evidence of fresh rupture, there was a small aperture that had been sealed with well-organised intraluminal thrombus with active fibroblast and neocapillary formation. Immediately adjacent to the sac and in the leptomeninges, blood pigment and phagocytic activity could be seen with local fibrosis. Retrospectively, therefore, the initial headache was attibuted to the minor leak. Examination of the CSF may often show no or scanty red cells in these cases.

Histopathological Features

Macroscopic Changes

After major haemorrhage the subarachnoid space is filled with a mixture of cerebrospinal fluid and clotted blood. The subarachnoid blood spreads to a variable extent depending upon the site of the aneurysm and the degree of haemorrhage, although in severe cases the entire brain and spinal cord may be covered with blood. The presence of this extravasated blood in the subarachnoid space causes an aseptic inflammatory reaction in the arachnoid mater. The thickening of pia and arachnoid mater, together with unabsorbed clot, results in adhesions between the pia, arachnoid and neighbouring structures. This resulting membrane is pigmented (with haemosiderin) and the process is most patchy at the base of the brain, especially after repeated haemorrhage (Fig. 3.1).

Microscopic Findings

Blood in the subarachnoid space provokes an inflammatory reaction in the meninges with a varying degree of subsequent fibrosis. A previous or old SAH may be recognised by blood pigments (haemosiderin) within macrophages situated in the pia arachnoid (Christensen 1956). In fact, blood products (bilirubin and biliverdin) are considered to be more irritant than blood itself. Hammes (1944) studied the reaction of meninges to blood in 53 patients dying at variable periods after SAH, and in 26 patients whose deaths were due to other causes. Patients with any infective process were excluded from the study and he observed the following.

1. *Sudden death (within 10 min).* In this series nine patients died immediately after, or within 10 min of, the SAH. Blood was in the basal cisterns and on the convexity of the brain, but there was no meningeal reaction.

2. *Death within 1–4 h.* The earliest histological evidence or reaction was observed at 2 h, with collections of polymorphonuclear leucocytes around blood vessels and pia arachnoid. There was no meningeal reaction.

3. *Death at 4–16 h.* More intense polymorphonuclear reaction was observed, tending to become diffuse throughout the pia arachnoid. After 4 h, lymphocyte accumulation around the pial vessels was noted. There was no constant relation between the severity of reaction and the anatomical location in the brain or the amount of blood.

4. *Death between 16 and 32 h.* Both polymorphonucleocytes and lymphocytes increased in numbers and were diffusely distributed.

By 24 h the mesothelial cells lining the subarachnoid space (which are normally flat and elongated) became swollen, rounded and actively phagocytic. Active phagocytes were also seen in the subarachnoid space. The first evidence of breakdown of haemoglobin to haem and globin was noted in the cytoplasm of phagocytes.

5. *Death within 3 days.* All the inflammatory cells increased in number and there was fairly intense meningitic reaction. The mesothelial cells and mononuclear phagocytes were very active and contained red cells and iron pigment.

6. *Death within 3–7 days.* This marked the peak of cellular reaction with lymphocytes and phagocytes taking an equal part. The polymorphonuclear reaction had subsided.

7. *Death within 7–10 days.* By the tenth day, there was evidence of an early fibrotic reaction in the leptomeninges (Fig. 3.8). This had three characteristics:
   a) It was seen in contact with blood in the subarachnoid space.
   b) It was patchy.
   c) In the final stage the pia arachnoid was bound with fibrosis, thus obliterating the subarachnoid space.

8. *Death after 2 or more weeks.* Variable amounts of blood pigment, leucocytes, iron and phagocytes were seen, in addition to fibrosis. At no time were changes noted in the blood vessels of the pia. Viewed as a whole, there was a good correlation between the clinical signs of meningeal reactions and pathological changes during the first few weeks of SAH.

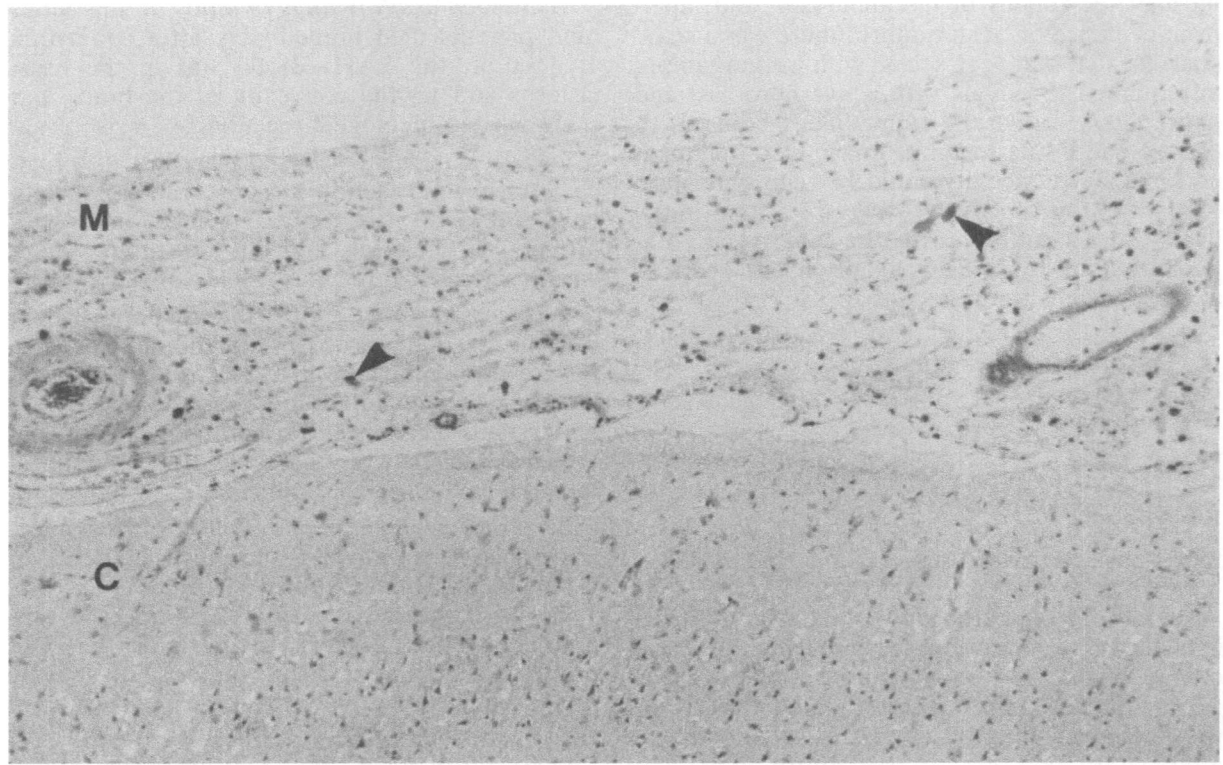

Fig. 3.8. Meningeal (*M*) thickening and fibrosis over surface cerebral gyri (C, cortex) has resulted from a previous subarachnoid haemorrhage. Haemosiderin pigment is present in macrophages (*arrowheads*).

Aetiology of Subarachnoid Haemorrhage

Subarachnoid bleeding may be found in various conditions. Spontaneous SAH as a clinical syndrome usually occurs from a specific cause. There are four major routes by which blood enters the subarachnoid space in non-traumatic SAH (Symonds 1923).

1. An effusion originating within the subdural space may disrupt the arachnoid membranes and gain entrance to the subarachnoid space.
2. Haemorrhage into the superficial parts of the brain may break through the pia mater into the subarachnoid space.
3. A deeply situated cerebral haemorrhage may rupture into one of the ventricles and hence the blood may find its way into the subarachnoid space.
4. The haemorrhage may be derived from one of the larger vessels lying in the subarachnoid space itself.

The last route is the major cause of SAH, with ruptured intracranial aneurysms and arteriovenous malformations together being responsible for approximately 80% of the cases of spontaneous SAH, the remaining small proportion of SAH being due to a variety of other disease, while the source of bleeding remains undetermined in approximately 10%–15% of cases (see Chap. 5). Walton (1956) carefully analysed an autopsy series of 173 cases of spontaneous SAH, and confirmed that ruptured aneurysm was responsible in 72% of cases, while in a further 8% he suspected an aneurysmal origin. In clinical series reported over the years, the source of haemorrhage remained undisclosed in as many as 28%–49% of the cases (Krayenbuhl and Yasargil 1958; McKissock and Paine 1959). However, with improved angiographic techniques and the use of four-vessel angiography, the incidence of detectable aneurysms conforms more to Walton's autopsy findings. Arteriovenous malformations are responsible for approximately 5%–7% of cases of SAH.

A complete list of the causes of SAH can be found in Chap. 5 dealing with differential diagnosis. Most of these are, however, pathological curiosities, and the remainder of this chapter deals with the aetiology and pathology of the various forms of intracranial aneurysms. The pathology of arteriovenous malformations will be discussed in Chap. 13.

Intracranial Aneurysms

The word "aneurysm" is derived from classical Greek and means dilatation. The recognition of non-cerebral arterial aneurysms was made long before the Greco-Roman medical literature gave a name to it (Walton 1956; Heidrich 1972). (Further history regarding cerebral aneurysms can be found in Chap. 1.)

The incidence of cerebral aneurysms in the population is generally agreed to be approximately 1% (Locksley 1966). However, in over 2500 autopsy studies, Mertland (1939) found a 2% incidence of SAH. Jellinger (1979), in an analysis of almost 8500 cases of aneurysm collected from several published series, found that the most frequent sites were (1) the terminal portion of the internal carotid artery and the origin of the posterior communicating artery (32%), (2) the junction of the anterior cerebral and anterior communicating artery (31.4%), (3) the proximal part of the middle cerebral artery (23.5%) and (4) the vertebrobasilar system (13%). The site of aneurysms in our 500 operated cases is shown in Table 7.1. Aneurysms of the central nervous system are classified as follows (Yates 1976):

Saccular (berry) aneurysms

Atherosclerotic fusiform aneurysms

Mycotic aneurysms

Traumatic aneurysms

Dissecting aneurysms

Microaneurysms of Charcot-Bouchard

To these can be added oncotic aneurysms and aneurysms in Moya Moya disease.

Dissecting aneurysms, oncotic aneurysms, microaneurysms of Charcot-Bouchard and Moya Moya disease rarely cause SAH, and these will only be briefly alluded to. Saccular (or berry) aneurysms are the commonest type of intracranial aneurysm responsible for SAH.

Saccular Aneurysms

These are also known as congenital or berry aneurysms. They present as a saccular dilatation of the artery and are connected to the vessel by a variable area of attachment, usually arising at or very close to a branch or division of an artery (Fig. 3.9). Curiously, a slight predominance of females has been found in all the reported series. Incidental aneurysms are more common in women than in men (du Boulay 1965). However, the anatomical distribution of aneurysms showed sexual bias. Internal carotid aneurysms occur twice as often in females, especially in the second and third decades, and middle cerebral aneurysms are found more frequently in females (at the ratio of three to two). Anterior communicating aneurysms, however, are more frequent in males—58% (Locksley 1966). In our study multiple aneurysms have been found in nearly 25% of patients.

Size and Appearance

Berry aneurysms vary in size from a pin head to several centimetres in diameter. Small aneurysms are little more than filling out of the apical angle of branching arteries, whereas the largest sacs are dome-shaped swellings that have either a wide attachment to the parent vessel or a relative constriction at the base, forming a narrow stalk. Small aneurysms have extremely thin walls, and are generally difficult to see, being relatively transparent. In contrast, the stalk and its adjacent parts are often opaque. In larger aneurysms the sac itself often becomes partially or completely filled with organised laminated thrombus. Scattered atheromatous lesions and calcification may also be seen, and variation in the wall thickness may result in a multilocular aneurysm which is more susceptible to bleeding. Arterial branches are never found to arise from the sac of the aneurysm; however, if an aneurysm continues to grow and attains a giant size, the neck may occupy more and more of the arterial wall of the parent vessel, and thus the adjacent branches have the appearance of arising from the proximal part of the aneurysm.

Microscopic Appearance

Microscopically the wall of the aneurysmal sac varies in thickness and consists of a thin layer of fibrous connective tissue which is continuous with

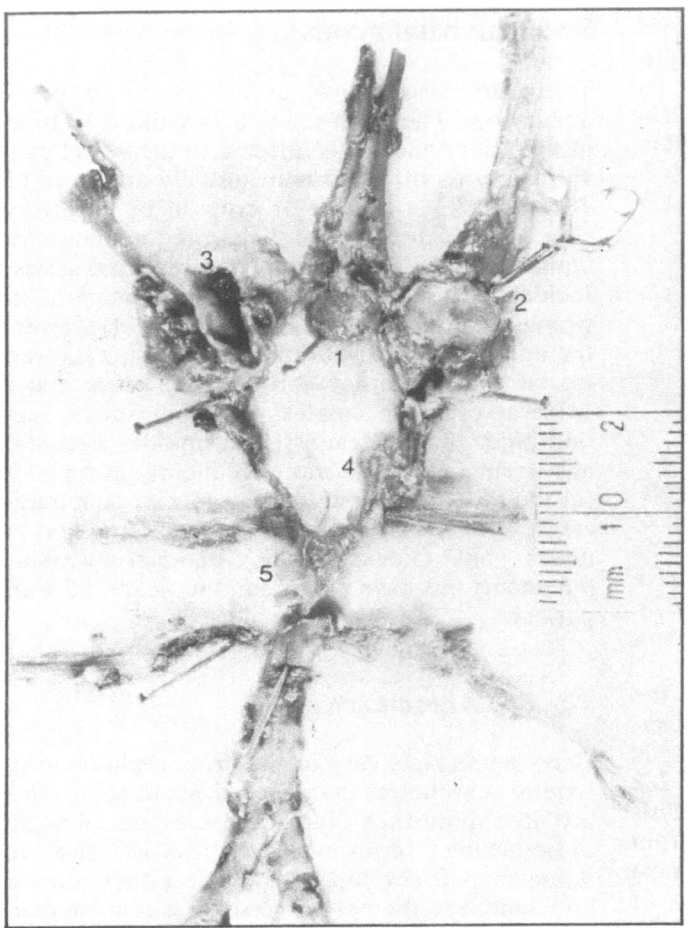

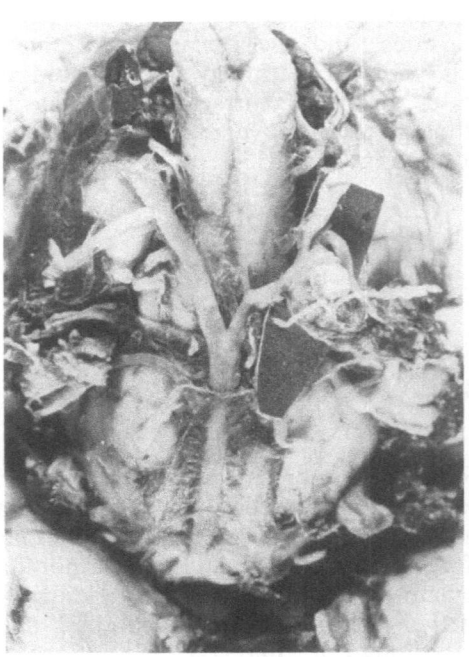

Fig. 3.9. a Dissected circle of Willis showing multiple berry aneurysms. *1*, anterior communicating aneurysm; *2*, previously clipped left middle cerebral aneurysm; *3*, ruptured right middle cerebral aneurysm; *4*, posterior communicating artery aneurysm; *5*, basilar bifurcation aneurysm. **b** A saccular (berry) aneurysm (partially elevated) arising from the right posterior inferior cerebellar artery. Subarachnoid blood over the ventral pons—which was 3–4 mm thick—was cleared prior to fixation, although a small quantity remains beneath the surface pontine meninges.

the adventitia of the parent vessel. The muscular layer ends abruptly at the neck of the aneurysm, and the internal elastic lamina is either fragmented or absent (Fig. 3.10). The intima is generally fragmented in places, and only the adventitia may remain in the thinnest part of the sac. Degenerative changes often occur in the wall, which may become loaded with cholesterol and foam cells. If a previous leakage from the aneurysm has occurred, haemosiderin-containing phagocytes may be seen.

Ultrastructurally, Nystrom (1963) found vacuolar swelling in the endothelium of aneurysms with lipid granules. The elastic lamina was split and the normal fibrillar structure lost. At the site of rupture, elastic tissue was totally absent. In other areas of the wall of the aneurysm the elastica was thickened and partially granular. Connective tis-

sue invaded the media separating the muscle cells, and the ground substance of the adventitia and media showed macrophages and lipid vacuoles. Collagen fibrils had a comparatively even distribution in the ground substance of the aneurysmal wall. Stehbens (1975) could not demonstrate internal elastic lamina in the aneurysmal wall. He found the media to be indistinct, and the muscle cells were degenerative and widely separated.

Pathogenesis

The pathogenesis of saccular aneurysms is controversial, and currently two opposing views are held. These propose on the one hand congenital and on the other hand acquired factors in the

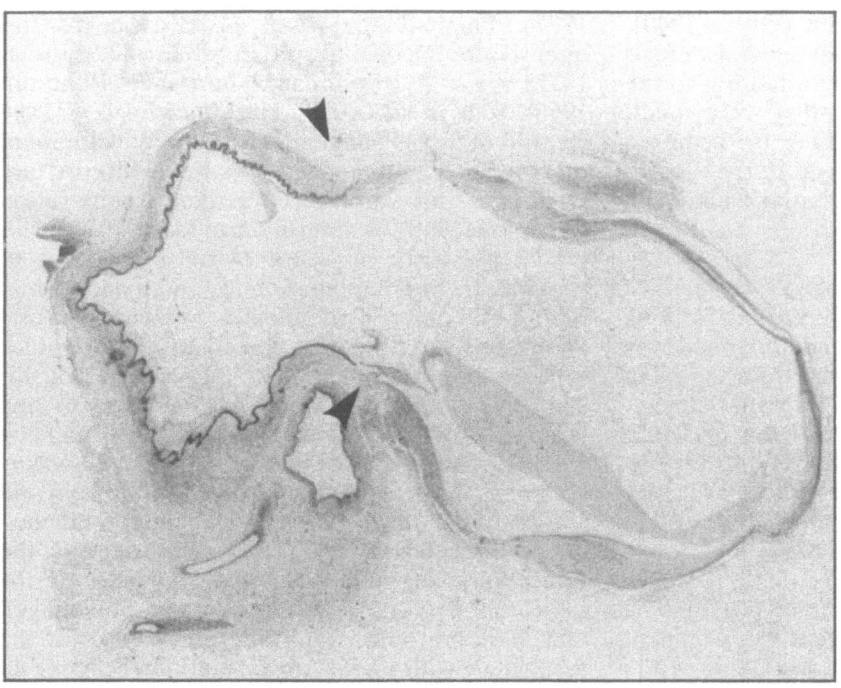

Fig. 3.10. In this photomicrograph a saccular aneurysm is attached to the parent vessel—the middle cerebral artery. The latter is identifiable by its inner elastic lamina and terminates at the origin of the aneurysm (*arrowheads*).

development of saccular aneurysms. This subject has been extensively reviewed recently by Sekhar and Heros (1981). It is known that cerebral arteries differ from extracranial vessels in the absence of the external elastic lamina. Since a vessel wall maintains its integrity by both the internal elastic lamina and the media, for an aneurysm to develop both of these should give way. More specific factors which have been cited as being associated with the two pathogenic mechanisms are listed below.

1. *Congenital factors*
   a) Defect in the muscular layer
   b) Dilatation of elastic pad
   c) Origin of small vessels
   d) Failure of involution of foetal vessels
   e) Genetic factors and familial aneurysms
2. *Acquired factors*
   a) Degeneration of the elastic lamina
   b) Pre-aneurysmal lesions of the arterial walls
   c) Atherosclerosis
   d) Hypertension
   e) Inflammation

Congenital Factors

The Medial Defect. Cerebral arterial walls have defects in the muscular layer at points of bifurcation. Developmentally, the muscle sheath of an artery derives from undifferentiated mesenchymal cells. These surround the branches, independent of the parent vessels. If the independently developing muscular coats fail to fuse at junction points, defects in the muscularis are apparent. Such defects are also found in other arteries such as the coronary and mesenteric. Forbus (1930) termed these defects "locus minoris resistentiae". To Eppinger (1887) belongs the credit for first recognising these defects and suggesting that herniation of the intima through this gap was responsible for the aneurysm formation. Though these defects were noted by other workers (Forbus 1930; Glynn 1940; Stehbens 1959), objections to this general theory have been raised.

In the presence of an intact elastic lamina, for instance, Forbus (1930) maintains that intima cannot herniate through the gap, and defects are found in the same proportion of normal arteries as in those bearing the aneurysm (Glynn 1940). Stehbens (1959) maintained that medial defects were acquired in origin, drawing attention to the increased incidence of defects with age. However, whether derived from congenital or acquired mechanisms, the presence of a gap in the muscular layer of the artery is an essential element in aneurysm formation (Fig. 3.10).

Elastic Pad. These structures arise from passive remoulding of the vessel wall by the blood flow. The elastic cushions occur in haemodynamically sheltered parts of the vessel, away from the main stream and often opposite the muscular defect. There is an associated increase in the muscular layer in the region of the cushions and this may be related to the nearby medial defect (Hassler 1961). Hassler gives credit to Rotter et al. (1955) for describing these intimal cushions.

Origin of Small Vessels. Drennan (1941) postulated that aneurysms arose from the origin of small vestigial vessels situated in the apices of the vessel bifurcation. Serial sections of the arterial bifurcations, however, have failed to detect such vessels (Stehbens 1972).

Failure of Involution of Primitive Vessels and Variations in the Circle of Willis. The location of aneurysms coincides with the site of the primitive vessels, and incomplete involution or atrophy of these arteries has been postulated as a cause of aneurysm formation (Padget 1944; Bisaria 1984). Although anterior communicating artery aneurysms coincides with the site of the primitive circle of Willis, the anatomical variations are not found significantly more in patients with aneurysms (Stehbens 1963).

Genetic Factors and Familial Aneurysms. The rarity of cerebral aneurysms in infancy and childhood disputes a congenital origin. Housepian and Pool (1958) could not find a single intracranial aneurysm in approximately 3000 brains examined at autopsy in children aged between 1 day and 12 years. These observations, however, cannot exclude the possibility of an inherited weakness of the vessel wall, which may predispose the individual to aneurysm formation in later years. Hashimoto (1977) reviewed the literature and found 46 families with more than one member having an aneurysm. The onset of symptoms occurred at a younger age in familial cases, and mirror image aneurysms were more frequent (Sakai et al. 1974). There were no detectable chromosomal abnormalities in the patients studied (Hashimoto

1977). Familial aneurysms occur twice as frequently in the same site in siblings (Andrews 1977) as a simple dominant inheritance (Beumont 1968; Kak et al. 1970; Hashimoto 1977). The arterial defect is congenital and the development of the aneurysm and its eventual rupture are attributed to variations in gene penetration (Beumont 1968). Bannermann et al. (1970) considered a polygenic or multifactorial inheritance to provide the best explanation for aneurysm formation. Four pairs of identical twins with cerebral aneurysms have been reported in the literature (Schon and Marshall 1984). Recently, in this centre, we have identified five children in one family with aneurysms (Patrick and Appleby 1983b). The association of hereditary disorders such as Ehlers–Danlos syndrome (Rubinstein and Cohen 1964; Graf 1965) and an increased incidence of cerebral aneurysm also suggests the importance of genetic factors. Further, at the molecular level, the different types of collagen and their variations in different sites may be associated with aneurysm formation (Pope et al. 1981). The proportion of type 3 collagen varies from 70% in the arteries to 10%–20% in the skin, and 0–1% in the bones. Type 3 collagen-deficient patients have abnormal collagen fibrils and this may influence the properties of arterial walls, and encourage aneurysm formation at points of known arterial weakness. Pope et al. (1981) found type 3 collagen deficiency in 7 out of 12 patients with congenital aneurysms. The association of cerebral aneurysms and other congenital anomalies, such as polycystic kidneys (Bigelow 1953) and coarctation of the aorta (Wright 1949), lends further support to advocates of congenital aetiological mechanisms, although hypertension may play a role in these patients.

Acquired Factors

Degeneration of the Internal Elastic Lamina. Forbus (1930), in a series of experiments, suggested that the elastic lamina, which gives significant strength to the vessel wall, degenerates due to mechanical overdistension. A combination of the congenital muscular defect and acquired degeneration of the elastic membrane results in the development of aneurysms. Glynn (1940) also stressed the importance of degeneration of the elastic layer in the development of aneurysms.

Pre-aneurysmal Lesions of the Arterial Walls. Stehbens (1963) studied 96 circles of Willis bearing saccular aneurysms, and noted funnel-shaped dilatations at the origin of the posterior communicating artery in 10%. Gradations of these dilatations to actual small aneurysms were also found, suggesting that the dilatations represented stages in the development of aneurysms. In another study, Hassler and Saltzman (1963) noticed infundibular dilatation in 10% of patients in whom the posterior communicating artery failed to fill at angiography. They examined seven cases for pathological changes. In most of the specimens the wall was much thinner than normal and consisted of connective tissue of intimal and adventitial type. The internal elastic lamina was split. In two cases no pathological changes were found. These infundibular dilatations have also been documented angiographically to lead to the formation of aneurysms (Patrick and Appleby 1983a).

Atherosclerosis. Although aneurysms are most common in adults with prevalent atherosclerosis, the exact role of this factor in the pathogenesis is difficult to assess. Carmichael (1950) proposed a combination of developmental defects and arterial degeneration (arteriosclerosis) in the developments of aneurysms. According to Walker and Allegre (1954), degenerative vascular changes play a major role in the formation of cerebral aneurysms, intimal changes being the early evidence of arteriosclerosis. It is postulated that a subintimal proliferation may lead to occlusion of the vasa vasorum, with consequential degeneration of the elastica and any remaining muscular layer. Frank generalised atherosclerosis is occasionally associated with fusiform dilatation of vertebral, basilar and internal carotid arteries (Walker and Allegre 1954). In these cases lipid-containing or calcified plaques are present in subintimal layers. According to Forbus (1930), Kerppola (1919), in a detailed study, noted degeneration of the media at the point of exit of small vessels, the connective tissue replacing the media with proliferation of intima and inducing further intimal proliferation. The plaque eventually penetrates the internal elastic lamina and weakens this important vessel-supporting layer.

Hypertension. Hypertension is an important factor in producing haemodynamic stress and intimal tensions, and acts against a background of elastic layer degeneration and the medial defect. These three factors play varying roles, depending upon the age at which the aneurysm forms (Crawford 1959). In old age it is suggested that atherosclerosis and hypertension play a significant role and the contribution of the medial defect is less, whereas in childhood and adolescence the medial defects are of greater importance. In early adult life it is the medial defect and blood pressure which are significant while atherosclerosis plays a minor role. In middle age all three factors are important (Crawford 1959).

In a recent study of a randomly selected group of patients compared with a control group, Andrews and Spiegel (1979) failed to find an association between hypertension and aneurysms. In certain subgroups, however, associations were apparent. A significantly higher number of females between the ages of 18 and 54 and males between the ages of 35 and 44 with aneurysms had hypertension. Under the age of 55 years, a hypertensive patient was twice as likely to have multiple aneurysms.

Inflammation. An inflammatory factor in the pathogenesis of intracranial aneurysms was proposed by Handler and Blumenthal (1954). They studied nine patients who showed varying stages of proliferative arteritis and suggested that inflammation results in the formation of gaps in the elastic lamina. In the first stage, the inflammation involves all the layers of the wall, including the elastic lamina. Resolving inflammation leaves gaps in the elastic layers, and the muscular layer is replaced by fibrous tissue, thus setting the stage for aneurysm formation. However, this hypothesis has not attracted much support.

In summary, there is still controversy regarding the origin of aneurysms, with both congenital and acquired mechanisms having their advocates. The arterial walls certainly have defects of the muscular coat (congenital) at the point of sacculation of the aneurysms. Such defects may be due to failure of embryonic fusion of the separate muscle coats of the main vessels and their branches. Subsequent degeneration of the internal elastic lamina (acquired lesion) may result in the development of aneurysm (Forbus 1930; Hassler 1961; Stehbens 1963). The age distribution of aneurysm formation favours an acquired rather than a congenital basis for the aetiology of the aneurysms (Stehbens 1963; Phillips et al. 1980). There is no overwhelming evidence to suggest that anatomical variations of the cerebral arteries are more frequent in patients with aneurysms than in the general population (Stehbens 1963). Funnel-shaped dilatations, especially at the origin of the posterior communicating artery, represent early stages of aneurysm formation.

Growth and Rupture

Small berry aneurysms apparently grow as a consequence of the haemodynamic stress imparted by pulse waves against a constraining wall that lacks elastic membrane and a muscular layer. The turbulent flow within the lumen may be a further factor inducing aneurysm dilatation. The velocity of blood flow in normal cerebral vessels is sufficient to produce turbulence at the bifurcation where aneurysms are seen (Ferguson 1972). In aneurysmal walls, fibrosis and infiltration with red and white blood cells are common features (Crompton 1964; Stehbens 1972), as are protruding defects or "blebs". These blebs may enlarge, thrombose, or rupture. Locules on the aneurysm surface produce enlargement of the aneurysm (Crawford 1959) and restricted silent bleeds result in local mesenchymal reaction (Sarwar et al. 1976). Both these factors may play a part in the growth of the aneurysm. Although bleeding may occur in the absence of loculation, when the latter is present it is almost invariably the result of previous haemorrhage (du Boulay 1965). Serial angiography has shown that while some aneurysms continue to enlarge (see Fig. 7.42), others may remain virtually unchanged, or occasionally decrease in size, or disappear (see Fig. 7.43). Mount and Taveras (1956) followed 16 patients with intracranial aneurysm and in only 3 was there evidence of enlargement of an aneurysm at subsequent angiography.

Bjorkesten and Troupp (1957) concluded from a study of 19 patients that internal carotid aneurysms are more likely to enlarge progressively because they lie free in the subarachnoid space, and thus are afforded better opportunity for growth. Middle cerebral aneurysms are less likely to enlarge because they are buried deep in the sylvian fissure. Moyes (1971), in a follow-up of 14 patients with unruptured aneurysms over 1 to 10 years, found progressive enlargement in only four patients. Winn et al. (1977) found increase in size of all aneurysms which had rebled. Zacks et al. (1980) followed ten patients with 12 incidentally discovered aneurysms for 2 to $7\frac{1}{2}$ years (mean 3 years). There was no evidence of SAH in any of these patients, nor was there increase in size in three patients who had undergone repeat angiography. Aneurysms which decrease in size or even disappear due to clotting were described by Bjorkesten and Troupp (1962), Hook et al. (1963) and Hayward (1977).

Rupture of an aneurysm is dependent upon the intense stress on its wall. The thinnest part of the aneurysm usually gives way and thus 84% of aneurysmal ruptures occur at the fundus, while only 2% take place at the neck of the aneurysm (Crawford 1959). The site of rupture is often close to a plaque of atheroma in the wall. The precise factors which influence the rupture are uncertain, but the aneurysmal size, hypertension, environmental stress, and pregnancy may be important.

The critical size at which most aneurysms become symptomatic is 7–10 mm (Locksley 1966; Weibers et al. 1981). Middle cerebral aneurysms may become symptomatic at a somewhat smaller size (3–6 mm), and, at the other end of the spectrum, unruptured carotico-ophthalmic aneurysms usually attain a size of 10 mm or more before they become symptomatic. If the aneurysm is more than 10 mm in diameter, there is a 50% chance of its rupture within $2\frac{1}{2}$ years (Weibers et al. 1981), the critical size being 7 mm. Aneurysms are liable to rupture or cause symptoms in those patients between the ages of 40 and 70 years (Stehbens 1963; Locksley 1966; Brewis et al. 1966). Housepian and Pool (1958) found aneurysms to be more frequent in the third, fourth and fifth decades, and extremely rare in infancy.

The role of environmental stress in precipitating aneurysmal haemorrhage is controversial and there is no consensus of opinion in the literature. If it does play a role, an increase in blood pressure is likely to be the main cause. In pregnancy, there is an increased incidence of SAH in the third trimester, during labour, and in the post-partum period.

There is no evidence to suggest that hypertension is a factor in the development of single or multiple aneurysms or in the rupture of the aneurysm (Housepian and Pool 1958; Locksley 1966; McCormick and Schmalstieg 1977; Jane et al. 1977; Phillips et al. 1980; Weibers et al. 1981).

Atherosclerotic Fusiform Aneurysms

Ectatic dilatation of the basilar or internal carotid artery is a frequent occurrence in patients with severe atherosclerosis (see Fig. 3.11). The basilar and vertebral arteries become elongated and tortuous, causing compression and distortion of the adjacent brain tissue and nerve roots. Histologically there is fibrosis of the elastic membrane, with hyaline degeneration, deposition of cholesterol, occasional inflammatory cells and intimal haemorrhage. Spontaneous thrombosis of fusiform aneurysms in the vertebrobasilar system may occur and produce acute brainstem or cerebellar infarction. Fusiform aneurysms of the

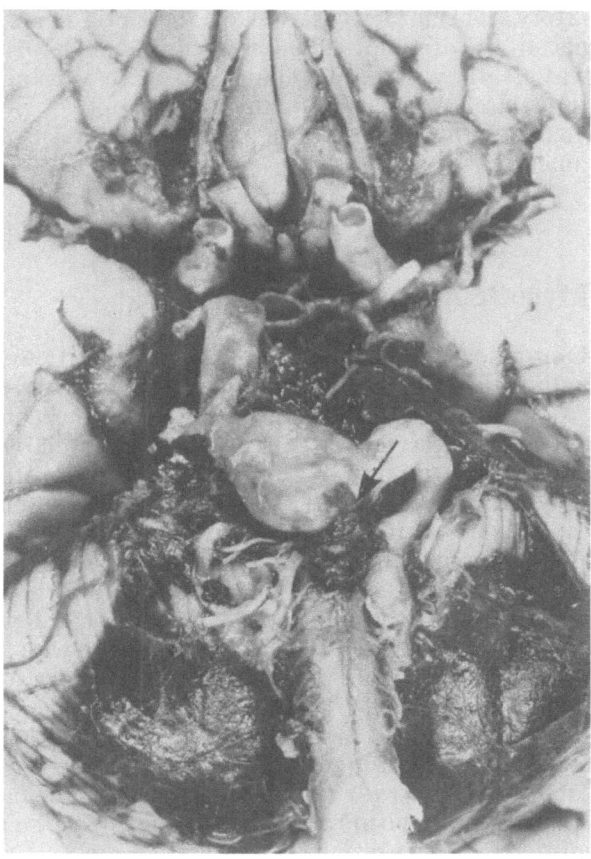

artery aneurysm may be suspected, but such a sequence of events has not been clearly documented previously. The following case demonstrates the origin of a fistula from such an aneurysm. Since the patient came to angiography and surgery within 3 days of rupture, the

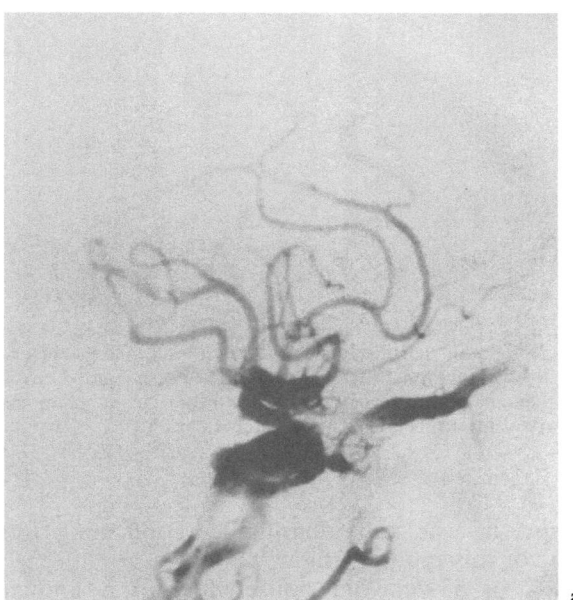

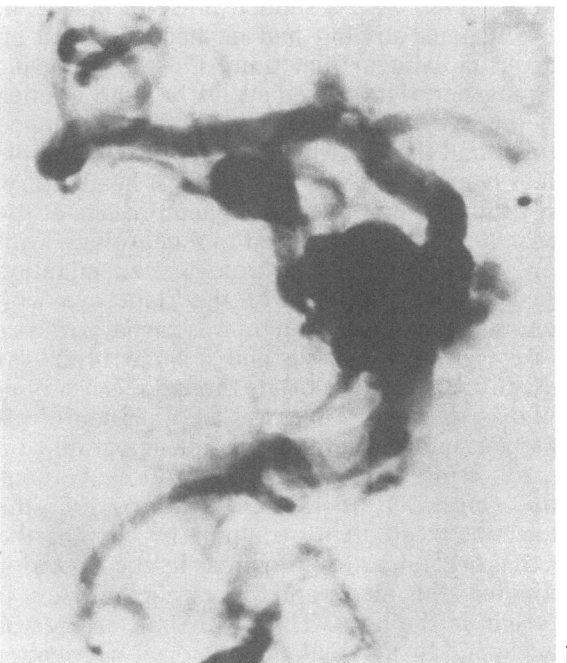

Fig. 3.11. This fusiform aneurysm has arisen in the midportion of the enlarged and tortuous basilar artery. Its rupture—site indicated with an *arrow*—was followed by massive subarachnoid haemorrhage around the ventral brain stem and cerebellum. As with the majority of cases showing such extensive subarachnoid haemorrhage over the brain stem, it proved rapidly fatal.

internal carotid artery usually involve the intracavernous portion, where expansion in all directions produces pressure symptoms. They rarely rupture.

Caroticocavernous Aneurysms

Caroticocavernous aneurysms are usually arteriovenous fistulae between the internal carotid artery and the cavernous sinus, though there are also aneurysms which arise from the internal carotid artery within the cavernous sinus. These aneurysms do not usually give rise to subarachnoid haemorrhage. The fistula may be secondary to mechanical trauma or may arise spontaneously. In cases with a spontaneous fistula, rupture of an undetected intracavernous internal carotid

Fig. 3.12. Right carotid angiogram (**a** lateral projection, **b** anteroposterior projection) showing a caroticocavernous fistula.

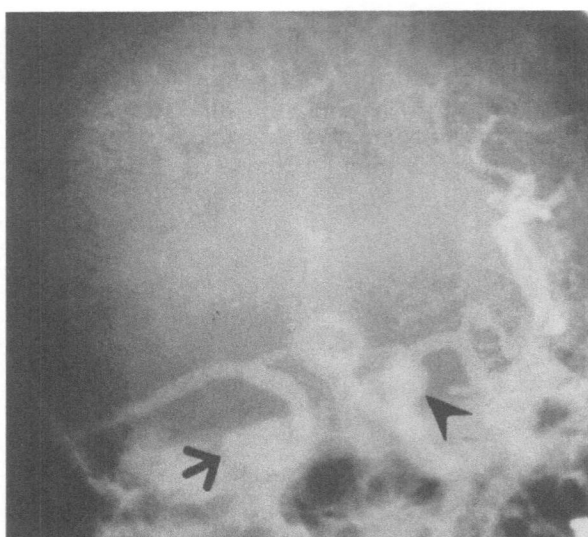

Fig. 3.13. Left carotid angiogram with compression of the right common carotid artery. A left ophthalmic artery aneurysm is demonstrated (*arrowhead*). There is good cross-flow, and part of the sac of the right internal carotid aneurysm observed at surgery is demonstrated (*arrow*).

aneurysm was still identifiable, confirming the view of this type of origin.

I.C. a 63-year-old housewife and a known hypertensive on therapy for 4 years, woke up on 3 March 1985 with a sudden noise in her head. She felt nauseous but had no headache and no other complaint at that time. On the following morning her right lower eyelid became swollen and the eye became congested. She developed pain behind the eye which radiated to the temple 2 days later. There was no history of head injury. Her brother died of cerebral haemorrhage at the age of 49. She was admitted to a neurology ward on 6 March 1985 and neurological examination revealed mild proptosis of the right eye with chemosis of the eyelid. There was partial paralysis of the right sixth nerve and a large bruit was present over both the orbits though more promi-nent over the right. There was no other neurologi-cal abnormality. Bilateral carotid angiography on the following day showed a caroticocavernous fistula (Figs. 3.12, 3.13). On 8 March 1985 the fistula was treated with trapping by clipping the internal carotid artery proximal to the posterior communicating artery and by ligating the artery at its origin in the neck. The ophthalmic artery was also clipped by manipulating the optic nerve after opening the optic canal with a high-speed drill. In addition a piece of muscle was used to embolise the fistula before ligating the cervical carotid

artery. During mobilisation on the optic nerve, part of the origin of the internal carotid aneurysm was clearly visible, extending into the cavernous sinus. Following surgery the bruit stopped im-mediately and the sixth nerve showed return of function.

Mycotic Aneurysms

Olmstead and McGee (1977) reviewed the pathogenesis of peripheral aneurysms and gave credit to Virchow for recognising embolism and destructive vascular lesions in cases of infective endocarditis. In 1885 Osler introduced the word "mycotic" to describe the lesion in the aortic arch in patients with endocarditis (Bohmfalk et al. 1978). Eppinger (1887) coined the term "mycotic-embolic aneurysm". He believed the infection spread from the intima to the adventitia (Richey and MacLachlan 1922). To avoid confusion with a true fungal infection, the term "bacterial intracra-nial aneurysm" was introduced by Bohmfalk et al. (1978). The common organisms involved are *Staphylococcus aureus*, *Staphylococcus albus* and *Streptococcus viridans*. The incidence of mycotic aneurysms has been reported as being 2.6% of all intracranial aneurysms (Roach and Drake 1965). "Spontaneous" SAH in patients with a cardiac murmur or other evidence of endocarditis, such as splenomegaly, petechiae, microscopic haema-turia, and a raised ESR, should enable a diagnosis of mycotic aneurysm to be made in life (Roach and Drake 1965). Such mycotic aneurysms may arise in unusual sites, and may be present in 4%–15% of patients with bacterial endocarditis (Bohmfalk et al. 1978). They are commoner in younger patients and rarely associated with warn-ing signs. The actual mechanisms involved in the spread of infection and the formation of mycotic aneurysm are still controversial (Olmstead and McGee 1977). Three modes of spread have been described.

1. Direct extension from the lumen through the wall.
2. Through the vasa vasorum.
3. By direct extension of an infective focus to the artery from a site external to the vessel wall.

Molinari et al. (1973) injected a pure growth of *Staphylococcus aureus* in 16 dogs and studied the development of aneurysm formation and the effect of antibiotic treatment. Aneurysmal dilatation could be identified in gross specimens as early as 24 hours after embolisation. The aneurysms were adherent to the leptomeninges with indurated and fibrotic walls. Abscess of deep cerebral structures was also found. Their observations suggested that organisms escaped the occluded lumen of the vessel through penetrating vessels in the Virchow–Robin spaces, and then reached the adventitia of parent vessels. The mortality is very high (80%) in patients with ruptured aneurysm associated with endocarditis (Bohmfalk et al. 1978). Because of the lack of specific symptoms during their development, the diagnosis is usually made after the haemorrhage. Some mycotic aneurysms may disappear spontaneously (see Fig. 7.55) and, if monitored by serial angiography, an increase in size is an indication for surgical treatment (Valadares et al. 1979). Aneurysms which fill and empty slowly pose less risk of rupture (Bohmfalk et al. 1978).

A rare case of phycotic intracranial middle cerebral aneurysm was reported by Steele et al. in 1972, in a $5\frac{1}{2}$-year-old boy. The major cause of the aneurysm was unquestionably the foreign body of plant origin embedded in the wall of the middle cerebral aneurysm. This was identified as an "awn of a grass inflorescence". The authors suggest that the awn entered via the retropharynx while the child was chewing dry grass.

Traumatic Aneurysms

Traumatic aneurysms account for 0.5% of all cerebral aneurysms found (Benoit and Wortzman 1973). They do not occur at the bifurcation of arteries. In a review, Burton et al. (1968) divided trauma into (a) direct penetrating injuries and iatrogenic injuries (Lassman et al. 1974), and (b) indirect closed head injuries. Traumatic aneurysms can be further classified into: (a) true, when the arterial wall is partially disrupted; (b) false, when the cavity of the aneurysm is encapsulated in a haematoma; and (c) mixed, where rupture of a true aneurysm gives rise to secondary false aneurysm. Mechanisms of trauma are given below.

1. *Direct trauma.* A vessel may be injured when it lies in the path of a penetrating object or in a surgical field.

2. *Indirect trauma.* Following closed head injury, aneurysms arise as a consequence of dynamic forces which disrupt the walls of an artery.

False aneurysms are always associated with direct trauma to the artery. These aneurysms may increase or decrease in size and even occasionally disappear (Burton et al. 1968; Benoit and Wortzman 1973). They are three times more common in males, and occur more often in young people (Fleischer et al. 1975). The majority of patients present with a syndrome of delayed traumatic haemorrhage 2–3 weeks following head injury. These aneurysms are irregular in contour and generally without a discrete neck. The mortality in surgically treated cases is 18%, and 41% in non-surgically treated cases (Fleischer et al. 1975).

Dissecting Aneurysms

Bigelow (1955b) defined dissecting aneurysm as "an arterial lesion in which, as a result of weakening, the vessel wall becomes split longitudinally into two layers, by leakage of blood beneath the weakened inner portion." The new channel is not lined by endothelium but by the tissues dissected. It is, therefore, a false aneurysm. Yonas et al. (1977) reviewed the literature and, depending upon the plain of dissection and the clinical manifestations, divided these aneurysms into two groups.

Group 1. A defect in the elastic lamina allows blood to force its way between the elastic membrane and the media, pushing the elastic membrane towards the lumen and occluding or narrowing it. These aneurysms are associated with headache and present as stroke. The CSF is normal in the majority of affected patients.

Group 2. In this group, blood travels between the media and adventitia or through the media, and there dissections may arise from the vasa vasorum. Such dissections are usually limited in length.

Subarachnoid haemorrhage is a rare presentation of dissecting intracranial aneurysms. Friedman and Drake (1984) reported 14 cases and found only 11 more in the literature which had presented with SAH. Though the dissecting aneurysm presents as a stroke in the anterior part of the circle of Willis, 20 of the 25 reported cases that presented as SAH involved the posterior circulation. Berger and Wilson (1984) have described six cases of intracranial dissecting aneurysm of the posterior circulation, four of which produced an SAH.

Microaneurysms of Charcot and Bouchard

Aneurysms often measuring less than 1 mm in diameter are frequently observed in small arterioles of the deep structures of cerebral tissue or superficial cerebral cortex. They are termed "miliary" as a result of their resemblance to a millet seed, and are usually found in considerable numbers although they produce isolated lesions. They are found most commonly in the basal ganglia, thalamus, pons and dentate nuclei. Though this type of aneurysm was noted by Cruveilhier (1935) and Gull (1859), it was Charcot and Bouchard (in 1868) who brought intracerebral miliary aneurysms into prominence (Bigelow 1955a). They contended that the majority of cases of intracerebral haemorrhage were due to rupture of miliary aneurysms. However, Bigelow (1955a) could not find many cases of miliary aneurysms associated with intracerebral haemorrhage. Russell (1963) examined 54 brains—38 normotensive and 16 hypertensive. Small saccular dilatations of the cerebral vessels supplying the putamen, pallidum, caudate nucleus, thalamus and cortical grey matter were found in all but one hypertensive patient, and in one-third of normotensive patients. A higher incidence of microaneurysms in hypertensive patients was also found in another controlled study (Cole and Yates 1976b). Poor development of the muscular and elastic coats may predispose to the development of such aneurysms. The formation of miliary aneurysms is a subacute process and they show a tendency to thrombose. The tendency to haemorrhage increases at a stage between rupture of the elastic lamina and the intimal thickening and thrombosis (Russell 1963), and ageing factors, such as change in the resilience of the arterial elastic lamina, may be responsible for the higher frequency of these aneurysms in older people (Cole and Yayes 1976b).

Oncotic Aneurysms

Tumour emboil from cardiac myxoma and choriocarcinoma have been documented to produce peripheral aneurysms (Vaughn and Howard 1962; Olmstead and McGee 1977). The tumour emboli, depending upon their size, lodge in small or large arteries. Fragmentation and distal migration may follow after a temporary circulatory arrest in major vessels. The tumour then penetrates the intact or damaged endothelium at the site of the final lodgement, with eventual destruction of the vessel wall. A spectrum of pathological process may be seen, depending upon the stage of involvement. There may be eventual stenosis or true aneurysmal formation (Stoane et al. 1966; New et al. 1970).

Moya Moya Disease

This is an acquired disease, in which an immunological vascular reaction and inflammation play an important role (Suzuki and Kodama 1971). In Japanese, Moya Moya translates as "something hazy, like a puff of cigarette smoke drifting in the air". This term was applied to the angiographic appearance of the intracranial vessels at the base of the brain (see Fig. 7.60). Though originally reported in Japan, similar cases have also been reported in the rest of the world. Recently, Suzuki and Kodama (1983) reviewed the literature. The disease is more common in females, in a ratio of 3:2, and there is usually a past history of inflammatory lesion in the neck. The clinical presentation is often of transient ischaemic attacks or hemiplegia in children and intracranial haemorrhage in adults. The Moya Moya vessels represent the collateral channels. The actual pathology is a progressive bilateral stenotic change in the internal carotid arteries. Depending upon the site of the collateral pathways, the disease is termed either ethmoidal or vault Moya Moya. Recently, Yamashita et al. (1983) studied the pathology in 22 patients with Moya Moya disease and 9 controlled patients who died of various other causes. They found stenosis or occlusion of the distal internal carotid artery bilaterally. There was fibrous thickening of the intima with laminated and reduplicated elastic lamina. The perforating arteries at the base of the brain formed complex channels connecting the anterior cerebral and middle cerebral arteries which were dilated and tortuous. They described two types of perforating arteries: (a) dilated with thin walls, and (b) stenosed with thick walls. In young patients the arteries were more dilated. In patients with Moya Moya disease the degree of stenosis was variable. There was also evidence of microaneurysm formation and dilatation of the vessels. In these dilated vessels, the media was fibrosed, the wall was attenuated and the elastic lamina was segmented. This attenuation of the vessel wall results in rupture of the Moya Moya vessels. The ischaemic events follow the stenotic process of the disease.

Moya Moya disease is also associated with saccular aneurysms of the circle of Willis (Debrun and Lacour 1974). Of the 12 cases of ruptured intracranial aneurysms associated with Moya Moya disease, 5 were located at the basilar bifurcation, signifying the haemodynamic stress on the posterior circulation (Suzuki and Kodama 1983). Moya Moya disease causes primary intracerebral and/or intraventricular haemorrhage, and when the patient presents with SAH, a saccular aneurysm should be suspected (Aoki and Mizutani 1984).

References

Andrews RJ (1977) Intracranial aneurysms: characteristics of aneurysms in siblings. N Engl J Med 297:115

Andrews RJ, Spiegel PK (1979) Intracranial aneurysms—age, sex, blood pressure and multiplicity in an unselected series of patients. J Neurosurg 51:27–32

Aoki N, Mizutani H (1984) Does Moya Moya disease cause SAH? Review of 54 cases with intracranial hemorrhage confirmed by computerised tomography. J Neurosurg 60:348–353

Bagley C (1928) Blood in the CSF; resultant functional and organic alterations in the central nervous system (a) experimental data, (b) clinical data. Arch Neurol 17:18–81

Ball MJ (1975) Pathogenesis of the 'sentinel headache' preceding berry aneurysm rupture. Can Med Ass J 112:78–79

Bannerman RM, Ingall GB, Graf CJ (1970) The familial occurrence of intracranial aneurysms. Neurology 20:283–292

Benoit BG, Wortzman G (1973) Traumatic cerebral aneurysms. Clinical features and natural history. J Neurol Neurosurg Psychiatry 36:127–138

Berger MS, Wilson CB, (1984) Intracranial dissecting aneurysms at the posterior circulation. Report of 6 cases and a review of the literature. J. Neurosurg 61:882–894

Beumont PJV (1968) The familial occurrence of berry aneurysms. J Neurol Neurosurg Psychiatry 31:399–402

Bigelow NH (1953) The association of polycystic kidneys with intracranial aneurysms and other related disorders. Am J Med Sci 225:485–494

Bigelow NH (1955a) Multiple intracranial arterial aneurysms. An analysis of their significance. Arch Neurol Psychiatry 73:76–79

Bigelow NH (1955b) Intracranial dissecting aneurysms. An analysis of their significance. Arch Pathol 60:271–275

Birse SH, Tom MI (1960) Incidence of cerebral infarction. A study of eight unoperated cases of anterior cerebral aneurysms. Neurology 10:101–106

Bisaria KK (1984) Anomalies of the posterior communicating artery and their potential clinical significance. J Neurosurg 60:572–576

Bjorkesten G, Troupp H (1957) Prognosis of subarachnoid haemorrhage: A comparison between patients with verified aneurysm and patients with normal angiograms. J Neurosurg 14:434–441

Bjorkesten G, Troupp H (1962) Changes in the size of intracranial arterial aneurysms. J Neurosurg 19:583–588

Bohmfalk GL, Storey JL, Wissinger JP, Brown WE Jr (1978) Bacterial intracranial aneurysms. J Neurosurg 48:369–382

Brewis M, Poskanzer DC, Rolland C, Miller H (1966) Neurological disease in an English city. Acta Neurol Scand (Suppl) 24:42

Burton C, Velasco F, Dorman J (1968) Traumatic aneurysm of a cerebral artery. J Neurosurg 28:468–474

Carmichael B (1950) The pathogenesis of non-inflammatory cerebral aneurysms. J Pathol 35:347–368

Charcot JM, Bouchard CH (1868) Nouvelles recherches sur la pathogénie de l'hémorrhagie cérébrale. Arch Physiol Paris 1:110

Christensen E (1956) Pathologie der intrakraniellen blutungen. In: Handbuch der Neurochirurgie, vol III. Springer, Berlin Heidelberg New York

Clarke ES, Walton JBN (1953) Subdural haematoma complicating intracranial aneurysm and angioma. Brain 76:378–404

Cole FM, Yates PO (1967a) Intracerebral microaneurysms and small cerebrovascular lesions. Brain 90:759–768

Cole FM, Yates PO (1967b) The occurrence and significance of intracerebral microaneurysms. J Pathol Bacteriol 93:393–411

Collier J (1931) Cerebral haemorrhage due to other causes than arteriosclerosis. Br Med J II:510–524

Courville CB (1965) Intracranial lesions secondary to congenital saccular aneurysm—A study of 387 cases with autopsy verification. Bull LA Neurol Soc (Suppl) 21:1–21

Crawford T (1959) Some observations on the pathogenesis and natural history of intracranial aneurysms. J Neurol Neurosurg Psychiatry 22:259–266

Crompton MR (1964) The pathogenesis of cerebral infarction following the rupture of cerebral berry aneurysms. Brain 87:491–510

Cruveilhier J (1835) Anatomie pathologique du corps humain. Baillière, Paris

Debrun J, Lacour P (1974) A new case of Moya Moya disease associated with several intracavernous aneurysms. Neuroradiology 7:277–282

Drennan AM (1941) Aneurysms of the larger cerebral vessels. NZ Med J 20:324–349

du Boulay GH (1965) Some observations on the natural history of intracranial aneurysms. Br J Radiol 38:721–757

Eppinger H (1887) Pathogenesis (Histogenesis and aetiologie) der aneurysmen einschliesslich des aneurysma equi verminosum. Arch Klin Chir 35 (Suppl. I):101–563

Fearnside ED (1916) Intracranial aneurysms. Brain 39:224–296

Ferguson G (1972) Physical factors in the initiation, growth and rupture of human intracranial aneurysms. J Neurosurg 37:666–677

Fisher CM, Kistler JP, Davis JM (1980) Relation of cerebral vasospasm to subarachnoid haemorrhage. Visualised by computerised tomographic scan. Neurosurgery 6:1–9

Fleischer AS, Patton JM, Tindall JM (1975) Cerebral aneurysms of traumatic origin. Surg Neurol 4:233–239

Foltz EL, Ward AA (1956) Communicating hydrocephalus from subarachnoid bleeding. J Neurosurg 13:546–566

Forbus WD (1930) On the origin of miliary aneurysms of the superficial cerebral arteries. Bull Johns Hopkins Hosp 47:239–284

Freytag E (1966) Fatal rupture of intracranial aneurysms. Survey of 250 medico-legal cases. Arch Pathol 81:418–424

Friedman AH, Drake CG (1984) Subarachnoid hemorrhage from intracranial dissecting aneurysms. J Neurosurg 60:325–334

Galera RG, Greitz T (1970) Hydrocephalus in the adult secondary to the rupture of intracranial arterial aneurysms. J Neurosurg 32:634–641

Gillingham FJ (1958) The management of ruptured intracranial aneurysms. Ann R Coll Surg Engl 23:89–117

Glynn LE (1940) Medial defects in the circle of Willis and their relation to aneurysm formation. J Pathol 51:213–222

Graf CJ (1965) Spontaneous carotico-cavernous fistulae, Ehlers–Danlos syndrome and related conditions. Arch Neurol 3:662–672

Gull W (1859) Cases of aneurysms of cerebral vessels. Guy's Hosp Rep 3:281

Hammes FM (1944) Reaction of the meninges to blood. Arch Neurol Psychiatry 52:505–514

Handler KP, Blumenthal HT (1954) Inflammatory factors in pathogenesis of cerebrovascular aneurysms. JAMA 155:1479–1483

Hashimoto I (1977) Familial intracranial aneurysms and cerebral vascular anomalies. J Neurosurg 46:419–427

Hassler O (1961) Morphological studies on the large cerebral arteries with reference to the etiology of subarachnoid haemorrhage. Acta Neurol Scand (Suppl) 154:1–145

Hassler O, Saltzman GF (1963) Angiographic and histological changes in infundibular widening of the posterior communicating artery. Acta Radiol 1:321–327

Hayward RD (1977) Subarachnoid hemorrhage of unknown etiology. A clinical and radiological study of 51 cases. J Neurol Neurosurg Psychiatry 40:926–931

Heidrich R (1972) Subarachnoid haemorrhage. In: Vinken PJ, Bruyn GW (eds) Handbook of clinical neurology, vol 12. North Holland, Amsterdam, pp 68–204

Hijdra A, Gijn JV (1982) Early death from rupture of an intracranial aneurysm. J Neurosurg 57:765–768

Hook O, Norlen G, Gusman J (1963) Saccular aneurysms of the vertebrobasilar arterial system. A report of 28 cases Acta Neurol Scand 39:271–304

Housepian EM, Pool JL (1958) A systematic analysis of intracranial aneurysms from the autopsy file of the Presbyterian Hospital 1914–1956. J Neuropathol Exp Neurol 17:409–423

Jane JA, Winn HR, Richardson AE (1977) The natural history of intracranial aneurysms: Rebleeding rates during the acute and long-term period and implication for surgical management. Clin Neurosurg 24:176–184

Kak VK, Gleadhill CA, Baily IC (1970) The familial incidence of intracranial aneurysms. J Neurol Neurosurg Psychiatry 33:29–33

Kerppola W (1919) Zur Kenntnis der Aneurysmen an den Basalarterien des Getvins mit besonderer Berücksichtigung der begleitenden Arteriosklerose in denselben Gefässen: Arb Path Inst Univ. Helsinki 2:115–185 (Quoted by Forbus 1930)

Kibler RF, Couch RSC, Crompton MR (1961) Hydrocephalus in the adult following spontaneous SAH. Brain 84:45–61

Krayenbuhl H, Yasargil MG (1958) Das Hirnaneurysma. JR Geigy, Basel, p 143

Lassman LP, Ramani PS, Sengupta RP (1974) Aneurysms of peripheral cerebral arteries due to surgical trauma. Vasc Surg 8:1–5

Locksley HB (1966) Report on the cooperative study of intracranial aneurysms and subarachnoid haemorrhage, Section V, Part I. J Neurosurg 25:219–239

McCormick WF, Schmalstieg EJ (1977) The relationship of arterial hypertension to intracranial aneurysms. Arch Neurol 34:285–287

McKissock W, Paine KWE (1959) Subarachnoid haemorrhage. Brain 82:356–366

Meadows SP (1951) Intracranial aneurysms. In: Feiling A (ed) Modern trends in neurology. Butterworth, London, pp 391–465

Mertland TS (1939) Spontaneous subarachnoid hemorrhage and congenital berry aneurysms. Am J Surg 43:10–19

Mizukami M, Takemae T, Tazawa T, Kawase T, Matenzaki T (1980) Value of computerised tomography in the prediction of cerebral vasospasm after aneurysm rupture. Neurosurgery 7:583–586

Molinari GF, Smith L, Goldstein MN, Satran R (1973) Pathogenesis of cerebral mycotic aneurysms. Neurology 23:325–332

Mount L, Taveras JM (1956) Cerebral angiographic studies following surgical treatment of intracranial aneurysms. Acta Radiol 46:333–340

Moyes PD (1971) Surgical treatment of multiple aneurysms and of incidentally discovered unruptured aneurysms. J Neurosurg 35:291–295

New PFJ, Price DL, Carter B (1970) Cerebral angiography in cardiac myxomas: Correlation of angiographic and histopathological findings. Radiology 96:335–345

Nornes H (1973) The role of intracranial pressure in the arrest of hemorrhage in patients with ruptured intracranial aneurysms. J Neurosurg 39:226–234

Nornes H, Magnaes B (1972) Intracranial pressure in patients with ruptured saccular aneurysms. J Neurosurg 36:537–547

Nystrom SHM (1963) Development of intracranial aneurysms as revealed by electron microscopy. J Neurosurg 20:329–337

Olmstead WW, McGee JP (1977) Pathogenesis of peripheral aneurysms of the central nervous system. A subject review for the AFIP. Radiology 123:6611–666

Padget DH (1944) The circle of Willis; Its morphology and anatomy. In: Dandy WE (ed) Intracranial arterial aneurysms. Comstock, Ithaca, New York, pp 67–90

Patrick D, Appleby A (1983a) Infundibular widening of the posterior communicating artery progressing to true aneurysm. Br J Radiol 56:59–60

Patrick D, Appleby A (1983b) Familial intracranial aneurysms and infundibular widening. Neuroradiology 25:329–334

Phillips LH, Whisnant JP, O'Fellon WM, Sundt JM Jr (1980) The unchanging pattern of SAH in a community. Neurology 30:1034–1040

Pope FM, Narcisi P, Neil-Dwyer G, Nicholls AC, Bartlett S, Doshi B (1981) Some patients with cerebral aneurysms are deficient in type III collagen. Lancet I:973–975

Raimondi A, Torres H (1973) Acute hydrocephalus as a complication of SAH. Surg Neurol 1:23–26

Richardson JC, Hyland HH (1941) Intracranial aneurysms. A clinical and pathological study of subarachnoid haemorrhage and intracerebral haemorrhage caused by berry aneurysms. Medicine (Baltimore) 20:1–83

Richey FAG, MacLachlan WG (1922) Mycotic embolic aneurysms of peripheral arteries. Arch Intern Med 29:139–140

Roach MR, Drake CG (1965) Ruptured cerebral aneurysms caused by micro-organisms. N Engl J Med 273:240–244

Robertson EG (1949) Cerebral lesions due to intracranial aneurysms. Brain 72:150–161

Rotter W, Wellmer HJ, Hinrichs A Muller W (1955). Zur Orthologie und Pathologie der Polsterarterien (sog. Verzweigungs und Spornpolster) des Gehirns. Beitr Pathol 115:253–294

Rubinstein MK, Cohen NH (1954) Ehlers–Danlos syndrome associated with multiple intracranial aneurysms. Neurology 14:125–132

Russell DS (1954) Discussions: The pathology of spontaneous intracranial haemorrhage. Proc R Soc Med 47:689–693

Russell RWR (1963) Observations of intracranial aneurysms. Brain 86:425–441

Sakai N, Sakata K, Yamada AH, Yamamoto M, Aiba T, Takeda F (1974) Familial occurrence of intracranial aneurysms. Surg Neurol 2:25–29

Sarwar M, Batnitzky S, Schecter MM et al. (1976) Growing intracranial aneurysms. Radiology 120:603–607

Schneck SA (1964) On the relationship between ruptured intracranial and cerebral infarction. Neurology 14:691–702

Schon P, Marshall J (1984) Subarachnoid hemorrhage in identical twins. J Neurol Neurosurg Psychiatry 47:81–83

Sekhar LN, Heros R (1981) Origin, growth and rupture of saccular aneurysms. A review. Neurosurgery 8:248–260

Schulman K, Martin BF, Popoff N, Ransohoff J (1963) Recognition of treatment of hydrocephalus following spontaneous SAH. J Neurosurg 20:1040–1049

Smith B (1963) Cerebral pathology in subarachnoid haemorrhage. J Neurol Neurosurg Psychiatry 26:535–539

Steele JJ, Kilburn HL, Leech AW (1972) Phytotic (mycotic) intracranial aneurysms with an unusual pathogenesis. Pediatrics 50:936–939

Stehbens WE (1959) Medial defects in the cerebral arteries of man. J Pathol Bacteriol 78:179–185

Stehbens WE (1963) Histopathology of cerebral aneurysms. Arch Neurol 8:272–285

Stehbens WE (1972) Pathology of the cerebral blood vessels. CV Mosby, St Louis, Miss., pp 351–470

Stehbens WE (1975) Ultrastructure of aneurysms. Arch Neurol 32:798–807

Stoane L, Allen J, Cohen H (1966) Radiological observations in cerebral embolisation of left heart myxomas. Radiology 87:262–266

Suzuki J, Kodama N (1971) Cerebrovascular Moya Moya disease—second report—collateral routes to forebrain via ethmoid sinus and superior nasal meatus. Angiology 22:223–236

Suzuki J, Kodama N (1983) Moya Moya disease. A review. Stroke 14:104–109

Symonds CP (1923) Contributions to the clinical study of intracranial aneurysms. Guy's Hosp Rep 73:139–158

Tomlinson BE (1959) Brain changes in ruptured intracranial aneurysms. J Clin Pathol 12:391–399

Valadares JB, De Souza MRK, Hankinson J, Hall K, Sengupta RP (1979) Multiplos aneurysmus micoticos intracranianos regist. de um. Caso. 37.3.311–318. Arquivas de Neuropsiquiatria

Vaughn HG Jr, Howard RG (1962) Intracranial haemorrhage due to metastatic chorionepithelioma. Neurology 12:771–777

Walker AE, Allegre GE (1954) The pathology and pathogenesis of cerebral aneurysms. J Neuropathol Exp Neurol 13:248–259

Walton JN (1956) Subarachnoid haemorrhage. ES Livingstone, Edinburgh London, pp 350

Weibers DO, Whisnant JP, O'Fellon WM (1981) The natural history of unruptured intracranial aneurysms. N Engl J Med 304:696–698

Wright TJE (1949) Coarctation of aorta with death from a cerebral aneurysm. Arch Pathol 48:382–486

Yamashita M, Oka K, Tanaka K (1983) Histopathology of the brain vascular network in Moya Moya disease. Stroke 14:50–58

Yasargil MG, Yonekawa Y, Zumstein B, Stahl HG (1973) Hydrocephalus following spontaneous subarachnoid haemorrhage; clinical features and treatment. J Neurosurg 39:474–479

Yates PO (1976) Vascular disease of central nervous system. In: Blackwood M, Corsellis JAN (eds) Greenfield's neuropathology, 3rd edn. Edward Arnold, London, pp 86–147

Yonas H, Agamanolis D, Takaoka Y, White AJ (1977) Dissecting intracranial aneurysms. Surg Neurol 8:407–415

Zacks DJ, Russel DB, Miller JDR (1980) Fortuitously discovered intracranial aneurysms. Arch Neurol 37:39–41

4 Clinical Features

Symptomatology

Introduction

Subarachnoid haemorrhage has assumed great clinical importance in recent years as it represents 10% of all vascular causes of death (Sahs et al. 1966). Nearly 28 000 Americans suffer from SAH due to ruptured intracranial aneurysm alone each year (Kassell and Drake 1982). It is not only an acute illness, but also a chronic process; when the diagnosis is delayed the result of treatment is often less than satisfactory. Recent advances in the management of SAH have resulted in a significant improvement in its prognosis and have also emphasised the importance of an early diagnosis. Advances in neuroradiology, with the advent of computerised tomography (CT), and the improvement of angiographic techniques, have meant that identification of the source of subarachnoid haemorrhage is now possible in over 80% of cases. Complications, such as intracerebral haematoma, cerebral ischaemia or hydrocephalus, can now be recognised and specific treatment instituted.

The commonest cause of SAH is a ruptured intracranial aneurysm and it may produce a minor leak some days or weeks prior to a major rupture. With a minor haemorrhage, the symptomatology more often seems trivial. However, if the condition can be diagnosed at this stage, some of the fatal or major debilitating haemorrhages may be prevented. The cerebral tissue is minimally affected by a minor leak, and surgical treatment usually results in an excellent outcome.

Subarachnoid haemorrhage may manifest itself in a variety of ways and unusual presentations may easily distract physicians from considering this diagnosis (Walton 1956; Adams et al. 1980). The symptomatology of SAH will be discussed under the following headings.

1. Classical clinical presentations as described by Collier (1922)
2. Clinical features in relation to the severity of haemorrhage
3. Atypical presentations

The clinical features of 500 patients with intracranial aneurysms operated on by one of the authors are analysed in this chapter.

Classical Clinical Features of Subarachnoid Haemorrhage

Collier (1922) described the clinical features of SAH long before surgical treatment for the condition was available, and he outlined five different modes of presentation.

Apoplectic

This is a form of presentation with loss of consciousness and significant involvement of the neuraxis. It is termed "apoplectic" as it simulates a stroke. The degree of coma and its duration vary with the severity of the haemorrhage.

Meningitic

This term is applied to an SAH presenting with features of meningitis, such as fever, photophobia, neck stiffness and delirium, due to irritation of the basal meninges by the subarachnoid blood.

Lumbosacral

This type of presentation is rare. It occurs when blood spreads along the nerve roots causing irritation with subsequent backache, leg pain and muscle stiffness.

Recurrent Coma

The patient who gives a history of several attacks of loss of consciousness before admission and during hospitalisation is in this category. The pathological basis is considered to be repeated haemorrhages from an aneurysm or intermittent blockage of the CSF pathways. This mode of presentation is extremely rare and we have only encountered two such cases. The first was that of a 26-year-old female, who, in the space of 7 days, had four episodes of transient loss of consciousness. She subsequently died from an anterior communicating artery aneurysm. The second case was that of a 20-year-old male, who, over a period of 6 weeks, suffered four episodes of loss of consciousness. Angiography demonstrated an internal carotid bifurcation aneurysm which was successfully clipped.

Migrainous

Collier (1922) considered that previous attacks of headache, like those in migraine, may be a premonitory symptom of SAH. The association of migraine and intracranial abnormalities, such as angioma, has been well described (Frankel 1950; Walton 1956). This association is not as frequent as previously thought. However, any change in the character of the headache should be investigated (Frankel 1950).

Clinical Features in Relation to the Severity of Haemorrhage

Whilst Collier's (1922) work still remains the classical description of SAH, the clinical presentation largely depends upon the severity of the haemorrhage.

Catastrophic

In a massive subarachnoid haemorrhage, there is a sudden onset of coma which deepens, the breathing becomes stertorous, and the blood pressure rises with a hectic swing of the pulse rate. The limbs are initially paralysed and flaccid, and later the patient may develop a decerebrate posture. The pupils become irregular and the patient dies within hours. Such a presentation is estimated to occur in approximately 30% of patients with aneurysmal SAH (Pakarinen 1967). Progressive deterioration and demise in these cases is usually due to massive intracerebral or intraventricular haemorrhage. The majority of patients dying within 72 h have an intracerebral, intracerebellar or subdural haematoma (Crompton 1962; Sahs et al. 1966; Hijdra and Gijn 1982).

Major Haemorrhage

A significant but non-fatal haemorrhage into the subarachnoid space is the commonly encountered presentation in a neurological centre. The presenting symptoms may include the following (Table 4.1):

1. *Headache*. This is abrupt in onset and is frequently described in such dramatic terms as "a bolt from the blue", "a blinding headache", "as if someone had hit me on the back of the head with an axe" or "as if something burst in my head". The site of the headache is variable and is no guide to the location of the offending lesion. Usually it starts in the occipital region and then spreads all over the head, neck and shoulders. The initial symptom was headache in 399 (80%) patients in a group of 500 cases in our series.

2. *Loss of consciousness*. Two hundred and twenty (44%) patients had lost consciousness at the time of ictus in this series. The patient usually regains consciousness after a short period.

3. *Convulsions*. Seizures at the onset are uncommon, even with a massive SAH. However,

Table 4.1. Initial symptoms (figures are percentages)

	Present series (500 cases)	Walton (312 cases)	Suzuki (1000 cases)
Headache	80	51	73
Loss of consciousness	44	21	35
Disturbance of vision	15	–	–
Convulsion	6	5	8
Dizziness	8.6	5	13.5
Confusion	8.4	1	–
Limb weakness	12	2	23.5
Sensory disturbance	4	–	8.7

they may develop later with the onset of complications, such as intracerebral haematoma or ischaemia from vasospasm. Only 31 patients (6%) had convulsion as the initial symptom.

4. *Vomiting.* This is a common feature of SAH, but it is of little diagnostic value.

5. *Disturbance of higher functions.* Confusion and impairment of memory are unusual modes of presentation. Forty-three patients (8%) presented with these symptoms. Speech disorders are occasionally seen and can be helpful in the localisation of the source of haemorrhage.

6. *Ocular symptoms.* Photophobia is a common complaint. Blurred vision may occur, particularly with subhyaloid haemorrhage in the region of the macula. Diplopia may result from direct involvement of the third nerve, or from a sixth nerve palsy as a false localising sign in raised intracranial pressure.

Minor Haemorrhage

In a minor haemorrhage the presenting symptoms are few and are frequently ignored by patients or their attending physician. A minor bleed is often followed by a major or a catastrophic haemorrhage (Strauss et al. 1932), and therefore should be considered as warning signs of a major haemorrhage (Frankel 1950; Gillingham 1958; Okawara 1973). Their recognition is important and potentially rewarding, and will be discussed in more detail later in the chapter.

Atypical Presentations

The unusual presentations of haemorrhage are due to variation in the severity of the haemorrhage, the degree of damage to the neuraxis, the development of complications, the localisation of haemorrhage within the cranium, and the cir-

cumstances under which the haemorrhage has occurred, e.g. a road traffic accident or head injury. The following unusual presentations have been seen in our experience:

Head Injury

The fall that accompanies the sudden loss of consciousness in SAH may lead to head injury. When evidence of external injury, e.g. scalp laceration or skull fracture, is seen on X-ray, the real nature of the problem can remain obscure. A similar situation arises in patients admitted comatose following a road traffic accident. In both of these situations careful eye-witness accounts of what happened may help alert one to the real problem. An underlying cause, such as SAH, should always be considered when a head injury or road traffic accident occurs under unusual circumstances.

In cases of SAH the extent of the trauma is often trivial compared to the clinical state of the patient. Retrograde amnesia is also a valuable guide in this context; in head injury, there is usually a retrograde amnesia, whilst in SAH the patient often has a clear recollection of the events up to and including the ictus. Finally, the CT scan may clarify the problem by showing subarachnoid blood or haematoma typical of SAH (Fig. 4.1). The following case illustrates the difficulty of the diagnosis in these circumstances:

O. S. was making a telephone call in a hotel in August, 1971, when she thought that someone had "hit her on the back of the head", causing her to fall on the ground. Her husband was nearby and came to help, and when she regained consciousness she was emphatic about her complaint. She even thought that she had seen someone rapidly disappearing. As there was a brawl in the hotel at the time, the husband and wife were insistent that it was a case of assault. She was admitted to the local hospital for observation with

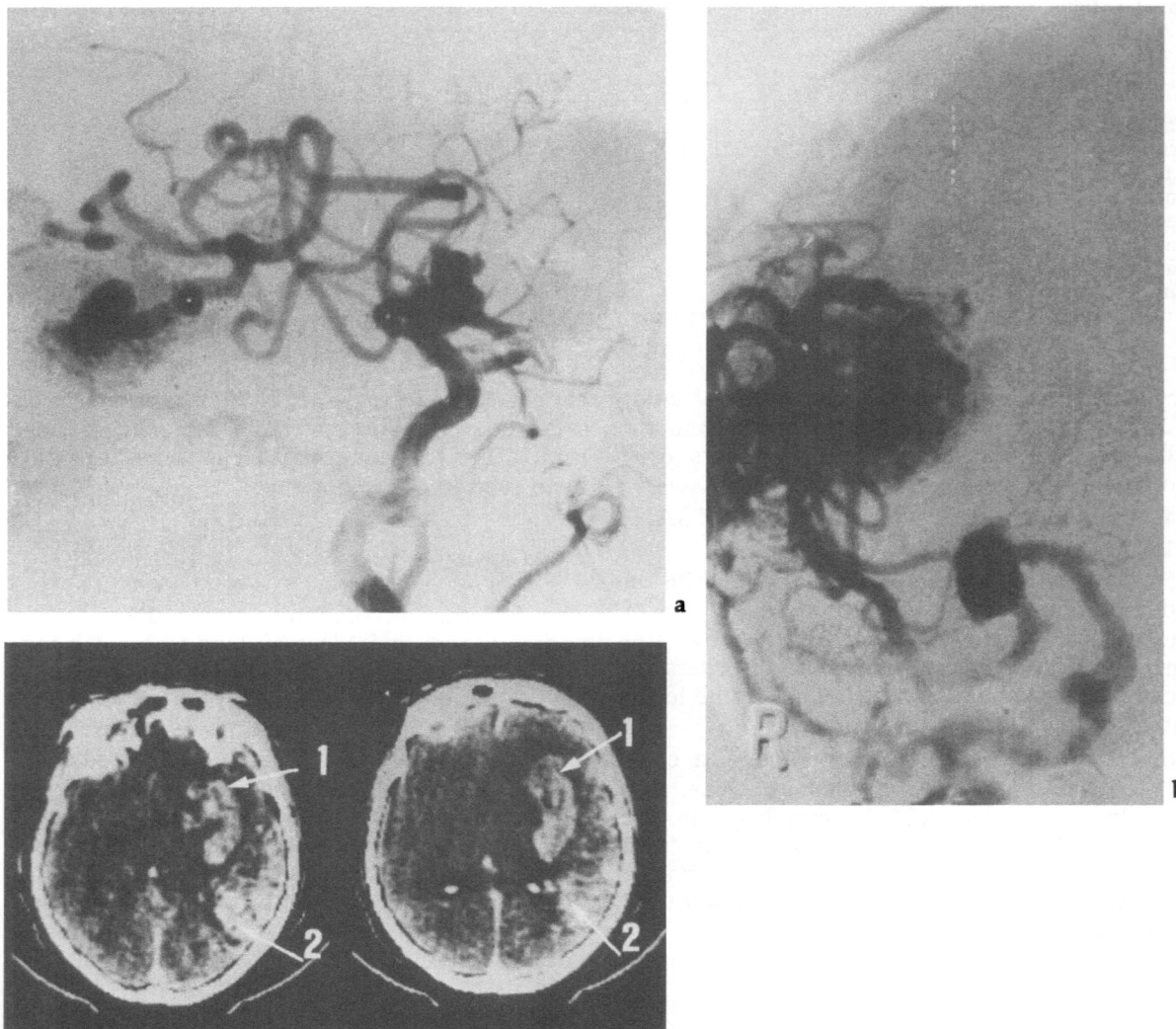

Fig. 4.1a–c. Patient with a history of head injury whose skull X-ray showed a fracture and in whom there was a clinical suspicion of an underlying subarachnoid haemorrhage. Right carotid angiogram (**a** lateral and **b** Townes projection) showed a middle cerebral artery aneurysm arising just beyond the ICA bifurcation and a right posterior temporal arteriovenous malformation. **c** CT showed a right temporal haematoma (*1*) together with enhancement of the AVM (*2*), thus indicating that it was the middle cerebral artery aneurysm which had bled.

a diagnosis of a head injury, and was discharged home 3 days later. She continued to have severe headache and was referred to the neuro-trauma unit for a further opinion. On detailed interview it became clear that she only felt as if someone had hit her on the head, but she did not actually see the alleged assailant. By this stage she had developed photophobia and neck stiffness, and a diagnosis of SAH was confirmed by lumbar puncture. Bilateral carotid angiography revealed an anterior communicating artery aneurysm which

was successfully clipped. (Ironically she was awarded substantial damages by the criminal compensation injuries board for her alleged assault!)

Neck Injury

When a patient seeks medical advice with pain in the neck or muscular spasm following a severe jolt, it is understandable that a diagnosis of neck injury rather than an SAH is made. In SAH the blood passes down the cervical canal and the upper cervical nerve roots are irritated, causing spasm of the suboccipital and cervical muscles. A clear history about the nature of the injury is essential in order to direct one's attention to the actual problem, as the following case illustrates:

F. M., a 60-year-old female, in September, 1975 experienced a severe headache associated with dizziness and vomiting, which she attributed to jarring of her neck whilst driving a car along a rough road. She did not lose consciousness but the headache persisted, and later that day she developed marked neck stiffness. She was taken to the local hospital, where she indicated having jarred her neck. As her main complaint was neck pain, a diagnosis of whiplash injury was made, and the patient was given a surgical collar. Two days later she was seen by her family doctor, but by this time she had developed photophobia and was referred to the neurosurgical unit at Newcastle General Hospital. On examination, marked neck stiffness and a positive Kernig's sign were present. There was no other focal neurological deficit. Lumbar puncture confirmed a diagnosis of SAH, and bilateral carotid angiography revealed an anterior communicating artery aneurysm. Seven days after the onset of her initial symptoms, the aneurysm was successfully clipped. It should be mentioned that in both of the above cases, when a careful history was obtained there was a definite suggestion of SAH.

Backache and Sciatica

Subarachnoid haemorrhage from an intracranial source may occasionally present as backache and sciatica. The following case is an example:

T. J., a 46-year-old man, developed sudden severe low backache in September, 1971. A similar episode had occurred 10 years earlier, and had been diagnosed as sciatica. The initial diagnosis on this occasion was also sciatica due to a disc prolapse. However, within 48 h of admission, he developed headache and photophobia, and lumbar puncture confirmed the diagnosis of SAH. On reviewing the history, the pain had radiated to the back of the neck and occiput at its onset, although back pain was his predominant symptom. Angiography demonstrated a right frontal arteriovenous malformation and an anterior communicating artery aneurysm. Both were successfully treated by separate surgical procedures. At surgery, there was clear evidence of recent haemorrhage from the arteriovenous malforma-

tion. A similar presentation may occur with a spinal SAH, and this is discussed in a separate chapter.

Cardiac and Respiratory Arrest

This type of presentation is exceptional. We have seen only one patient who presented in this unusual fashion:

D. G., a 54-year-old female, collapsed at work in January, 1980, and was rushed to the local hospital, where, on arrival, she was comatose. Whilst being examined in the casualty department, she had a cardiorespiratory arrest with apnoea and hypotension, from which she was successfully resuscitated. Over the ensuing 24 h her conscious level improved and she was transferred to the neurosurgical unit. On examination, the patient was drowsy but rousable, and was obeying simple verbal commands. There was marked neck stiffness and a positive Kernig's sign. The left pupil was larger than the right but reacted briskly to light, and there was a large subhyaloid haemorrhage in the right fundus. She also had a mild, left hemiparesis with bilateral extensor plantar responses. CT scan was normal. Four vessel angiography demonstrated a left posterior inferior cerebellar artery aneurysm, which was successfully clipped. At operation, a large haematoma over the brain stem was noted. The patient slowly improved postoperatively, and was discharged home 2 weeks later.

Cardiorespiratory arrest from cardiac arrythmias has also been reported in SAH without mass effect (Parizel 1979). Other unusual reported presentations include sudden deafness (Gussen 1976), intermittent deafness (Mori et al. 1978), and, very rarely, as a visible mass in the middle ear (Morantz et al. 1976). Epistaxis (Moore et al. 1979) and otorrhagia (Holtzman and Pariser 1979) are other unusual presentations. Priapism as a very unusual presentation of SAH was reported by Takaku et al. (1979).

Loss of Appetite and Cachexia

W. S., a 46-year-old unemployed labourer, developed pins and needles in the right foot in January 1983 which gradually spread up the right side of his body to the right arm and hand and also the right side of his face. These were constant and worsened on touching objects. From June 1983 he started to lose weight, from $11\frac{1}{2}$ to $8\frac{1}{2}$ stone. He had no appetite. In the area of pins and needles he developed gradual numbness. From December 1983 the paraesthesia changed to the left side, involving the left upper and lower limbs. He became progressively unsteady and dizzy upon sudden movement. There was also a feeling of vertigo.

From October 1984 he developed dysphagia for solid foods, sensation of food sticking in his throat, and often vomited undigested food. During extensive diagnostic investigations he developed diarrhoea. A provisional diagnosis of gastro-intestinal neoplasm was made, but all investigations, including barium meal and barium enema, endoscopy and pancreatic function proved normal. With continued weight loss and neurological symptoms he was referred to the Neurological Clinic in January 1985, where marked left cerebellar signs were noted. He had generalised grade 4 muscle weakness. All reflexes were brisk with equivocal plantar responses. There was no sensory deficit. The possibility of motor neurone disease was raised; however, a CT

scan showed a space-occupying lesion in the region of the fourth ventricle extending to the foramen magnum and left cerebellopontine angle (Fig. 4.2). The possibility of a large thrombosed aneurysm was considered. Four vessel angiography showed an irregular right PICA aneurysm (Fig. 4.3). The relationship of the right PICA aneurysm to the space-occupying lesion involving the left cerebellopontine angle mass was admittedly not entirely clear before operation, but a large thrombosed aneurysm was still thought likely.

On 15 February 1985, the posterior fossa was explored through a midline incision. At the foramen of Magendi a golf ball size, shape and colour mass was noted. This was in fact a thrombosed and calcified aneurysm which was extending through the fourth ventricle to the left cerebellopontine angle. It was a part of a small patent aneurysm of the right PICA. The floor of the fourth ventricle was stained yellow, suggesting previous haemorrhage. Using a Cavitron, the

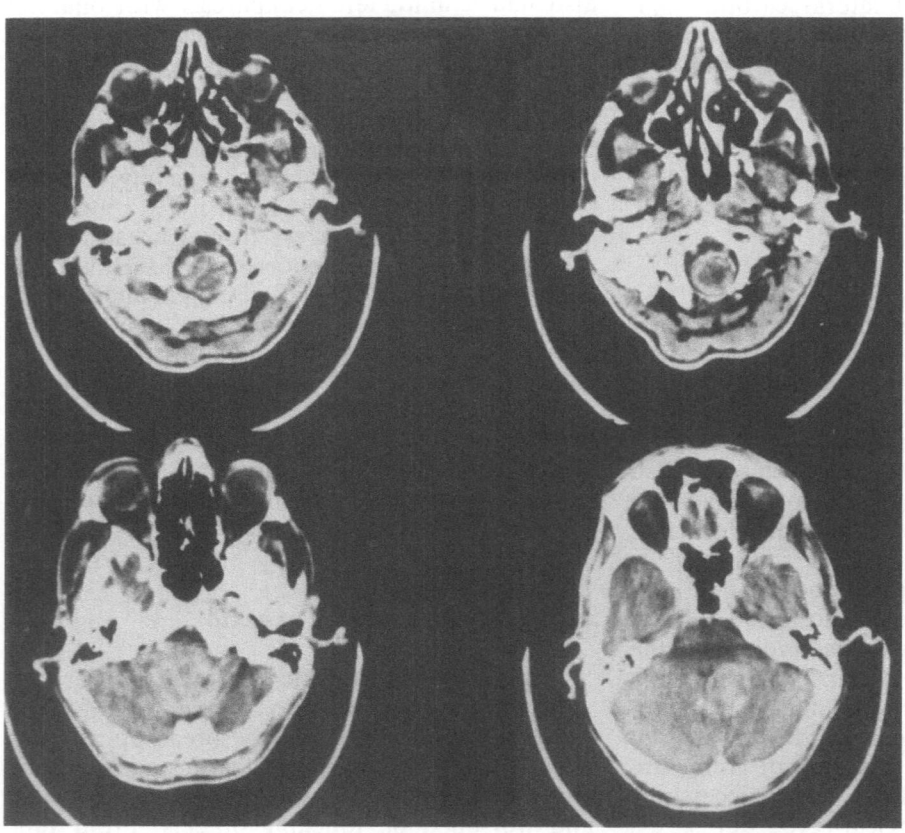

Fig. 4.2. CT scans showing a well defined ring enhancing lesion with peripheral calcification in the foramen magnum and extending up into the region of the fourth ventricle and left cerebellopontine angle.

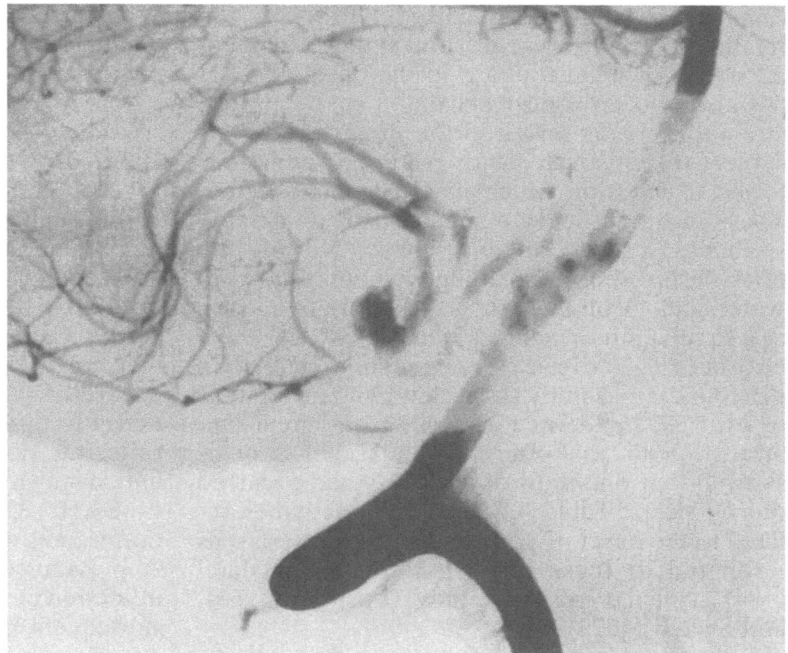

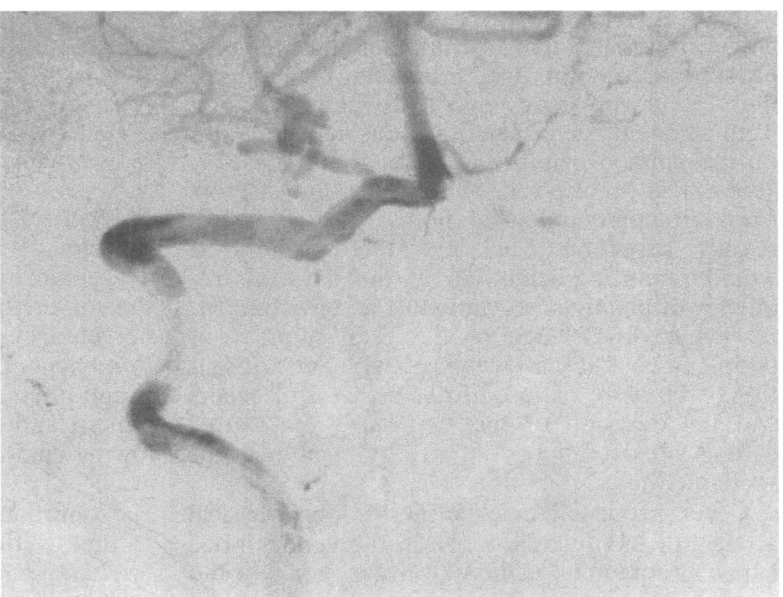

Fig. 4.3. Vertebral angiogram (a lateral and b anteroposterior projection) shows a loculated aneurysm arising from the posterior medullary segment of the right posterior inferior cerebellar artery.

calcified part of the aneurysm was excised and the rest clipped. He made an uneventful recovery and started to gain weight rapidly within 14 days of operation.

The interesting aspect of this case is the loss of appetite with severe weight loss resulting from compression of the appetite centre around the fourth ventricle.

Activities or Events Relating to the Onset of Subarachnoid Haemorrhage

Patients with SAH often give a history of exertion or strenuous circumstances at the onset of symptoms. The role of environmental stress in the causation of SAH is well recognised, and is of importance both medicolegally and in the prevention of recurrent haemorrhage. However, the relationship of physical exertion and environmental stress, or head trauma, to the onset of SAH has always been controversial.

Walton (1956) reviewed the literature on this subject exhaustively and recorded numerous forms of exertion which have been implicated. These included heavy manual labour, coughing, straining at stool, running, coitus, blowing the nose, lacing shoes, wrestling, jumping into cold water and alcoholic excess. Mild trauma, such as a sudden jolt, heading a football, or a fall, have also been considered as precipitating factors. In the cooperative study (Locksley 1966) an analysis of over 6000 patients with SAH from aneurysm, arteriovenous malformation and other sources showed that one-third of all SAHs had occurred during sleep. Table 4.2 shows the activities related to the onset of SAH in the present series, as compared to those of Richardson and Hyland (1941), the cooperative study (Locksley 1966), and Suzuki (1979).

Subarachnoid haemorrhage can occur at rest without any apparent precipitating factors. It is, however, possible that any form of strain, whether physical or mental, that momentarily increases the blood pressure may provoke bleeding from an aneurysm or arteriovenous malformation on the point of rupture (Walton 1956; Locksley 1966). The precise role of environmental factors from an epidemiological point of view is not readily apparent. Locksley (1966) states "It would require, in addition to the data on frequency of positive association of an environmental event, knowledge of the total number of people in each disease category with and without SAH who were exposed to such stressful events and the duration of this exposure. This latter data is almost impossible to obtain and is not available."

Other proposed mechanisms linking physical strain to SAH include a rise in the venous pressure consequent upon the Valsalva manoeuvre and mechanical shift of the brain and the circle of Willis with respect to other fixed structures in the cranium (Locksley 1966). We were not able to detect any seasonal variation in the onset of SAH.

Past Medical History

A thorough history of past medical records should be obtained in all patients because, although the great majority of cases of SAH result from rupture of a berry aneurysm, the clinician should always be on the look-out for rarer causes, e.g. mycotic aneurysm associated with bacterial endocarditis. A history of easy bruising or a tendency to prolonged bleeding from minor wounds raises the possibility of a bleeding diathesis, and anticoagulant therapy is a well-recognised cause of SAH. The intake of drugs, such as phenothiazines or amphetamines, can produce SAH. A previous history of hypertension, myocardial infarction or other major illness can also influence subsequent management.

Physical Examination

Introduction

The majority of patients with SAH will have as the underlying cause a berry aneurysm; a small percentage may have an arteriovenous malformation, hypertension or a rarer condition. A thorough physical examination is necessary in every patient and should be directed towards the following goals:

1. Confirmation of the clinical diagnosis of SAH, that is the presence of subhyaloid haemorrhage and/or neck rigidity and a positive Kernig's sign.

Table 4.2. Activities related to the onset of SAH (figures are percentages)

Type of event	Richardson and Hyland (1941)	Coop. study (Locksley 1966)	Suzuki (1979)	Present series
Sleep	16	27.4	6	8
Lifting weight	14	9.1	24	9.2
Intercourse	–	2.9	0.1	2
Other times	70	38	70	73
Data not available	–	23	–	8

2. Identification of the underlying aetiology, e.g. evidence of pre-existing hypertension with fundal changes and stroke or left ventricular hypertrophy, signs of bacterial endocarditis, bruising or trauma.

3. Localisation of the primary site of haemorrhage, e.g. the third nerve palsy seen in patients with a posterior communicating artery aneurysm or leg weakness, consistent with rupture of an aneurysm of the anterior communicating artery.

4. Assessment of fitness for angiography and subsequent surgery from a medical and neurological point of view, i.e. severity of SAH and evidence of cardiopulmonary insufficiency.

5. Detection of any complications of SAH that may require urgent treatment, i.e. hydrocephalus, haematoma or cerebral ischaemia due to vasospasm.

The widespread neurological and autonomic disturbances that may occur in SAH are discussed below.

The commonest picture we have encountered in recent years is of a fully conscious, well-orientated person with neck stiffness plus or minus a positive Kernig's sign (Tables 4.3, 4.4), which we feel reflects the increased awareness of the early symptoms and signs of SAH in the Newcastle region.

Table 4.3. Conscious level on admission   (%)

Fully conscious	71
Obtunded	8.5
Drowsy	16.5
Barely responds to commands	1.5
Unconscious	2.5

Table 4.4. Neurological signs on admission

	Yes (%)	No (%)	Data not recorded
Disturbance of memory	23	77	–
Disturbance of speech	10	88	2
Neck stiffness	86	14	–
Papilloedema	10	88	2
Cranial nerve involvement	23	75	2
Limb weakness	16	84	–
Extensor plantar response	29	71	–

Neurological Signs

The presence of abnormal neurological signs in a patient with an SAH depends upon several factors:

1. The severity of haemorrhage. Massive haemorrhage leads to a severe neurological deficit whereas a modest or minimal haemorrhage without complication produces very little in the way of neurological signs (Falconer 1954).

2. The presence of complications, such as intracerebral haematoma or hydrocephalus.

3. The source of haemorrhage. The destruction of cerebral tissue is greater in aneurysmal SAH than in haemorrhage arising from an arteriovenous malformation (Sahs et al. 1966).

4. The location of the haemorrhage. Severe haemorrhage in the posterior fossa or within the ventricles is likely to produce a greater deficit or depression of the conscious level than that in other areas.

5. Patient selection. Thirty per cent of patients will rapidly succumb to catastrophic haemorrhage and in these patients a detailed physical examination is not possible. Some patients will not reach the neurological centre for assessment and thus any analysis of the neurological signs in SAH will be influenced by patient selection.

6. Timing of the examination. At the onset of SAH some patients may show little in the way of abnormal signs, only to develop them later with the onset of complications.

Disturbance of Higher Functions

State of Consciousness. Following a massive haemorrhage the patient remains deeply comatose without ever regaining consciousness. In a moderate haemorrhage, consciousness may be lost transiently at the onset. With the development of brain stem compression from haematoma or hydrocephalus, the conscious level deteriorates. Fluctuating consciousness may occur in patients with a subdural haematoma or communicating hydrocephalus. In our series, at the time of admission 71% of the patients were conscious, 8.5% obtunded, and 16.5% drowsy (Table 4.3).

Memory. Disturbance of memory does not usually occur early but may be seen in the later stages of SAH. Korsakoff's syndrome, which is a state of profound, organic amnesia with impairment of recent memory and subsequent confabulation, similar to that seen in alcoholics, is also occasionally encountered in SAH (Hall 1929; Lindquist and Norlen 1966). Hall (1932) gives credit to Goldflam for describing this condition in patients with SAH in 1923. Ischaemic lesions are found in the mamillary bodies, fornices and the dorsal medial and anteroventral nuclei of the thalamus. Ischaemic damage to the hypothalamic area can be seen occasionally at the time of surgery for anterior communicating artery aneurysm. Memory disturbance was noted in 116 (23%) patients on admission in our group.

Disorders of Speech. Dysphasia is rarely seen in an uncomplicated SAH. Its presence indicates focal damage to the neuraxis and helps localise the site of haemorrhage. In 50 patients (10%) some degree of dysphasia was detected.

Dysarthria is extremely rare and we have seen only one such patient, a man 32 years of age, with SAH and a cerebellar haematoma due to an arteriovenous malformation. The haematoma was evacuated and the AVM subsequently excised but he remained dysarthric. We suspect that prior to the advent of the CT scan such patients rapidly deteriorated before appropriate treatment could be instigated, and thus such disorders were rarely recognised. Walton (1956) described two cases of dysarthria of cortical origin.

Parietal Lobe Dysfunction. Signs of parietal lobe dysfunction in patients with SAH are noted infrequently. However, an angioma may occur in this region, and it should be considered in the presence of these signs.

Personality Disorders. Dementia and emotional lability are well known, especially with bilateral frontal lobe damage from an anterior communicating artery aneurysm (Sengupta et al. 1975). Patients with normal pressure hydrocephalus secondary to an SAH (either unrecognised or which occurred in the past) may also present with dementia. Barnett (1968) described such a case— a 64-year-old widower who presented with dementia and attributed his hydrocephalus to an SAH diagnosed as "flu" some 2 months previously. SAH can result in adhesive arachnoiditis with delayed and progressive hydrocephalus, leading to an impaired mental state (Foltz and Ward 1956). A severe form of personality disorder resembling the Klüver-Bucy syndrome, from bilateral temporal lobe lesions, has been seen in one patient who underwent surgery for a basilar artery aneurysm, initially by a right subtemporal and subsequently a left subtemporal approach.

Cranial Nerve Dysfunction

Involvement of the cranial nerves can be caused by the following mechanisms:

1. The direct pressure of an aneurysm
2. Direct pressure by extravasated blood
3. A rise in intracranial pressure
4. Compression by an intracerebral haematoma

Olfactory Nerve

Anosmia due to spontaneous SAH is extremely rare. This nerve is not usually examined carefully in patients with SAH and thus its true incidence remains unknown. Heidrich (1972) reported two cases of verified anosmia in a series of 300 patients.

Optic Nerve and Its Connections

Momentary disturbance of vision may be the presenting symptom in some cases, due to a sudden rise in intracranial pressure. It occurred in 75 patients (15%) in our study. Jefferson (1937), in an excellent review, divided the internal carotid trunk aneurysms into infraclinoid and supraclinoid, and found that visual disturbance was common with supraclinoid aneurysms. He further subdivided them into those involving the optic radiation, the optic tract, the chiasm and the optic nerve.

The optic radiation is usually compromised by posterior cerebral artery aneurysms, and the optic tract by internal carotid or large middle cerebral artery aneurysms. Anterior communicating artery aneurysms may compress the chiasm, whilst internal carotid artery aneurysms may involve the optic nerve. This is at variance with the finding of Peiris and Russell (1980), but our experience would support the views of Jefferson. Poppen (1948) described nine cases of optic pallor due to a direct compression of the optic nerves by an aneurysm. Bird et al. (1970) described five cases of supraclinoid aneurysms presenting with visual failure. There was a long interval between the involvement of the two eyes, and he suggested that the delay may be due to the involvement of individual optic nerves, rather than the chiasm. He also suggested that aneurysms may grow intermittently, or less constantly, than a neoplasm, and that the visual loss occurs during a period of rapid growth. In a series of 32 carotid ophthalmic aneurysms, of which 22 had caused

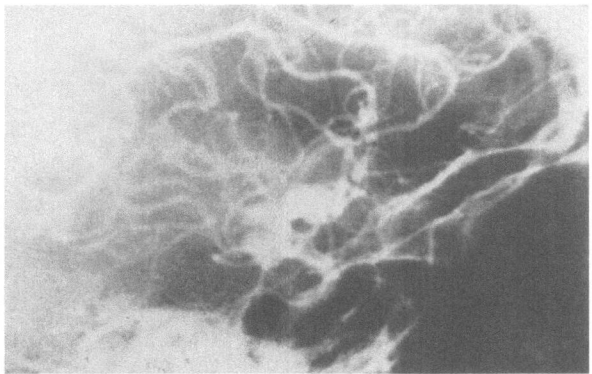

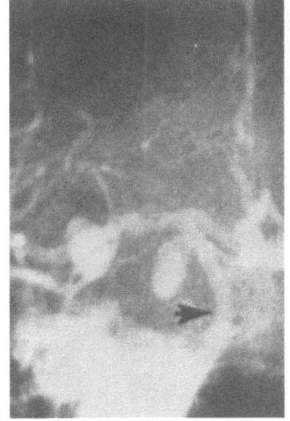 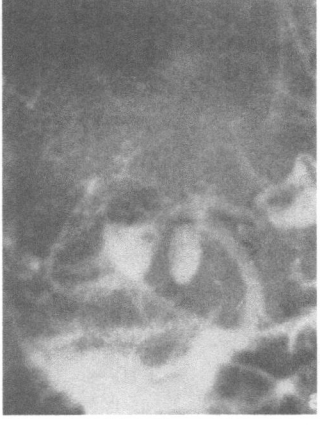

a

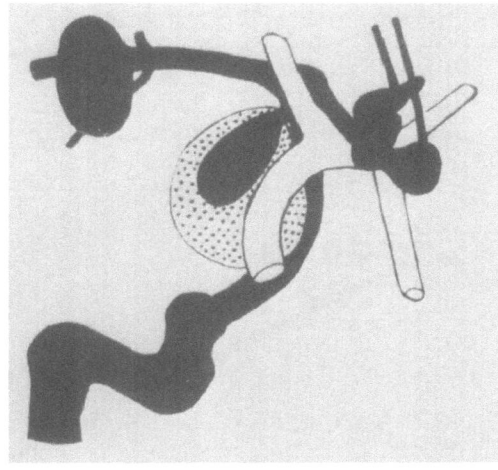

b

Fig. 4.4. a Right carotid angiogram showing a middle cerebral aneurysm, anterior communicating artery aneurysm and posterior communicating artery aneurysm. The posterior communicating artery aneurysm at surgery was considerably larger than shown in the angiogram. Notice the displacement of the internal carotid artery medially (*arrowhead*).
b Diagrammatic representation of the operative findings. This shows that the large aneurysm of the internal carotid artery, which contained mural clot, has pushed the artery medially to the optic nerve.

SAH, four cases of optic nerve compression were reported (Sengupta et al. 1976). In one patient in the present series, a carotid bifurcation aneurysm causing SAH produced optic nerve compression. We have also described optic nerve compression in a patient with a giant posterior communicating artery aneurysm (Sengupta and Hankinson 1979), in which the aneurysm displaced the internal carotid artery medially beneath the optic nerve (Fig. 4.4). Aneurysmal compression of the visual pathways is rarely considered early in patients presenting with visual failure or field defects. The following case illustrates this particular point well:

N. L., a 50-year-old woman, was admitted in July, 1971. She had suffered from typical migrainous attacks for 6 years. In October, 1970, she suddenly experienced pain over the left eye, and 5 min later found that she was completely blind in that eye. Over the following few days perception of light returned. Two weeks later, when seen by an ophthalmologist, only a rim of peripheral vision remained in the left eye, but the fundus was normal. The optic disc became pale within 3 weeks, and a diagnosis of ischaemic optic neuritis,

associated with migraine, was made. In April, 1971, she noticed a gradual painless deterioration of vision in her right eye, and within 6 weeks the acuity had deteriorated to 6/60. She did not seek medical advice until she had become virtually blind. When admitted to the Regional Neurological Centre, the patient had gross left optic atrophy. The visual acuity was 6/60 on the right, while on the left there was perception of hand movement only (Fig. 4.5a). Neurological examination was otherwise normal. The patient was normotensive and in sinus rhythm. Plain X-rays of the skull were normal. Bilateral carotid angiography revealed a large saccular aneurysm arising at the origin of the left ophthalmic artery (Fig. 4.5b). Through a left frontotemporal craniotomy the aneurysm was trapped and excised. The patient developed dysphasia and mild right hemiparesis which gradually improved. The vision in the right eye at the time of discharge from hospital 2 months later had returned to normal.

Delayed referral in the above case resulted in the loss of vision in one eye. Timely intervention may help in the rapid recovery of vision, as is seen in the following patient:

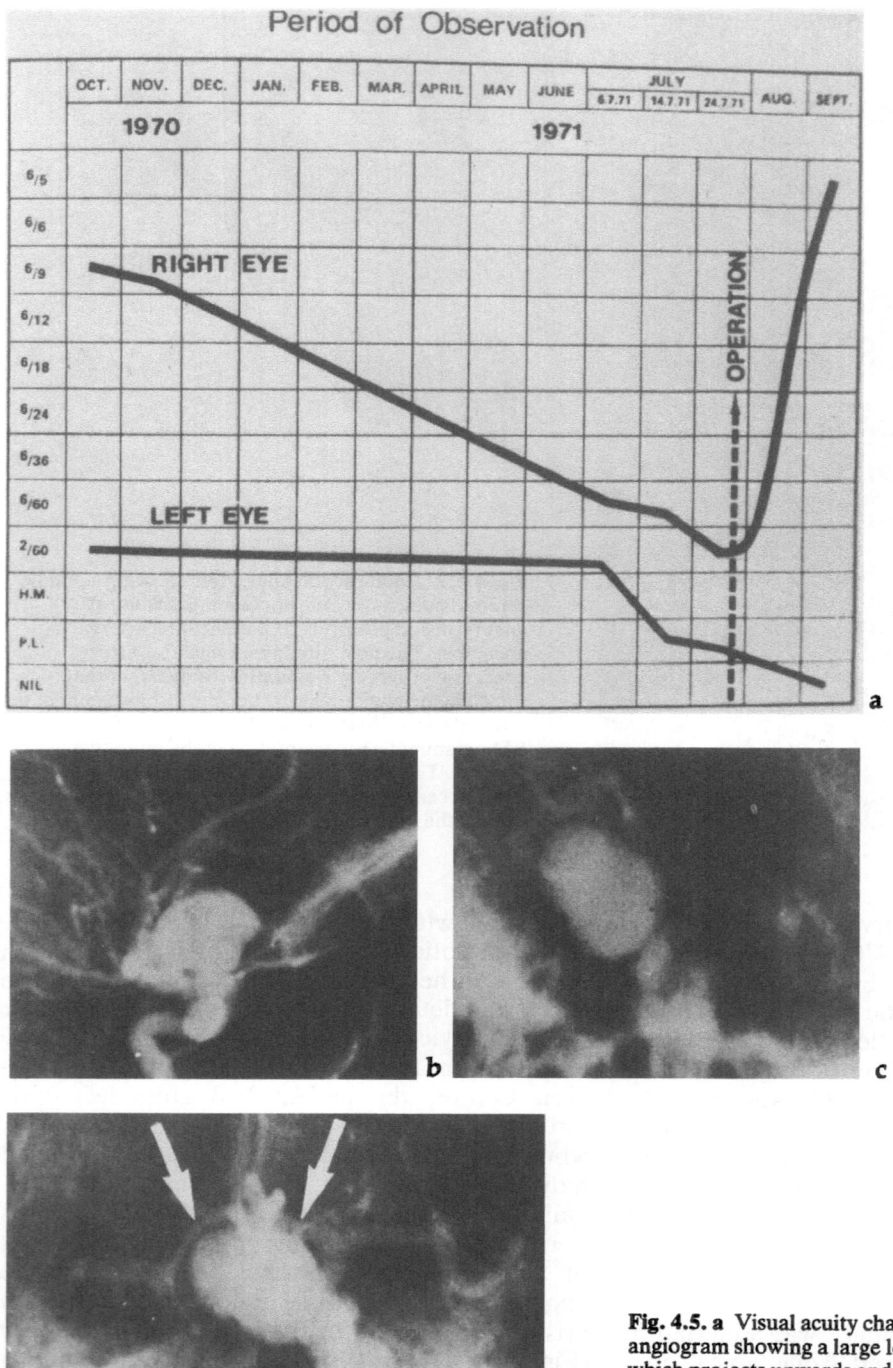

Fig. 4.5. a Visual acuity chart of patient N. L. **b, c** Left carotid angiogram showing a large left carotid ophthalmic aneurysm, which projects upwards and medially into the suprasellar region. **d** Right carotid compression showing good cross-flow and elevation of the anterior part of the circle of Willis.

T. A., an 18-year-old female, was admitted to a peripheral hospital because she had experienced frequent fainting spells three to four times per year for the preceding 2 years. She had also suffered from right frontal headaches every 2–3 weeks, associated with nausea and vomiting, and the severity of the headaches had increased. Two weeks prior to admission she suffered a generalised seizure, with a recurrence whilst in hospital. Following the second seizure she completely lost the vision in her right eye. On emergency admission to the neurosurgical unit she was conscious, there was no evidence of neck stiffness, and Kernig's sign was negative. She had total loss of vision in the right eye, although the fundus was normal. The corneal reflex was diminished on the right, but otherwise neurological examination was unremarkable. A diagnosis of pituitary apoplexy was made, but plain X-ray of the skull and CT scan did not reveal any abnormality. Lumbar CSF was also normal. However, an angiogram revealed two aneurysms of the right internal carotid artery, one in the intracavernous portion, and the other at the carotid ophthalmic junction (Fig. 4.6). The latter was successfully clipped, and at surgery it was found to be buried within the optic nerve, with no evidence of SAH. Four days postoperatively the patient began to regain vision in the right eye, and at discharge 10 days later it was normal (6/6).

Visual field defects can also occur from destruction of the optic radiation in the temporal or occipital lobes due to haematoma from rupture of an aneurysm or arteriovenous malformation.

A further cause of visual impairment is intraocular haemorrhage or secondary optic atrophy due to papilloedema. These are discussed later.

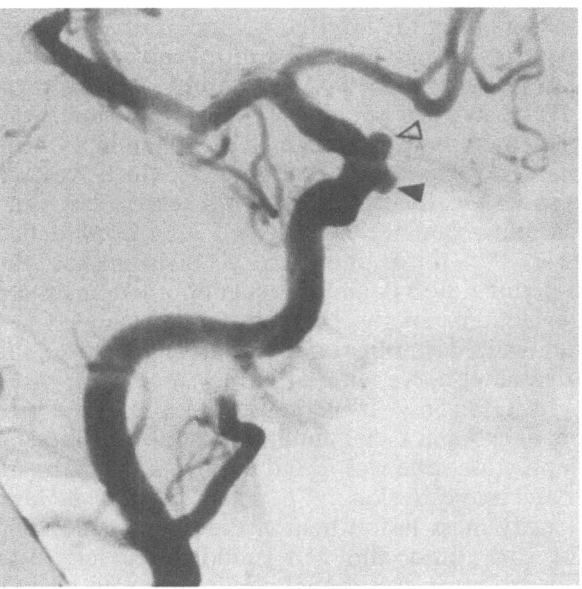

Fig. 4.6. Right carotid angiogram showing carotid ophthalmic aneurysm which projects upwards and medially (*open arrowhead*) and an intracavernous aneurysm (*black arrowhead*) which projects downwards and medially.

Ocular Haemorrhage. The presence of subhyaloid haemorrhages is pathognomonic of SAH. They are described as prominent, brick-red swellings around the optic disc, and are believed to be caused by rapid venous engorgement. Following SAH, the cerebrospinal fluid, or blood, may be forced along the optic nerve sheath with sufficient force to transiently occlude the central retinal vein as it traverses along the optic nerve, whilst at the same time there is a significant rise in the retinal artery pressure, reflecting the generalised hypertension that occurs with raised intracranial pressure. These changes result in rupture of the capillaries, causing subhyaloid haemorrhages (Manschot 1954). Manschot found intraocular haemorrhages in 20% of 225 patients studied.

Intraocular haemorrhages are usually asymptomatic and do not interfere with visual acuity unless the haemorrhage encroaches upon the macula region. Late impairment of vision may occur when the subhyaloid haemorrhage has ruptured into the vitreous space with subsequent scar formation and retinal detachment (Carruthers and Black 1976). Shaw et al. (1977) found vitreous haemorrhages in 2.6% of patients with SAH and the mortality in these patients was above average.

Papilloedema. Swelling of the optic disc in cases of SAH is well known, and yet, considering the fact that the intracranial pressure is often raised, the incidence of papilloedema is surprisingly low. The fact that its occurrence is rare is thought to be due to compression of the optic nerve sheath by the sudden rise in intracranial pressure, which prevents transmission of the intracranial pressure into the optic disc (Griffith et al. 1938).

Poppen (1948) described eight patients with papilloedema, while reviewing 114 with acute SAH. Richardson and Hyland (1941) thought that early papilloedema was due either to a profuse and rapid SAH or to a less severe haemorrhage close to the optic nerves. Walton (1956) attributed its early appearance to the direct compression of the venous return from the retina by a diffusion of blood into the optic nerve sheath. In the present series, the incidence of papilloedema was 10% and it was more commonly encountered in patients with anterior communicating artery aneurysms than in patients with aneurysms in other locations. ($P < 0.01$). In an analysis of 225 patients, Manschot (1954) found papilloedema in 15%. The late appearance of papilloedema should alert one to the presence of complications, such as hydrocephalus, a space-occupying haematoma or cerebral oedema.

Oculomotor Nerve

This is the most commonly involved cranial nerve in SAH. Hyland and Barnett (1954) described the following possible modes of involvement:

1. Direct compression of the nerve by an aneurysm, either during enlargement or at the time of rupture.
2. A midbrain haemorrhage secondary to raised intracranial pressure.
3. Kinking and compression of the contralateral third nerve through the displacement of the posterior cerebral artery (resulting from venous displacement).
4. Compression of the nerve against the edge of the tentorium (reflecting uncal herniation).
5. Stretching and compression of the brain stem by a sudden intracerebral or intraventricular haemorrhage.

We have seen a young man of 32 years with an SAH and a third nerve palsy resulting from a chordoma. The pathogenesis of his third nerve palsy was a localised haematoma within the temporal lobe causing compression of the third nerve at the tentorial hiatus.

The commonest mechanism of involvement is direct compression of the third nerve by a rupturing or enlarging aneurysm. In an analysis of 42 patients with aneurysmal third nerve palsy in our centre, Raja (1972) found a posterior communicating artery aneurysm in 37, an internal carotid, intracavernous aneurysm in four and a carotid bifurcation aneurysm in one. In 22 of the 42 patients third nerve palsy presented in the absence of clinically overt SAH.

As the pupilloconstrictor fibres and the fibres to the levator palprebrae superioris lie superficially beneath the epineurium (Kerr and Hollowell 1964), third nerve palsy in the presence of an aneurysm is usually associated with a dilated pupil and ptosis. Pupillary sparing was reported by Kasoff and Kelly (1975), and they suggested that this was due to a variability in the location of the parasympathetic fibres around the optic nerve. Soni (1974) found that the return of third nerve function follows a somewhat constant course. The levator palprebrae superioris improves first, and subsequently the medial and inferior recti. The superior rectus shows the least recovery of function. Persistent abnormalities of the pupil were also common in his patients. Third nerve function does not recover completely if the palsy is present for more than 10 days. Aberrant regeneration

may lead to abnormal movements of the eyelids and globe, the commonest being abduction of the eye on attempted elevation.

Bilateral third nerve palsy can occur with haemorrhage around the quadrigeminal plate or from a large basilar artery aneurysm. We have not seen a case of third nerve palsy due to an aneurysm of the posterior circulation, though such cases were described by Timberlake and Kubik (1952).

Trochlear Nerve

The trochlear nerve is rarely involved in SAH because of its circuitous course away from the circle of Willis. Dysfunction has been reported as an isolated finding in a small number of cases (Dandy 1944). In the region of the superior orbital fissure it is closely approximated to the internal carotid artery, as are the third and sixth nerves, and in this situation a large aneurysm can result in complete ophthalmoplegia. Under such circumstances detecting a fourth nerve palsy can be difficult.

Trigeminal Nerve

Involvement of the trigeminal nerve occurs as an isolated symptom with facial pain and objective sensory loss, including a depressed corneal reflex. A more common presentation is periodic neuralgic pain from an unruptured infraclinoid aneurysm on the internal carotid artery. Involvement of the nerve by an arteriovenous aneurysm has been described by Eisenbrey and Hegarty (1956). We have seen a 27-year-old woman who presented with paroxysms of trigeminal facial pain, resembling tic douloureux, which was unresponsive to treatment with carbamazepine. Careful examination revealed a sensory deficit over the third and second divisions of the trigeminal nerve, and investigation demonstrated an angioma in the cerebellopontine angle. The following case illustrates the involvement of the trigeminal nerve with an intracranial aneurysm.

M. G., a 56-year-old housewife, presented with headache, left facial numbness, double vision and depression. She was found to have a left fifth and sixth nerve lesion. CT scan showed a high density mass lesion behind the clivus, extending forwards into the left middle cranial fossa (Fig. 4.7a). Carotid angiography showed a small aneurysm arising from the left internal carotid artery at the origin of the posterior communicating artery (Fig. 4.7b). Vertebral angiography showed a large space-occupying lesion (Fig. 4.7c)

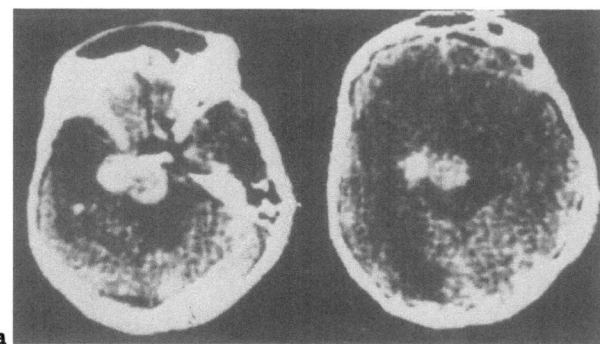

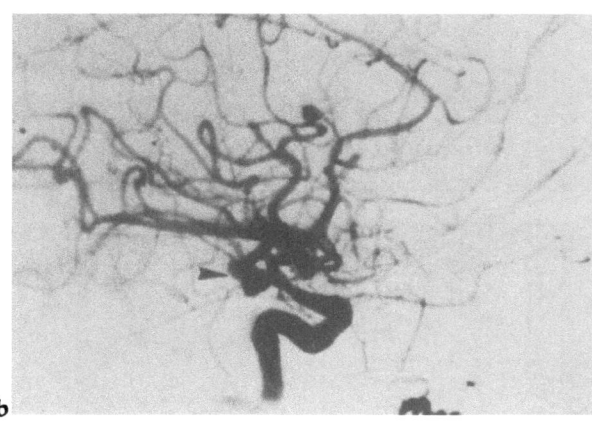

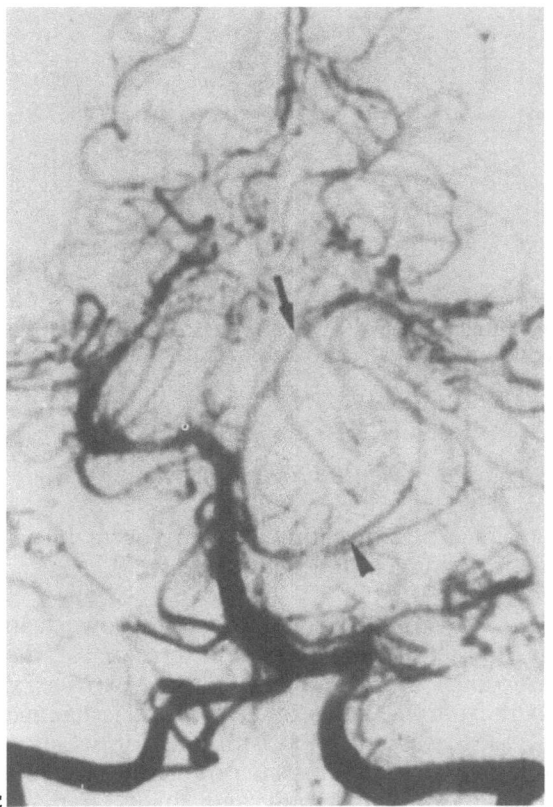

Fig. 4.7. **a** Contrast-enhanced CT scan showing a high density mass behind the dorsum sellae and upper clivus which extends forwards into the middle cranial fossa on the left side. **b** Left carotid angiogram showing a bilocular posterior communicating artery aneurysm. **c** A vertebral angiogram showing elevation of the posterior cerebral artery (*arrow*) and depression of the superior cerebellar arteries (*arrowhead*). There is some displacement of the basilar artery to the right side.

and at operation a giant, mainly thrombosed aneurysm with a small lumen was found. After clipping the aneurysm the clot within the sac was removed. The patient made a good recovery.

Abducent Nerve

Owing to its position, length and course, the abducent nerve is the most common cranial nerve affected by raised intracranial pressure, and it is often a false localising sign. Its occurrence in SAH, however, is infrequent. Compression of the abducent nerve in isolation or in combination with other cranial nerves by large aneurysms is well known. An isolated sixth nerve palsy commonly occurs from an unruptured infraclinoid aneurysm. Bilateral involvement by a large basilar aneurysm has also been reported (Dandy 1944). Crevits et al. (1975) described a case of a right lateral gaze palsy with an internuclear ophthalmoplegia following SAH. At autopsy there was a small infarct involving the pontine radicular formation, the tectospinal tract and the ventral part of the right median longitudinal fasciculus.

Nystagmus has rarely been reported (Richardson and Hyland 1941) and should alert one to the possibility of a vascular lesion in the posterior cranial fossa, including a cerebellar haemangioblastoma or an angioma of the brain stem. Ocular bobbing is a rare disorder characterised by abrupt, spontaneous conjugate downward deviation of the eyes, with a slow return to the mid position (Fisher 1964; Daroff and Waldman 1965). It is seen with destructive lesions of the pontine tegmentum, and hence is helpful in localisation of the lesion, although Bosch et al. (1975) dispute this. Sherman and Salmon (1977) described such a case with a superior cerebellar artery aneurysm.

Facial Nerve

Upper motor neurone facial weakness is seen in complicated SAH where there is hemispheric damage. This is often associated with a hemiparesis. Compression of the facial nerve by a superior cerebellar artery aneurysm has been reported by Fearnsides (1916) and Walton (1956). Unilateral loss of taste sensation, with compression of the superficial petrosal nerve by a large infraclinoid aneurysm, has also been described (Walton 1956).

Acoustic Nerve

Sensations such as buzzing, ringing or vertigo are often described by patients with SAH as part of their presenting symptoms. They are due to irritation of the central connections of the eighth nerve by the sudden rise of intracranial pressure. More rarely, disturbances of the temporal lobes by a severe haemorrhage can affect function of the auditory area. In our series 44 patients (9%) complained of dizziness at the time of ictus. The eighth nerve can also be directly compressed by an aneurysm of the superior cerebellar artery, the internal auditory artery or the basilar artery (Hori et al. 1971).

Glossopharyngeal, Vagus, Accessory and Hypoglossal Nerves

These four lower cranial nerves lie close together in the posterior fossa in relation to the posterior inferior cerebellar artery. Direct involvement of them by an aneurysm in this region is, however, uncommon. Poppen (1948) described involvement of the lower five cranial nerves by a large basilar aneurysm. In one case he attributed glossopharyngeal neuralgia to an infraclinoid aneurysm. Guta et al. (1979) reported a case of a giant internal carotid artery aneurysm in the carotid canal with erosion of the petrous temporal bone and resultant sixth, seventh, eighth, ninth and tenth cranial nerve palsies in an 8-year-old. We have seen a patient recently with a similar presentation.

   T. S., a 67-year-old medical practitioner, presented in August, 1982, with progressive difficulty in swallowing for 18 months. He was found to have paralysis of the right eighth, ninth and tenth cranial nerves. CT scan showed a space-occupying lesion in the posterior cranial fossa. Vertebral angiography demonstrated a giant right vertebrobasilar aneurysm (Fig. 4.8). It is interesting that 10 years previously he had been treated for "meningitis". Presumably he suffered an unrecognised SAH from the aneurysm at that time.

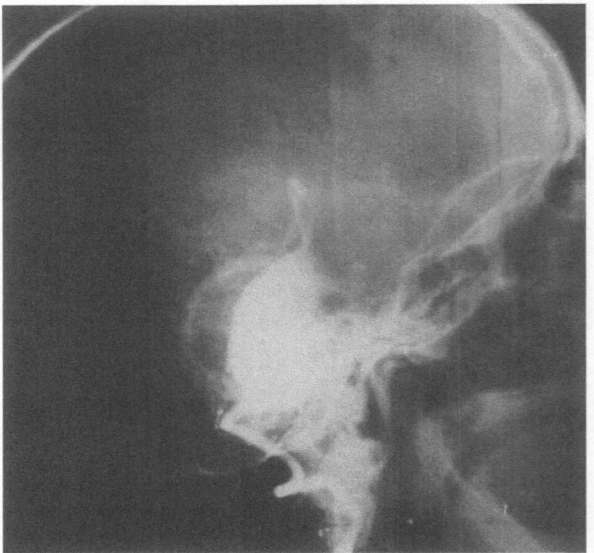

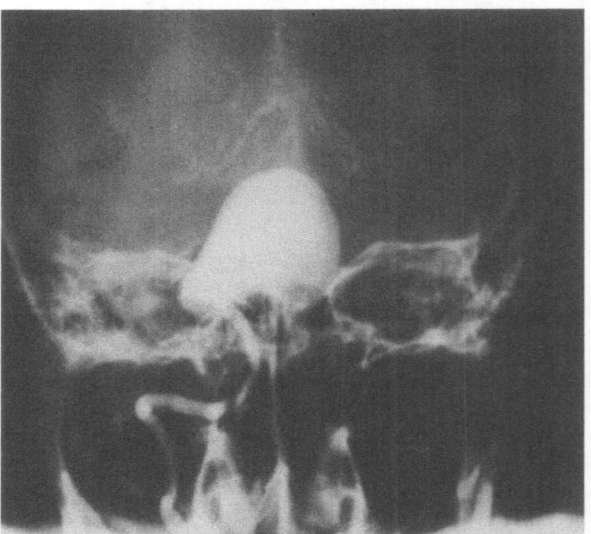

Fig. 4.8. Right vertebral angiogram (a lateral and b Townes projection) showing a giant vertebrobasilar aneurysm.

Disturbance of Motor Function

Disturbance of motor function may occur in patients presenting with a major SAH.

Power. A variable degree of loss of power can occur in the following ways: extension of the haemorrhage into the white matter, extra-axial pressure from the haematoma, cerebral ischaemia from vasospasm, thrombosis of a major vessel, a giant unruptured aneurysm producing a space-occupying lesion or emboli, and, finally, damage to the spinal motor roots by the spread of blood throughout the subarachnoid space. The type of weakness, either partial or complete, depends upon the location of the lesion. Unilateral pathology will produce contralateral weakness, and a paraparesis can be seen with anterior communicating or pericallosal aneurysms. Collections of blood in the posterior fossa or upper cervical canal may produce bilateral loss of power from pressure on the pyramidal tracts. A variable degree of motor weakness was noted in 83 patients (21%) in our series. As would be expected, limb weakness was more common in patients with rupture of middle cerebral artery aneurysm ($P < 0.01$).

Tone. Alterations in tone, like power, reflect the clinical circumstances. In a severe SAH the patient may be flaccid throughout but usually decerebrate posturing occurs, due to pressure on the brain stem with massive intracerebral or intraventricular haemorrhage.

Wasting. Wasting of the muscles may be seen after prolonged illness or due to chemical polyradiculopathy (produced by blood in the subarachnoid space). We have seen three such cases of extreme wasting of limb muscles following SAH.

Coordination. This is often impossible to examine in seriously ill patients. Vascular lesions in the posterior fossa can give rise to a cerebellar type of incoordination.

Reflex Activity. With a catastrophic bleed more reflex activity is abolished but in a minor haemorrhage there may be no abnormality at all. Reflex changes are variable. The presence of an extensor plantar response is not only of localising value but also indicates significant disturbance of the neuraxis, which influences the timing of surgical intervention. In 145 patients (29%) in our series there was an extensor plantar response.

Disturbance of Sensory Function

Tingling, numbness and peculiar sensation in the limbs have occasionally been described by patients as premonitory or initial symptoms. Less than 5% of our patients experienced these symptoms at the onset of SAH. Detailed testing in the acute stage of SAH, when patients are often obtunded or uncooperative, is unreliable and unnecessary. In an alert, cooperative patient

cortical sensory loss indicates parietal lobe dysfunction, whilst a sensory radiculopathy from irritation of the spinal nerve roots may give rise to a disc-like syndrome.

Signs of Meningeal or Cerebral Irritation

Cerebral irritation often follows a major haemorrhage, and is considered to be due to irritation of the sensory dural nerves and congestion of the pia-arachnoid. The patient becomes irritable, confused, disorientated and uncooperative.

Neck stiffness is one of the most frequent and important diagnostic signs of SAH (86% in our series). Although it may occur in other diseases of the meninges, the presence of this sign in a patient with abrupt onset of headache is virtually pathognomonic of SAH. In this series it was more common in patients with anterior communicating artery aneurysm than in those with middle cerebral or internal carotid artery aneurysms ($P < 0.025$). In its extreme form the head may become opisthotonic (Fig. 4.9). Neck stiffness is caused by excitation of the cervical sensory nerve roots in the subarachnoid space. The absence of neck stiffness may be seen under the following circumstances:

1. Catastrophic haemorrhage: The severity of the haemorrhage abolishes all reflex activity in the muscles of the neck, as it does in other parts of the body.
2. Very minor haemorrhage: Inflammation of the meninges may not be severe enough to cause sufficient irritation to produce neck stiffness.

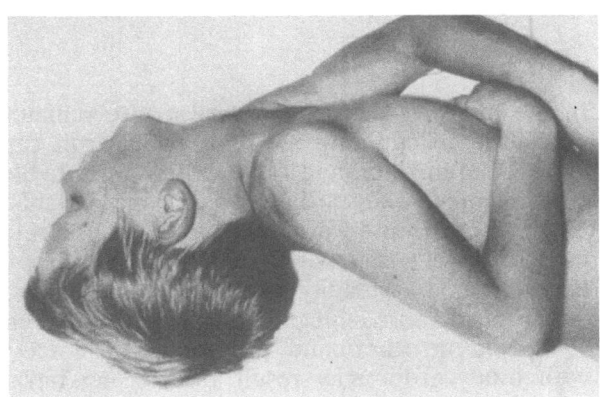

Fig. 4.9. Patient with opisthotonus.

3. Sudden enlargement of an aneurysm or a localised haematoma may preclude the spread of blood into the cervical region. Early on in an SAH, examination may not reveal neck stiffness (14% of the current series) as the blood has not had time to spread to the cervical meninges.

4. In spinal SAH below the level of the cervical region, neck rigidity may be absent.

Disturbance of Autonomic Activity and Visceral Function

Disorders of autonomic activity and visceral function are frequent associates of SAH. In their minor form they are due to meningeal irritation. Severe disturbances are associated with lesions in the diencephalic area of the floor of the third ventricle. This area may be disturbed by direct extension of the haemorrhage or by vasospastic ischaemia of the hypothalamus. Careful monitoring of these vital functions can indicate deterioration or the development of complications in SAH.

Temperature

In most cases there is a rise in temperature (to 38°–39°C), generally on the second or third day, but it returns to normal within a few days. A secondary rise in temperature may indicate fresh bleeding (Dekaban and McEachern 1952). A temperature above 39°C usually indicates extension of the haemorrhage within the cerebrum or ventricular system. An abnormally high temperature with failure of the central regulatory mechanism is seen in the moribund patient and signals impending demise.

Pulse

In the majority of cases the pulse rate remains within the normal range. A slight tachycardia can result from anxiety, and vagal irritation probably explains mild bradycardia seen in some patients. However, extreme variations in the pulse rate may indicate a significant pathological process; for example, a steadily rising pulse may occur with central neurogenic pulmonary oedema (Weir 1978). On the other hand, progressive drowsiness with bradycardia may result from rising intracranial pressure, which needs to be corrected by appropriate treatment.

Respiration

Disturbances of the respiratory rate are frequently noticed in patients with severe SAH (Weir 1978). Pulmonary oedema after massive SAH may develop occasionally. Maire and Patton (1956) described an "oedemagenic centre" in the rostral hypothalamus 1–2 mm caudal to the preoptic nucleus. Lesions in this region produce pulmonary oedema by overloading the pulmonary circulation via splanchnic-mediated constriction of the visceral venous reservoir. Ducker and Simmons (1968) were of the view that rising intracranial pressure not only increases the diastolic pressure but also the pulmonary venous and arterial pressure, the sequence of physiological events being the elevation of intracranial pressure with subsequent systemic vasoconstriction and systemic arterial hypertension. The latter leads to an increase in the left atrial pressure, whilst the former results in a shift in the blood from the systemic to the pulmonary circulation. Both factors, combined with the raised pulmonary vasoconstriction, result in increased pulmonary venous pressure above oncotic pressure, with the resultant pulmonary oedema.

Blood Pressure

A transitory rise in blood pressure is a frequent finding at the onset of SAH. It is considered to be a physiological response to raised intracranial pressure in order to maintain cerebral perfusion. However, it is essential to enquire about the patient's previous blood pressure and to search for evidence of pre-existing hypertension, such as left ventricular hypertrophy, retinal vascular changes or renal impairment. In the absence of such findings one must be cautious about diagnosing hypertensive SAH, even if the blood pressure is significantly raised. Excessive hypertension with a systolic blood pressure above 250 mmHg in critically ill patients often denotes a fatal outcome.

Vomiting

This is a common manifestation with SAH. Excessive vomiting and haematemesis can occur with hypothalamic disturbances. Alteration of the gastric mucosa has been documented in hypothalamic lesions with subsequent haematemesis.

Sweating

Profuse sweating in patients with SAH is seen in the moribund state in which central failure of the autonomic centre has occurred.

Other Autonomic and Endocrine Disturbances

Hyperaemia of the face, urticaria and insomnia can be features of autonomic dysfunction. Gradual involvement of the sella or pituitary stalk by a slowly enlarging aneurysm can give rise to endocrine hypofunction. Hoff et al. (1961) reported three cases with evidence of hypopituitarism and suggested that interference of the blood supply to the hypothalamus was the underlying cause.

Warning Signs of Impending Subarachnoid Haemorrhage

Warning signs have been reported in retrospective analysis to occur in 48.2% of patients (Okawara 1973). Some of these are useful, whilst others are so totally non-specific to be of no value at all. Such warning signs can be discussed along the following lines:

1. Pathogenesis
2. Non-specific and non-neurological
3. Non-specific and neurological
4. Specific and neurological
5. Warning signs specific to the nature and location of the lesion

Pathogenesis

The majority of symptoms are a result of either recurrent small leakages from or direct enlargement of the aneurysm, and the symptoms vary, depending upon the size of the aneurysm (Richardson and Hyland 1941). Confirmation of recurrent small leaks can be seen at surgery in patients not considered to have a ruptured aneurysm, when haemosiderin or a small haematoma may be observed in relation to the aneurysm.

Okawara (1973) suggested three possible aetiological mechanisms, which, however, are not universally accepted:

1. Vascular factors—in which small haemorrhages into the wall of the aneurysm cause referred pain by stimulating nerve endings, both mechanically and chemically.
2. Minor leakages of blood into the subarachnoid space.
3. Ischaemic lesions due to arterial spasm or small local haematomas. Ischaemia is also felt by others (Mullen et al. 1964) to result from small thromboembolic clots which have formed in the aneurysm.

Non-specific and Non-neurological

Symptoms such as neck pain, nausea, back pain, lethargy, diarrhoea, insomnia, depression and a feverish feeling have been recorded (Okawara 1973) but are clearly so non-specific as to be of no value as warning signs.

Non-specific and Neurological

Dizziness, visual hallucinations, photophobia and motor or sensory impairment have also been noted (Okawara 1973; Waga et al. 1973). Again, these symptoms are unlikely to lead to an earlier diagnosis of impending SAH. A prior history of significant headache occurred in 19.4% of patients in the present series.

Specific and Neurological

The sudden onset of a painful third nerve palsy with dilatation of the pupil (Fig. 4.10) is perhaps the most clear-cut example of an early warning sign. Although there are many causes of a third nerve palsy, a valuable clinical aphorism is that "a painful third nerve palsy with pupillary dilatation is due to an aneurysm until proven otherwise".

The sudden onset of severe non-paroxysmal facial pain should also alert one to the possibility of an aneurysm of the internal carotid artery, particularly if a trigeminal sensory deficit can be demonstrated. Absence of the latter finding certainly does not exclude an underlying aneurysm. The most frequently ignored warning sign is the abrupt onset of a severe explosive headache, with or without loss of consciousness. Prompt referral

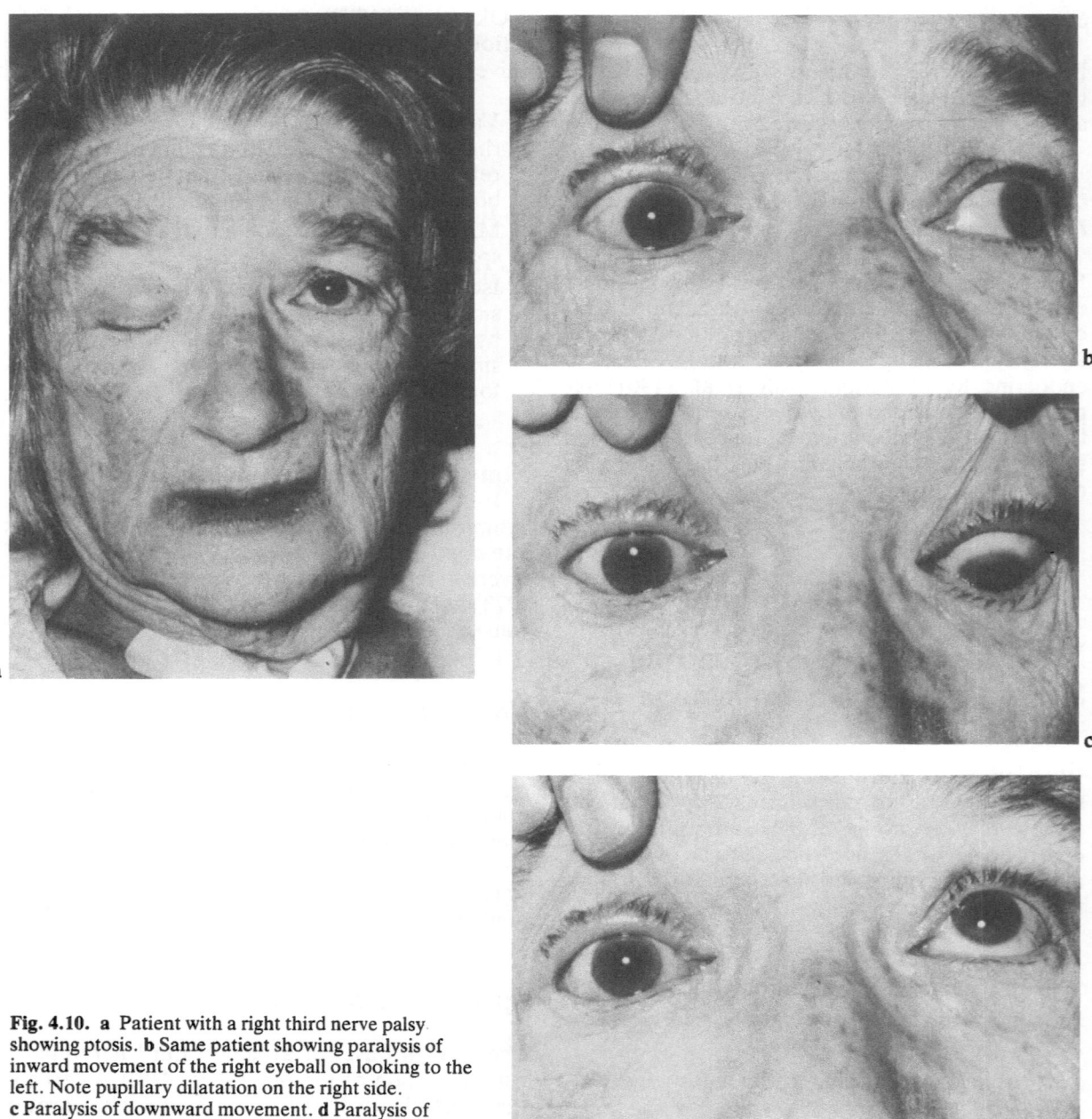

Fig. 4.10. a Patient with a right third nerve palsy showing ptosis. **b** Same patient showing paralysis of inward movement of the right eyeball on looking to the left. Note pupillary dilatation on the right side. **c** Paralysis of downward movement. **d** Paralysis of upward movement.

at this stage, and a simple lumbar puncture, will quickly establish true cases of SAH. Gillingham (1958) stressed the importance of this symptom.

Visual field defects can be a premonitory sign of impending SAH (Walsh 1964). Peiris and Russell (1980) have recently reviewed 19 patients who presented with visual field loss (often of a fluctuating nature) due to a large intracranial carotid aneurysm. They observed that carotid ophthalmic aneurysms mostly caused pure unilateral visual loss consistent with optic nerve compression. A lateral chiasmal syndrome was seen with supraclinoid aneurysms, and anterior communicating artery aneurysms caused asymmetric compression of one or both nerves. Periorbital pain or frontal headache was common. There was no discussion of the risk of SAH in this group.

Warning Signs Specific to the Nature and Location of the Lesion

Specific warning signs may also be useful for detecting the site and underlying nature of the causative lesion in a patient with SAH (Table 4.5). Such examples include epilepsy (Sengupta et al. 1978), a third nerve palsy and a transient ischaemic attack (TIA). This latter presentation is illustrated by the following example:

A 35-year-old man was admitted following sudden onset of severe headache, nausea and vomiting accompanied by neck stiffness. Lumbar puneture confirmed SAH, and carotid angiography demonstrated an anterior communicating artery aneurysm which was subsequently clipped. Two weeks prior to his admission he had had transient left leg weakness, without any associated symptoms.

Focal warning signs or symptoms are of particular value in detecting the source of haemorrhage in patients wth multiple lesions (Sengupta and Lassman 1974).

In patients with an arteriovenous malformation the symptoms of focal or generalised epilepsy and transient ischaemic attacks have been reported to precede subsequent SAH (Walton 1956). In an analysis of 100 cases of anterior communicating artery aneurysms, Sengupta (1977) found various signs of a minor leak before a major haemorrhage in 25% of cases. Patients with loss of consciousness were usually referred to hospital promptly, whilst those presenting with other symptoms were treated at home, some even being considered hysterical or depressive. The consequences of

ignoring warning signs is vividly illustrated by the following two cases:

A. C., a 16-year-old schoolgirl, complained of sudden headache. Her family doctor treated her as a case of migraine. She continued to complain of headache and was then thought to be suffering from depression. One month after her original complaint, she was found unconscious in the toilet by her mother. On admission to hospital she was deeply comatose, with spontaneous decerebrate posturing and bilaterally fixed dilated pupils. An emergency CT scan showed a massive intraventricular haemorrhage (Fig. 4.11a), and she died a few hours later. At postmortem a ruptured carotid bifurcation aneurysm was found (Fig. 4.11b).

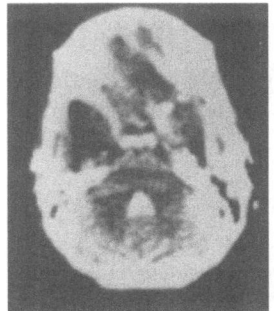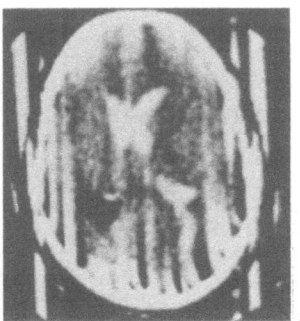

a

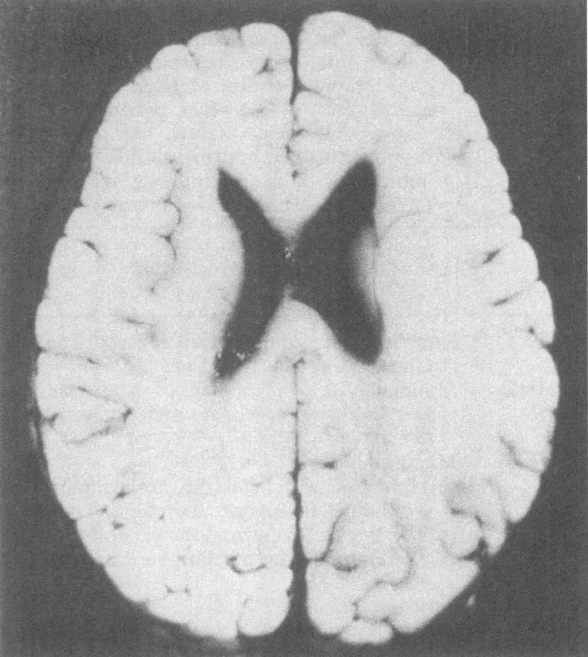

b

Fig. 4.11. a CT scan showing extensive blood in both lateral ventricles and in the fourth ventricle. **b** The same case as in **a**. Section through the brain showing extensive intraventricular haematoma which is similar in appearance to the CT scan.

Table 4.5. The relationship between the site of aneurysm and focal disturbance

Site of aneurysm	Focal disturbance
Anterior communicating artery	Sensory motor disturbance in lower limbs
	Visual field defects
	Endocrine dysfunction
	Localised frontal headache or pain
Internal carotid artery	Localised facial pain
	Impaired visual acuity
	Visual field defect
	Oculomotor paresis
Middle cerebellar artery	Dysphasia
	Focal arm weakness or numbness
	Visual hallucinations
Basilar bifurcation	Dizziness (vertigo)
	Oculomotor paresis[a]

[a] This has not been seen by the author but has been reported by Dandy (1944).

P. R., a 24-year-old army officer, suddenly developed headache while on leave at home. His family doctor treated him with analgesics, but, as he continued to complain of headaches, the doctor thought he was malingering in order to delay his return to camp. A few weeks after his original complaint, he was found unconscious on the floor of his bedroom. On admission to hospital he was unresponsive, with bilateral papilloedema. An external ventricular drain revealed haemorrhage into the ventricle. The patient died a few days later. Postmortem was refused.

Grading of Severity of Subarachnoid Haemorrhage

Complete information regarding the patient's condition from the onset of the ictus to the time of

Table 4.6. Classification of patients according to Botterell et al. (1956)

Grade 1	A patient who is conscious with or without signs of blood in the subarachnoid space
Grade 2	A drowsy patient without significant neurological deficit
Grade 3	A drowsy patient with a neurological deficit and probably an intracerebral haematoma
Grade 4	A patient with a major neurological deficit and deteriorating because of large intracerebral haematoma, or an older patient with less severe neurological deficit, but pre-existing degenerative cerebral or vascular disease
Grade 5	A moribund, or near moribund, patient with failing vital centres and extensor rigidity

Table 4.7. Classification of patients according to Nishioka (1966)

Grade 1	Symptom-free, completely recovered from the effects of last haemorrhage
Grade 2	Minimally ill, complaining of headache, but alert and responsive; no major neurological deficit
Grade 3	Moderately ill (a) Lethargic with headache, neck stiffness, but without hemispheric neurological deficit (b) Alert, recovered from the general effects of SAH, but having a hemispheric neurological deficit
Grade 4	Seriously ill (a) Severely obtunded without major neurological deficit (b) Lethargic, with hemispheric deficit (hemiparesis, dysphasia, mental confusion)
Grade 5	Moribund, decerebrate or unresponsive to all stimuli

admission and the subsequent course has an important bearing on the final outcome. As mentioned before, a history of major illness in the past influences the management. Taking these facts into consideration, the clinical condition of patients has been classified into various grades (Botterell et al. 1956; Nishioka 1966; Hunt and Hess 1968; Hunt and Kosnik 1974; Nibbelink et al. 1977). These grading systems also serve as

Table 4.8. Classification of patients according to Hunt and Hess (1968)

Grade 1	Asymptomatic or minimal headache and slight nuchal rigidity
Grade 2	Moderate severe headache, nuchal rigidity, no neurological deficit other than cranial nerve palsy
Grade 3	Drowsiness, confusion or mild focal deficit
Grade 4	Stupor, moderate to severe hemiparesis, possibly early decerebrate rigidity, and vegetative disturbances
Grade 5	Deep coma, decerebrate ridigity, moribund appearance

Table 4.9. Classification of patients according to Hunt and Kosnik (1974)

Grade 0	Unruptured aneurysm
Grade 1	Asymptomatic or minimal headache and slight nuchal rigidity
Grade 1a	No acute meningeal or brain reaction, but fixed neurological deficit
Grade 2	Moderate to severe headache, nuchal rigidity, no neurological deficit other than cranial nerve palsy
Grade 3	Drowsiness, confusion or mild focal deficit
Grade 4	Stupor, moderate to severe hemiparesis, possibly early decerebrate rigidity, and vegetative disturbances
Grade 5	Deep coma, decerebrate rigidity, moribund appearance

N.B. Serious systemic disease, such as hypertension, diabetes, severe atherosclerosis or chronic pulmonary disease, or severe intracranial arterial spasm, seen on arteriography, results in placement of the patient in the next less favourable category. This also applies to the classification described by Hunt and Hess (1968).

Table 4.10. Classification of patients according to Nibbelink et al. (1977)

Grade 1	Symptom-free
Grade 2	Minor symptoms, headache, meningeal irritation, diplopia
Grade 3	Major neurological deficit, but fully responsive
Grade 4	Impaired state of alertness, but capable of predictive or other adapted responses to noxious stimuli
Grade 5	Poorly responsive but with stable vital signs
Grade 6	No response to address or shaking, non-adaptive response to noxious stimuli and progressive instability of vital signs

a yardstick to assess the result of a particular method of management in a group of patients. There may, however, be observer variability in assigning the patient to a particular grade (Lindsay et al. 1980). One should also bear in mind the fluctuation of grades often seen in these patients. We use the Hunt and Hess (1968) classification in our analysis. However, systemic illness was not taken into consideration for grading the patients. Tables 4.6–4.10 describe the criteria used in different grading systems.

References

Adams HP Jr, Jergenson DD, Kassell NF, Sahs AL (1980) Pitfalls in the recognition of SAH. JAMA 244:794–796

Barnett HJM (1968) Some clinical features of intracranial aneurysms. Clin Neurosurg 16:43–72

Bird AC, Nolan B, Gargano FP, David NJ (1970) Unruptured aneurysms of the supraclinoid carotid artery. A treatable cause of blindness. Neurology 20:445–454

Bosch EP, Kennedy SS, Aschenbrener CA (1975) Ocular bobbing. The myth of its localising value. Neurology 25:949–953

Botterell WM, Lougheed WM, Scott JW, Vandewater SL (1956) Hypothermia and interruption of the carotid and vertebral circulation in the surgical management of intracranial aneurysms. J Neurosurg 13:1–42

Carruthers J, Black RK (1976) Vitrectomy in SAH. Br Med J II: 404

Collier J (1922) Spontaneous SAH. In: Price FW (ed) A text book of the practice of medicine. Oxford University Press, London, p 1351

Crevits L, Reuck JD, Edcken VH (1975) Paralytic pontine exotropia in subarachnoid haemorrhage. A clinicopathological correlation. Clin Neurol Neurosurg 78 (4): 269–276

Crompton MR (1962) Intracerebral haematoma complicating ruptured cerebral berry aneurysm. J Neurol Neurosurg Psychiatry, 25:378–386

Dandy WE (1944) I.C. arterial aneurysms. Comstock, Ithaca, New York

Daroff RB, Waldman AL (1965) Ocular bobbing. J Neurol Neurosurg Psychiatry 28:375–377

Dekaban A, McEachern D (1952) Subarachnoid haemorrhage, intracerebral haemorrhage and intracranial aneurysm. Arch Neurol Psychiatry 67:641–649

Ducker TB, Simmons RL (1968) Increased intracranial pressure and pulmonary oedema. Part 2. The haemodynamic response of dogs and monkeys to increased intracranial pressure. J Neurosurg 28:118–128

Eisenbrey A, Hegarty WM (1956) Trigeminal neuralgia and aneurysms of the cerebello-pontine angle. J Neurosurg 13:647–649

Falconer MA (1954) Surgical pathology of spontaneous intracranial haemorrhage due to aneurysm and A.V.M. Proc R Soc Med 47:693–700

Fearnsides EG (1916) Intracranial aneurysms. Brain 39:224–296

Fisher CM (1964) Ocular bobbing. Arch Neurol 11:543–546

Foltz EL, Ward AA Jr (1956) Communicating hydrocephalus from subarachnoid bleeding. J Neurosurg 13:546–566

Frankel K (1950) Relation of migraine to cerebral aneurysm. Arch Neurol Psychiatry 63:195–204

Gillingham FJ (1958) The management of ruptured intracranial aneurysms. Ann R Coll Surg Engl 23:89–117

Griffith JQ, Jeffers WA, Fry WE (1938) Papilloedema associated with subarachnoid haemorrhage. An experimental and clinical study. Arch Intern Med 61:880–890

Gupta SK, Gupta OP, Singh MM et al. (1979) Giant aneurysms of the internal carotid artery in the carotid canal. J Laryngol Otol 93:299–305

Gussen R (1976) Sudden deafness of vascular origin. A human temporal bone study. Ann Otol Rhinol Laryngol 85:94–100

Hall AJ (1929) Lecture on three cases of spontaneous subarachnoid haemorrhage with special reference to the occurrence of massive albuminuria and Korsakoff's syndrome. Br Med J I:1025–1028

Hall AJ (1932) Spontaneous subarachnoid haemorrhage. Lancet I:1135–1139

Heidrich R (1972) SAH In: Vinken PJ, Bruyn GW (eds) Vascular diseases of the nervous system. Part II: Handbook of Clinical Neurology. Elsevier, New York, pp 68–204

Hijdra A, Gijn JV (1982) Early death from rupture of an intracranial aneurysm. J Neurosurg 57:765–768

Hoff W, Hornabook RW, Marks V (1961) Hypopituitarism associated with intracranial aneurysm. Br Med J II:1190–1194

Holtzman RN, Parisier S (1979) Acute spontaneous otorrhagia resulting from a ruptured petrous carotid aneurysm. J Neurosurg 51:258–261

Hori T, Hirakawa K, Ishima B, Manaka S, Fukushima T, Shimizu N, Sato T (1971) Aneurysm in the internal auditory meatus. Case report. J Neurosurg 35:605–609

Hunt WE, Hess RM (1968) Surgical risk as related to time of intervention in the repair of intracranial aneurysm. J Neurosurg 28:14–19

Hunt WE, Kosnik EJ (1974) Timing and pre-operative care in intracranial aneurysm surgery. Congr Neurol Surg 21: 79–89

Hyland HH, Barnett HJM (1954) The pathogenesis of cranial nerve palsies associated with intracranial aneurysms. Proc R Soc Med 47:141–146

Jefferson G (1937) Compression of the chiasma, optic nerve and optic tract by intracranial aneurysms. Brain 60:444–497

Kasoff I, Kelly DL (1975) Pupillary sparing in oculomotor palsy from internal carotid aneurysm. J Neurosurg 42:713–717

Kassell NF, Drake CG (1982) Timing of aneurysm surgery. Neurosurgery 10:514–519

Kerr FWL, Hollowell OW (1964) Location of pupillomotor and accommodation fibres in the oculomotor nerve: Experimental observations on paralytic mydriasis. J Neurol Neurosurg Psychiatry 27:473–481

Lindquist G, Norlen G (1966) Korsakoff's syndrome after operation on ruptured aneurysm of anterior communicating artery. Acta Psychiatry Scand 42:24–34

Lindsay KW, Teasdale GM, Murray L, Knill-Jones R (1980) Observer variability in grading patients with subarachnoid haemorrhage. Proceedings of the Autumn Meeting of the Society of British Neurological Surgeons, pp 61–67

Locksley HB (1966) Natural history of subarachnoid haemorrhage, intracranial aneurysms and arteriovenous malformations. Based on 6368 cases in the Cooperative Study. J Neurosurg 25:219–242

Maire FW, Patton HD (1956) Neural structure involved in the genesis of "preoptic pulmonary odema". Gastric erosions and behaviour changes. Am J Physiol 184:345–350

Manschot WA (1954) Subarachnoid haemorrhage—intra-ocular symptoms and their pathogenesis. Am J Ophthalmol 38:501–505

Moore D, Budde RB, Hunter CR, Mayfield FH (1979) Massive epistaxis from aneurysm of the carotid artery. Surg Neurol 11:115–117

Morantz RA, Kirchner FR, Kishore P (1976) Aneurysms of the petrous portion of the internal carotid artery. Surg Neurol 6:313–318

Mori K, Miyazaki H, Ono H (1978) Aneurysm of the anterior inferior cerebellar artery at the internal auditory meatus. Surg Neurol 10:297–300

Nibbelink BW, Torner JC, Henderson WC (1977) Intracranial aneurysm and SAH. A report on a randomised treatment study. Stroke 8:200–218

Nishioka H (1966) Evaluation of the conservative management of ruptured intracranial aneurysm. J Neurosurg 25:574–592

Okawara S (1973) Warning signs prior to rupture of an intracranial aneurysm. J Neurosurg 38:575–580

Pakarinen S (1967) Incidence, aetiology and prognosis of primary subarachnoid haemorrhage. A study based on 589 cases diagnosed in a defined urban population during a defined period. Acta Neurol Scand 43 [Suppl 29]:1–28

Parizel G (1979) On the mechanism of sudden death with subarachnoid haemorrhage. J Neurol 220:71–76

Peiris JB, Russell RWR (1980) Giant aneurysms of the carotid system presenting as visual field defect. J Neurol Neurosurg Psychiatry 43:1053–1064

Poppen JL (1948) Diagnosis of intracranial aneurysms. Am J Surg 75:178–186

Raja IA (1972) Aneurysm induced third nerve palsy. J Neurosurg 36:548–551

Richardson JC, Hyland HH (1941) Intracranial aneurysm (a clinical and pathological study of subarachnoid and intracerebral haemorrhage caused by berry aneurysms). Medicine 20:1–88

Sahs AL, Perret GE, Locksley HB, Nishioka H (1966) Intracranial aneurysms and subarachnoid haemorrhage. A cooperative study. Lippincott, Philadelphia Toronto

Sengupta RP (1977) Anterior communicating aneurysms. M.Sc. Thesis, University of Newcastle upon Tyne

Sengupta RP, Hankinson J (1979) An unusual case of multiple intracranial aneurysms. Acta Neurochir 45:259–275

Sengupta RP, Lassman LP (1974) Identification of the source of bleeding in multiple intracranial aneurysms. Vasc Surg 8:177–183

Sengupta RP, Chiu JSP, Brierley H (1975) Quality of survival following direct surgery for anterior communicating artery aneurysms. J Neurosurg 43:58–64

Sengupta RP, Gryspeerdt GL, Hankinson J (1976) Carotico-ophthalmic aneurysms. J Neurol Neurosurg Psychiatry 39:837–853

Sengupta RP, Saunders M, Clarke PRR (1978) Unruptured intracranial aneurysms—an unusual source of epilepsy. Acta Neurochir 40:45–53

Shaw HE, Landers MB, Sydnor LF (1977) The significance of intraocular haemorrhages due to subarachnoid haemorrhage. Ann Ophthalmol 9:1403–1405

Sherman DG, Salmon JH (1977) Ocular bobbing with superior cerebellar artery aneurysm. A case report. J Neurosurg 47:596–598

Soni SR (1974) Aneurysm of the posterior communicating artery and oculomotor paresis. J Neurol Neurosurg Psychiatry 37:475–484

Strauss I, Globus JH, Ginsburg SW (1932) Spontaneous subarachnoid haemorrhage. Its relation to aneurysms of cerebral blood vessels. Arch Neurol Psychiatry 27:1080–1132

Suzuki J (1979) Cerebral aneurysm. Experience with 1000 directly operated cases. Neuron, Tokyo, pp 35–50

Takaku A, Fukawa O, Suzuki J (1979) A case of priapism with ruptured intracranial aneurysm. Suzuki J (ed) In: Cerebral aneurysm. Neuron, Tokyo, pp 132–135

Timberlake WH, Kubik CS (1952) Follow-up report with clinical and anatomical notes on 280 cases with subarachnoid haemorrhage. Trans Am Neurosurg Assoc 77:26–30

Waga S, Ohtsubok K, Handa H (1973) Warning signs in intracranial aneurysms. Surg Neurol 3:15–20

Walsh FB (1964) Visual field defects due to aneurysms at the circle of Willis. Arch Ophthalmol 71:15–27

Walton JN (1956) Subarachnoid haemorrhage. Livingstone, London Edinburgh, pp 30–36

Weir BK (1978) Pulmonary oedema following fatal aneurysmal rupture. J Neurosurg 49:502–507

5 Differential Diagnosis

Written in conjunction with P. Gates

Introduction

The clinical manifestations of SAH are varied, and the causes of haemorrhage into the subarachnoid space are numerous. The diagnosis has often been missed when a patient is first seen. The rarity of SAH, an inadequate or uncertain history, and the variable clinical features probably account for the difficulty with the diagnosis.

Subarachnoid haemorrhage may present in a number of ways, the commonest being headache, coma and focal neurological deficits. The possible alternative diagnoses that must be considered clearly depend upon the mode of presentation.

The first section of this chapter discusses the three common modes of presentation, and the alternative diagnoses to be considered. This is followed by a discussion of the CSF findings in SAH. Once the diagnosis of SAH is firmly established, the underlying cause needs to be elicited. The second half of the chapter deals with this aspect.

Modes of Presentation

(Table 5.1)

Headache

The abrupt onset of severe headache associated with nausea and vomiting, with or without loss of consciousness or focal neurological signs, should

Table 5.1. The three common modes of presentation of SAH and the more commonly considered alternative diagnoses

Headache	Loss of consciousness		Acute focal deficit
	Transient	Persistent	
Migraine	Epilepsy	*Without focal signs:*	Cerebral haemorrhage
Meningitis	Myocardial infarction	Meningitis	or infarction
Hypertensive encephalopathy		Drugs	Cerebellar haemorrhage
Encephalitis		Metabolic	Oculomotor palsy
Intracerebral haemorrhage			
Cerebral venous thrombosis		*With focal signs:*	
Cavernous sinus thrombosis		Encephalitis	
Pituitary apoplexy		Intracerebral haemorrhage	
Temporal arteritis			
Cluster headache			
Lymphocytic meningitis			
Benign coital headache			
Immersion headache			

be considered to be due to an SAH until proven otherwise. The instantaneous onset is characteristic, with the patient frequently able to recall the precise moment. Neck rigidity may not appear for some hours, and in patients with a minimal bleed it may not be present at all.

Subarachnoid haemorrhage is, however, not the only cause of headache, and the following conditions, discussed in order of frequency, should be considered.

Migraine

The visual fortification phenomena, nausea, vomiting, photophobia, and a strong family history of classical migraine help to differentiate migraine from SAH. However, a migraine headache may be abrupt in onset, with neck stiffness and vomiting, and thus virtually indistinguishable from SAH (Pearce and Foster 1965). A lumbar puncture or a CT scan may be necessary to establish the correct diagnosis. Ophthalmoplegic migraine, causing a third nerve palsy, is a diagnosis which is established only by the exclusion of an aneurysm by cerebral angiography.

Meningitis

When a reliable history as to the precise onset of symptoms is not available, or the onset is not instantaneous, in the presence of headache, neck stiffness and fever the patient is often thought to be suffering from meningitis. Subhyaloid haemorrhages, when present, point to the correct diagnosis. The other differentiating feature is the nature of the progression of illness. Subarachnoid haemorrhage is worst at its onset, with a tendency to improve subsequently unless complications arise, whilst meningitis is characterised by progressive worsening. In rare instances the CSF may be haemorrhagic or xanthochromic in meningitis, but the differential white cell count, Gram stain and culture will establish the correct diagnosis. Rarely lymphocytic meningitis may be ushered in by an abrupt onset of headache, particularly in children. Examination of the CSF will quickly establish the correct diagnosis.

Hypertensive Encephalopathy

These patients present with subacute onset and impaired consciousness on the background of longstanding hypertension with evidence of hypertensive retinopathy and left ventricular hypertrophy. The CSF is clear unless parenchymal haemorrhage has occurred.

Encephalitis

Encephalitis may present with a relatively benign picture of headache, fever, nausea, vomiting and neck stiffness. Lumbar puncture reveals a mononuclear pleocytosis in the CSF.

Intracerebral Haemorrhage

Primary intracerebral haemorrhage may present with a sudden onset of headache, but is associated with focal neurological signs. Signs may, however, be absent when the haemorrhage is small or located in a silent area, e.g. frontal lobes. Meningism may occur if there is associated haemorrhage into the subarachnoid space. A CT scan and, on occasions, angiography, is necessary to establish the correct diagnosis.

Cerebral Venous Thrombosis

Cerebral venous thrombosis often presents with the acute onset of headache, fever and meningism. Epilepsy, either focal or generalised, impairment of the conscious state, and hemiparesis or paraparesis are frequently seen. Clinically, it may be difficult at times to differentiate cerebral venous thrombosis from SAH. Venous thrombosis usually progresses over a period of days, whilst SAH has a tendency to improve unless complications supervene. The CSF is either blood-stained or xanthochromic in approximately 50% of cases of cerebral venous thrombosis (Kalbag and Woolf 1967). The severity of the illness is out of proportion to the degree of haemorrhage into the subarachnoid space. The majority of patients have a CSF red cell count of less than $1500/mm^3$. The CT scan can be normal or may show multiple intracerebral haemorrhages or areas of haemorrhagic infarction, either unilateral or at times bilateral (Brismar 1980). Cerebral angiography may show occlusion of the cerebral veins. Digital subtraction angiography reveals the anatomy of the cerebral veins (Meaney et al. 1980) and is a useful aid in the diagnosis of cerebral venous thrombosis.

Cavernous Sinus Thrombosis

Proptosis, chemosis and orbital swelling, initially unilateral, associated with headache, fever, neck rigidity and clouding of consciousness, are the features of thrombosis of the cavernous sinus. The CSF shows an increase in the white cell count, usually polymorphs, with a raised protein and a slightly reduced glucose (Clifford-Jones et al. 1982).

Pituitary Apoplexy

Pituitary apoplexy due to haemorrhagic infarction of the pituitary gland presents with sudden headache, nausea and vomiting, depression of the conscious level and meningism. If there is a significant haemorrhagic component the cerebrospinal fluid may be blood-stained or xanthochromic. Ophthalmoplegia, either unilateral or bilateral, and visual field impairment are usually present. Prior evidence of endocrine dysfunction is infrequent (Rovit and Fein 1972). Skull X-rays usually but not invariably reveal an enlarged pituitary fossa. Wakai et al. (1979) described haemorrhage into pituitary adenomas in 16.6% of 560 cases. In approximately three-quarters of the patients the haemorrhage was asymptomatic and discovered at the time of surgery. Subarachnoid haemorrhage was the presenting feature in only three of their cases—approximately 0.5%.

Temporal Arteritis

Temporal arteritis presents with the subacute onset of severe headache in the elderly. The patient is generally unwell, with muscle aches and pain of polymyalgia rheumatica, and tender swollen temporal arteries may be present. The ESR is usually raised. Temporal artery biopsy, although the definitive procedure, may be negative because of the segmental involvement.

Cluster Headache

The headache is usually unilateral, involving the eye and one side of the face. In most cases the headache lasts for 10–15 min, though sometimes its duration is several hours. The attacks come in clusters for 2–3 months with remission. They are mostly nocturnal, and occur three to four times per day. The severity of the headache may resemble that of SAH. The headache often recurs at the same time every day. Unilateral rhinorrhoea, lacrimation, conjunctival injection and nasal congestion are the frequent features associated with this type of headache. Occasionally, ptosis and miosis are also noticed, due to oculosympathetic paralysis. Cluster headaches are more frequent in men.

Lymphocytic Meningitis

Lymphocytic meningitis may be ushered in by an abrupt onset of headache, especially in children. Examination of the CSF will quickly establish the correct diagnosis.

Benign Coital Headache

Benign sex or coital headache is probably a variant of migraine. It is abrupt in onset, occurring at the time of orgasm (Lundberg and Osterman 1974). The lack of associated features, such as vomiting, impairment of consciousness and neck rigidity, and the brief duration of the headache—in the great majority the duration is less than 1 h (Paulson and Klawans 1974)—help to distinguish it from headache of SAH. In the absence of previous similar episodes, the CSF should be examined in order not to overlook a case of SAH occurring during intercourse.

Immersion Headache

Headache may occur when a water-skier plunges into icy water, or as he arises out of the water. This is termed "immersion headache". It is brief in duration and not associated with other symptoms, such as vomiting or loss of consciousness. The pathogenesis is unknown.

Loss of Consciousness

Loss of consciousness may be transient or persistent by the time the patient is seen by the first attending doctor. Depending upon the duration of disturbance of conscious level, the differential diagnosis may vary.

Transient Impairment of Consciousness

Epilepsy. Both convulsions and transient loss of consciousness are common in SAH. Prolonged drowsiness or severe headache and vomiting on awakening should alert the clinician to an underlying diagnosis of SAH. The interictal fluctuations of conscious level differentiate tonic epilepsy from the decerebrate rigidity that occurs with transtentorial herniation, and patients are very occasionally seen who are thought to be suffering from epilepsy when they have repeated episodes of decerebrate posturing, reflecting transtentorial herniation.

"Sustained coma in patients with epilepsy is nearly always due to underlying structural pathology or a metabolic disturbance" (Plum and Posner 1980).

Myocardial Infarction. Occasionally patients with SAH associated with loss of consciousness are incorrectly diagnosed as suffering from myocardial infarction or ischaemia. This is because an ECG has shown ST-T wave changes suggestive of ischaemic heart disease and the cardiac enzymes are raised. In patients with SAH, ECG changes of transmural infarction may be seen in the absence of demonstrable cardiac pathology (Pfister and de Pando 1962). Other ECG abnormalities include peaked T waves, short P-R interval, prolonged QT segments and tall U waves (Cruickshank 1974) Raised cardiac enzymes, including the myocardial iso-enzyme CKMB, may occur in SAH, (Fabinyi et al. 1977) One helpful clue is that the ECG changes of myocardial infarction evolve over a few days whilst in SAH Q waves are often present on the initial ECG. The diagnosis is usually evident once the patient regains consciousness and complains of headache, nausea and vomiting. An earlier diagnosis is possible if subhyaloid haemorrhages or neck rigidity are present.

Persistent Loss of Consciousness

Coma is seen in the presence of massive SAH or when complications such as intracerebral haemorrhage or hydrocephalus occur. Localising neurological signs may occur, but are not a constant feature. Therefore, the differential diagnosis will be of coma with or without a focal deficit.

In the absence of neck rigidity or fundal haemorrhages, coma resulting from uncomplicated SAH is difficult to differentiate from other causes of an impaired conscious state, i.e. coma due to metabolic disturbances, drugs or meningitis. The final diagnosis will often depend upon the results of investigations, particularly CT scan and lumbar puncture. The presence of

hypotension is extremely rare in subarachnoid haemorrhage, and strongly suggests an alternative diagnosis.

The common metabolic causes of coma are hyper- or hypoglycaemia, whilst alcohol or barbiturates and other sedative overdoses are the major exogenous causes of coma.

Focal neurologcal signs present from the outset in patients with SAH are usually due to associated haemorrhage into the parenchyma. The site of haemorrhage within the neuro axis is valuable in making an underlying pathological diagnosis. Hypertensive haemorrhages usually occur in the region of the internal capsule and basal ganglia. Intracerebral haematomas, due to an aneurysm or AVM, are generally located more superficially, or in the region of the aneurysms more commonly found, e.g. the Sylvian fissure or interhemispheric fissure.

Major pontine haemorrhage presents with a sudden loss of consciousness and blood-stained CSF. This condition is almost invariably associated with pre-existing hypertension and the presence of pin-point pupils, apneustic breathing and impaired oculocephalic and oculovestibular reflexes (Dinsdale 1964).

On rare occasions, coma is attributed to head injury, when in fact the head injury is the result of the SAH. The unusual circumstances of the accident should lead the clinician to consider an underlying cause for the accident.

Acute haemorrhagic leucoencephalitis and herpes simplex encephalitis often present with headache, fever, neck rigidity and impairment of the conscious state (Hurst 1941; Drachman and Adams 1962). Epilepsy and focal neurological deficits commonly occur. In the CSF only a small number of red cells are found. Extensive haemorrhage into the subarachnoid space has been reported with encephalitis (Sands 1941).

Sudden Onset of a Focal Neurological Deficit

When a patient presents with the acute onset of a focal neurological deficit, the commonest causes include cerebral infarction, SAH complicated by intracerebral haemorrhage or ischaemia, and primary (parenchymal) intracerebral haemorrhage with or without subsequent haemorrhage into the subarachnoid space. Clinically, it is often difficult to differentiate between cerebral infarction and haemorrhage and between primary parenchymal haemorrhage and that secondary to

SAH. Headache and vomiting are more common with haemorrhage than infarction, as is the onset of coma within the first 24 h. A visual field defect is extremely rare in SAH. The CT scan and angiogram are often necessary to establish the correct diagnosis.

In cerebellar haemorrhage the clinical picture in its early stages is distinctive and should present little difficulty with the diagnosis. The patient is usually 40 years of age or older, and hypertensive. The diagnostic features are the sudden onset of severe nausea and vomiting with an inability to walk, with true vertigo (i.e. a sensation of rotation) occurring in less than a third of patients (Ott et al. 1974). This is often, but not invariably, associated with headache, ipsilateral facial weakness and gaze palsy, dysarthria, nystagmus and neck rigidity (Fisher et al. 1965; Ott et al. 1974). The diagnosis is difficult if the patient presents in coma due to brain-stem compression.

Oculomotor Palsy Due to Diabetes. In oculomotor palsy due to diabetes, the pupil is usually spared because the periphery of the nerve is not involved in the pathological process (Weber et al. 1970). In Goldstein and Cogan's (1960) series of 22 diabetic patients with a third nerve palsy, the pupil was involved in five patients. More recently, Kissel et al. (1983) reported that the pupil was spared in as many as 14% of cases. Cerebral aneurysms account for approximately 20% of isolated third nerve palsies, the pupil being involved in more than 90% of these (Rucker 1966). Angiography should be considered in patients with third nerve palsy when the pupil is dilated and in the absence of an obvious aetiology when the pupil is spared.

Confirmation of Subarachnoid Haemorrhage

Examination of CSF

Lumbar puncture and examination of CSF has been the corner-stone in the diagnosis of SAH. However, on occasions, traumatic lumbar puncture may make the diagnosis of true SAH difficult. In these conditions, the observations made by McMenemy (1954) over 30 years ago cannot be improved upon. Frank clotting of the specimen virtually never occurs with SAH. Perhaps the most important guide is to collect three successive

tubes and note whether the specimens become progressively less blood-stained, thus indicating a traumatic puncture. Xanthochromia is usually seen in true cases of SAH, but may rarely occur in a traumatic lumbar puncture if the red cell count exceeds 200 000.

Further difficulty is encountered in correlating the CSF findings in patients with a history suggestive of SAH some days to weeks prior to admission, e.g. patients who present with a typical history of SAH but for one reason or another are referred late. Matthews and Frommeyer (1955) demonstrated (in vitro) that red blood cells crenated immediately on contact with the CSF, and disappeared within 60 h. Xanthochromia was evident within 4 h if more than 1000 red cells were added to the CSF. The CSF may remain clear if there are less than 360 red cells (Tourtellotte et al. 1958). Xanthochromia is initially due to oxyhaemoglobin and subsequently to bilirubin (Barrows et al. 1955).

The duration of "abnormal CSF" is variable. Froin (1904) found that haemolysis was complete by 5 days, which is in keeping with the experimental work of Matthews and Frommeyer (1955). Richardson and Hyland (1941) and Walton (1956) described patients in whom (in the absence of any "clinically evident re-bleed") the CSF was blood-stained after 19 and 24 days respectively. Walton (1956) described three patients in whom the CSF was found not to be blood-stained when examined within 24 hours, which he interpreted as representing rapid clearing of the CSF. Clear CSF may occur with a ruptured aneurysm where the bleeding is largely into the parenchyma (Robertson 1949) or associated with coning of the tonsils through the foramen magnum, which prevents spread of blood into the spinal canal (Taylor and Whitfield 1936).

Xanthochromia is usually seen after 4–6 h and lasts on an average 3–4 weeks (Richardson and Hyland 1941; McMenemy 1954; Walton 1956).

Tourtellotte et al. (1964) have arbitrarily defined three rates of clearing of the CSF in a study based on 62 patients: (a) rapid, i.e. within 1 week, (b) intermediate, i.e. between 10 and 20 days and (c) slow, i.e. longer than 20 days. They found that a slower rate of clearance was associated with older age and extensive brain damage (cerebral infarction or parenchymal haemorrhage). Rapid clearing was, however, occasionally seen in patients of advanced years.

Thus, in patients with a history suggestive of uncomplicated SAH it is possible that the CSF may clear within 1–2 weeks and therefore a negative lumbar puncture at this stage does not exclude the necessity of further investigation, such as cerebral angiography.

In a study at the Newcastle General Hospital between January, 1980, and March, 1983, 11 patients with a history very suggestive of SAH some weeks prior to admission, were submitted to four vessel angiography. These patients suffered abrupt onset of severe headache associated with nausea and vomiting 2–10 weeks prior to admission, with a mean duration of 5 weeks. CSF was invariably normal, although on two occasions the CSF protein level was found to be elevated. These two cases were investigated 2–3 weeks after the onset of headache. In nine patients, four vessel angiography failed to reveal an underlying vascular abnormality. In one patient a posterior communicating artery aneurysm was found, whilst in another a frontal arteriovenous malformation was detected. There was nothing to differentiate the patients in whom the angiography had been rewarding.

Computerised Tomography

With the routine use of computerised tomography, especially immediately after the onset of symptoms, a probable diagnosis of SAH can be made in 80%–90% of patients. Computerised tomography will also help in making a provisional diagnosis as to the aetiology of the SAH, in accordance with the location and extent of the subarachnoid and intraparenchymal blood.

Aetiology of Subarachnoid Haemorrhage

Once the diagnosis of SAH is established, the next step is to find the underlying cause.

The list of causes of SAH is lengthy (see Tables 5.5–5.9). However, when the reports of "unusual" causes of SAH are carefully scrutinised, an underlying berry aneurysm frequently cannot be excluded. This is particularly so for publications appearing prior to the widespread introduction of angiography.

From a practical point of view, the majority of patients with SAH will fall into the diagnostic categories listed in Table 5.2. Berry aneurysm is the commonest cause of SAH. The reported percentage of patients suffering from aneurysmal SAH has varied a great deal from one author to another (Table 5.3). This largely reflects the method of establishing the diagnosis.

The records of all patients admitted to the Regional Neurological Centre, Newcastle General Hospital, between January, 1980, and April, 1983, with a confirmed diagnosis of SAH, were examined. This is a secondary referral centre and thus there is some bias in the figures, in that the patients with more severe SAH are unlikely to

Table 5.2. Causes of SAH in order of frequency

Berry aneurysm
Arteriovenous malformation
Hypertensive intracerebral haemorrhage with secondary SAH
Traumatic
Unknown

Table 5.3. Reported incidences (in percentages) of the more common causes of SAH in different published series. The studies of Courville, Walton and Heidrich are autopsy series; the remainder are clinical and radiological

Aetiology	Courville 1937 $n = 107$	Walton 1956 $n = 173$[a]	Coop. study 1966 $n = 5836$	Heidrich 1972 $n = 646$[b]	West et al. 1977 $n = 98$	Illingworth 1979 $n = 232$	Burrows and Leeds 1981 $n = 1588$	Newcastle study Unpublished $n = 534$
Traumatic	–	–	–	29.9 (–)	–	–	–	–
Aneurysm	15	71.7	51	8.8 (14.1)	74.5	73.3	58.6	73.4
Arteriovenous malformation	–	2.9	6	0.9 (1.5)	12.2	6.9	9.9	6.4
Hypertensive, atherosclerotic	30	4.6	43	21.8 (34.9)	3	–	9.5	5.9
Normal angiography (or unknown)	19	8.1		6.6 (10.6)	9.1	19.8	21.7	13.1
Miscellaneous	36	13.3		3.2 (38.9)	3	–	–	1.3

[a] 177 cases studied at post-mortem
[b] Adjusted figure excluding cases of traumatic SAH = 404

reach the hospital. In this period of time 574 patients with proven SAH were admitted to the Regional Neurological Centre. Of these, 40 were too ill to undergo angiography and are excluded. In 12 of this group, a probable diagnosis of aneurysmal SAH could be made on the basis of the CT scan, which also demonstrated a tumour in another patient.

In the remaining 534 patients, the diagnosis was established by angiography in 519, and at post-mortem in 15 patients. Our policy is to perform four vessel angiography in patients with SAH. The extent of initial angiography was varied, on the basis of the clinical picture and the CT scan findings. In some, bilateral carotid angiography was initially performed, and the posterior cerebral circulation studied at the time of check angiography in the postoperative period. When the site of haemorrhage was unknown, four vessel angiography or three vessel angiography with reflux down the opposite vertebral artery at the time of the initial study was performed. This includes the routine use of subtraction films and magnification views.

Table 5.4 shows that aneurysmal (berry) SAH accounted for 73.4% of cases, whilst arteriovenous malformations were responsible for 6.4%. There remained 13.1% of cases in which CT scan and four vessel angiography failed to reveal an underlying cause for the SAH, and to date none of these patients has returned with a second SAH. Primary intracerebral haemorrhage with subsequent SAH accounted for 5.2% of cases. This may reflect the known trend towards a reduction in hypertensive cerebrovascular disease. The problem of differentiating the cause of SAH in patients with multiple potential sources of

haemorrhage, e.g. multiple intracranial aneurysms, is discussed elsewhere.

Tables 5.5–5.9 list a large number of documented causes of SAH. These lists have been compiled by carefully reviewing the literature, and accepting only those cases which fulfil the following criteria:

1. Post-mortem confirmation of SAH and its aetiology, or
2. A clinical and radiological diagnosis in which (a) the patient has suffered an ictus, (b) in the absence of a localising haematoma, vertebral and carotid angiography have been performed, or (c) in the presence of a localising haematoma, appropriate angiography has been done.

Angiography was not performed, however, in all the patients suffering from a bleeding diathesis.

A brief discussion of some of the rarer causes of SAH which are listed in Tables 5.5–5.9 will follow.

Tumours Associated with Subarachnoid Haemorrhage

Almost every tumour known to involve the central nervous system has been reported as being associated with SAH (see Table 5.5). Haemorrhage, not necessarily subarachnoid, was found in 95 (5.1%) of 1861 cases studied by Wakai et al. (1982). In an earlier publication of 560 patients with pituitary tumour, the same authors described 51 patients with symptomatic haemorrhage, rep-

Table 5.4. A detailed analysis of 534 patients with proven SAH admitted to the Regional Neurological Centre between January, 1980, and 30 April, 1983

Berry aneurysm	392[a,b]	(73.4%)
Arteriovenous malformation	34[a]	(6.4%)
Normal angiography	70	(13.1%)
Intracerebral haemorrhage with secondary SAH	28	(5.2%)
Atherosclerosis	4	(0.7%)
Mycotic aneurysm	2	(proven endocarditis)
Thrombocytopenia	2	(1 gold induced, 1 in association with disseminated maligancy)
Pinealoma	1	
Secondary carcinoma	2	(1 lung, 1 unknown primary)

[a] In six patients coexistent arteriovenous malformation and aneurysm were present. The latter was felt to be responsible for the SAH in four cases, and the former in the remaining two.
[b] In one patient in whom Moya Moya disease was present, the aneurysm was found to be the cause of the SAH.

Table 5.5. Neoplasms that have been reported to cause SAH

Neoplasm	Author(s)
Primary	
Oligodendroglioma	Harper (1977)
Astrocytoma	Glass and Abbot (1955)
Medulloblastoma	Glass and Abbot (1955)
Ependymoma	Changaris et al. (1981)
Neurolemmoma	Kubota et al. (1981)
Meningioma	Yasargil and So (1976)
Pineocytoma	Steinbok et al. (1977)
Pituitary adenoma	Kirschbaum and Chapman (1948)
Choroid plexus papilloma	Abbott et al. (1957)
Chordoma	Simonsen (1963)
Osteochondroma of skull	Northfield and Russell (1951)
Perivascular sarcoma	Glass and Abbott (1955)
Primary melanoma	Glass and Abbott (1955)
Haemangioma	Meadows (1951)
Secondary	
Secondary melanoma	Clifford et al. (1975)
Secondary choriocarcinoma	Dagi and Macabe (1980)
Secondary cardiac myxoma	Price et al. (1970)
Secondary carcinoma	Unpublished Newcastle study

resenting 9.1% of the total. In 1955 Glass and Abbott collected 33 cases of SAH, including eight of their own, associated with a tumour, and two-thirds of these were grade four gliomas or pituitary adenomas. Melanoma is associated with xanthochromic or blood-stained CSF in about 50% of cases (Madonick and Savitsky 1951). Meningiomas can result in subdural, parenchymal or subarachnoid haemorrhage (Lazaro et al. 1981). In these patients, the histological type of meningioma bore no relationship to the incidence or severity of the haemorrhage.

It is thus clear that SAH can occur with intracranial tumours, but this is extremely rare. Haemorrhage usually arises from the substance of the tumour, though rarely a tumour may invade a cerebral vessel (Hart and Byer 1974). Undifferentiated carcinoma (Helmer 1976), choriocarcinoma (Dagi and Macabe 1980) and cardiac myxoma (Price et al. 1970) embolise to peripheral branches of the cerebral vessels and result in an "oncotic aneurysm" that radiologically may resemble a mycotic aneurysm.

Patients presenting with SAH (due to a berry aneurysm) may be found to also have a tumour of the central nervous system. The association of berry aneurysms and tumours occurs in approximately 1% of patients (Wakai et al. 1979), but in patients with a pituitary tumour the incidence is greater (Jakubowski and Kendall 1978). In patients with both a pituitary tumour and an aneurysm, it may be difficult to decide which has caused the SAH; this has been discussed by

Wakai et al. (1979, 1981). Subarachnoid haemorrhage occurred in three of the 250 patients with meningiomas seen at Newcastle General Hospital between 1962 and 1983 (unpublished data). In one patient the haemorrhage was due to an aneurysm, whilst in two the tumour was responsible for the SAH.

Tumours are occasionally associated with repeated episodes of SAH (Kalbag 1964; Steinbok et al. 1977; Latchaw et al. 1981), although with CT scanning such tumours can now be diagnosed earlier. In Latchaw et al.'s patient, the clivus meningioma was finally diagnosed by CT scan; this was also the means of diagnosis in the patient with a chordoma in the region of the clivus, described elsewhere in this textbook (Figs. 6.30, 6.31).

Unusual Aneurysms Producing Subarachnoid Haemorrhage

The great majority of aneurysms responsible for SAH are saccular (so-called congenital or berry) in nature, but unusual aneurysms account for a small percentage of cases. The most important of these are mycotic aneurysms. The incidence of mycotic aneurysms has declined over the years, and in the 1960s represented 2.6% of all aneurysms (McDonald and Korb 1939; Roach and Drake 1965). This figure may now be lower because of the dramatic decline in the incidence of rheumatic heart disease.

Table 5.6. Abnormalities of the cerebral vasculature associated with SAH[a]

Abnormality	Author(s)
Cerebral vascular malformations	
Capillary telangiectases	Quinckel and Whaley (1967)
Cavernous angioma	Voigt and Yasargil (1976)
Arteriovenous malformations	McKenzie (1953)
Sturge-Weber disease	Anderson and Duncan (1974)
Intracranial aneurysms	
Berry	
Dissecting	Yonas et al. (1977)
Malignant—Cardiac myxoma	Price et al. (1970)
Choriocarcinoma	Dagi and Macabe (1980)
Unknown primary	Helmer (1976)
Mycotic —Bacterial	Roach and Drake (1965)
Fungal	Horten et al. (1976)
Phytotic	Steele et al. (1972)
Arteriosclerotic	Taylor and Whitfield (1936)
Syphilitic	Taylor and Whitfield (1936)
Traumatic	Fleischer et al. (1975)
Inherited disorders of connective tissue	
Ehlers-Danlos	Rubinstein and Cohen (1964)
Pseudoxanthoma elasticum	Scheie and Hogan (1957)
Marfan's syndrome	Finney et al. (1976)
Other vascular abnormalities	
Moya Moya	Kowada et al. (1979)
Cerebral vein thrombosis	Kalbag and Woolf (1967)
Cerebral Vasculitis	
Polyarteritis nodosa group	
Polyarteritis nodosa	Ford and Siekert (1965)
Allergic granulomatosis	Magidson et al. (1978)
Wegener's granulomatosis	Tuhy et al. (1958)
Hypersensitivity vasculitis	
Systemic lupus erythematosus	Gonzalez-Scarano et al. (1979)
Rheumatoid arthritis	Watson et al. (1977)
Drug induced (amphetamines)	Chynn (1975)
Ulcerative colitis	Edwards (1977)
Giant cell arteritis	Kozuka et al. (1979)
Atherosclerosis	Hamby (1948)
Hypertension	Russell (1954)
Cerebral artery rupture	Taylor and Whitfield (1936)

[a] The classification of vasculitis is taken from Fauci et al. (1978) and the classification of vascular malformations from Russell and Rubinstein (1977).

Table 5.7. Subarachnoid haemorrhage associated with infections in the absence of aneurysm formation

Infection	Author(s)
Septicaemia, bacterial	De Reuck et al. (1979)
Meningitis—Bacterial	Suwanwela et al. (1972)
Syphilis	Strauss et al. (1932)
Schistosoma	Pompeu and de Lacerda (1979)
Encephalitis	Sands (1941)
Brain abscess	Sands (1941)

The majority of mycotic aneurysms are bacterial and are associated with endocarditis (Bohmfalk et al. 1978). Approximately 2%–10% of patients with endocarditis develop mycotic aneurysms (Weinstein and Rubin 1973), and SAH may be the presenting feature of bacterial endocarditis (Roach and Drake 1965). Bacterial mycotic aneurysms are usually small and situated in the more peripheral branches of the cerebral vessels. A unique case of septic embolus to the fundus of a berry aneurysm has been described (Ray and Wahal 1957). Mycotic aneurysms of fungal origin are extremely rare. They are large and arise from major cerebral arterial trunks. *Candida albicans* is usually the cause, and they are almost invariably fatal (Horten et al. 1976; Ahuja et al. 1978).

Table 5.8. Blood dyscrasias reported to be associated with SAH (in most of these cases angiography was not performed)

Blood dyscrasia	Author(s)
Platelet abnormalities	
Idiopathic thrombocytopenic purpura	Humphreys et al. (1976)
Defects of coagulation	
Hageman deficiency	Kovalainen et al. (1979)
Haemophilia	Kerr (1964)
Prothrombin complex deficiency (infants)	Bhanchet et al. (1977)
Warfarin	Barron and Fergusson (1959)
DIC	Heron et al. (1974)
Waldenström's macroglobulinaemia	Logethetis et al. (1960)
Sickle cell anaemia	Adeloye and Ogbeide (1970)
Henoch-Schönlein purpura	Lewis and Philpott (1956)

Table 5.9. Miscellaneous unusual causes of SAH[a]

Cause	Author(s)
Trauma—cervical	Dymock (1977)
Intranasal polypectomy	Sachdev et al. (1977)
Conn's syndrome	Sterling (1965)
Monoamine oxidase inhibitors	Villiers (1966)

[a] Many additional unusual causes have been described by Heidrich (1972)

Subarachnoid Haemorrhage and Infection

Subarachnoid haemorrhage may complicate septicaemia (de Reuck et al. 1979), bacterial meningitis (Heidelberger et al. 1968; Suwanwela et al. 1972) or brain abscess in which the abscess has eroded into a vessel (Sands 1941). Although multiple aneurysms due to tuberculous meningitis have been described (Suwanwela et al. 1972), they are not associated with SAH.

Bleeding Diathesis

Intracranial haemorrhage occurred in approximately 14% of patients with haemophilia followed for a 5-year period (Kerr 1964). In these 15 patients, 19 episodes of haemorrhage occurred, of which 10 were subarachnoid. Occasionally SAH can be the presenting feature of haemophilia (Visconti and Hilgartner 1980).

In patients suffering from leukaemia, intracranial haemorrhage is usually associated with thrombocytopenia. Approximately one-third to one-half of the haemorrhages are subarachnoid (Groch et al. 1960; Moore et al. 1960).

Intracranial haemorrhage may arise as a complication of anticoagulant therapy, even when the clotting profile is within the accepted therapeutic range (Silverstein 1979). It is usually intracerebral or subdural (Snyder and Renaudin 1977). Subarachnoid haemorrhage has also been reported (Barron and Fergusson 1969). Aneurysmal SAH can also occur in patients on anticoagulants. We have recently encountered a female patient who had undergone mitral valve surgery and was on warfarin. She developed an SAH with a third nerve palsy. Her clotting profile showed a markedly prolonged prothrombin time, consistent with excessive anticoagulant dosage. Carotid angiography was performed because of the presence of a third nerve palsy, and revealed a posterior communicating artery aneurysm which at surgery was found to be the cause of the SAH.

Subarachnoid haemorrhage has been described in two patients on the basis of Hageman factor deficiency (Slade and Rabiner 1973; Kovalainen et al. 1979). The deficiency was only discovered when detailed clotting studies were performed. Kovalainen et al.'s patient had suffered from recurrent epistaxes, suggesting an underlying bleeding diathesis. On the other hand, the patient of Slade and Rabiner had not suffered from any previous episode of abnormal bleeding. This suggests that patients in whom no obvious aetiology for their SAH is found, should be submitted to detailed clotting studies.

Subarachnoid Haemorrhage and Vascular Abnormalities

A large number of vascular abnormalities may rarely be associated with SAH (Table 5.6). In a review of 549 cases of arteriovenous malformation, Perret and Nishioka (1966) found 307, (61%) with a history of SAH. They also found that SAH due to arteriovenous malformations occurred in a younger age group, with approximately 70% occurring in those less than 40 years old. Fifty-three per cent of their patients who suffered SAH developed a focal deficit, suggesting co-existent parenchymal haemorrhage. CT scanning reveals intracerebral haematoma in 90% of cases in which the SAH is due to an arteriovenous malformation (Hayward 1976).

In a small percentage of patients an arteriovenous malformation may coexist with an intracranial aneurysm. Under these circumstances, it may be difficult to establish which is the causative lesion. Perret and Nishioka (1966) reviewed the literature and, on the basis of morbid anatomical studies, found the arteriovenous malformation to be the more likely cause of SAH. In the cooperative study's own material of 37 patients with coexistent aneurysm and arteriovenous malformation, 29 suffered an SAH; in nine cases the SAH was thought to be due to the arteriovenous malformation, in seven to the aneurysm, and in 13 the cause could not be decided (Sahs et al. 1966). The diagnostic criteria used to establish the causative lesion were not discussed. Haywood (1976) reported that in two patients in whom both an aneurysm and an arteriovenous malformation were present, at surgery the aneurysm was found to be the cause of SAH.

A similar problem arises when intracranial aneurysms coexist with Moya Moya disease. Adams et al. (1979) felt that the aneurysm was the cause of the haemorrhage in two out of three patients with Moya Moya disease associated with an intracranial aneurysm. The source of the haemorrhage was confirmed in one patient at autopsy, and in another at surgical exploration. In 13 cases collected by Kowada et al. (1979), seven of the aneurysms were located on the vertebrobasilar system, representing a very atypical distribution of aneurysms in patients with Moya Moya disease.

In our analysis of 534 cases (Table 5.4), six patients had a coexistent aneurysm and an arteriovenous malformation, whilst one had an aneurysm coexistent with Moya Moya disease. In this latter patient, the origin of the SAH was due to the aneurysm. In the patients with a coexistent aneurysm and arteriovenous malformation, on the basis of the CT scan and/or operative findings the aneurysm was considered to be the cause in four cases.

When multiple pathology exists, unless there is a focal neurological deficit, a localised haematoma on the CT scan or vascular changes, such as vasospasm at angiography, it may be impossible to define clinically the site of origin of the SAH.

Subarachnoid Haemorrhage and Vasculitis

Most of the reports of SAH associated with vasculitis consist of isolated cases. Vasculitis affects small vessels and therefore almost invariably is associated with parenchymal haemorrhage. Vasculitis is usually diagnosed from the typical beaded appearance of the cerebral arteries seen at angiography. It can cause aneurysm formation in peripheral vessels (Kozuka et al. 1979) and even multiple aneurysms (Griffin et al. 1973), and thus is easily confused with mycotic aneurysms. Subarachnoid haemorrhage may occur in cerebral vasculitis in the absence of aneurysm formation (Ford and Siekert 1965).

Subarachnoid Haemorrhage of Unknown Aetiology

There is a group of patients with a typical clinical picture of SAH, confirmed by lumbar puncture, in whom investigations fail to reveal an underlying cause. This group has been labelled with various titles, including "subarachnoid haemorrhage of unknown aetiology" (Hayward 1977) or "subarachnoid haemorrhage without arteriographic vascular abnormality" (Levy 1960). With the advent of CT scanning, it is now possible to identify those patients with SAH secondary to primary hypertensive intracerebral haemorrhage, who in the past may have been included in the group with a normal angiogram (Hayward and O'Reilly 1976). The percentage of patients with proven SAH of unknown aetiology varies considerably from one series to another, depending upon the nature of the study, i.e. clinical versus radiological or post-mortem. Furthermore, the extent of radiological investigation also influences the results. In autopsy series, between 6.6% (Courville 1937) and 19% (Heidreich 1972) of patients with SAH have no obvious underlying cause. In clinicoradiological studies (most of which suffer from incomplete angiography), the figures are somewhat higher. In our series of 534 patients, 13.1% of the patients had normal four vessel angiography, and no definable cause for the SAH.

In summary, SAH may mimic many diseases and should be considered whenever a patient presents with headache of sudden onset. Once clinically suspected, the diagnosis can usually be confirmed by lumbar puncture and/or CT scan. Although there are a large number of causes of SAH, the commonest are aneurysms and arteriovenous malformations.

References

Abbott KH, Rollas ZH, Meagher JN (1957) Choroid plexus papilloma causing spontaneous subarachnoid haemorrhage. Report of case and review of literature. J Neurosurg 14:566–570

Adams HP, Kassell NF, Wisoff HS, Drake CG (1979) Intracranial saccular aneurysm and Moya Moya disease. Stroke 10:174–179

Adeloye A, Ogbeide MI (1970) Massive intracranial haemorrhage in sickle cell anaemia. Neurology 20:1165–1170

Ahuja GK, Jain N, Vijayaraghavan M, Roy S (1978) Cerebral mycotic aneurysm of fungal origin, case report. J Neurosurg 49:107–110

Anderson FH, Duncan GW (1974) Sturge-Weber disease with subarachnoid haemorrhage. Stroke 5:509–511

Barron KD, Fergusson G (1959) Intracranial haemorrhage as a complication of anticoagulant therapy, Neurology 9:447–455

Barrows LJ, Hunter FT, Banker BQ (1955) The nature and signficance of pigmented cerebrospinal fluid. Brain 78:59–80

Bhanchet P, Tuchinda S, Hathirat P, Visudhiphan P (1977) A bleeding syndrome in infants due to acquired prothrombin complex deficiency: A survey of 93 affected infants. Clin Pediatr 16:992–998

Bohmfalk GL, Story JL, Wissinger JP, Brown WE (1978) Bacterial intracranial aneurysm. J Neurosurg 48:369–382

Brismar J (1980) Computer tomography in superior sagittal sinus thrombosis. Acta Radiol [Diagn] 21:321–326

Burrows EH, Leeds NE (1981) Subarachnoid haemorrhage in neuroradiology I. Churchill Livingstone, New York Edinburgh London Melbourne

Changaris DG, Powers JM, Perot PL Jr, Hungerford GD, Neal GB (1981) Subependymoma presenting as subarachnoid haemorrhage. Case report. J Neurosurg 55:643–645

Chester EM, Agamonolis DP, Barker BQ, Victor M (1978) Hypertensive encephalopathy: A clinicopathological study of 20 cases. Neurology 28:928–939.

Chynn KY (1975) Acute subarachnoid haemorrhage. JAMA 233:55–56

Clifford JR, Kirgis HD, Connolly ES (1975) Metastatic melanoma of the brain presenting as subarachnoid haemorrhage. South Med J 68:206–208

Clifford-Jones RE, Ellis CJK, Stevens JM, Turner A (1982) Cavernous sinus thrombosis. J Neurol Neurosurg Psychiatry 45:1092–1097

Cogan DG, Mount HT (1963) Intracranial aneurysms causing ophthalmoplegia. Arch Ophthalmol 70:757–771

Cookson H (1933) Spontaneous subarachnoid haemorrhage. Br Med J I:555–558

Courville CB (1937) Pathology of the central nervous system. Pacific Press Publishing Association, Mountain View California

Cruickshank JM, Neil-Dwyer G, Brice J (1974) Electrocardiographic changes and their prognostic significance in subarachnoid haemorrhage. J Neurol Neurosurg Psychiatry 37:755–759

Dagi TF, Macabe JJ (1980) Metastatic trophoblastic disease presenting as a subarachnoid haemorrhage. Report of two cases and review of literature. Surg Neurol 14:175–184

De Reuck J, Eeckhaut W, De Coster W, Vander Eecken H (1979) Subarachnoid haematoma in staphylococcal septicemia. A report of two cases. Acta Neurol Belg 79:22–29

Dinsdale HB (1964) Spontaneous haemorrhage in the posterior fossa. Arch Neurol 10:200–217

Drachman DA, Adams RD (1962) Herpes simplex encephalitis and acute inclusion body encephalitis. Arch Neurol 7:45–63

Dymock RB (1977) Traumatic basal subarachnoid haemorrhage. Med J Aust 2:216–218

Edwards KR (1977) Haemorrhagic complications of cerebral arteritis. Arch Neurol 34:549–552

Fabinyi G, Hunt O, McKinley L (1977) Myocardial creatine kinase isoenzyme in serum after subarachnoid haemorrhage. J Neurol Neurosurg Psychiatry 40:818–820

Fauci AS, Hayes BF, Katz P (1978) The spectrum of vasculitis. Clinical, pathologic, immunologic and therapeutic considerations. Ann Intern Med 89:660–676

Finney HL, Roberts TS, Anderson RE (1976) Giant intracranial aneurysm associated with Marfan's syndrome. J Neurosurg 45:342–347

Fisher CM, Picard EH, Polak A, Dalal P, Ojemamm RG (1965) Acute hypertensive cerebellar haemorrhage. Diagnosis and surgical treatment. J Nerv Ment Dis 1, 140:38–57

Fleischer S, Patton JM, Tindall GT (1975) Cerebral aneurysms of traumatic origin. Surg Neurol 4:233–239

Ford RG, Siekert RG (1965) C.N.S. manifestations of periarteritis nedosa. Neurology 15:114–122

Froin G (1904) Les hemorragies sous-arachnoidiennes et le mécanisme de l'hématolyse en general. Thèse de Paris. Steinheil, Paris

Glass B, Abbott KH (1955) Subarachnoid haemorrhage consequent to intracranial tumours. Arch Neurol Psychiatry 73:369–379

Goldstein JE, Cogan DG (1960) Diabetic ophthalmoplegia with special reference to the pupil. Arch Ophthalmol 64:529–600

Goldzieher JW, Lisa JR (1947) Gross cerebral haemorrhage and vascular lesions in acute tuberculous meningitis and meningoencephalitis. Am J Pathol 23:133–146

Gonzalez-Scarano F, Lisak RP, Bilaniuk LT, Zimmerman PA, Atkins PE, Zweiman B (1979) Cranial computed tomography in the diagnosis of systemic lupus eythematosus. Ann Neurol 5:158–165

Greenhoot JH, Reichenbach DD (1969) Cardiac injury and subarachnoid haemorrhage: A clinical, pathological and physiological correlation. J Neurosurg 30:521–531

Griffin J, Price DL, Davis L (1973) Granulomatous angiitis of the central nervous system with aneurysms of multiple cerebral arteries. Trans Am Neurol Assoc 98:145–148

Groch SN, Sayre GP, Heck FJ (1960) Cerebral haemorrhage in leukaemia. Arch Neurol 2:439–451

Hamby WB (1948) Spontaneous subarachnoid haemorrhage of aneurysmal origin: Factors influencing prognosis. JAMA 136:522–528

Harper CG (1977) Recurrent subarachnoid naemorrhage and obesity. Med J Aust 2:865–867

Hart MN, Byer JA (1974) Rupture of middle cerebral artery by invasive astrocytoma. Neurology 24:1171–1174

Hayward RD (1976) Intracranial arterio-venous malformations: Observations after experience with computerised tomography. J Neurol Neurosurg Psychiatry 39:1027–1033

Hayward RD (1977) Subarachnoid haemorrhage of unknown aetiology. J Neurol Neurosurg Psychiatry 40:926–931

Hayward RD, O'Reilly GVA (1976) Intracerebral haemorrhage. Lancet I: 1–4

Heidelberger KP, Layton WM, Fisher RG (1968) Multiple mycotic aneurysms complicating post-traumatic pseudomonas meningitis. J Neurosurg 29: 631–635

Heidrich R (1972) Subarachnoid haemorrhage. In: Vinken PJ, Bruyn GW (eds) Handbook of clinical neurology, vol 12, Chap 5. North Holland Publishing Co., Amsterdam

Helmer FA (1976) Oncotic aneurysm: case report. J Neurosurg 45: 98–100

Heron JR, Hutchinson EC, Boyd WN, Aber GM (1974) Pregnancy subarachnoid haemorrhage and the intravascular coagulation syndrome. J Neurol Neurosurg Psychiatry 37: 521–525

Horten BC, Abbott GF, Porro RS (1976) Fungal aneurysms of intracranial vessels. Arch Neurol 33: 577–579

Humphreys RP, Hockley AD, Freedman MH, Saunders EF (1976) Management of intracerebral hemorrhage in idiopathic thrombocytopenic purpura. J Neurosurg 45: 700–704

Hurst EW (1941) Acute haemorrhagic leucoencephalitis: A previously undefined entity. Med J Aust 2: 1–6

Illingworth RD (1979) Surgical management of subarachnoid haemorrhage due to ruptured intracranial aneurysm. In: Greenhalgh RM, Rose FC (eds) Progress in stroke research. Pitman Medical, London, pp 377–386

Ito V, Inaba Y (1979) Cerebrospinal fluid cytology after subarachnoid haemorrhage J Neurosurg 51: 352–354

Jakubowski J, Kendall B (1978) Coincidental aneurysms with tumours of pituitary origin. J Neurol Neurosurg Psychiatry 41: 972–979

Kalbag RM (1964) Recurrent subarachnoid haemorrhage from paraventricular lesions with normal angiography. J Neurol Neurosurg Psychiatry 27: 435–439

Kalbag RM, Woolf AL (1967) Cerebral venous thrombosis with special reference to primary aseptic thrombosis. Oxford University Press, London

Kasoff I, Kelly DL Jr (1975) Pupillary sparing in oculomotor palsy from internal carotid aneurysms. J Neurosurg 42: 713–717

Kerr CB (1964) Intracranial haemorrhage in haemophilia. J Neurol Neurosurg Psychiatry 27: 166–173

Kirschbaum JD, Chapman BM (1948) Subarachnoid haemorrhage secondary to a tumour of the hypophysis with acromegaly. Ann Intern Med 29: 536–540

Kissel JT, Burde RM, Klingele TG, Zeiger HE (1983) Pupil-sparing oculomotor palsies with internal carotid-posterior communicating artery aneurysms. Ann Neurol 13: 149–154

Kovalainen S, Myllyla VV, Tolonen V, Hokkanen E (1979) Recurrent subarachnoid haemorrhages in patient with Hageman factor deficiency. Lancet I: 1035–1036

Kowada M, Momma F, Kikuchi K (1979) Intracranial aneurysms associated with cerebrovascular Moya Moya disease. Report of a case and review of 13 cases. Br J Radiol 52: 236–237

Kozuka S, Iguchi I, Furuse M, Nakaya T, Taki T (1979) Cerebral aneurysm induced by giant cell arteritis. Angiology 30: 131–137

Kubota T, Hayashi M, Yamamoto S (1981) Subarachnoid haemorrhage due to trigeminal neurinoma. Surg Neurol 16: 157–160

Latchaw JP Jr, Dohn DF, Hahn JP, Von Der Luft E (1981) Subarachnoid haemorrhage from an intracranial meningioma. Neurosurgery 9: 433–435

Lazaro RP, Messer HD, Brinker RA (1981) Intracranial hemorrhage associated with meningioma. Neurosurgery 8: 96–101

Levy LF (1960) Subarachnoid haemorrhage without arteriographic vascular abnormality. J Neurosurg 17: 252–258

Lewis IC, Philpott MG (1956) Neurological complications in the Schönlein-Henoch syndrome. Arch Dis Child 31: 369–371

Logethetis J, Silverstein P, Coe J (1960) Neurological aspects of Waldenström's macroglobulinemia. Arch Neurol 3: 564–573

Lundberg PO, Osterman PO (1974) The benign and malignant forms of orgasmic cephalgia. Headache 14: 164–165

Madonick MJ, Savitsky N (1951) Subarachnoid haemorrhage in melanoma of the brain. Arch Neurol Psychiatry 65: 628–636

Magidson MA, Rajendran MM, Leutcher WM (1978) Granulomatous angitis of the central nervous system with an unusual angiographic feature. Surg Neurol 10: 355–360

Matthews WF, Frommeyer WB Jr (1955) The in vitro behaviour of erythrocytes in human C.S.F. J Lab Clin Med 45: 508–515

McDonald CA, Korb M (1939) Intracranial aneurysms. Arch Neurol Psychiatry 42: 298–328

McKenzie I (1953) The clinical presentation of the cerebral angioma. A review of 50 cases. Brain 76: 184–214

McMenemy WH (1954) The significance of subarachnoid bleeding. Proc R Soc Med 47: 701–704

Meadows SP (1951) Intracranial aneurysms. In: Fieling A (ed) Modern trends in neurology. Butterworth, London

Meadows SP (1959) Intracavernous aneurysms of the internal carotid artery. Arch Ophthalmol 62: 566–574

Meaney TF, Weinstein MA, Buonocone E, Pavlicek W, Borkowski GP, Gallagher SH, Sufka B, MacIntyre WS (1980) Digital subtraction angiography of the cardiovascular system. Am J Radiol 135: 1153–1159

Moore EW, Thomas LB, Shaw RK, Freireich EJ (1960) The central nervous system in acute leukemia. Arch Intern Med 105: 451–468

Northfield DWC, Russell DS (1951) Intracranial tumors. In: Fieling A (ed) Modern trends in neurology. Butterworth, London

Osler W (1885) 'The Gulstonian Lectures' on malignant endocarditis. Br Med J I: 467–470

Ott KH, Kase CS, Ojemann RG, Mohr JP (1974) Cerebellar haemorrhage: diagnosis and treatment. Arch Neurol 31: 160–167

Paulson GW, Klawans HL Jr (1974) Benign orgasmic cephalgia. Headache 13: 181–187

Pearce JMS, Foster JB (1965) An investigation of complicated migraine. Neurology 15: 333–340

Perret G, Nishioka H (1966) Arterio-venous malformations. In: Sahs AL et al. (eds) Intracranial aneurysms and subarachnoid haemorrhage. A cooperative study. J.B. Lippincott, Philadelphia Toronto, pp 200–222

Pfister CW, de Pando B (1962) Cerebral haemorrhage simulating acute myocardial infarction. Dis Chest 42: 206–207

Plum F, Posner JB (1980) The diagnosis of stupor and coma. F.A. Davis, Philadelphia

Pompeu F, Sampaio de Lacerda PR (1979) Subarachnoid haemorrhage due to S. mansoni. A rare aetiology. J Neurology 221: 203–207

Price DL, Harris JL, New PFJ, Cantu RC (1970) Cardiac myxoma. A clinico-pathologic and angiographic study. Arch Neurol 23: 558–567

Quinckel KE, Whaley ARJ (1967) Subarachnoid haemorrhage in a patient with hereditary haemorrhagic telangiectasia. Neurology 17: 716–719

Ray H, Wahal KM (1957) Subarachnoid haemorrhage in subacute bacterial endocarditis. Neurology 7: 265–269

Richardson JC, Hyland HH (1941) Intracranial aneurysms. A clinical and pathological study of subarachnoid and intracerebral haemorrhage caused by berry aneurysms. Medicine (Baltimore) 20:1–88

Roach MR, Drake CG (1965) Ruptured cerebral aneurysms caused by micro-organisms. N Engl J Med 273:240–244

Robertson EG (1949) Cerebral lesions due to intracranial aneurysms. Brain 72:150–185

Rovit RL, Fein JM (1972) Pituitary apoplexy: A review of and reappraisal. J Neurosurg 37:280–288

Rubinstein MK, Cohen NH (1964) Ehlers-Danlos syndrome associated with multiple intracranial aneurysms. Neurology 14:125–132

Rucker CW (1966) The causes of paralysis of the 3rd, 4th and 6th cranial nerves. Am J Ophthalmol 61:1293–1298

Russell DS (1954) Discussion: The pathology of spontaneous intracranial haemorrhage. Proc Soc Med 47:689–693

Russell DS, Rubinstein LJ (1977) Pathology of tumours of the nervous system, 4th edn. Edward Arnold, London, pp. 116–146

Sachdev VP, Drapkin AJ, Hollin SA, Malis LI (1977) Subarachnoid haemorrhage following intranasal procedure. Surg Neurol 8:122–125

Sahs AL, Perret GE, Locksley HB, Nishioka H (1966) Intracranial aneurysms and subarachnoid haemorrhage: A cooperative study, J.B. Lippincott, Philadelphia Toronto

Sands IJ (1941) Diagnosis and management of subarachnoid haemorrhage. Arch Neurol Psychiatry 46:973–1005

Scheie HG, Hogan TF (1957) Angioid streaks and generalised arterial disease. Arch Ophthalmol 57:855–868

Scott M (1975) Spontaneous intracerebral haematoma caused by cerebral neoplasms. Report of eight verified cases. J Neurosurg 42:338–342

Silverstein A (1979) Neurological complications of anticoagulation therapy. A neurologist's review. Arch Intern Med 139:217–220

Simonsen J (1963) Fatal subarachnoid haemorrhage originating in an intracranial chordoma. Acta Path Microbiol Scand 59:13–20

Slade WR, Rabiner AM (1973) Plasma thromboplastin antecedent deficiency and subarachnoid haemorrhage. Angiology 24:533–537

Smith RO (1968) Ice cream headache. In: Vinken PJ, Bruyn GW (eds) Handbook of clinical neurology, vol 5. North Holland Publishing Co., Amsterdam

Snyder M, Renaudin J (1977) Intracranial haemorrhage associated with anticoagulation therapy. Surg Neurol 7:31–34

Steele JJ, Kilburn HL, Leech RW (1972) Phytotic (mycotic) intracranial aneurysms with an unusual pathogenesis. Pediatrics 50:936–939

Steinbok P, Dolman CL, Kaan K (1977) Pineocytomas presenting as subarachnoid haemorrhage. Report of two cases. J Neurosurg 47:776–780

Sterling GM (1965) Conn's syndrome and subarachnoid haemorrhage. Br Med J I:839–840

Strauss I, Globus JH, Ginsburg SW (1932) Spontaneous subarachnoid haemorrhage. Its relation to aneurysms of

cerebral blood vessels. Arch Neurol Psychiatry 27:1080–1132

Suwanwela C, Suwanwela N, Charuchinda S, Hongsaprabhas C (1972) Intracranial mycotic aneurysms of extravascular origin. J Neurosurg 36:552–559

Suzuki J (1979) Cerebral aneurysm. Experience with 1000 directly operated cases. Neuron, Toyko

Taylor AB, Whitfield AGW (1936) Subarachnoid haemorrhage based on observations of 81 cases. Quart J Med 5:461–472

Tourtellotte WW, Somer JF, Parker JA, Itabashi HH, De Jong RN (1958) A study on traumatic lumbar puncture. Neurology 8:129–134

Tourtellotte WW, Metz LN, Bryan ER, De Jong RN (1964) Spontaneous subarachnoid haemorrhage. Factors affecting the rate of clearing of the C.S.F. Neurology 14:301–306

Tuhy JE, Maurice GL, Niles NR (1958) Wegener's granulomatosis. Am J Med 25:638–646

Villiers JC (1966) Intracranial haemorrhage in patients treated with monoamine oxidate inhibitors. Br J Psychiatry 112:109–118

Visconti EB, Hilgartner MW (1980) Recognition and management of C.N.S. haemorrhage in haemophilia. Paediatrician 9:127–137

Voigt K, Yasargil MG (1976) Cerebral cavernous haemangiomas or cavernomas. Neurochirurgia 19:59–68

Wakai S, Fukushima T, Furihata T, Sano K (1979) Association of cerebral aneurysm with pituitary adenoma. Surg Neurol 12:503–507

Wakai S, Fukushima T, Teramoto A, Sano K (1981) Pituitary apoplexy. Its incidence and clinical significance. J Neurosurg 55:187–193

Wakai S, Yamakawa K, Manaka S, Takakura K (1982) Spontaneous intracranial haemorrhage caused by brain tumor. Its incidence and clinical significance. Neurosurgery 10:437–444

Watson P, Fekete J, Deck J (1977) Central nervous system vasculitis in rheumatoid arthritis. Le Journal Canadien des Sciences Neurologiques 4:269–272

Weber RB, Daroff RB, Mackey EA (1970) Pathology of oculomotor palsy in diabetics. Neurology 20:835–838

Weidler DJ (1974) Myocardial damage and cardiac arrhythmias after intracranial haemorrhage. A critical review. Stroke 5:759–764

Weinstein L, Rubin RH (1973) Infective endocarditis. Prog Cardiovasc Dis 16:239–274

West HH, Mani RL, Eisenberg RL, Tuerk K, Stucker TB (1977) Normal cerebral arteriography in patients with spontaneous subarachnoid haemorrhage. Neurology 27:592–594

Yasargil MG, So SC (1976) Cerebellopontine angle meningioma presenting as subarachnoid haemorrhage. Surg Neurol 6:3–6

Yonas H, Agamanolis D, Takaoka Y, White RJ (1977) Dissecting intracranial aneurysms. Surg Neurol 8:407–415

6 Computerised Tomography

Introduction

The technique of computerised tomography (CT) was developed by Godfrey Hounsfield (1973). This major achievement earned him a knighthood and the award of the Nobel Prize for Medicine in 1979.

The CT findings of intracerebral haemorrhage were first described by Paxton and Ambrose (1974) at the Atkinson Morley Hospital, where the first prototype CT scanner was installed in 1972. Hayward and O'Reilly (1976) showed that the accuracy of CT scanning in identifying the cause of the bleed (e.g. aneurysm rupture or primary spontaneous haemorrhage) approached 90%. Reports of the CT scan findings in SAH due to ruptured aneurysms (Kendall et al. 1976; Liliequist et al. 1977), spontaneous haemorrhage (Hayward and O'Reilly 1976) and arteriovenous malformations (Hayward 1976) quickly followed.

Cerebral angiography still remains the definitive investigative tool in the assessment of the cause of SAH. However, in the practical management of patients with a ruptured aneurysm or arteriovenous malformation it is important to understand the pathological changes produced within the brain (e.g. haematoma, infarction, cerebral oedema and hydrocephalus). Demonstration of these pathological changes which contribute to patient morbidity and mortality, and the initiation of appropriate therapy, has been revolutionised by the advent of CT.

Material

The contents of this chapter are based on an analysis of the CT scan findings in 500 proven, but not consecutive, cases of SAH. In this group, SAH was due to a ruptured aneurysm in 308 cases (single 245 and multiple 63), an arteriovenous malformation in 46 cases, spontaneous haemorrhage (no cause found or related to atheroma or hypertension) in 64 cases, and a tumour in 7 cases. In 75 cases no cause for the SAH could be found on four vessel angiography.

CT Scan Appearances

The typical findings resulting from an SAH which can be demonstrated on CT scan are outlined in Table 6.1.

Blood in the Subarachnoid Cisterns

Clotted blood characteristically shows as a high attenuation lesion in the subarachnoid cisterns (Fig. 6.1). The contribution of the various constituents of the blood to this high attenuation at CT

Table 6.1. CT scan findings in SAH

Blood in subarachnoid cisterns
Haematoma
  Intracerebral
  Intraventricular
  Subdural
Low density lesions
  Oedema
  Infarct
Hydrocephalus
  Early
  Late
Calcification
  Giant aneurysm and AVMs
Contrast enhancement
  Demonstration of aneurysms
  Demonstration of AVM
  Occult AVMs
  Cisternal enhancement
  Enhancement around haematoma
Serial Studies
  Complications of SAH pre- and postoperatively

Abbreviation: AVM, arteriovenous malformation

has been shown to be mainly due to its haemoglobin content (New and Arinow 1976; Norman et al. 1977). As clotted blood retracts, serum is extruded, the haemoglobin concentration increases, and with it the attenuation of the blood. The length of time that the high attenuation persists at CT is dependent on the amount of blood in a given part of the subarachnoid space, but usually it lasts for about a week, although rarely it may be seen for up to 13 days. After 5–7 days, blood becomes isodense, with a density similar to the surrounding brain, so that the involved cisterns are no longer visualised at CT. The cisterns then resume their previous low density after about 14 days, as the CSF replaces blood.

The majority of workers (Hayward and O'Reilly 1976; Kendall et al. 1976; Scott et al. 1977; Brismar 1979; Liliequist and Lindqvist 1980) are in agreement that in 80%–90% of patients scan-

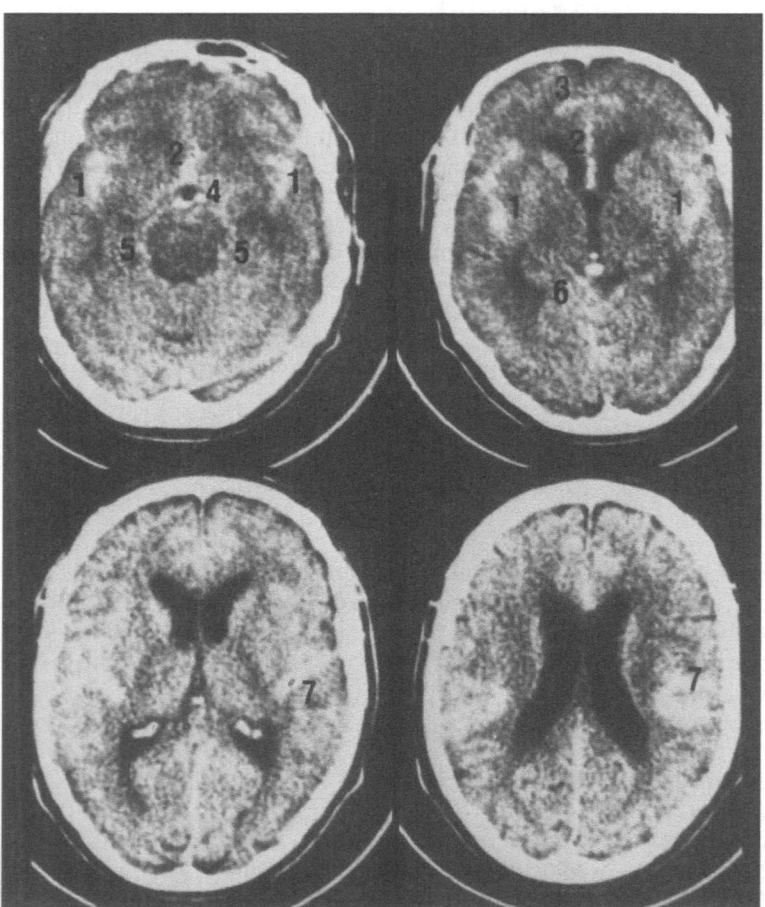

Fig. 6.1. Generalised blood of high attenutation in the basal subarachnoid cisterns. *Key: 1*, sylvian fissure; *2*, interhemispheric fissure; *3*, pericallosal cistern; *4*, suprasellar cistern; *5*, ambient cistern; *6*, quadrigeminal cistern, *7*, cerebral sulci.

Table 6.2. CT scan site of blood in subarachnoid cisterns in relation to aneurysm site in 245 cases of SAH with a single aneurysm

Aneurysm site	No.	IH	SF	SF bilat	Sup	Amb	Peric	Pont	Quad	No. SAH blood
Anterior communicating	77	51	10	8	7	5	2	0	0	7
Middle cerebral	61	9	41	2	4	1	0	0	0	16
Posterior communicating	47	15	17	8	14	12	0	2	0	12
ICA bifurcation	20	2	3	1	4	1	0	0	0	14
Pericallosal	10	4	0	0	2	0	6	0	0	3
Ophthalmic	3	2	1	0	1	0	0	0	0	1
PICA	14	0	1	0	1	2	0	0	0	16
Basilar tip	13	0	1	0	2	2	0	4	0	6

Abbreviations: IH, interhemispheric fissure; SF, sylvian fissure; SF bilat, bilateral sylvian fissure; Sup, suprasellar cistern; Amb, ambient cistern; Peric, pericallosal cistern; Pont, pontine cistern; Quad, quadrigeminal cistern

ned within the first 5–7 days after an SAH, blood can be demonstrated in the subarachnoid space. In this series, CT detection of subarachnoid blood occurred in 88.2% of cases scanned within 5 days of the bleed, and in 57% of cases scanned 6–14 days after the bleed. CT evidence of subarachnoid blood was not found in any of the cases scanned after 14 days.

The pattern of distribution of blood in the subarachnoid cisterns in relationship to different aneurysm sites is shown in Table 6.2. In many cases the pattern is non-specific with blood involving most of the subarachnoid cisterns (Fig. 6.1), but the location of the cistern with the largest collection of blood is a good guide as to the approximate site of the aneurysm, especially with an anterior communicating artery aneurysm. If one cannot precisely localise the site of the bleed, it is often possible to lateralise it, and this is of value in planning the type and extent of angiography.

Anterior communicating artery aneurysms frequently show blood in the midline interhemis-pheric cistern (Fig. 6.2), but in many cases one or both sylvian fissures are also involved and the diagnosis depends on showing a maximal concentration of blood in the interhemispheric fissure (Fig. 6.3). Anterior communicating aneurysms, as will be discussed, frequently also show a small localised haematoma in the septum pellucidum which further aids localisation (Fig. 6.8). Blood largely confined to the sylvian fissure is suggestive of a middle cerebral artery or posterior communicating artery aneurysm (Fig. 6.4). Posterior communicating artery aneurysms more frequently show generalised blood involving the sylvian fissure, suprasellar and ambient cisterns, and less commonly give rise to localised haematoma formation compared with middle cerebral artery aneurysms. Basilar tip aneurysms may show blood in the pontine, and occasionally the ambient and suprasellar cisterns. More characteristically, however, one may see a small area of high density

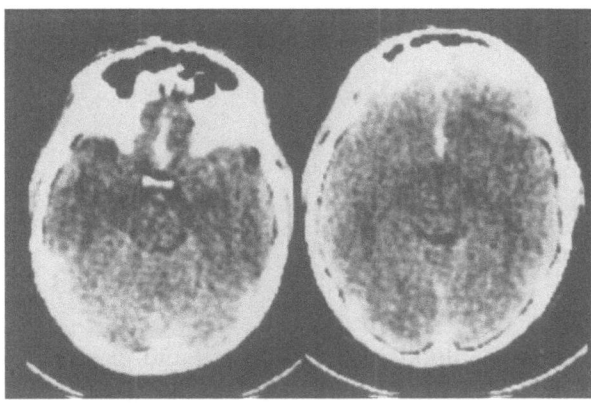

Fig. 6.2. Subarachnoid blood confined to the interhemispheric fissure in a patient with a ruptured anterior communicating artery aneurysm.

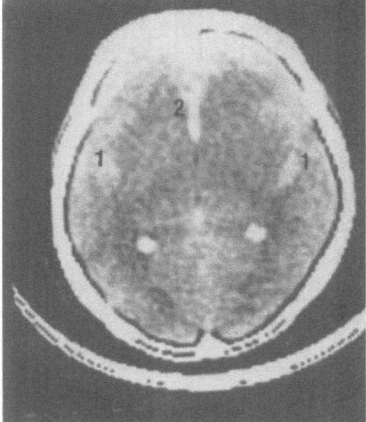

Fig. 6.3. Subarachnoid blood is demonstrated in both sylvian fissures (*1*) and the interhemispheric fissure (*2*). The maximal concentration of blood is in the interhemispheric cistern however, indicating that the bleed is most likely to have been due to an anterior communicating artery aneurysm.

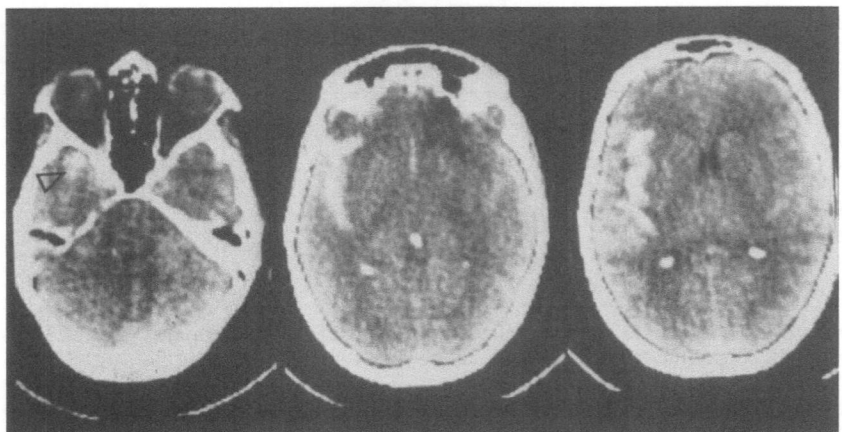

Fig. 6.4. Subarachnoid blood is largely confined to the left sylvian fissure. A small amount of blood is also present in the interhemispheric and right sylvian fissure. There is a small haematoma in the tip of the left temporal lobe (*open arrrowhead*). This patient had a ruptured left middle cerebral trifurcation aneurysm.

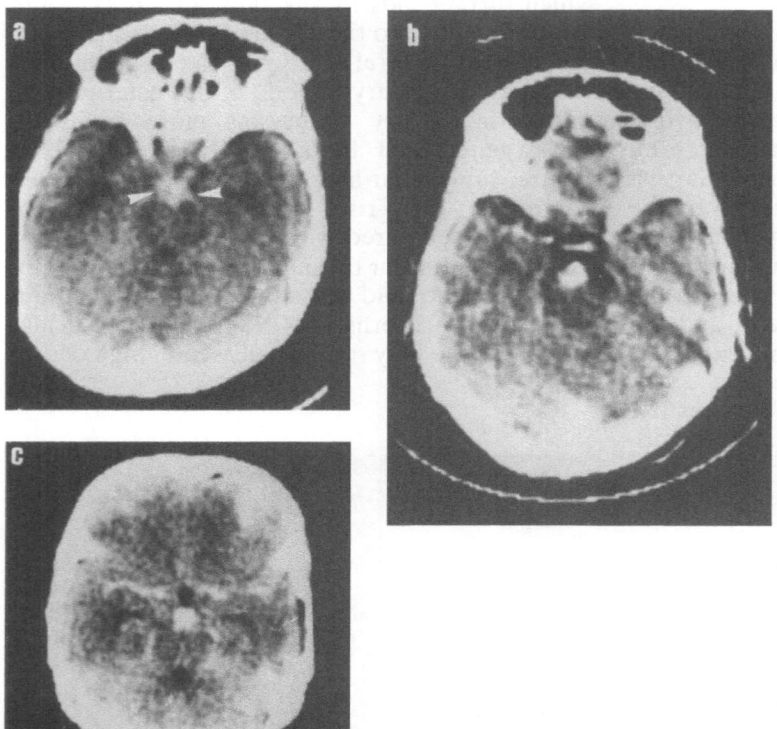

Fig. 6.5. a A basilar tip aneurysm, shown as a small high density lesion in the front of the pons and in the posterior part of the suprasellar cistern (*arrowhead*). **b, c** There is uniform contrast enhancement of the aneurysm sac.

due to the aneurysm sac situated in the posterior part of the suprasellar cistern, in front of the brain stem, which demonstrates contrast enhancement (Fig. 6.5). None of our patients with posterior inferior cerebellar artery aneurysms had CT evidence of blood in the subarachnoid cisterns. A small area of haemorrhage in the pericallosal cistern may be found with pericallosal artery aneurysms but more frequently they show a haematoma in the corpus callosum (Fig. 6.6).

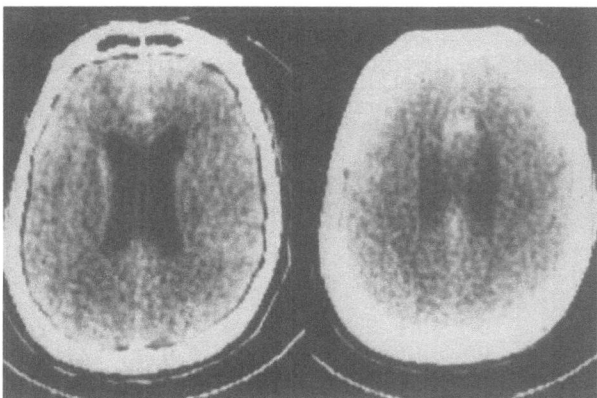

Fig. 6.6. CT scan in a patient with a bleed due to a pericallosal artery aneurysm, showing blood in the pericallosal cistern and a small haematoma in the corpus callosum.

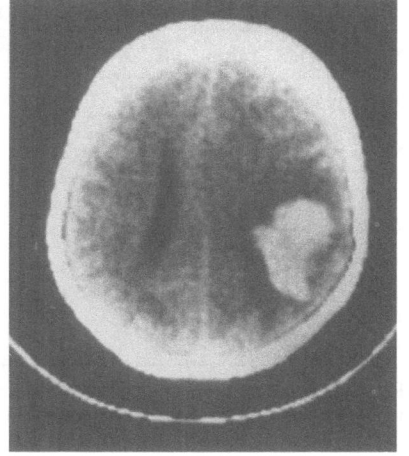

Fig. 6.7. CT scan in a patient with spontaneous hypertensive haemorrhage showing a haematoma of homogeneous high attenuation in the right parietal region, with typical low density halos surrounding it.

The high accuracy of CT in detecting subarachnoid blood has meant that painful and potentially dangerous lumbar puncture in those patients with space-occupying haematoma may be avoided. However, the majority of cases of SAH are first seen in the peripheral referring hospital where CT scan facilities may not be available, and therefore diagnostic lumbar puncture is required for early diagnosis. A negative or equivocal CT scan does not exclude an SAH.

Intracerebral Haematoma

CT is superior to angiography in demonstrating a haematoma, showing its extent and any intraventricular extension. CT allows rapid identification of large, life-threatening haematoma, which is potentially amenable to emergency surgical evacuation. The typical CT appearances of a haematoma consist of a homogeneous region of increased attenuation, usually with a small, low density halo (Fig. 6.7), which, it is believed, corresponds to a zone of ischaemic necrosis (Kendall and Radue 1978). Serial CT scans will show a progressive reduction of the increased attenuation at the periphery of the lesion, until eventually a final CT picture resembling an old infarct is produced.

A review of the literature suggests that the frequency with which CT will demonstrate an intracerebral haematoma following aneurysm rupture is in the order of 30%–40% of cases (Kendall et al. 1976; Weir et al. 1977; Modesti and Binet 1978; Brismar 1979; Imanaga et al. 1980). In this series, haematoma formation was demonstrated in 36.7% of cases of aneurysm rupture. Haematomas were frequently found in association with anterior communicating and middle cerebral artery aneurysms. Posterior communicating and posterior circulation aneurysms relatively infrequently produced haematomas (Table 6.3).

The pattern of distribution of intracerebral haematomas is more specific than that of subarachnoid cistern haemorrhage for aneurysm location. Table 6.4 outlines the position of haematoma found at CT and its relationship to aneurysm site.

Anterior communicating aneurysms produce a highly characteristic haematoma in the septum pellucidum (Weisberg 1979; Silver et al. 1981)

Table 6.3. CT scan demonstration of intracerebral haematoma and aneurysm site

Aneurysm site	No.	No. of haematomas	%
Anterior communicating	77	35	45.5
Middle cerebral	61	27	44.3
Posterior communicating	47	5	10.6
ICA bifurcation	20	14	70.0
Pericallosal	10	7	70.0
Ophthalmic	3	2	66.6
PICA	14	0	0
Basilar tip	13	0	0
Total aneurysms	245	90	36.7

Table 6.4. CT scan site of haematoma in relation to aneurysm site in 245 cases of SAH with a single aneurysm

Aneurysm site	No.	SP-IH	Temp	SF	FT	FR	CC	Bg-Thal	Par	Occip	Pont	Cereb	SDH	IV	Normal
Anterior communicating	77	19	2	0	0	12	2	0	0	0	0	0	0	11	42
Middle cerebral	61	0	17	4	4	2	0	0	0	0	0	0	1	5	34
Posterior communicating	47	0	5	0	0	0	0	0	0	0	0	0	1	0	42
ICA bifurcation	20	1	2	0	2	1	0	8	0	0	0	0	0	7	6
Pericallosal	10	2	0	0	0	3	2	0	0	0	0	0	0	0	3
Ophthalmic	3	1	0	0	0	1	0	0	0	0	0	0	0	0	1
PICA	14	0	0	0	0	0	0	0	0	0	0	0	0	0	14
Basilar tip	13	0	0	0	0	0	0	0	0	0	0	0	0	2	11

Abbreviations: SP-IH, septum pellucidum–interhemispheric fissure; Temp, temporal; SF, sylvian fissure; FT, frontotemporal; FR, frontal; CC, corpus callosum; Bg-Thal, basal ganglia–thalamus; Par, parietal; Occip, occipital; Pont, pontine; Cereb, cerebellar; SDH, subdural haematoma; IV, intraventricular

(Fig. 6.8) and/or the inferior medial part of the frontal lobe (Fig. 6.9). Unilateral flame-like haematomas involving the medial part of the frontal lobe may also occur (Fig. 6.10). In two cases in this series pericallosal artery aneurysms produced a septum pellucidum haematoma.

Haematomas in the corpus callosum may occur with pericallosal aneurysms but may also be present as a direct extension from an anterior communicating artery aneurysm (two cases). Internal carotid bifurcation aneurysms may produce frontal or temporal haematomas but a significant number (40%) occurred in the basal ganglia and thalamus and, therefore, distinction from a hypertensive haemorrhage proved difficult on CT alone.

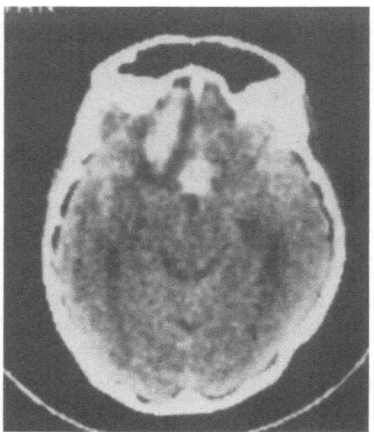

Fig. 6.9. CT scan in a patient with an anterior communicating artery aneurysm showing a haematoma in the inferomedial part of the left frontal lobe and in the septal region.

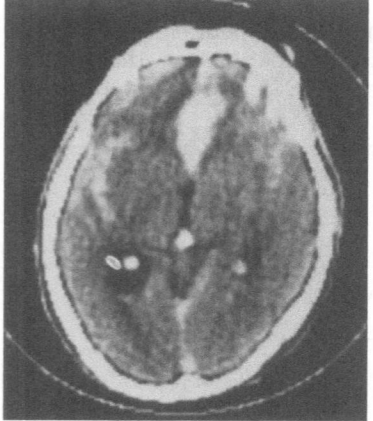

Fig. 6.8. A highly characteristic septal haematoma; septal haematomas are frequently seen with a ruptured anterior communicating artery aneurysm.

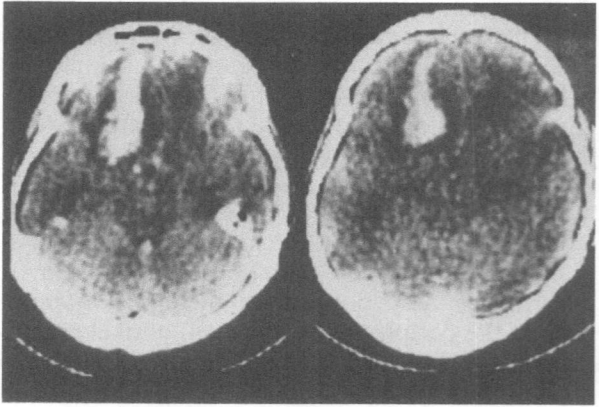

Fig. 6.10. Anterior communicating artery aneurysm with a flame-shaped haematoma involving the medial part of the left frontal lobe.

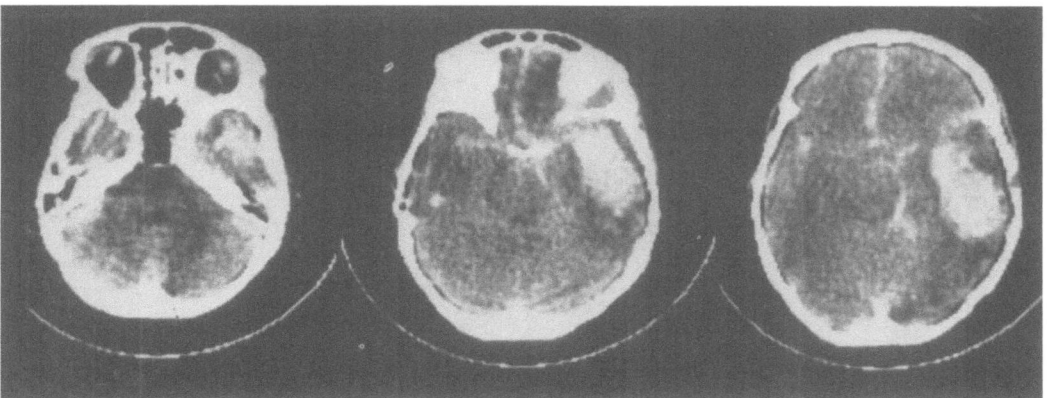

Fig. 6.11. Patient with a ruptured middle cerebral artery aneurysm in which the CT scan shows a haematoma in the temporal lobe. There is also extensive subarachnoid blood in the interhemispheric fissure and the suprasellar and ambient cisterns.

Middle cerebral artery aneurysms may rupture directly into the brain substance, producing a temporal lobe haematoma (Fig. 6.11), or, less commonly, a pure sylvian fissure haematoma (Fig. 6.12). Frontal lobe haematomas, however, were observed in four cases. Posterior communicating artery aneurysms in this series produced intracerebral haematomas in only 10.6% of cases, but when present, they were usually in the temporal lobe. In this series, none of the posterior circulation aneurysms produced a haematoma. In Table 6.5, localisation of the site of haematoma due to aneurysm rupture is compared with those due to arteriovenous malformation or spontaneous (hypertensive or arteriosclerotic) haemorrhage. Primary spontaneous intracerebral haematomas tend to produce haematomas in the parietal lobe (29.7%), basal ganglia and thalamus (14.6%), cerebellar hemisphere (11%) and pons (4.7%) (Fig. 6.13). Haematomas due to arteriovenous malformations produce haematomas in

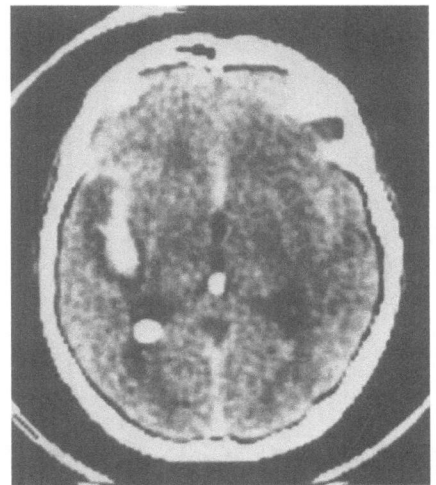

Fig. 6.12. CT scan in a case of ruptured middle cerebral artery aneurysm, showing a haematoma confined to the right sylvian fissure.

Table 6.5. CT scan comparison of haematoma site in aneurysm, arteriovenous malformation (AVM) and spontaneous haemorrhage groups

Haematoma site	Aneurysms (245)	AVM (46)	Spont. haemorrhage (64)
Septal	23 (9.4%)	0 (0%)	1 (1.56%)
Temporal	26 (10.6%)	3 (6.5%)	2 (2.1%)
Sylvian fissure	4 (1.6%)	0 (0%)	0 (0%)
Frontal	19 (7.75%)	1 (2.1%)	0 (0%)
Frontotemporal	6 (2.4%)	0 (0%)	0 (0%)
Corpus callosum	4 (1.6%)	0 (0%)	0 (0%)
Basal ganglia/thalamus	8 (3.2%)	7 (15.2%)	26 (40.6%)
Parietal	0 (0%)	17 (36.9%)	19 (29.7%)
Occipital	0 (0%)	6 (12.6%)	8 (12.5%)
Pontine	0 (0%)	2 (4.2%)	3 (4.7%)
Cerebellar	0 (0%)	8 (17.3%)	7 (11.0%)
Intraventricular	25 (10.2%)	18 (39.0%)	20 (31.25%)

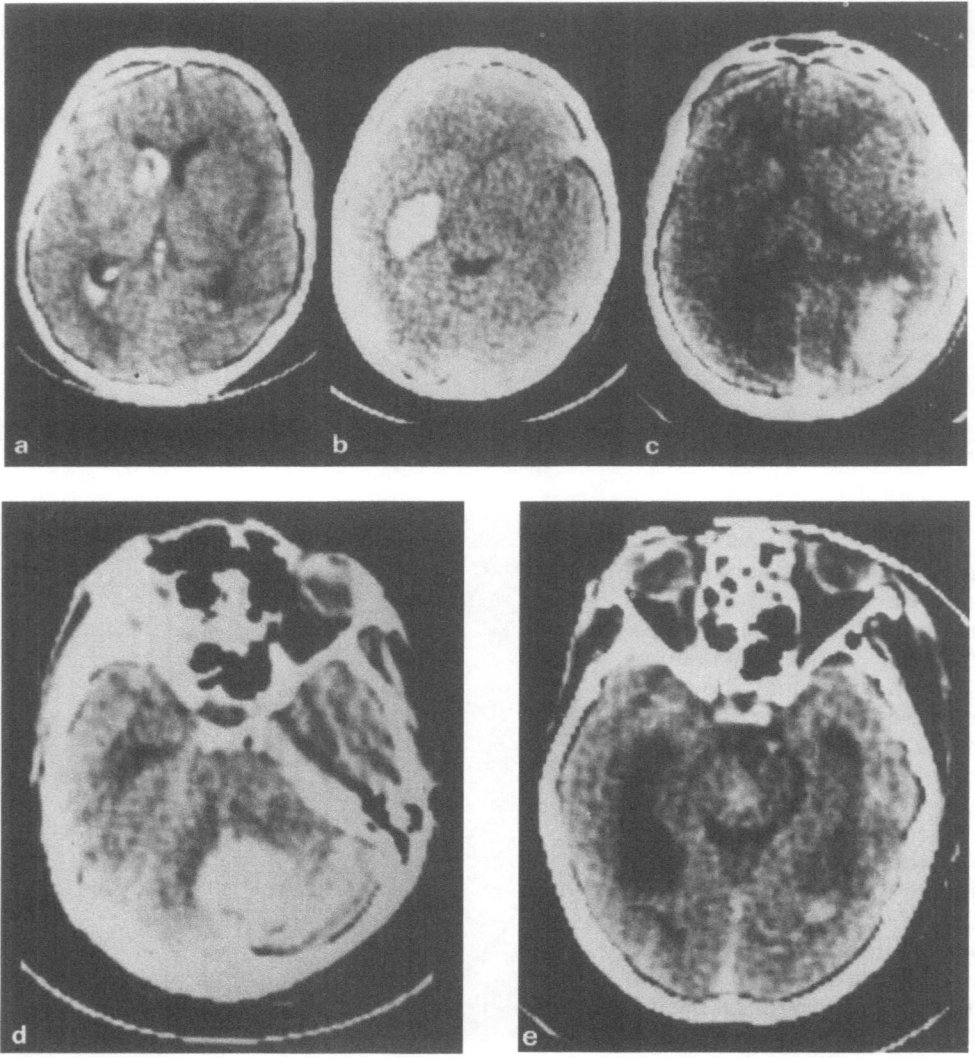

Fig. 6.13a–e. Common sites for spontaneous intracerebral haematomas. **a** caudate nucleus; **b** basal ganglia and thalamus; **c** parietal lobe; **d** cerebellum; **e** pons

similar sites, including the parietal lobe (36.9%), cerebellar hemisphere (17.3%), basal ganglia and thalamus (15.2%) and occipital lobes (12.6%).

The features which may help to distinguish between a haematoma produced by an arteriovenous malformation and one due to spontaneous haemorrhage include the demonstration of serpiginous areas of enhancement related to feeding arteries and draining veins (Fig. 6.21). However, clinical features, including the patient's age and the presence of hypertension or generalised atheroma, are also useful for making a correct diagnosis.

Intraventricular Haematoma

Intraventricular haematoma (IVH) most commonly results from extension of an intracerebral or subarachnoid haematoma (Fig. 6.14) rather than retrograde passage of blood through the fourth ventricular foramina from the subarachnoid space. Since the introduction of CT scanning, IVH has been more frequently diagnosed and does not necessarily indicate a fatal outcome. Silver et al. (1981) reported CT evidence of IVH in 17% of 81 cases of ruptured aneurysm. Vassi-

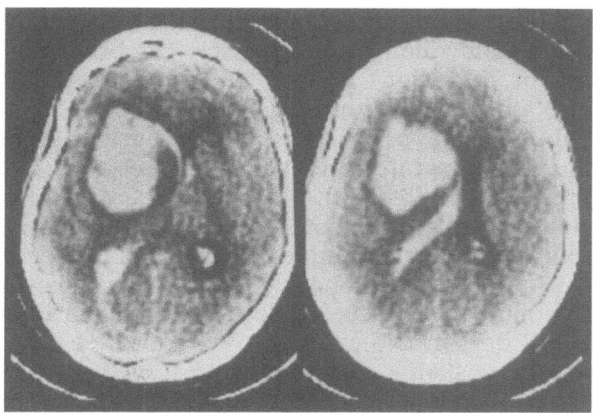

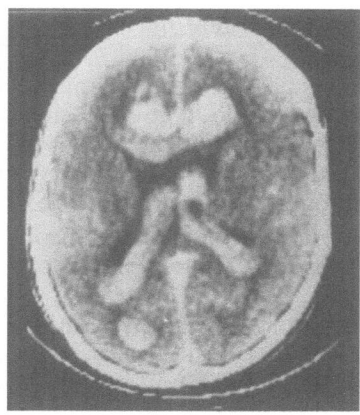

Fig. 6.14. A very large haematoma in the left frontotemporal region with deep extension into the basal ganglia and thalamus and rupture into the left lateral ventricle.

Fig. 6.15. There is extensive haematoma in both lateral ventricles, which show moderate hydrocephalus.

louthis and Richardson (1979) reported a 13% incidence of IVH in 200 cases of SAH (80% of which were due to ruptured aneurysm). Intraventricular haematoma associated with aneurysmal rupture was usually related to either anterior communicating artery or internal carotid bifurcation aneurysms.

In this series 63 patients (12%) showed IVH. It occurred in 18 out of 46 cases of arteriovenous malformations (39%), 20 out of 64 cases of spontaneous haemorrhage (31.25%), and 25 out of 245 cases of ruptured aneurysm (10.2%).

Patients with CT evidence of IVH may show evidence of early acute hydrocephalus (Fig. 6.15). Intraventricular haematoma may produce acute hydrocephalus in about 35% of cases (Vassilouthis and Richardson 1979). The presence of IVH does not seem to influence the development of communicating hydrocephalus.

The size of the IVH is probably not of prognostic significance, but the ventriculocranial ratio (VCR) is a more sensitive index in predicting survival (Mohr et al. 1983). The VCR is the ratio of the width of the ventricles behind the frontal horns between the caudate nucleus to the width of the brain at the same level. Vassilouthis and Richardson (1979) established the normal range and the mean VCR plus two standard deviations was 0.155. In the series of Mohr et al. (1983), no patient with a VCR of 0.25 or more survived.

Subdural Haematoma

CT evidence of a subdural haematoma was demonstrated in only two cases of SAH due to aneurysmal rupture in this series. One further case of subdural haematoma was not demonstrated by CT but shown at surgery. The overall incidence was therefore about 1%. Adams et al. (1983) have reported a 1% incidence of CT-demonstrated subdural haematoma associated with rupture of aneurysms.

Weir et al. (1984) found 18 cases of subdural haematoma (incidence 2%) in an analysis of 897 cases of ruptured aneurysm. At CT the subdural haematomas were unilateral and hyperdense of variable thickness. In 72% of cases the ruptured aneurysm was on the internal carotid artery. In 17 cases (94%) there was evidence of blood in other locations. Death occurred in 50% of cases and these were the cases showing a greater midline shift, larger haematomas and a higher percentage of pre-operative herniation. These authors suggest that early evacuation of the haematoma with clipping of the aneurysm should be carried out since the not infrequent development of tentorial herniation has such an adverse effect on outcome.

To differentiate subdural haematoma due to ruptured aneurysm from trauma on the CT scan, the following CT criteria are important (Weir et al. 1984):

1. Subdural haematomas due to ruptured aneurysms are unilateral and hyperdense and usually crescentic in convexity or triangular over the lower sylvian fissure. Traumatic subdural haematomas are more likely to be iso- or

hypodense, may be bilateral, and may be lentiform as well as crescentic.

2. In subdural haematoma from ruptured aneurysm there is frequently blood at other sites, e.g. subarachnoid, intracerebral or intraventricular. In trauma only the subdural haematoma or perhaps an associated contusion will be shown.

3. Direct visualisation of the aneurysm on contrast-enhanced CT scans may be helpful.

If there is no history of significant head injury then angiography should be considered.

Low Attenuation Areas

Low density areas on the CT scan may be due to ischaemic oedema or infarction (Fig. 6.16). In the presence of vasospasm there is a reduced perfusion pressure in the territory affected, which, if not augmented by an adequate collateral circulation, leads to impairment of the blood–brain barrier, with the production of cerebral oedema. If the perfusion pressure is further reduced, and autoregulation is lost, a definitive area of infarction is produced.

Various authors (Bryan et al. 1979; Weisberg 1979; Saito et al. 1979; Silver et al. 1981) have observed a high degree of association between low density on CT scan and spasm at angiography. Adams et al. (1983) found CT evidence of areas of low density (presumably cerebral oedema or infarction) in only 18 of 1378 patients (1.3%) scanned within 3 days of the SAH.

In our series of 245 cases of SAH due to a single aneurysm rupture, pre-operative vasospasm was present in 73 (29.8%). CT at the time of admission showed evidence of a low density area consistent with oedema or infarction in only 11 of these cases. In three further cases, an infarct was shown on follow-up CT. The CT scan interval after SAH was 3 days in two cases, 4–6 days in three cases and more than 7 days in nine cases. All patients were grade three or four and CT evidence of infarction occurred only in those patients with clinical features suggesting ischaemia. Evidence of infarction was always accompanied by angiographic evidence of vasospasm, e.g. severe generalised spasm in seven cases, moderate segmental spasm in five cases and localised spasm in two cases. The latter two cases showed evidence of infarction only on follow-up CT; however, it is possible that spasm may have become more severe in these cases. The low incidence of CT changes suggesting infarction in this series is perhaps explained by the fact that 78% of our cases were scanned within 6 days of the bleed before the onset of vasospasm. It is generally accepted that vasospasm is maximal at 6–13 days, and usually neurological symptoms (and CT evidence of infarction) develop 1 or 2 days later. Repeat CT scans after a week in this series would no doubt have shown a higher proportion of low attenuation areas due to infarction.

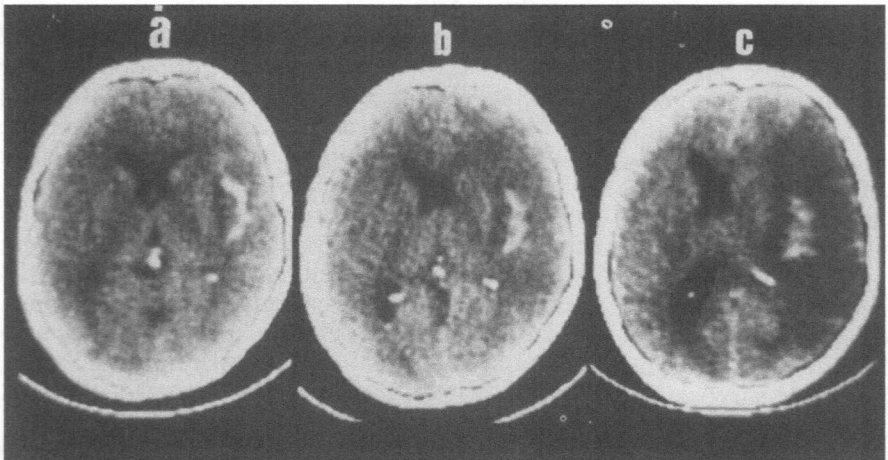

Fig. 6.16. a, b. Blood is present in the right sylvian fissure. In **b** there is a suggestion of low density in the right middle cerebral artery distribution, with some compression of the right frontal horn. **c** Repeat CT scan 2 days later now shows an extensive area of low density in the right middle cerebral artery territory, consistent with cerebral infarction. There is displacement of the ventricular system to the left side.

Hydrocephalus

The reported incidence of hydrocephalus following SAH has varied between 10% (Yasargil et al. 1973) and 34% (Galera and Greitz 1970), depending on whether radiological or clinical criteria were used. Foltz and Ward (1956) recognise two phases of hydrocephalus following SAH: an acute phase resulting from blood in the basal cisterns or ventricular system, producing a mechanical obstruction to the flow of CSF, and a chronic phase which may occur any time between 2 and 6 weeks following the bleed and is explained on the basis of the development of leptomeningeal fibrosis, producing obstruction of the CSF pathways at the tentorial hiatus and/or arachnoidal granulations.

CT scanning provides a non-invasive method of demonstrating acute hydrocephalus (Fig. 6.15) and has proved very valuable in defining chronic progressive hydrocephalus (communicating hydrocephalus) (Fig. 6.17), which is often very subtle in its clinical presentation and requires a high index of clinical suspicion for diagnosis. The reported CT incidence of hydrocephalus has been very variable. Vassilouthis and Richardson (1979), using the VCR on the CT scan, reported that 12.4% of patients with an SAH would develop ventricular enlargement. Silver et al. (1981) demonstrated evidence of hydrocephalus at CT in 47 (58%) out of 81 patients with SAH due to ruptured aneurysm. Yamamoto et al. (1983), accepting a VCR of 1:5 or more as representing hydrocephalus, showed CT evidence of ventricu-

lar enlargement in 29.2% of their cases. Adams et al. (1983) found hydrocephalus on CT in about 16% of their patients who were scanned within 3 days of the bleed.

CT scans in our series of 245 cases of SAH with a single aneurysm showed hydrocephalus in 36 cases (14.2%). We made use of the VCR to assess ventricular size. A VCR below 1:6.4 was considered normal. Ratios between 1:5 and 1:6.5 were considered to represent minimal enlargement, 1:4 to 1:5 moderate enlargement, and above 1:4 marked ventricular dilatation (Vassilouthis and Richardson 1979). Using these criteria, hydrocephalus was assessed as mild in 64%, moderate in 32% and marked in 4% of cases. In the majority of cases it was not clinically significant and did not require shunting.

Vassilouthis and Richardson (1979) reported delayed significant ventricular enlargement (communicating hydrocephalus) in 7% of cases. Symon (1979) reported significant hydrocephalus requiring shunting in 6% of a group of 200 cases of aneurysm rupture. The diagnosis is made on the basis of clinical features and CT scan findings. A CT diagnosis of communicating hydrocephalus is considered highly probable in the presence of (a) moderate to severe hydrocephalus (Fig. 6.17), (b) rounding of the frontal horns, (c) evidence of periventricular lucency (Fig. 6.20) and (d) small or obliterated cerebral sulci (Gunasekera and Richardson 1977).

We confirm previous reports (Vassilouthis and Richardson 1979; Yamamoto et al. 1983) that there is a significantly higher incidence of hydrocephalus associated with anterior communicating artery aneurysms. We found a low incidence with middle cerebral artery aneurysms.

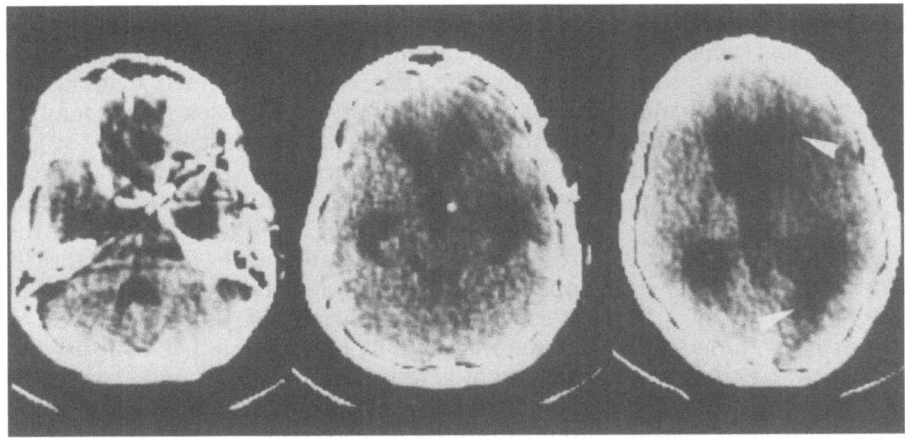

Fig. 6.17. Communicating hydrocephalus. The lateral ventricles, third ventricle and fourth ventricle show moderate enlargement. There is evidence of periventricular lucency.

Galera and Greitz (1970) and Yasargil et al. (1973), unlike Griffith et al. (1972), found a strong correlation between the presence of arterial spasm and the occurrence of hydrocephalus. Galera and Greitz observed spasm in 78% of those patients developing hydrocephalus and in 41% of patients who did not develop hydrocephalus. In our series of 245 patients with single aneurysm rupture, spasm occurred in 31 out of the 64 cases with CT evidence of hydrocephalus (48.4%) compared with 41 out of 181 cases (22.6%) without CT evidence of hydrocephalus. Cerebral infarct diagnosed clinically and radiologically preceded the development of chronic ventricular enlargement in 45% of cases reported by Vassilouthis and Richardson (1979).

Contrast Enhancement

In the majority of cases of SAH, contrast-enhanced scans are not required, since plain CT scans will confirm the diagnosis and help localise or lateralise the site of the bleed prior to definitive angiographic investigations. Contrast-enhanced CT scans were carried out in 120 cases in this series, so that we have been able to analyse what additional information it provides.

Demonstration of Aneurysms

Contrast-enhanced scans demonstrated an aneurysm in a third of the cases (Figs. 6.5, 6.18). This may be complementary information to localisation of the aneurysm site, as suggested by the distribution of blood in the basal subarachnoid cisterns, but angiography is still necessary to define precise anatomical details. Contrast enhancement demonstrated aneurysms which at angiography varied from 6 to 30 mm in size, with a mean of 13 mm. It has proved of particular value in demonstrating basilar tip aneurysms, which on the plain CT scan often appear normal (Fig. 6.5).

Arteriovenous Malformations

The CT scan appearances in arteriovenous malformations has been described by Kendall and Claveria (1976) and Leblanc et al. (1979). CT provides a much better demonstration of associated pathological features, e.g. haematoma, oedema, infarction and hydrocephalus, than

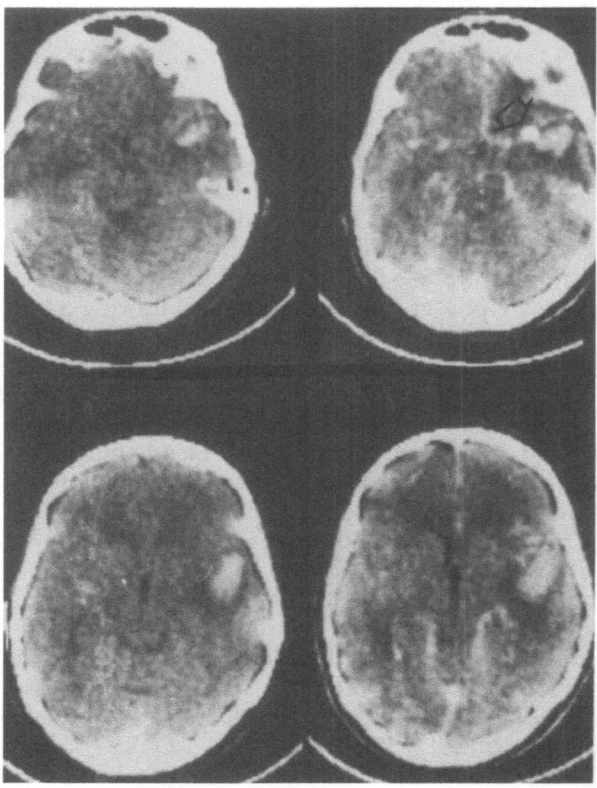

Fig. 6.18. CT scans show a haematoma in the right temporal region. After contrast administration there is definite enhancement of a middle cerebral aneurysm (*open arrow*) adjacent to the haematoma.

angiography. Plain CT scans demonstrated a haematoma in 95.6% of our cases (Table 6.5); they were supratentorial in 79.5% of cases and infratentorial in 21.5%. Intraventricular extension of the haematoma occurred in 39% of cases. Hydrocephalus may be due to obstruction within the ventricular system produced by enlarged veins or be of a communicating type following repeated haemorrhage (Fig. 6.19). CT shows evidence of calcification in about 6% of cases, but it may be obscured by the dense haematoma.

Contrast enhancement may show typical vascular enhancement and demonstration of feeding arteries or of draining veins (Fig. 6.20). In the presence of a haematoma these characteristic appearances may, however, be obscured. An arteriovenous malformation associated with a haematoma should be suspected if contrast enhancement is more diffuse within and around the haematoma or is associated with adjacent serpiginous or tubular densities due to enlarged bleeding or draining vessels (Kendall and Claveria 1976) (Fig. 6.21).

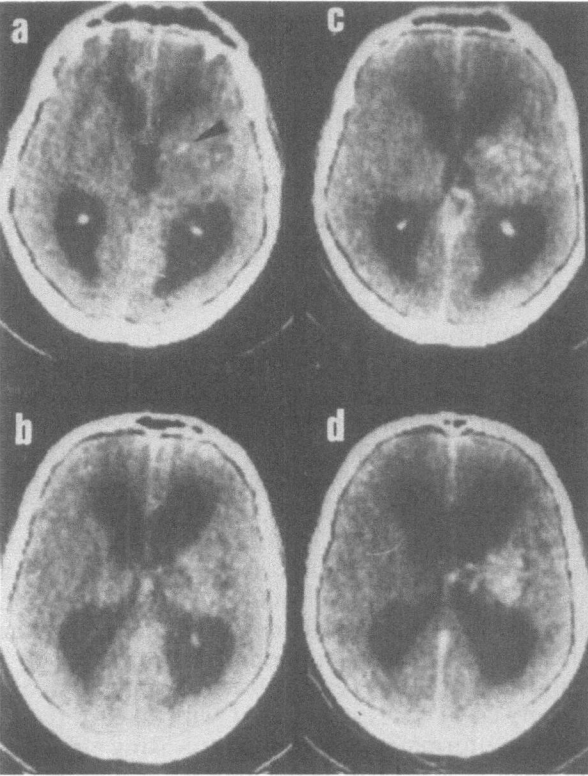

Fig. 6.19. a,b CT scans showing hydrocephalus with periventricular lucency in a patient with repeated episodes of SAH from an arteriovenous malformation. The malformation shows faint flecks of calcification and projects into the body of the right lateral ventricle. c, d After contrast administration there was slight enhancement.

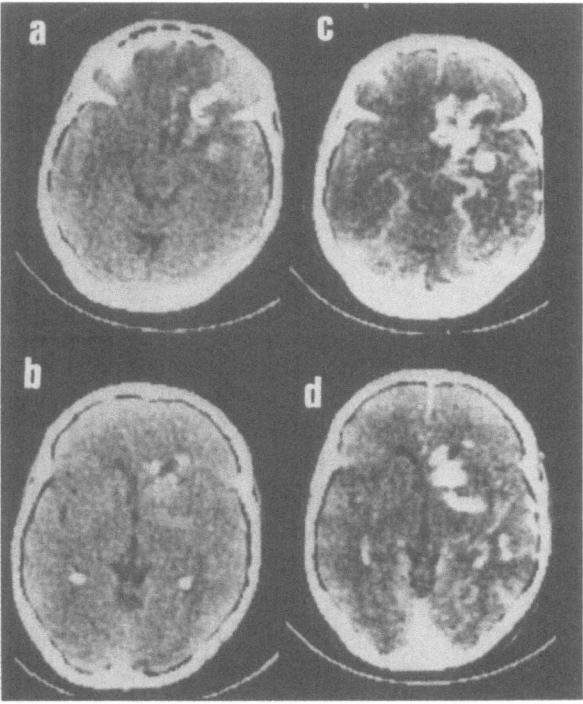

Fig. 6.20. a, b Plain CT scans of an arteriovenous malformation showing curvilinear and irregular calcification in the right frontal region. c, d After contrast administration there is a large serpiginous area of enhancement with prominence of the basal vein of Rosenthal.

Occult Arteriovenous Malformations

CT abnormalities have been described in a group of patients with angiographically occult arteriovenous malformations (Kramer and Wing 1977). CT usually demonstrates a high density lesion which invariably shows contrast enhancement. A case of angiographic occult arteriovenous malformation diagnosed by CT which at operation was proven to be a thrombosed cavernous angioma is described and illustrated in Chap. 15 (Fig. 15.6).

Cisternal Enhancement

Dense contrast enhancement of the basal subarachnoid cisterns and cerebral sulci may be observed in patients with SAH (Fig. 6.22). It is believed that this abnormal cisternal enhancement initially may be due to leakage caused by increased vascular permeability, and later to increased vascularity associated with developing arachnoiditis. We have observed such dense contrast enhancement in 24 of the 120 cases (20%) who had contrast-enhanced CT scans. Abnormal enhancement correlated closely with the poorer clinical grades, the presence of extensive blood in the basal cisterns and the subsequent demonstration of spasm at angiography. Sobel et al. (1981) observed abnormal enhancement of the basal cisterns in 21 out of 42 patients with SAH. They showed that enhancement was associated with an increased incidence of hydrocephalus but did not correlate with clinical grade, arterial spasm, location of bleed or temporal relation to the bleed. Tazawa et al. (1983), however, have recently provided evidence that prominent enhancement may be a useful predictor of vasospasm. Doczi et al. (1984) report abnormal enhancement in 26 out of 80 patients (29.5%) examined by contrast-

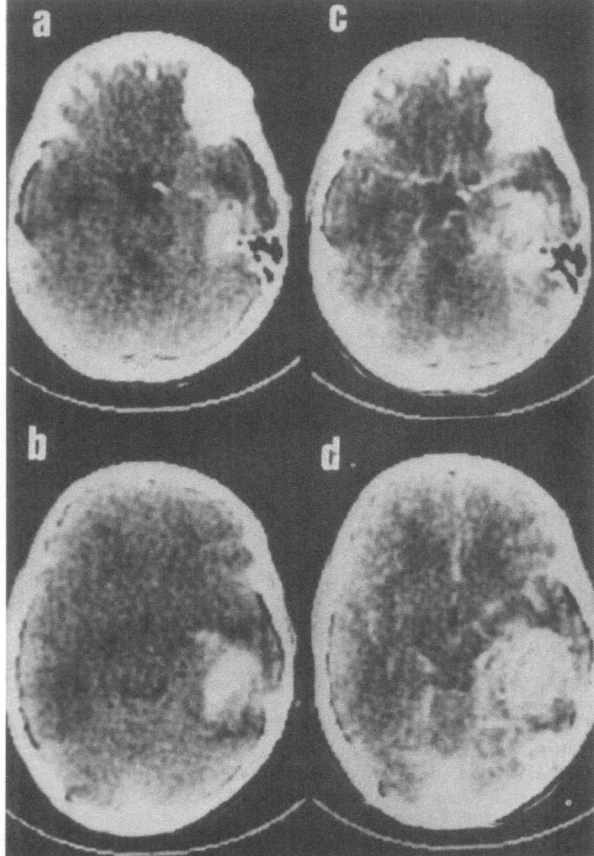

enhanced CT. Abnormal enhancement was associated with a poor clinical condition, angiographic spasm and a poor outcome. These authors suggest that abnormal enhancement is parenchymal and not subarachnoid. They propose that it is due to gyral hyperaemia or extravasation of contrast material into the cortex resulting from breakdown of the blood–brain barrier or a combination of both factors.

Haematoma Enhancement

A ring of contrast enhancement is occasionally seen in resolving intracranial haematomas (Fig. 6.23) (Messina 1976). This ring enhancement can be modified by steroid administration in the early stages. However, enhancement seen in the later stages is not affected. Early contrast enhancement is probably due to breakdown of the blood–brain barrier, and late enhancement to vascular granulation tissue which forms at the periphery of the haematoma. CT findings of a ring enhancement could lead to an erroneous diagnosis of SAH associated with an arteriovenous malformation or a neoplasm. Ring enhancement associated with a haematoma is not usually seen for 6 days following haemorrhage, so that early enhancement on the CT scan should raise the possibility of some other underlying pathology, such as an arteriovenous malformation or a tumour.

Fig. 6.21. a,b Plain CT scan showing a right posterior temporal haematoma. **c, d** After i.v. Conray there is prominent enhancement around the haematoma together with tubular densities suggestive of associated vessels.

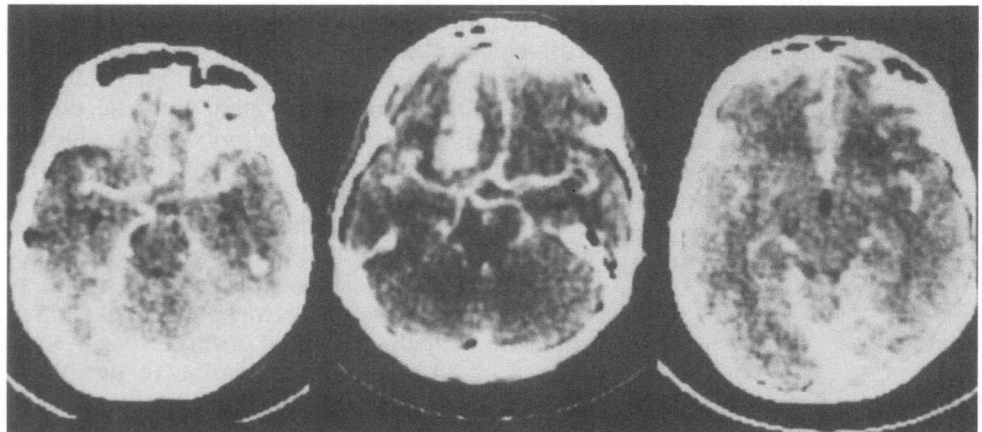

Fig. 6.22. Contrast-enhanced scans in a patient with a ruptured anterior communicating artery aneurysm. There is a haematoma in the left frontal lobe together with marked generalised enhancement of the basal subarachnoid cisterns and around the tentorium.

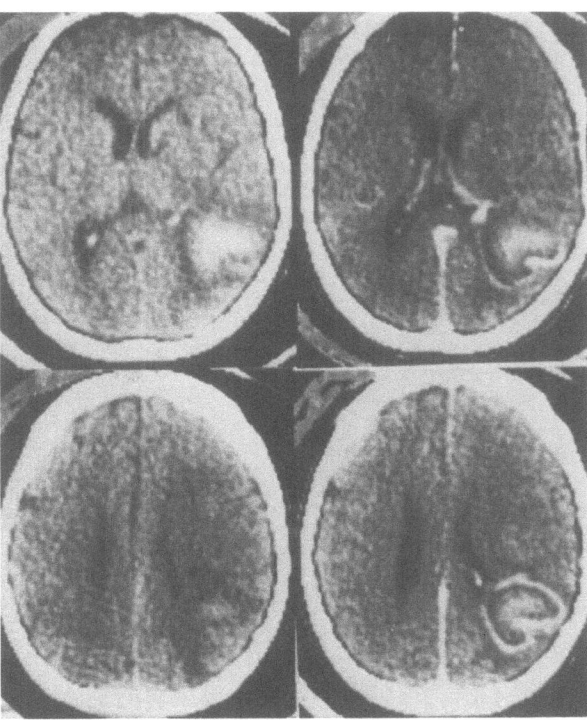

Fig. 6.23. Contrast-enhanced CT scan showing ring enhancement around a resolving intracranial haematoma. Distinction from a tumour could be difficult but the central area of increased attenuation and a history suggestive of subarachnoid haemorrhage helps avoid diagnostic difficulties.

Indications

Contrast enhancement is considered unnecessary in the majority of cases when angiography will in any case be carried out. It is indicated in suspected arteriovenous malformations. In patients with a normal scan, or when localisation of the site of the bleed is not possible, clinically or at CT, the demonstration of an aneurysm on contrast-enhanced CT scans may help in planning subsequent angiography.

CT in Multiple Aneurysms

CT scanning can be extremely helpful in patients with multiple aneurysms to decide which has

bled. Although angiographic criteria, such as size, loculation of the aneurysm, localised spasm and vessel displacement associated with a haematoma, can be helpful in deciding which aneurysm has bled, these features are not always reliable. CT scan can show an area of increased density indicative of a bleed in the vicinity of one of the aneurysms, thereby indicating the site of the haemorrhage. In the case illustrated in Fig. 6.24, bilateral carotid angiography showed multiple aneurysms involving both the middle cerebral arteries and also a pericallosal artery aneurysm. There were no specific features to assess which aneurysm had bled, the vessel spasm being fairly generalised. The CT scan, however, showed a midline haematoma extending into the corpus callosum, which indicated that it was a pericallosal artery aneurysm which had bled.

Multiple aneurysms occurred in 63 patients in this series. Clinical features suggested the site of the aneurysm or lateralised the site of the bleed in 12 cases (19%). Cerebral angiography indicated correctly the offending aneurysm in 36 cases (57.1%), but was doubtful in six cases (9.6%) and uninformative in 21 cases (33.3%). CT scans indicated correctly the site of the bleed in 48 cases (76.2%) but were doubtful in six cases (9.6%) and uninformative in nine (14.2%). Silver et al. (1981) reported a 77% accuracy of CT in predicting the aneurysm which bled in the presence of multiple aneurysms.

When the information from both the CT scan and the angiogram was used, a correct localisation of the offending aneurysm was possible in 57 cases (90.4%), doubtful in three (4.8%) and uninformative in three (4.8%). Definite angiographic localising features were significantly less in this series (57.1%) compared with the accuracy of 95% reported by McKissock et al. (1964), but were very similar to recent reports by Kendall et al. (1976) and Almaani and Richardson (1978).

The unique ability of CT scanning to demonstrate the site and aetiology of a subarachnoid haemorrhage was illustrated in Fig. 4.1. In Fig. 6.25 the CT findings are illustrated in a patient who has a right parietal arteriovenous malformation and a right middle cerebral artery aneurysm and left carotico-ophthalmic artery aneurysm. CT showed a large, partly calcified, right parietal arteriovenous malformation projecting into the body of the right lateral ventricle. There was extensive blood in both lateral ventricles and in the third ventricle, but no blood in the vicinity of either aneurysm. CT indicated, therefore, that it was the parietal arteriovenous malformation which had bled.

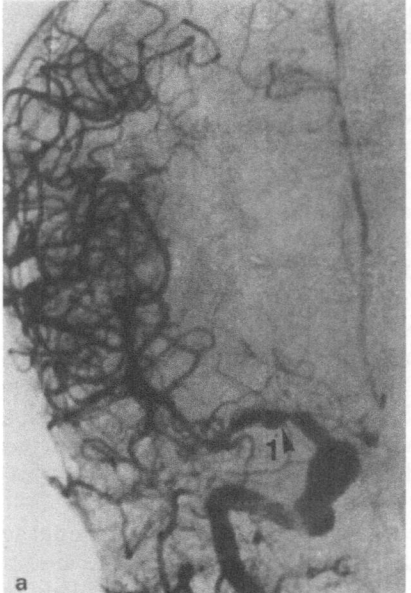
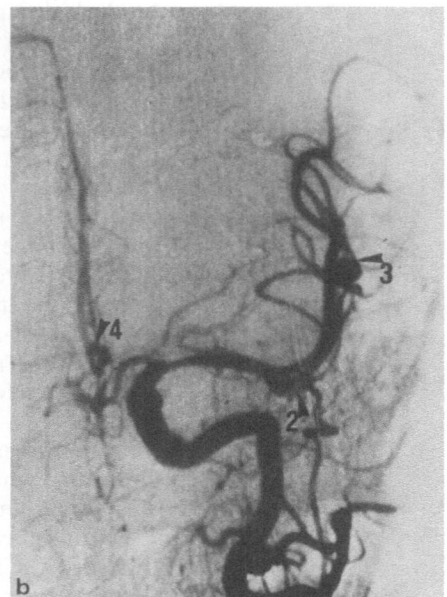

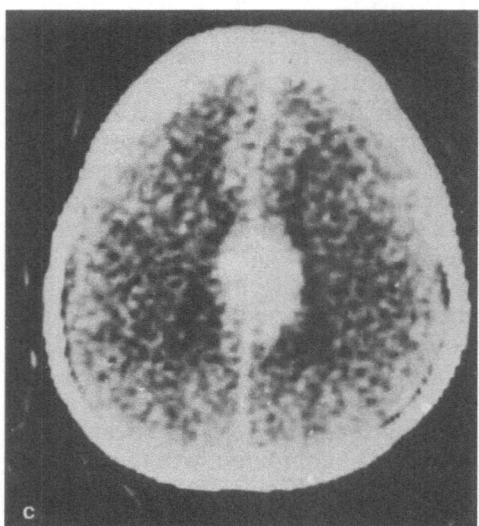

Fig. 6.24a–c. Value of CT scan in patients with multiple aneurysms. **a, b** In this patient **a** a right carotid angiogram showed an aneurysm arising from the M1 segment of the middle cerebral artery (*1*) and **b** a left carotid angiogram showed a further aneurysm arising near the bifurcation of the left middle cerebral artery (*2*), a peripheral middle cerebral artery aneurysm (*3*) and a pericallosal artery aneurysm (*4*). There was generalised vessel spasm. There were no distinguishing features on the angiogram to decide which of these aneurysms had bled. **c** CT scan in the same patient, however, showed an extensive haematoma in the corpus callosum, thus indicating that it was the pericallosal artery aneurysm that had bled.

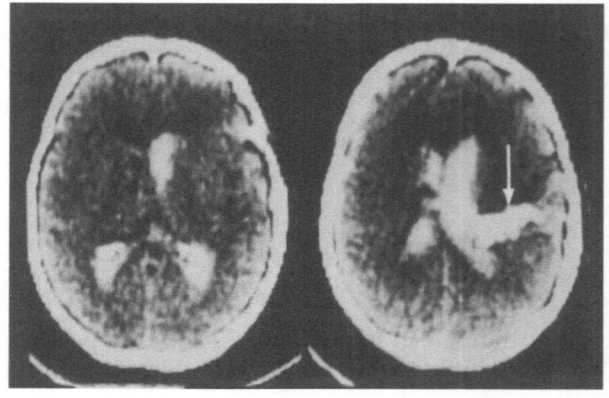

Fig. 6.25. CT scans in a patient with a calcified right parietal arteriovenous malformation (*arrow*), a right middle cerebral artery aneurysm, and a left carotico-ophthalmic aneurysm. There is extensive blood in both lateral ventricles and in the third ventricle. No blood was seen in the vicinity of either aneurysm, indicating that it was the arteriovenous malformation that had bled.

CT Scan Findings and Patient Grade

Davis et al. (1976) reported that grade 1 patients (as classified by Botterell's criteria) had a normal CT scan, whilst grade 4 or 5 patients frequently had intracerebral haematomas, intraventricular haemorrhage and hydrocephalus on CT. Hori et al. (1979) also showed that grade 1 patients usually showed no significant abnormality as regards evidence of subarachnoid blood, whereas grade 3 and 4 patients showed marked and widespread haemorrhage or acute hydrocephalus.

In 231 cases of single aneurysm rupture the CT scan findings were correlated with the patient's clinical grade at the time of CT scanning (Table 6.6). In the 65 cases in grade 1 the CT scan was typically normal (22 cases) or simply demonstrated blood confined to the subarachnoid space (37 cases). The higher incidence of demonstration of subarachnoid blood in this series probably reflects earlier scanning compared with the series reported above. Intracerebral haematoma was demonstrated in only three cases (4.6%). These were two small septum pellucidum haematomas associated with anterior communicating artery aneurysms and one small sylvian fissure haematoma associated with a middle cerebral artery aneurysm. The one subdural haematoma demonstrated was small and required no treatment. Of the 78 grade 2 patients, the CT scan was normal in 22 cases and demonstrated blood confined to the

subarachnoid space in 30 cases. Intracerebral haematoma was demonstrated in 24 cases (30%). In 20 cases, however, they were small in size, arising from an anterior communicating artery aneurysm rupture, and involved the septum pellucidum or medial part of the frontal lobe. The remaining four haematomas were also small in size, involving the temporal lobe, and resulted from middle cerebral artery aneurysm.

In the 60 grade 3 patients, CT scans were normal in only nine cases and demonstrated blood confined to the subarachnoid space in 24 cases. Intracerebral haematomas were shown in 28 cases (46.7%). Intraventricular haemorrhage occurred in nine cases (15%). There was CT evidence of infarction in 18.3% of cases and of hydrocephalus in 38.3%.

The 28 grade 4 patients showed an intracerebral haematoma in 26 cases (93%), and intraventricular haemorrhage occurred in 14 cases (50%). There were no normal scans, and blood confined only to the subarachnoid space occurred in only three cases.

It is clear that grade 1 and 2 patients tend to have either a normal CT scan or one that shows blood confined to the subarachnoid space. Whilst 30% of grade 2 patients demonstrated a haematoma, all of them were small in size and did not warrant consideration of surgical evacuation.

Patients in grades 3–5 rarely had a normal CT scan and frequently showed evidence of intracerebral or intraventricular haematoma.

The majority of infarcts demonstrated at CT were shown in grade 3 and 4 patients.

Table 6.6. Comparison of clinical grade at time of CT and CT findings in 231 cases of SAH with a single aneurysm

CT findings	Grade 1	Grade 2	Grade 3	Grade 4	Grade 5
No. of cases	65	78	60	28	0
Normal	22	22	9	0	
Subarachnoid blood (SAH)	37	30	24	3	
Intracerebral haematoma	3	24	28	26	
Intraventricular blood	0	2	9	14	
Infarct	1	0	10	1	
Hydrocephalus	3	11	14	6	
Subdural haematoma	1	0	1	0	
Small ventricles (oedema)	1	1	1	0	

Note: In 14 cases of the 245 single aneurysm group details of the patient's grade were not available.
Grades (Hunt and Hess)—see table 4.8.

CT Scan Findings and Prognosis

Turnbull (1980) noted the CT scans of 93 patients as regards features which might influence prognosis. In his series, a normal scan pointed to a complete recovery. Only three out of 20 patients who showed an area of low attenuation consistent with an infarct recovered completely, nine did badly, and eight died. Prognosis was also influenced by the size of the haematoma. Over 80% of patients with a haematoma smaller than 2.5 cm made a full recovery, while only 20% of patients recovered fully if the haematoma was greater than 2.5 cm. In 13 patients with intraventricular haemorrhage, five recovered completely, five partially and three died. Mohr et al. (1983) have previously studied 91 cases of intraventricular haemorrhage retrospectively, and found an overall mortality of 64%.

Accuracy of CT

In the 500 cases of SAH examined by CT, 375 cases (75%) had a positive scan, confirming the presence of an SAH, whilst 125 cases (25%) had normal scans. The latter consisted of 55 patients in the single aneurysm group, 10 with multiple aneurysms, and 60 with no vascular lesion demonstrated on four vessel angiography.

Analysis of the 65 normal scans in the aneurysm group revealed that 44 cases were scanned more than 6 days after the bleed, when the CT scan is less likely to demonstrate blood in the subarachnoid space, so that earlier scanning would probably have been more rewarding in this group. Of the 21 cases scanned within the first 5 days of the bleed, 8 involved posterior circulation aneurysms, which because of their very low position are difficult to demonstrate on CT, and 13 supratentorial aneurysms. As indicated above, there were 60 patients who had a typical history of SAH and uniformly blood-stained CSF at lumbar puncture in whom CT and four vessel angiography were normal. In our experience, a normal CT scan performed 1–3 days after a definite SAH implies strongly that either the subsequent four vessel angiogram will be normal or one will find a posterior circulation aneurysm.

CT Scan Findings and Subarachnoid Haemorrhage of Unknown Cause

In 75 patients (15%) with SAH in this series, no causative lesion was found at four vessel angiography. In 60 cases (75%) CT scan was normal, but in 15 cases (20%) the CT scan showed definite evidence of blood in the subarachnoid space. There has been only a short follow-up of this group, but two patients returned with a recurrent bleed, and on this occasion CT showed evidence of a haematoma in the external capsule and occipital lobes respectively, consistent with a spontaneous bleed. In the group of patients with normal CT scans we could have been misled with the diagnosis; it is more likely that they represent patients who have had minor bleeds, perhaps related to hypertension or atherosclerosis. Eskesen et al. (1984), in an analysis of 308 proven cases of SAH, found 44 patients (14%) in whom no cause for the SAH could be identified. These patients were followed up for 3–64 months (mean, 36 months) and it was found that the mortality (two patients dead) after SAH of unknown aetiology was 5% and the risk of rebleeding (three patients), 7%. In the three patients who had a rebleed, one was fatal (no autopsy obtained) and two were diagnosed on clinical grounds and had no further investigations. In the other patient who died in the series, autopsy showed no cause for the SAH.

Shephard (1984) followed up 254 cases of SAH of unknown cause (mean follow-up, 4.7 years) and reported a more favourable outcome as regards the late rebleed rate (1.5%). The mortality was 3% in normotensive patients, 20% in hypertensive patients, and 8.7% overall. In the 20 patients who died, there were 18 deaths from ruptured aneurysm proved at autopsy. It should be emphasised that only 113 patients in this series underwent carotid and vertebral angiography. There was no mention of how many of the aneurysms shown at autopsy were on the vertebrobasilar system. His results confirm the favourable prognosis in normotensive patients with SAH. However, patients who are hypertensive tend to have a poorer prognosis.

CT Scan Findings and Vasospasm

Several authors (Fisher et al. 1980; Mizukami et al. 1980; Yamamoto et al. 1983) have indicated that if a thick layer of subarachnoid blood is demonstrated at CT, then there is a high probability that clinically significant vasospasm would develop in nearby vessels in relationship to the blood clot. Patients who show no significant accumulation of subarachnoid blood probably would not suffer severe vasospasm. Further information can be found in Chap. 12.

CT and Brain Haemorrhage Due to Intracranial Tumours

Spontaneous haemorrhage from intracranial tumours is rare but is more frequently recognised since the advent of CT. Little et al. (1979) reported haemorrhage originating from an intracranial tumour in 6% of patients with brain haemorrhage diagnosed by CT. Wakai et al. (1982) reported haemorrhage associated with intracranial tumours (other than pituitary adenomas) in 45 cases out of 1550 brain tumours (2.9%). Haemorrhage was intratumoural in 30 cases, intracerebral in seven cases, subdural in one case and subarachnoid, without detectable haemorrhage in the tumour site, in only seven cases (0.45%). There were seven cases of tumour in this series which, on the CT scan, could be confused with an SAH from an arteriovenous malformation. They included metastases (three cases), glioblastoma multiforme (one case), pinealoma (one case) (Fig. 6.26), choroid plexus

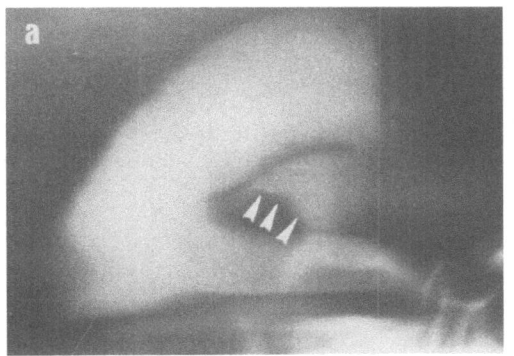
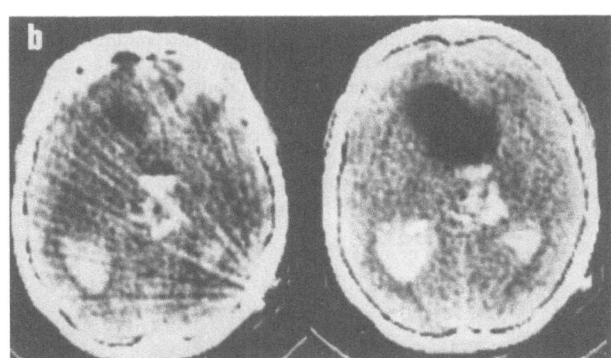
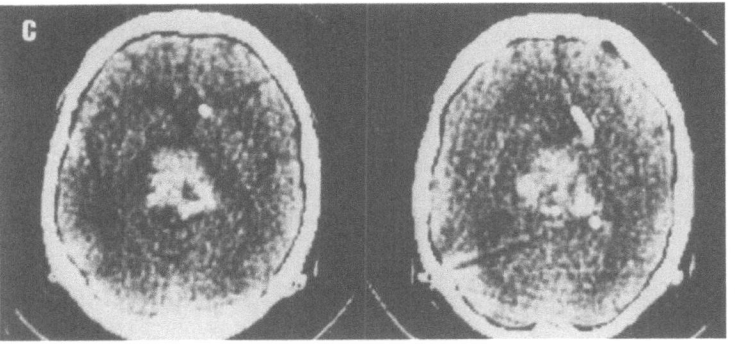

Fig. 6.26. a A 22-year-old female patient with a pinealoma (*arrows*) diagnosed by Conray ventriculogram in 1976, and treated by shunting and radiotherapy. **b** CT scan in January, 1982 after the patient had a sudden onset of headache and neck stiffness associated with blood in the shunt fluid. There is extensive blood in the region of the pineal gland, in the ventricle, and in the trigone of both lateral ventricles. Four-vessel angiography failed to disclose another cause of the haemorrhage. **c** Follow-up CT scan after haemorrhage had cleared showed a large calcified pineal tumour.

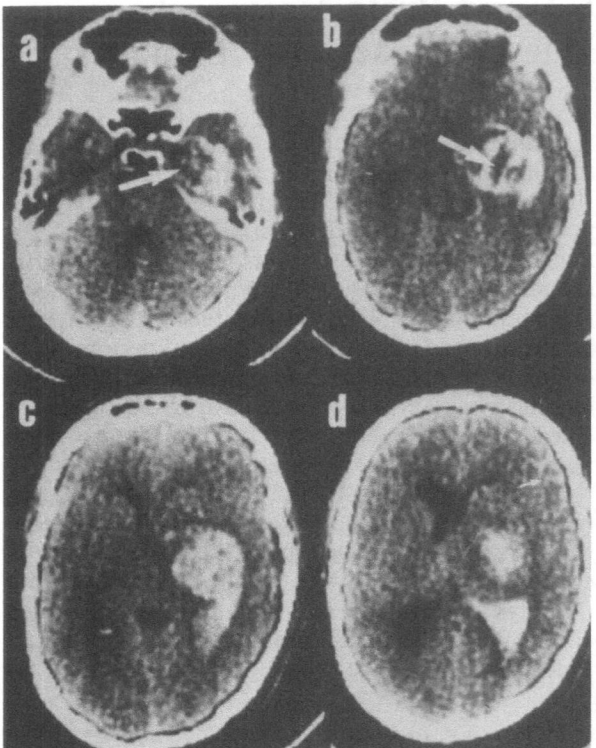

Fig. 6.27. CT demonstrates a right parasellar and middle fossa lesion, consisting of central areas of low density surrounded by high density, consistent with haematoma (**a, b**). The haematoma extends upwards into the medial temporal region and external capsule, and there is blood in the trigone of the right lateral ventricle (**c, d**). At surgery, haematoma was confirmed and evacuated. In addition, tumour tissue was removed which, at histology, was shown to be a chordoma.

papilloma (one case) (see Fig. 15.9, Chap. 15) and chordoma (one case) (Fig. 6.27).

The diagnosis of intracranial haemorrhage associated with a tumour will depend on the CT scan findings. The diagnosis should be considered when:

1. Haematomas occur in non-hypertensive patients in unusual locations not typical of a hypertensive haemorrhage.
2. CT demonstrates a low density neoplastic core with haematoma at its periphery (Little et al. 1979). In addition with a tumour there is often more extensive surrounding oedema.
3. CT demonstrates early contrast enhancement resulting from abnormal tumour vascularity distinguishable from the serpiginous-type enhancement of an arteriovenous malformation or the later ring enhancement previously described in association with an ageing haematoma.

Follow-up CT after the haematoma has resolved may finally disclose the underlying neoplasm (Fig. 6.28).

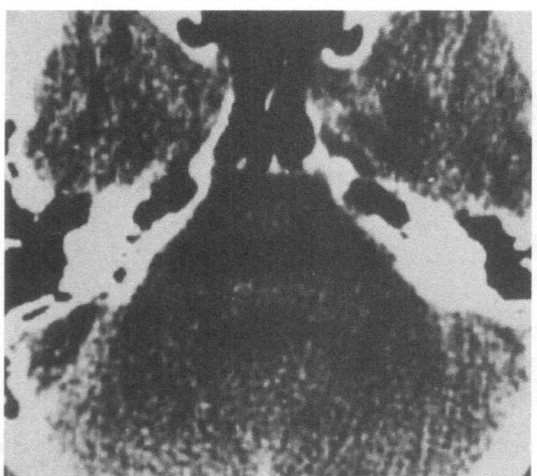
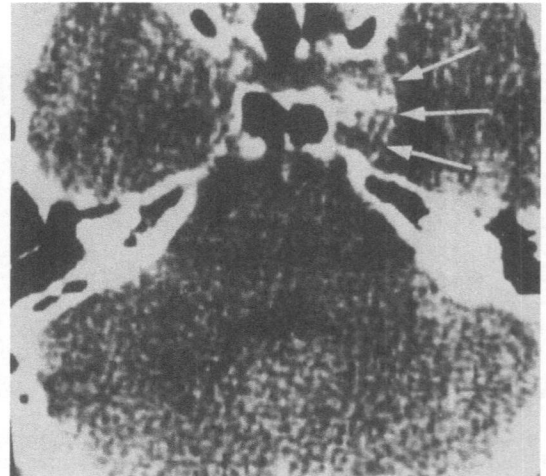

Fig. 6.28a, b. Same case as Fig. 6.27. Repeat CT scan after removal of haematoma. **a** Plain scan. **b** Contrast-enhanced scan. Showing residual right parasellar enhancing tumour (*arrows*). (Compare with Fig. 6.27a).

CT and Giant Aneurysms

Giant intracranial aneurysms are defined as those
over 2.5 cm at their maximum diameter. Five per
cent of all verified intracranial aneurysms have
reached this size when they present clinically.
They frequently present as a space-occupying
lesion, but in our experience 25% of giant
aneurysms presented as an SAH. Giant
aneurysms appear on CT as a round or globular
mass, usually of slightly increased attenuation.
They may show ring calcification (Fig. 6.29). A
peripheral ring of increased density is present
when there is intraluminal thrombosis. Non-
thrombosed aneurysms enhance uniformly but
partially thrombosed aneurysms may show a central area of enhancement (target sign) (Fig. 6.29).

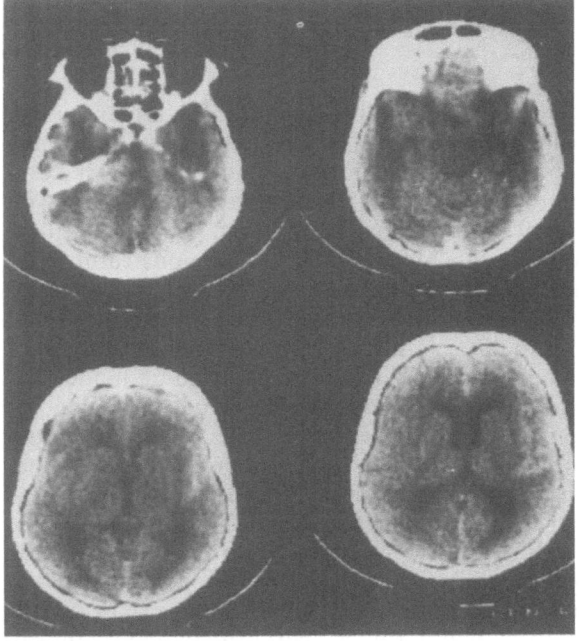

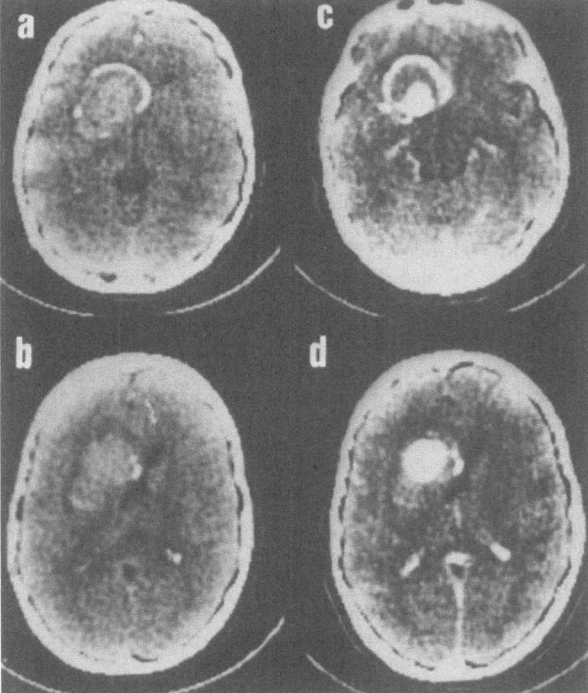

Fig. 6.29a–d. CT scans in a patient with giant carotid ophthalmic aneurysm. **a, b** Plain CT scan showing a rounded mass of
increased attenuation with peripheral ring calcification. **c, d**
Contrast-enhanced scan showing central areas of enhancement (target sign).

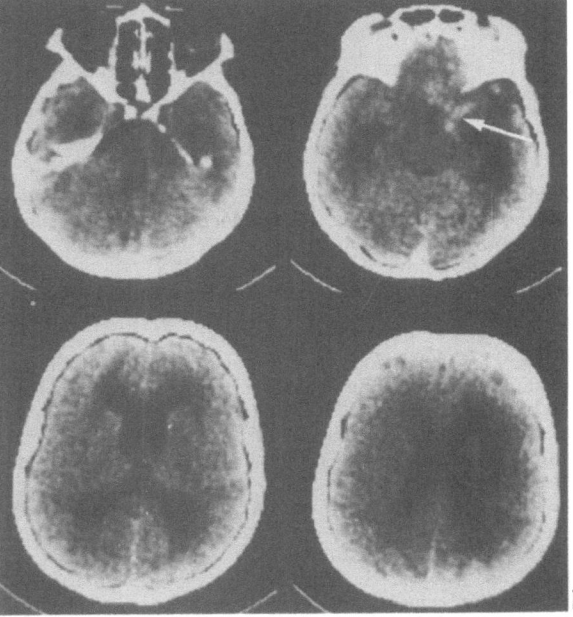

Fig. 6.30. a CT scan 4 days after an SAH shows blood in the
RT sylvian fissure. There is slight ventricular enlargement.
The patient was not fit for surgery but gradually improved in
condition. **b** A repeat CT was carried out 9 days later, after the
patient became drowsy with fluctuating hemiparesis. It
showed evidence of a rebleed, with blood now present in the
suprasellar cistern (*arrow*). In addition there was now evidence of hydrocephalus with periventricular lucencies.

CT and Patient Deterioration

CT is the safest and most valuable technique for evaluating the cause of a patient's deterioration in the pre-operative period. The three most common causes of a deterioration are recurrent SAH, hydrocephalus and vasospasm. CT is an ideal non-invasive technique for demonstrating hydrocephalus. In most cases CT scanning will identify those patients who have had a rebleed (Fig. 6.30). A strong presumptive diagnosis of ischaemia from vasospasm can also be made by a process of elimination if CT excludes a rebleed or developing hydrocephalus. The CT scan is often initially normal in such patients, but a repeat study 1 or 2 days later may demonstrate a low density area consistent with infarction (Fig. 6.16).

CT is also now used as the primary diagnostic procedure in the postoperative period for evaluation of complications, such as intra- or extracerebral haematomas, cerebral oedema, infarction or infection.

References

Adams HP, Kassell NF, Torner JC, Sahs AL (1983) CT and clinical correlations in recent aneurysmal subarachnoid haemorrhage: A preliminary report of the Cooperative Aneurysm Study. Neurology 33:981–988

Almaani WS, Richardson AE (1978) Multiple intracranial aneurysms. Identifying the ruptured lesion. Surg Neurol 9:303–305

Brismar J (1979) Computed tomography as the primary radiological procedure in acute subarachnoid haemorrhage. Acta Radiol [Diagn] 20:849–864

Bryan RN, Shah CP, Hilal SK (1979) Evaluation of subarachnoid haemorrhage and cerebral vaso-spasm by computed tomography. CT 3:144–152

Davis KR, New PFJ, Ojemann RG (1976) Computed tomographic evaluation of haemorrhage secondary to intracranial aneurysm. AJR 127:143–153

Doczi T, Ambrose J, O'Laoire S (1984) Significance of contrast enhancement in cranial computerized tomography after subarachnoid haemorrhage. J Neurosurg 60:335–342

Eskesen V, Sorensen EB, Rosen J, Schmidt K (1984) The prognosis in SAH of unknown aetiology. J Neurosurg 61:1029–1031

Fisher CM, Kistler JP, Davis JM (1980) Relation of cerebral vaso-spasm to subarachnoid haemorrhage visualised by computerised tomographic scanning. Neurosurgery 6:1–9

Foltz EL, Ward AA (1956) Communicating hydrocephalus from subarachnoid bleeding. J Neurosurg 13:546–566

Galera RG, Greitz T (1970) Hydrocephalus in the adult secondary to the rupture of intracranial arterial aneurysm. J Neurosurg 32:634–641

Griffith HB, Cummins BH, Thomson JLG (1972) Cerebral arterial spasm and hydrocephalus in leaking arterial aneurysms. Neuroradiology 4:212–214

Gunasekera L, Richardson AE (1977) Computerized axial tomography in idiopathic hydrocephalus. Brain 100:749–754

Hayward RD (1976) Intracranial arterio-venous malformations. Observations after experience with computerised tomography. J Neurol Neurosurg Psychiatry 39:1027–1033

Hayward RD, O'Reilly GVA (1976) Intracerebral haemorrhage: accuracy of computerised transverse axial scanning in predicting the underlying aetiology. Lancet I:1–4

Hori S, Fujiwara S, Mori T, Suzuki J (1979) Computed tomography in ruptured intracranial aneurysms. In: Suzuki J (ed) Cerebral aneurysms. Neuron, Tokyo, pp 199–207

Hounsfield GN (1973) Computerised transverse axial scanning (tomography). Part 1. Description of system. Br J Radiol 46:1023–1047

Imanaga H, Yamamoto M, Jimbo M, Kitamura K, Kobayashi N, Saito Y (1980) Computed tomography in the diagnosis of haemorrhage secondary to intracranial aneuryrms. Neurol Surg (Tokyo) 8:623–631

Kendall BE, Claveria LE (1976) The use of computed axial tomography (CAT) for the diagnosis and management of intracranial angiomas. Neuroradiology 12:141–160

Kendall BE, Radue EW (1978) Computed tomography in spontaneous intracerebral haematomas. Br J Radiol 51:563–573

Kendall BE, Lee BCP, Claveria E (1976) Computerised tomography and angiography in subarachnoid haemorrhage. Br J Radiol 49:483–501

Kramer RA, Wing SD (1977) Computed tomography of angiographically occult cerebral vascular malformation. Radiology 123:649–652

Leblanc R, Ethier R, Little JR (1979) Computerized tomography findings in arterio-venous malformations of the brain. J Neurosurg 51:765–772

Liliequist B, Lindqvist M (1980) Computer tomography in the evaluation of subarachnoid haemorrhage. Acta Radiol [Diagn] 21:327–331

Liliequist B, Lindqvist M, Valdimarsson E (1977) Computed tomography and subarachnoid haemorrhage. Neuroradiology 14:21–26

Little JR, Dial B, Belanger G, Carpenter S (1979) Brain haemorrhage from intracranial tumour. Stroke 10:283–288

Messina AV (1976) Computed tomography: contrast enhancement in resolving intracerebral haemorrhage. AJR 127:1050–1052

Mizukami M, Takemal T, Tazawa T, Kawase T, Matsuzaki T (1980) Value of computed tomography in the prediction of verebral vaso-spasm after aneurysm rupture. Neurosurgery 7:583–586

Modesti LM, Binet EF (1978) Value of computed tomography in the diagnosis and management of subarachnoid haemorrhage. Neurosurgery 3:151–156

Mohr G, Ferguson G, Khan M, Malloy D, Watts R, Benoit B, Weir B (1983) Intraventricular hemorrhage from ruptured aneurysm. J Neurosurg 58:482–487

New PFJ, Arinow S (1976) Attenuation measurements of whole blood and blood fractions in computed tomography. Radiology 121:635–640

Norman D, Price D, Bayd D, Fishman R, Newton TH (1977) Quantitative aspects of computed tomography of the blood and cerebro-spinal fluid. Radiology 123:335–338

Paxton R, Ambrose J (1974) The EMI scanner. A brief review of the first 650 patients. Br J Radiol 47:530–565

Saito I, Shigeno T, Aritake K, Tanishima T, Sano K (1979) Vaso-spasm assessed by angiography and computerised tomography. J Neurosurg 51:466–475

Scott IG, Ethier R, Malancon D, Terburgge K, Tchang S

(1977) Computed tomography in the evaluation of intracranial aneurysms and subarachnoid haemorrhage. Radiology 123:85–90

Shephard RH (1984) Prognosis of spontaneous (nontraumatic) subarachnoid haemorrhage of unknown cause. A personal series 1958–1980. Lancet I:777–779

Silver AJ, Pederson ME Jr, Ganti SR, Hilal SK, Jost Michelson W (1981) CT of subarachnoid haemorrhage due to ruptured aneurysm. Am J Neuroradiol 2:13–22

Sobel D, Chaney LF, Norman D, Newton TH (1981) Cisternal enhancement after subarachnoid haemorrhage. Am J Neuroradiol 2:549–552

Symon L (1979) Hydrocephalus following subarachnoid haemorrhage In: Pia HS, Langmaid C, Zierski J (eds) Cerebral aneurysms. Advances in diagnosis and therapy. Springer, Berlin Heidelberg New York, pp 162–168

Tazawa T, Mizukami M, Kawase T, Usami T, Togashi O, Hyodo A, Eguchi T (1983) Relationship between contrast enhancement on computed tomography and cerebral vasospasm in patients with subarachnoid haemorrhage. Neurosurgery 12:643–648

Turnbull IW (1980) Computed tomographic points to the prognosis of subarachnoid haemorrhage. Br J Radiol 53:416–420

Vassilouthis J, Richardson AE (1979) Ventricular dilatation and communicating hydrocephalus following spontaneous subarachnoid haemorrhage. J Neurosurg 51:341–351

Wakai S, Yamakawa K, Manaka S, Takakurl K (1982) Spontaneous intracranial haemorrhage caused by brain tumour. Its incidence and clinical significance. Neurosurgery 10:437–444

Weir B, Miller J, Russell D (1977) Intracranial aneurysms. A clinical angiographic and computerised tomographic study. Can J Neurol Sci 4:99–105

Weir B, Myles T, Kahn M, Maroun F, Malloy D, Benoit B, McDermott M, Cochrane D, Mohr G, Ferguson G, Durity F (1984) Management of acute subdural hematomas from aneurysmal rupture. Can J Neurol Sci 11:371–376

Weisberg LA (1979) Computed tomography in aneurysmal subarachnoid haemorrhage. Neurology 29:802–808

Yamamoto I, Hara M, Ogura K, Suzuki Y, Nakane T, Kageyama N (1983) Early operation from rupture of intracranial aneurysms: Comparative study with computed tomography. Neurosurgery 12:169–174

Yasargil MG, Yonekawa Y, Zumstein B, Stahl HG (1973) Hydrocephalus following spontaneous subarachnoid haemorrhage; clinical features and treatment. J Neurosurg 39:474–499

7 Cerebral Angiography

Introduction

Egaz Moniz and his colleague Almeida Lima introduced the technique of cerebral angiography in 1927. Their first successful case involved surgical exposure of the carotid artery and the direct injection of a 25% solution of sodium iodide. The technique initially did not gain wide acceptance, mainly owing to the toxicity of the contrast medium used and the fact that a surgical cut down on the carotid artery was necessary.

Percutaneous cerebral angiography was subsequently developed by Loman and Myerson in 1936 and Shimidzu in 1937.

Seldinger in 1953 introduced the technique of femoral artery catheterisation. The femoral catheter approach provided the advantage that one could carry out a four vessel cerebral angiogram at one study with one arterial puncture. The technique of subtraction (Ziedses des Plantes 1963) by which bony structures are eliminated from the angiographic film by a photographic method resulted in a significant improvement in detail of vascular anatomy and pathology. Magnification techniques further improved the visualisation of the intracranial vascular anatomy and increased the diagnostic accuracy of the neuroradiologist. The use of subtraction and magnification techniques have developed pari passu with the use of the operating microscope, enabling the neurosurgeon to plan more safely an operative approach to aneurysms and arteriovenous malformations (AVMs).

Recent improvements in angiographic technique, including better equipment, catheter and guide wire design as well as increased safety of the current contrast media, mean that angiography now has an acceptably low complication rate in patients with SAH.

CT scanning often helps to localise the site of the bleed and has meant that the neuroradiologist can then carry out more detailed angiographic study of the relevant cerebral vessels by subtraction and magnification techniques. (Kendall et al. 1976).

Indications

The aims of angiography are to:

1. Define the cause of the SAH (e.g. aneurysm, AVM, Moya Moya disease, etc)
2. Provide information about the anatomy of an aneurysm, its location, its size, its relationship to surrounding vessels and the configuration of its neck; in AVMs to demonstrate feeding vessels and outline venous drainage
3. Provide information about the complications of aneurysm rupture, e.g. vasospasm

4. Detect whether multiple aneurysms are present and if so, help indicate which has bled
5. Study the collateral circulation and demonstrate whether any anomalies of the circle of Willis are present (e.g. hypoplastic anterior cerebral artery, foetal posterior cerebral artery) which may influence surgical technique
6. Check the effectiveness of surgical treatment of aneurysms or AVMs postoperatively

Contraindications

There are no absolute contraindications to cerebral angiography in SAH. In each individual case one must balance the risks of angiography against the potential risks of the known natural history of the disease. Relative contraindications to angiography include a past history of anaphylaxis associated with contrast media, serious cardiac or pulmonary disease, severe hypertension and the rare case of bleeding diathesis.

The age limit for angiography is a rather controversial subject. Some surgeons have suggested that surgical treatment of patients over the age of 60 years will give no better results than the natural history of the disease, but others report successful results (Sengupta et al. 1978).

Timing

The fundamental principle of aneurysm surgery is to protect the patient from the dangers of recurrent haemorrhage, the peak incidence of which is 7–10 days after the initial rupture (Locksley 1966). In recent years the trend has been towards the earliest possible surgical treatment of patients in grades 1–3. Our policy is to carry out angiography as soon as possible in patients of grades 1–3, preferably within 24 h of admission. Limited angiography may be required as an emergency measure in seriously ill patients requiring life-saving evacuation of a haematoma demonstrated by CT.

In patients with haemorrhage from a known AVM there is probably less urgency for angiography to be carried out in the acute stage. In the cooperative study (Perret and Nishioka 1966a), 23% of patients had a second haemorrhage occurring from a few days to many years after the first

haemorrhage. Forster et al. (1972) also indicated that the risk of recurrent haemorrhage from AVM is significantly less compared with aneurysms. They quoted a rebleed rate of 29% in a conservatively managed group with an average period of follow-up of 12 years. In addition, vasospasm is not a consideration in delaying surgery.

Technique

Anaesthesia

The reader is referred to Chap. 9 for a full discussion on this topic. In the past we have tended to use a general anaesthetic. It is less painful for the patient and assures better quality films, particularly in uncooperative patients. The recent introduction of lower cost non-ionic contrast media has encouraged many neuroradiologists to alter to local anaesthesia. Local anaesthesia is also used in postoperative check angiography, making use of non-ionic contrast media.

Advocates of local anaesthesia point out that it is less time consuming and any deterioration in the neurological condition of the patient may be recognised immediately.

Many neuroradiologists still prefer to use general anaesthesia for the following reasons.

1. General anaesthesia, by eliminating patient movements, ensures optimal quality films, including subtractions.
2. Under general anaesthetic the risk of serious contrast media reactions is much less. In addition, sympathetic stimulation accompanying fear and anxiety which could result in further constriction of spastic vessels is avoided.
3. General anaesthesia provides optimal control of the $PaCO_2$ (ideally 25–30 Torr). This helps ensure optimal radiographic contrast in the cerebral vessels. It also avoids possible adverse effects of altered $PaCO_2$ on cerebral vessels, which in SAH are very sensitive to changes in $PaCO_2$. There is evidence that a rise in $PaCO_2$ may make arteries already narrowed by vasospasm constrict further (du Boulay et al. 1973).

A recent questionnaire was carried out concerning the use of general anaesthesia in cerebral angiography for SAH since the advent of the new non-ionic contrast media. Replies were received from 27 centres. In 14 (52%) angiography was carried out under local anaesthesia with sedation in all patients, with the exception of young children and unco-operative patients. In 12 centres (44%) all or almost all angiograms were carried out under general anaesthesia. In one centre both local and general anaesthesia were used. Hospitals in both groups were occasionally spontaneously vehement about their points of view, saying either "there is virtually no place for an anaesthetist in neuroradiology" or "all the investigations must be carried out under general anaesthesia if acceptable films are to be obtained" (Dr. C. K. McKnight, personal communication, 1984).

Type of Angiography

Either direct puncture or catheter femoral cerebral angiography may be used. The choice of method will depend on the age of the patient and the condition of the arterial tree, the type of apparatus available for performing angiography, and the skill and preference of the radiologist. A recent trend has been to use femoral catheter technique, especially in younger patients and particularly if there is no clinical or CT clue of the site of the haemorrhage. This is simple to perform and allows a rapid demonstration of four vessel anatomy in the course of one examination. In older patients (over 55 years), vessel tortuosity and atheromatous disease may make this technique more difficult or impossible. Direct puncture is used in older patients where the site of the bleed has been localised at CT. Whichever technique is employed, ideally it should be carried out by an experienced neuroradiologist.

Mani and Eisenberg (1978) showed clearly that the complication rate of catheter cerebral arteriography is closely related to operator proficiency. They showed that in SAH the complication rate was 1.3% in the non-training hospital, compared with 2.6% in training hospitals where the majority of the angiograms were carried out by junior medical staff.

Type of Equipment

Direct puncture carotid angiography is carried out in our unit using a disposable angiogram set (Travenol Laboratories) which consists of an 18 gauge needle attached to plastic tubing suitable for connection to a Luer syringe. Catheter cerebral angiography is carried out following percutaneous puncture of the femoral artery using a Cook Mani catheter (5 French). With this catheter carotid and vertebral arteries can be easily selectively catheterised and the failure rate is extremely low. The neuroscope (angioscope, Siemens) enables angiography to be carried out quickly without having to move the patient's head to obtain the necessary projections (especially valuable for direct puncture techniques) and provides facilities for magnification angiography. 9 cc of Conray 280 or non-ionic contrast media, e.g. iopamidol 300 or iohexol 300, is used for such injections.

Non-ionic contrast media are less neurotoxic and their low osmolality means that patient movement (due to a painful hot sensation in the face and head) is reduced and this results in better film quality when the procedure is carried out under local anaesthesia.

Extent of Angiography

The extent of angiography will depend on the age of the patient, the clinical grade and the attitude and local expertise of one's neurosurgical colleagues. In young patients (under 55 years of age) in grades 1–3, four vessel angiography is carried out since multiple aneurysms are common (25% in our series). In the majority of cases this means that both common or internal carotid arteries and one vertebral artery (usually the left, which is more readily catheterised) are injected, as in most cases the other vertebral artery fills in a retrograde fashion owing to reflux of contrast beyond the origin of the posterior inferior cerebellar artery.

In patients over 55 years old in whom the CT scan has definitely localised the site of the haemorrhage, we may limit the extent of angiography to the relevant vessels. In a patient with a definite unilateral sylvian fissure haematoma or a cerebellar haematoma, for example, we usually limit angiography to the relevant carotid or vertebral artery respectively, because we do not in general operate on incidental aneurysms in this age group. Anterior communicating aneurysms require bilateral carotid angiography to determine the type of circle of Willis. If CT is negative we usually carry out bilateral carotid angiography initially. Vertebral angiography will be carried out as well if the bilateral carotid angiogram is negative. Patients (of any age) who have had limited angiography may have the remaining vessels examined at the time of check angiography following clipping of the offending aneurysm.

Angiographic Projections

There are few aneurysms which cannot be treated by direct surgical attack, so that a clear delineation of the neck of the aneurysm and its relationship to surrounding vessels must be shown at angiography.

Four standard projections are carried out for anterior circulation aneurysms: (a) lateral, (b) Townes, (c) Townes oblique and (d) AP oblique projection through the orbit. For the latter projection the Frankfurter base line (lower border of orbit to external auditory meatus) is used. The tube is angled 5–10° cranially and 20° oblique to the RT or LT for RT and LT carotid AP oblique projections respectively. Centering is through the pupil. A reverse AP oblique projection through the orbit is also occasionally useful.

For posterior circulation aneurysms three standard projections are carried out: (a) lateral, (b) Townes with a tube tilt of 30–33° to show more clearly the posterior fossa structures, and (c) vertebral oblique to show more clearly the origin of the posterior inferior cerebellar arteries. For the vertebral oblique projection the Frankfurter base line is used. The tube is angled 10° caudally and 40° oblique to either side from the vertical. Centering is 1 in. in front of and 1.5 in. above the external auditory meatus. A control film is always obtained prior to injection of contrast so that subtraction studies are possible.

The standard views are supplemented by additional projections which may be required to show anatomical details more clearly or to distinguish between a vessel loop and aneurysm. Magnification studies with subtraction in the projections which optimally show the aneurysm or AVM anatomy are routinely carried out. Fluoroscopy can be used to determine the optimal projection in difficult cases.

Aneurysm Sites

The distribution of aneurysm sites in 500 operated patients is shown in Table 7.1.

Table 7.1. Distribution of aneurysm sites (500 operated patients)

	No.	%
Anterior cerebral artery	174	34.8
Anterior communicating	160	32.0
A$_1$ segment	4	0.8
Pericallosal	10	2.0
Middle cerebral artery	99	19.8
Internal carotid artery	197	39.4
Posterior communicating	116	23.2
Bifurcation	32	6.4
Carotid-ophthalmic	24	4.8
Anterior choroidal	10	2.0
Cavernous	3	0.6
Non-specific	12	2.4
Posterior circulation	30	6.0
Basilar bifurcation	14	2.8
PICA	10	2.0
Vertebrobasilar junction	2	0.4
Superior cerebellar	2	0.4
Posterior cerebral	2	0.4

Anterior Cerebral Artery Aneurysms

Anterior cerebral artery aneurysms are conveniently classified into three groups (Pia 1979).

1. Aneurysms of the anterior cerebral artery and anterior communicating artery junction; these constitute about 90% of cases
2. Aneurysms of the peripheral anterior cerebral artery, which are usually called pericallosal artery aneurysms (9%)
3. Aneurysms of the main branch (A$_1$ segment of the anterior cerebral artery); these are rare and account for approximately 1.3% of cases

Anterior Communicating Artery Aneurysms

The anterior communicating artery is orientated in a strictly transverse plane in only 18% of cases (Rhoton et al. 1979), which explains the potential difficulty of demonstrating it at angiography on the conventional lateral and AP projections and the necessity for oblique projections. The oblique projection through the orbit provides most information about the anatomy of the anterior communicating artery region (Fig. 7.1). This view is useful for planning the surgical approach as the angiographic outline of the vessels and aneurysm correspond closely to the view obtained at operation through the subfrontal gyrus rectus approach.

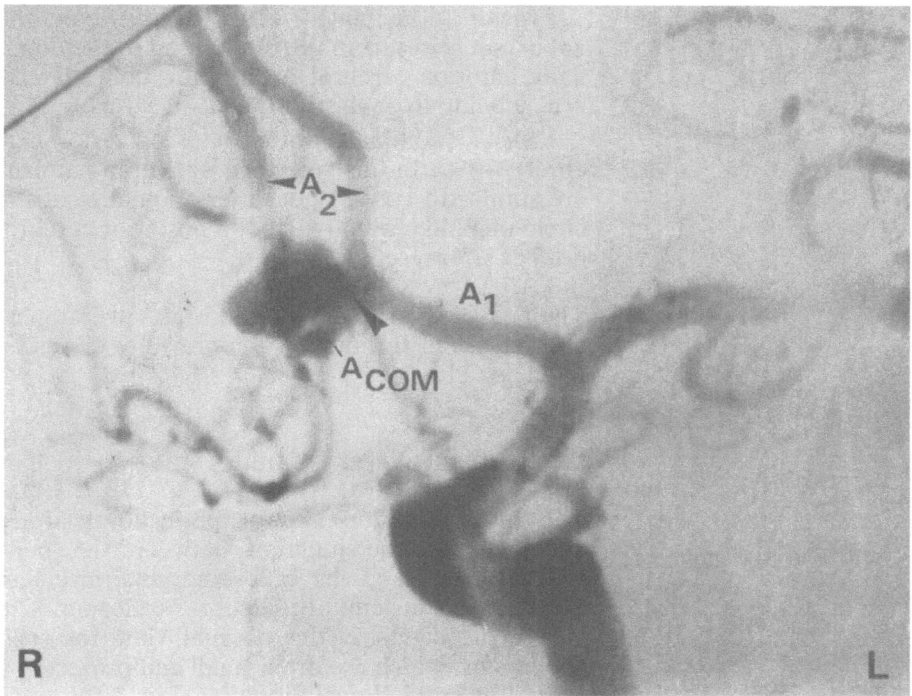

Fig. 7.1. Oblique projection through the orbit showing an anterior communicating artery aneurysm. The neck of the aneurysm is shown clearly to arise near the junction of the A_2 segment of the left anterior cerebral artery and the anterior communicating artery (A_{com}) (*arrowhead*). The sac of the aneurysm projects to the right side and lies in close relationship to the A_2 segment of the right anterior cerebral artery.

Anterior communicating aneurysms may project forward or backward (Figs. 7.2, 7.3). This is important information for the surgeon as he tries to avoid exposing the fundus of the aneurysm before the neck. Aneurysms projecting backward are approached from below through the longitudinal fissure, and those projecting forward from above by removing a small area of the gyrus rectus. In the majority of cases this information is provided by the lateral projection but occasionally a modified basal view will be found valuable, especially if the aneurysm is small (Fig. 7.4).

Norlen and Barnum (1953) drew attention to the different patterns of circulation through the anterior part of the circle of Willis in patients with anterior communicating aneurysms, stressing their importance for different surgical procedures. The circulatory pattern in patients with anterior communicating aneurysms has been analysed and classified into four types:

Type 1 (ipsilateral)—66%. In this type the aneurysm and distal anterior cerebral artery fill from one proximal anterior cerebral artery (Fig. 7.5).

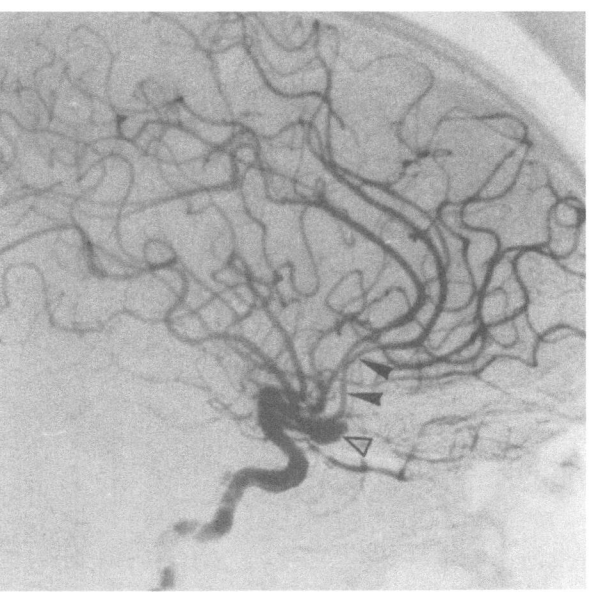

Fig. 7.2. Anterior communicating artery aneurysm (*open arrowhead*) projecting forwards and slightly downwards. There is some spasm of both anterior cerebral arteries (*black arrowheads*).

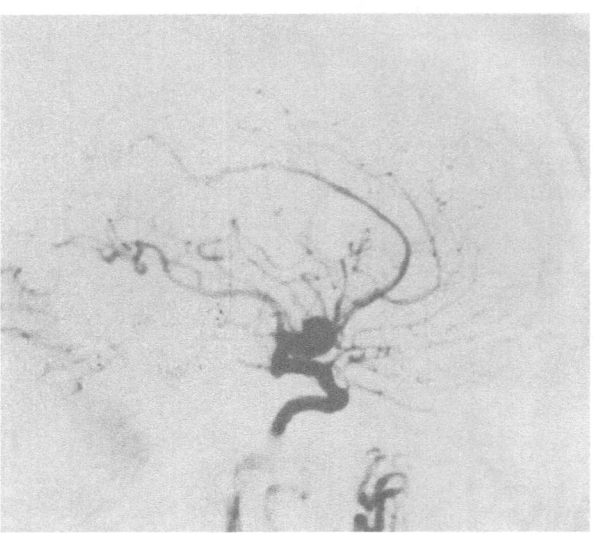

Fig. 7.3. Anterior communicating artery aneurysm projecting upwards and backwards.

Type 2 (bilateral)—14%. In this type the aneurysm, as well as both anterior cerebral arteries, fills from both carotid injections. The anterior communicating artery on the angiogram may appear rudimentary or prominent (Fig. 7.6).

Type 3 (dominant)—12%. In this type the aneurysm arises from the bifurcation of the dominant anterior cerebral artery, the contralateral artery being hypoplastic (Fig. 7.7).

Type 4 (dominant with foetal posterior cerebral)—8%. In this type the circulation patterns are similar to type 3, but other anomalies of the circle of Willis (usually a foetal posterior cerebral artery) are present (Fig. 7.8).

Their significance in relationship to surgical approach and techniques is more fully discussed in Chap. 11.

Pericallosal Artery Aneurysms

The most common site of pericallosal artery aneurysms is the junction between the pericallosal artery and the callosomarginal artery at the level of the genu of the corpus callosum. The lateral projection is the optimal view for such aneurysms, which are often small and project in a cranial or craniodorsal direction (Fig. 7.9).

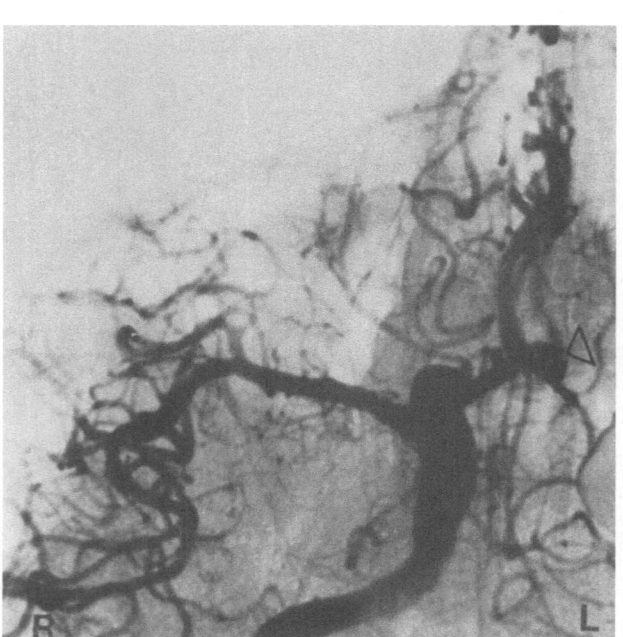

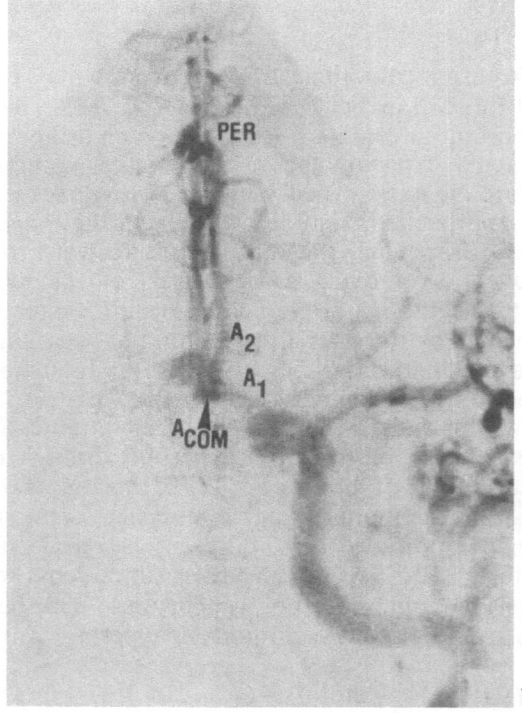

Fig. 7.4. a Modified basal projection clearly shows a small anterior communicating artery aneurysm, which projects forwards and to the left side (*open arrowhead*). **b** Modified basal projection showing anterior communicating aneurysm projecting forwards to the right side. *PER*, pericallosal artery.

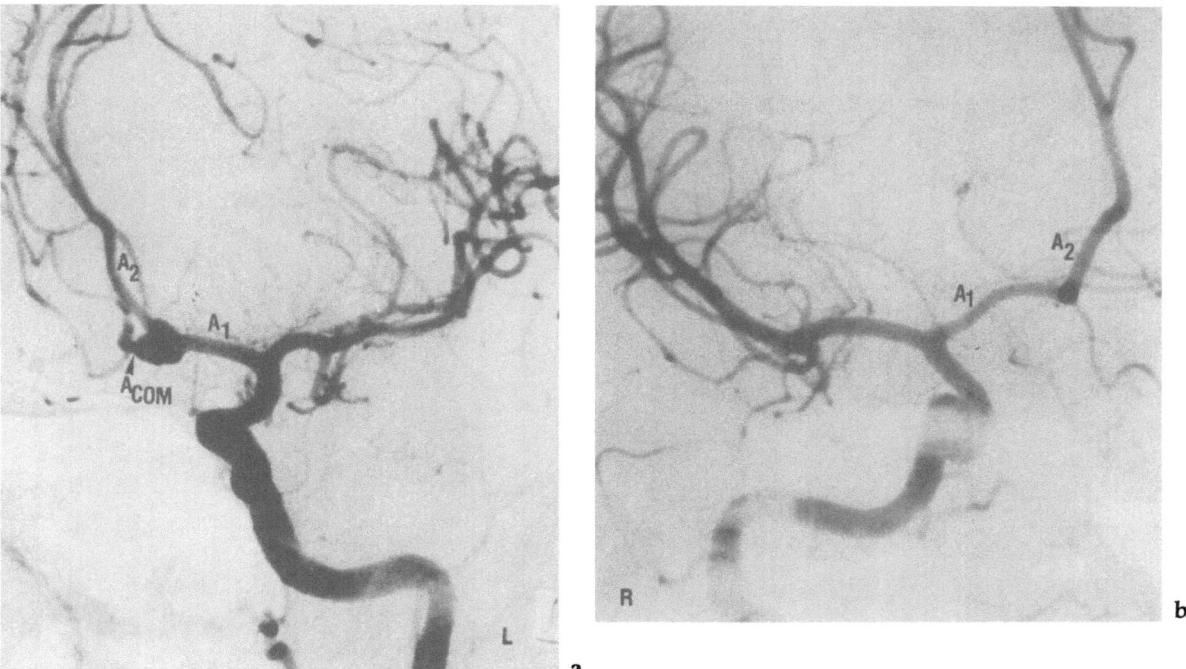

Fig. 7.5. a Left carotid injection showed filling of the anterior cerebral artery and an anterior communicating artery aneurysm. **b** Right carotid injection failed to fill the anterior communicating artery aneurysm (type 1 circulation).

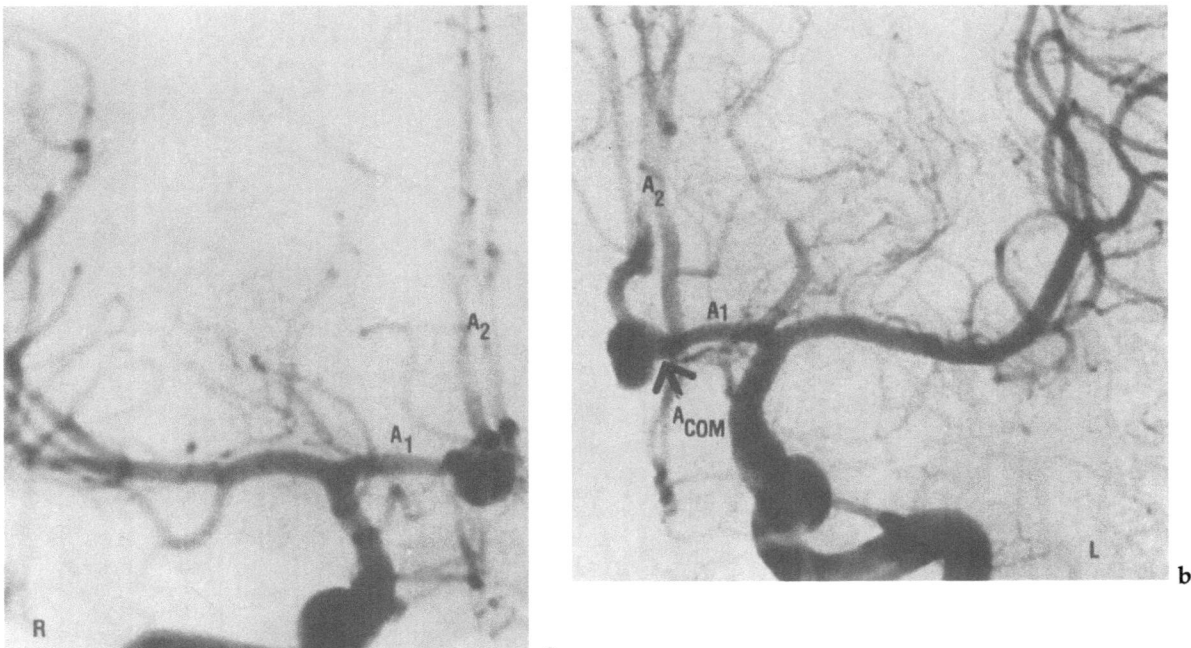

Fig. 7.6a, b. Both anterior cerebral arteries and an anterior communicating artery aneurysm fill from both the right and left carotid injections. The anterior communicating artery appears prominent (*arrow*).

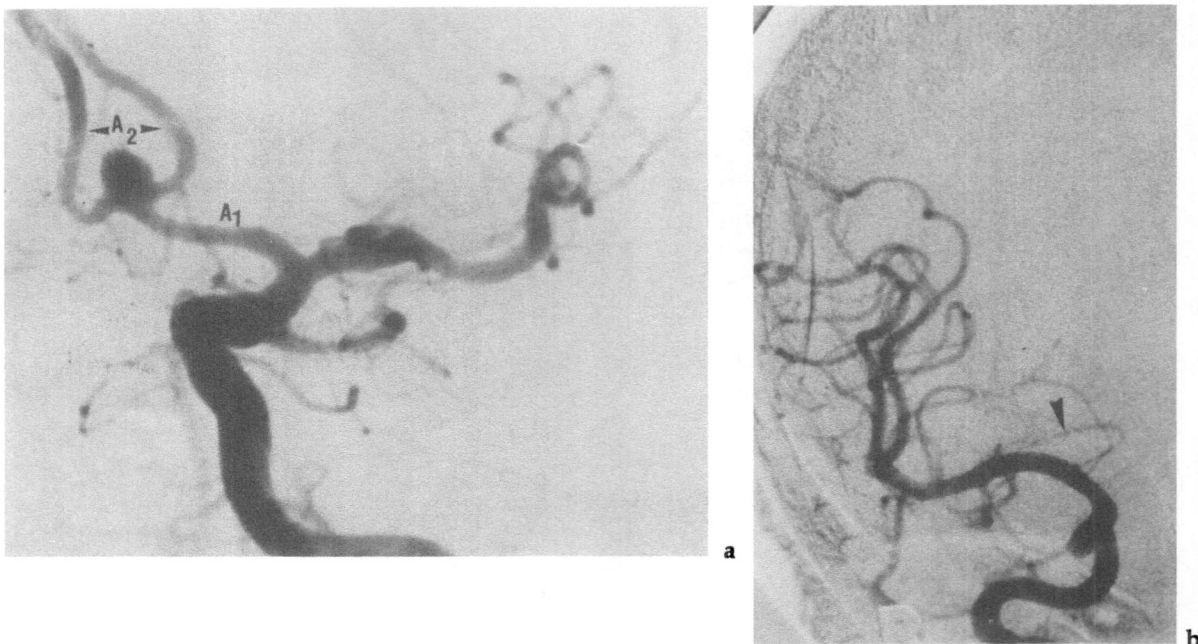

Fig. 7.7a, b. Left carotid injection shows filling of the anterior communicating artery aneurysm and both anterior cerebral arteries. Right carotid injection shows that the left A₁ segment of the anterior cerebral artery is hypoplastic (*arrowhead*).

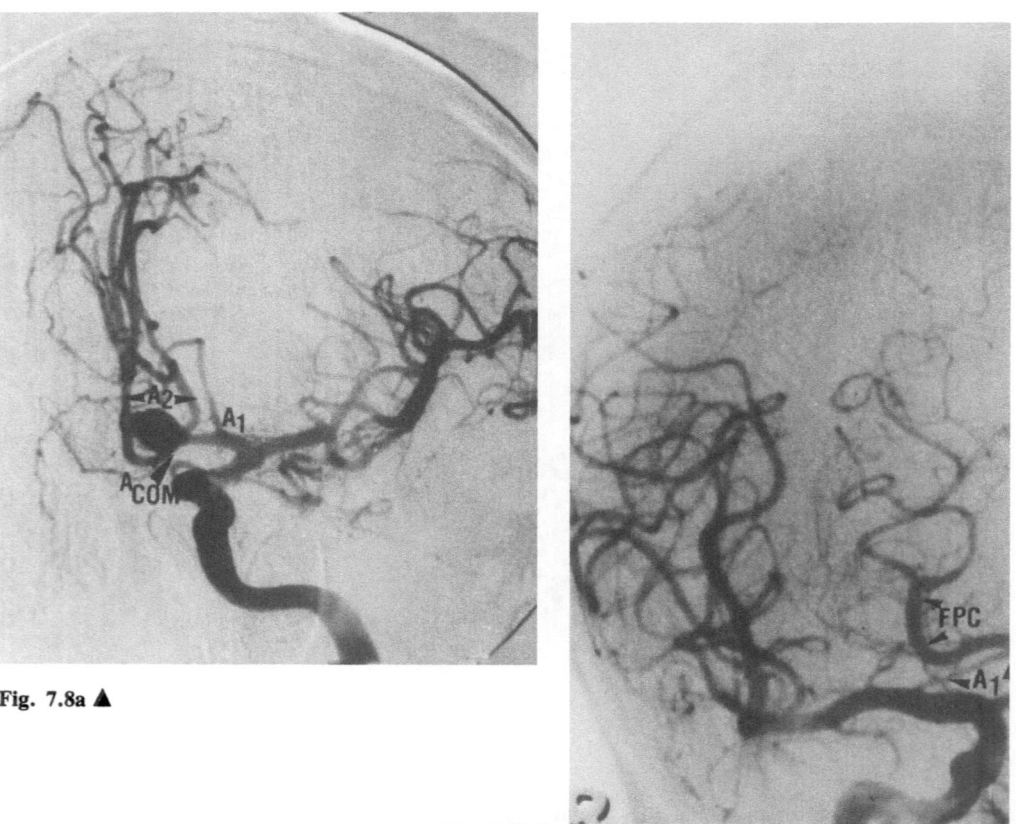

Fig. 7.8a ▲

Fig. 7.8b ▶

Fig. 7.8c ▶

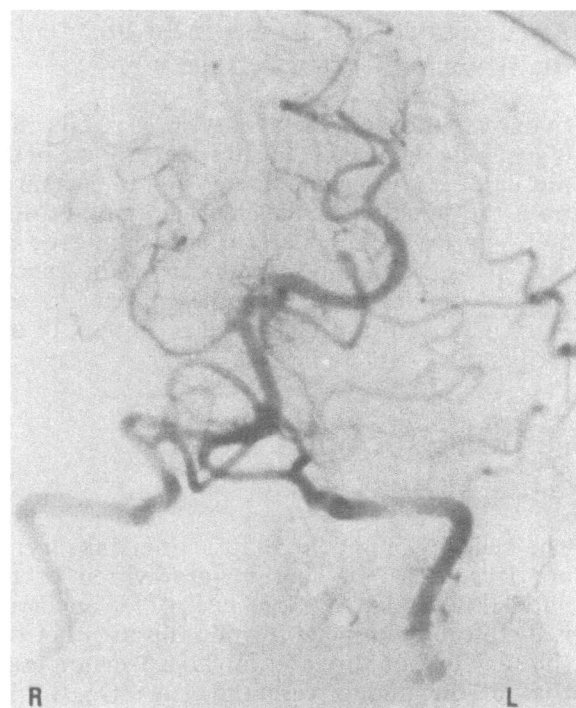

Fig. 7.8. a Left carotid injection shows filling of an anterior communicating artery aneurysm and both anterior cerebral arteries. **b** Right carotid injection shows that the A_1 segment of the anterior cerebral artery is hypoplastic (*arrowheads*). In addition there is a foetal origin of the posterior cerebral artery from the internal carotid artery (*FPC*). **c** Vertebral angiography confirms that there is no filling of the right posterior cerebral artery from the vertebrobasilar system.

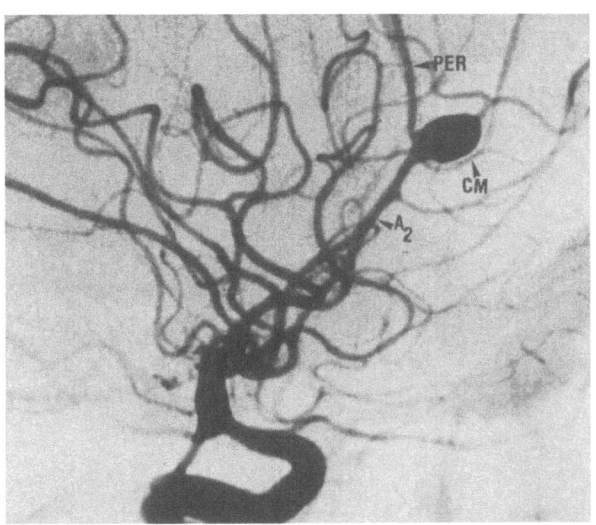

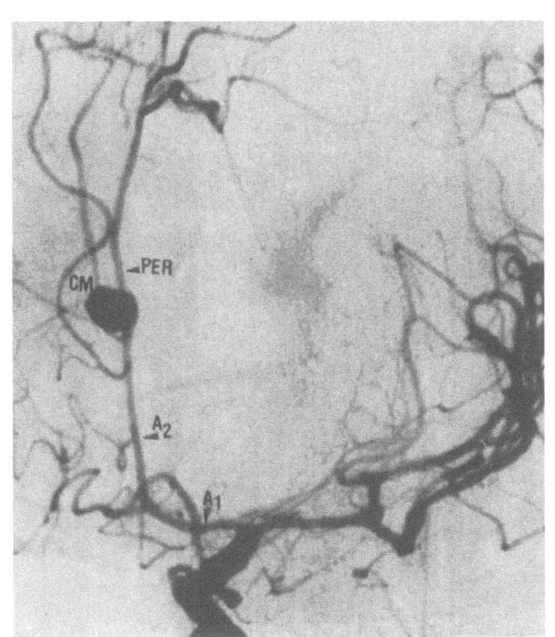

Fig. 7.9a, b. Pericallosal artery (*PER*) aneurysm. *CM*, callosomarginal artery.

Aneurysms of the A_1 Segment of the Anterior Cerebral Artery

In our experience these aneurysms are rarer than is generally reported in the literature. Some of the presumed A_1 segment aneurysms in fact arise from the junction of the internal carotid artery and anterior cerebral artery and should be regarded as bifurcation aneurysms with specific surgical implications. Examples of the A_1 segment aneurysm are illustrated in Figs. 7.10 and 7.36.

Middle Cerebral Artery Aneurysms

The majority of middle cerebral artery aneurysms are located at the first major division of the middle cerebral artery. The neck of the aneurysm is therefore in intimate relationship to either two (bifurcation) or three (trifurcation) major branches of the middle cerebral artery (Figs. 7.11, 7.12). Careful analysis of the preoperative angiogram in Townes oblique and oblique projection through the orbit will provide identification of branches arising from the middle cerebral artery proximal to and at the site of the aneurysm. A modified basal view may be of further value in separating the aneurysm from surrounding branches, clearly defining its neck and indicating whether the aneurysm projects anteriorly or posteriorly (Fig. 7.13).

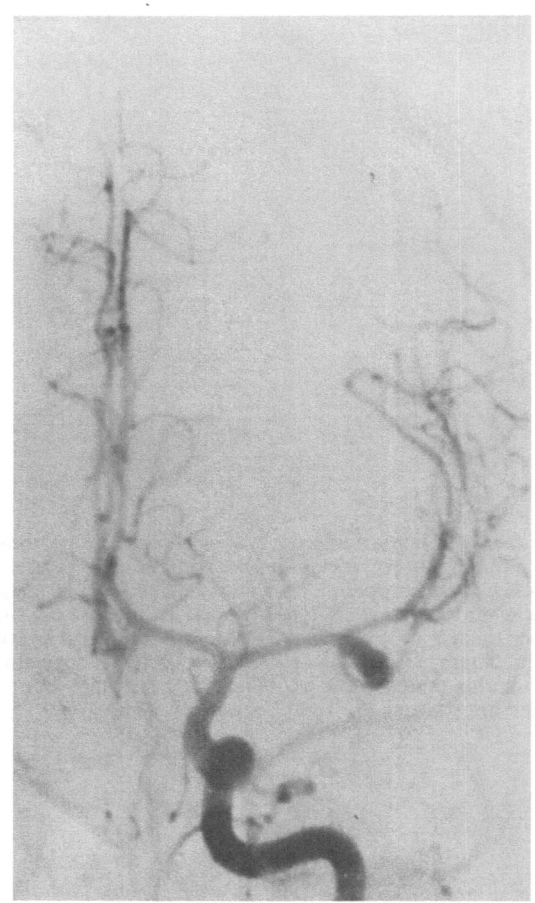

Fig. 7.11. Cerebral artery aneurysm arising near the major bifurcation of the middle cerebral artery trunk.

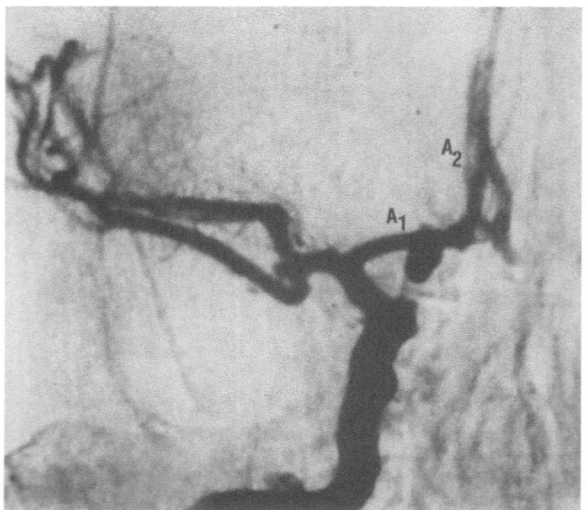

Fig. 7.10. Aneurysm arising from the A_1 segment of the right anterior cerebral artery.

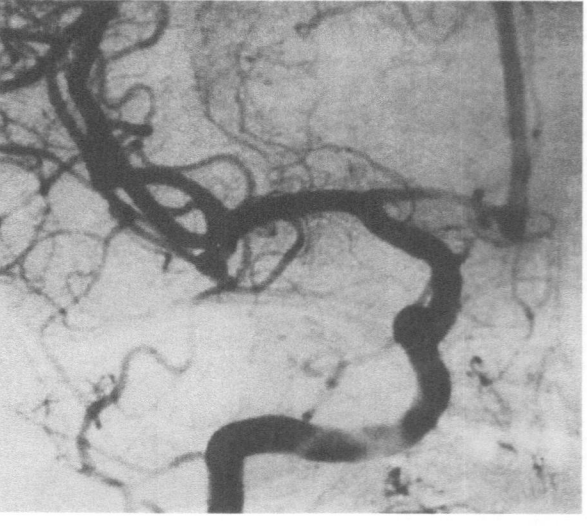

Fig. 7.12. Cerebral artery aneurysm arising near the major trifurcation of the middle cerebral artery trunk.

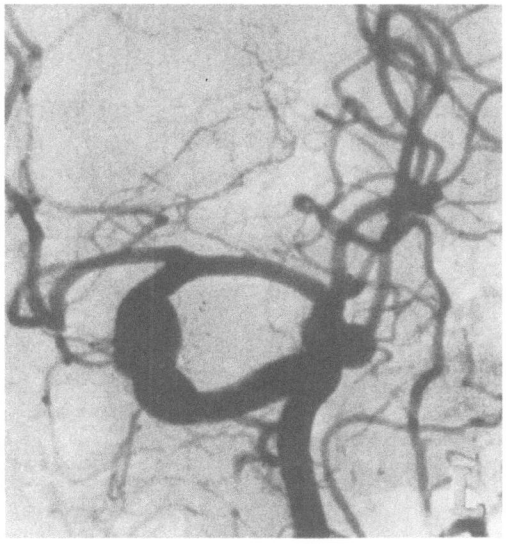
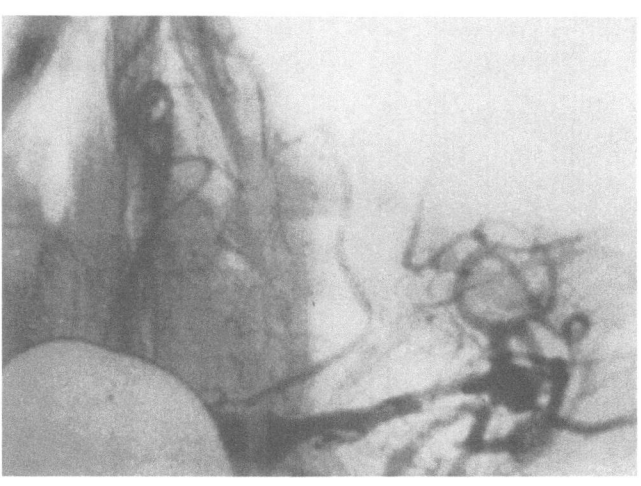

Fig. 7.13. a Aneurysm arising near the trifurcation of the middle cerebral artery. In this projection (Townes) the relationship of the aneurysm to the surrounding vessels and its neck is not clearly demonstrated. **b** A modified basal projection shows more clearly that the aneurysm has a neck and its relationship to the surrounding vessels.

The majority of middle cerebral artery aneurysms are not closely related anatomically to the lenticulostriate arteries, but when the aneurysm arises at a proximal bifurcation or trifurcation of the middle cerebral artery they may be intimately related (Fig. 7.14). Aneurysms may arise from the M_1 segment of the middle cerebral artery, in which case they are usually related to the lenticulostriate arteries. Aneurysms of the peripheral branches of the middle cerebral artery are rare, and of unusual aetiology (e.g. mycotic).

Posterior Communicating Artery Aneurysms

Posterior communicating artery aneurysms in fact arise from the junction of the internal carotid artery with the posterior communicating artery. Aneurysms involving the posterior communicating arteries alone are extremely rare, but when they do occur they are usually associated with a foetal posterior cerebral artery. The lateral projection will clearly define the aneurysm and show its relationship to the posterior communicating artery and anterior choroidal artery (Fig. 7.15). It will also indicate whether there is an anomalous

(foetal) origin of the posterior cerebral artery, which has an important bearing on the results of surgery (Sengupta 1975).(Fig. 7.16).

In some cases a waist-like deformity of the aneurysm sac produced by the tentorial edge may be seen (Fig. 7.17).

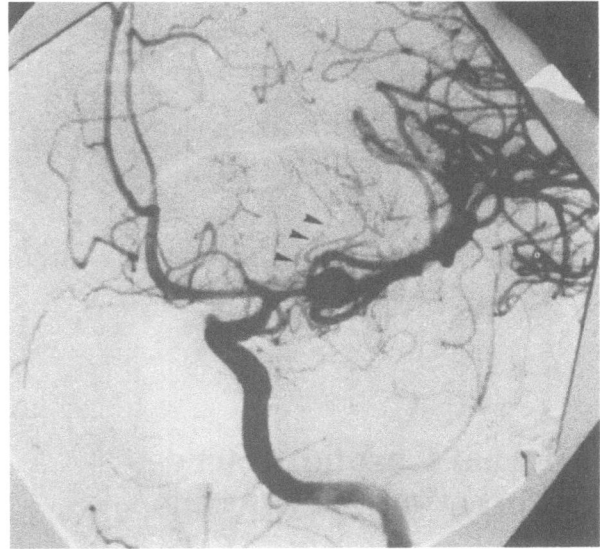

Fig. 7.14. Middle cerebral artery aneurysm arising at a proximal bifurcation and intimately related to the lenticulostriate arteries (*arrowheads*).

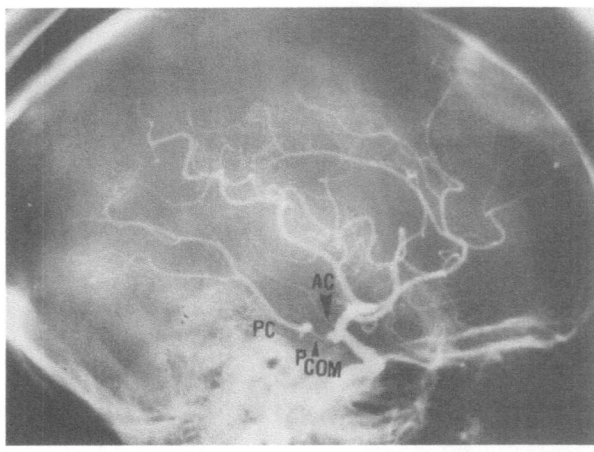

Fig. 7.15. A small posterior communicating artery aneurysm has been demonstrated, arising near the junction of the internal carotid artery and the posterior communicating artery (*P_{com}*). *AC*, anterior choroidal artery; *PC*, posterior cerebral artery.

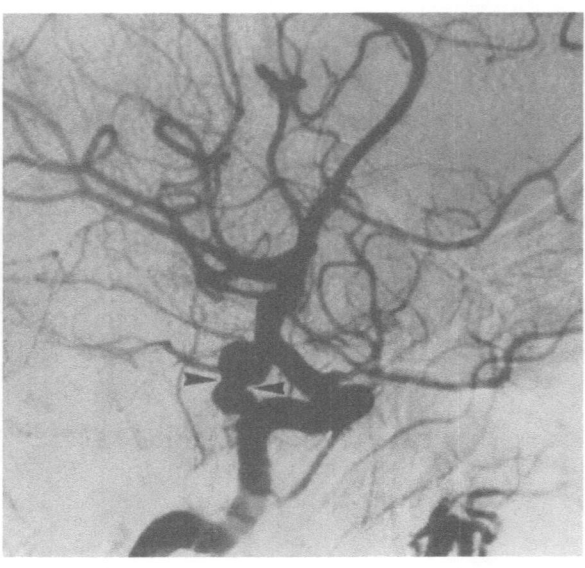

Fig. 7.17. Posterior communicating artery showing a waist-like constriction of its sac (*arrowheads*) produced by the tentorial edge. The lower portion of the sac below the constriction will be hidden by the tentorium at surgery.

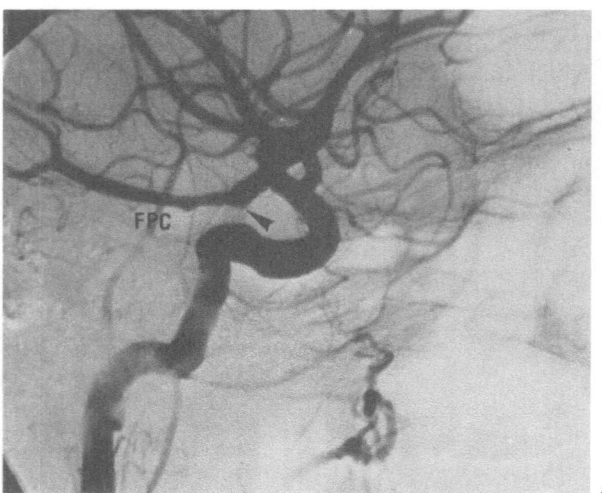

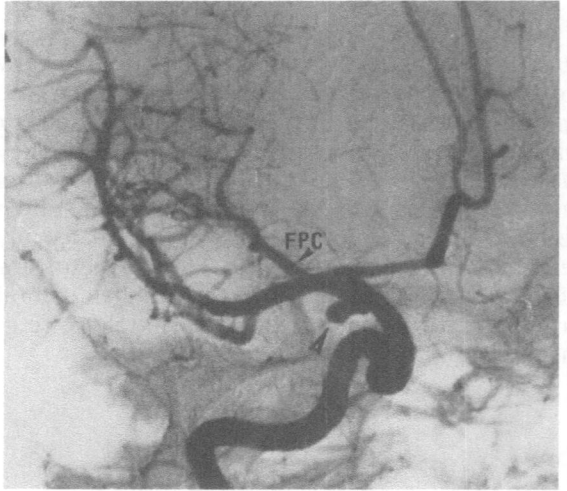

Fig. 7.16a, b. Posterior communicating artery aneurysm (*arrowheads*) associated with a foetal-type posterior cerebral artery (*FPC*).

Internal Carotid Artery (Bifurcation) Aneurysms

Bifurcation aneurysms are often difficult to demonstrate angiographically since most are small (less than 25 mm), and when they project in an anterior or posterior direction they tend to be superimposed on the internal carotid artery (Fig. 7.18). Multiple oblique projections may be necessary to confirm definitely the presence of a bifurcation aneurysm. A straight AP view through the orbit may be valuable.

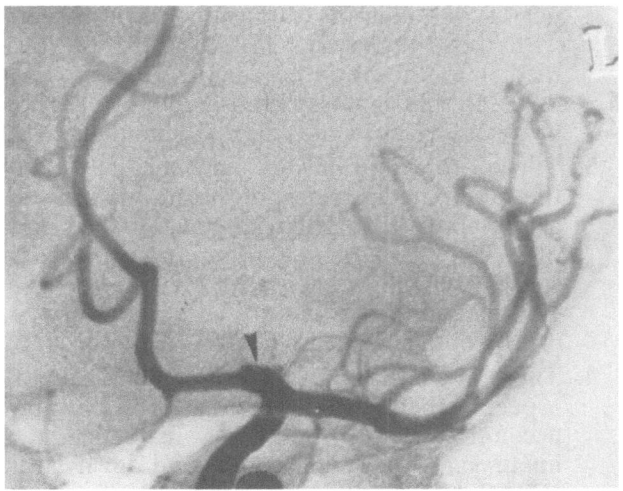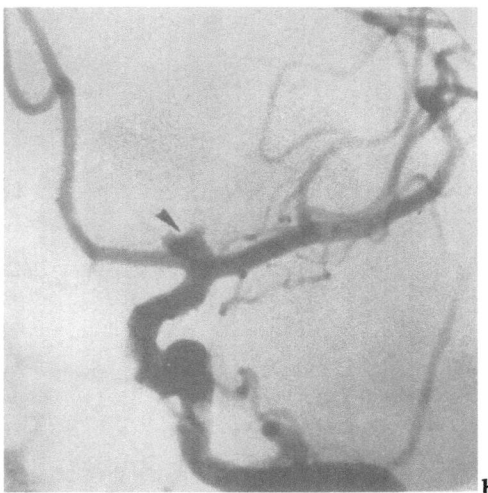

Fig. 7.18. **a** Internal carotid artery bifurcation aneurysm sac is largely obscured by overlapping on the bifurcation and anterior cerebral artery. **b** Oblique projection through the orbit more clearly demonstrates the presence of the bifurcation aneurysm.

Anterior Choroidal Aneurysms

Anterior choroidal aneurysms arise at the superior angle between the anterior choroidal artery and the internal carotid artery. They may easily be misdiagnosed as posterior communicating artery aneurysms, especially when the posterior communicating artery and anterior choroidal artery cannot be visualised. In most cases they are defined by the fact that they arise from the internal carotid artery distal to the origin of the posterior communicating artery but proximal to the bifurcation of the internal carotid artery (Fig. 7.19).

Carotid Ophthalmic Aneurysms

We use the term "carotid ophthalmic aneurysms" only for those aneurysms which arise from the internal carotid artery in the region of the ophthalmic artery (Drake et al. 1968). The relationship of the aneurysm to the anterior clinoid process and the configuration of the neck of the aneurysm are especially important features to demonstrate angiographically prior to surgery.

The ophthalmic artery most commonly arises from the superomedial aspect of the internal carotid artery. At angiography carotid ophthalmic aneurysms can be classified into four types:

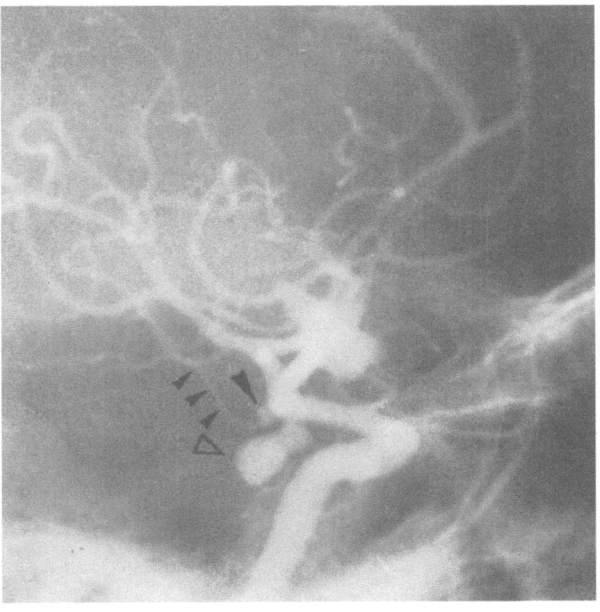

Fig. 7.19. Anterior choroidal artery aneurysm (*large black arrowhead*). The anterior choroidal artery is outlined (*small black arrowheads*). There is in addition a posterior communicating aneurysm (*open arrowhead*).

1. Those arising from the superior wall of the internal carotid artery and projecting upwards and above the anterior clinoid process.
2. Those projecting horizontally and medially from the superomedial internal carotid artery and if sufficiently large, passing under the optic

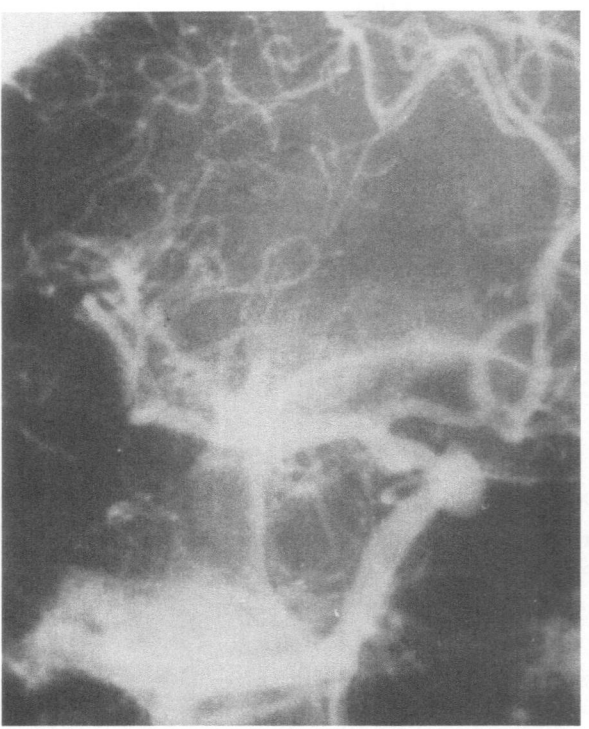

Fig. 7.20. Carotid ophthalmic artery aneurysm projecting medial to the anterior clinoid process.

nerves and chiasm. Surgery is more difficult with those aneurysms in which the sac lies medial to the anterior clinoid process (Fig. 7.20), for the anatomy is obscured by the optic nerve as well as by the anterior clinoid process.

3. Those projecting upwards and medially from the superomedial aspect of the internal carotid artery above the optic tract towards the circle of Willis. This type may produce a suprasellar space-occupying effect, with elevation of the A_1 segment of the anterior cerebral artery on one or both sides (Fig. 7.21).

4. Those arising from the inferomedial or lateral aspect of the internal carotid artery. This may account for the few cases in which the aneurysm projects backwards and downwards (Fig. 7.22). Aneurysms of this group may be mistaken for a posterior communicating artery aneurysm. The majority of carotid ophthalmic aneurysms, however, project anterior and medial to the internal carotid artery on the AP projection, whilst posterior communicating aneurysms generally project laterally (Fig. 7.23).

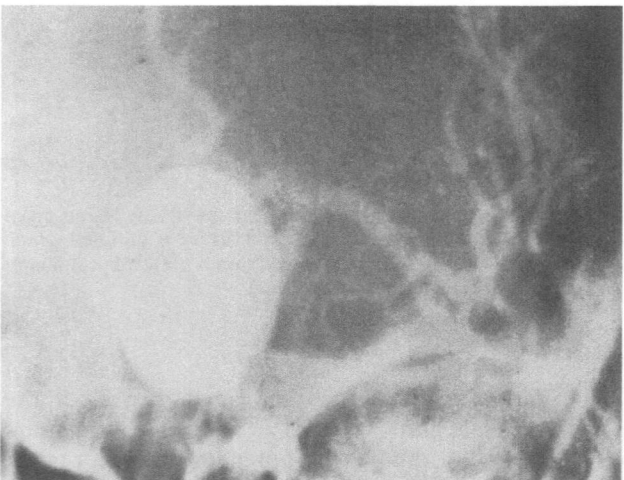
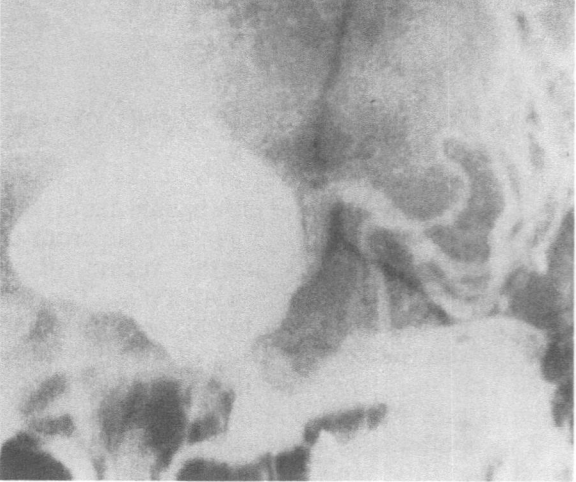

Fig. 7.21. Carotid ophthalmic artery aneurysm projecting upwards and medially to produce a suprasellar space-occupying effect. There is elevation of the A_1 segment of the anterior cerebral artery on both sides.

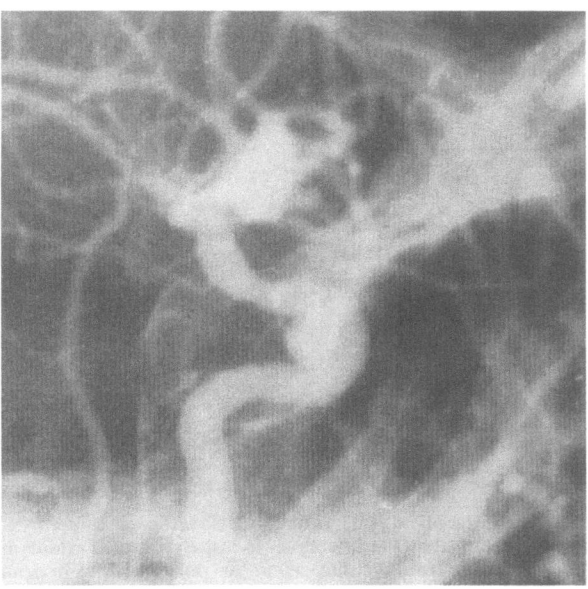

Fig. 7.22. Carotid ophthalmic artery aneurysm projecting backwards and downwards.

Intracavernous Aneurysms

Aneurysms arising from the intracavernous portion of the internal carotid artery usually do not give rise to SAH; if they do rupture, a caroticocavernous fistula is produced. In the context of SAH, however, they are important for two reasons:

1. They may be confused angiographically with ophthalmic artery aneurysms, which may lead the surgeon to carry out a direct intracranial approach.
2. These aneurysms lie within the cavernous sinus, so that they cannot be treated directly by the intracranial approach and the only methods of treatment available are carotid ligation in the neck, nowadays combined with an EC/IC anastomosis or a detachable catheter balloon technique. The following angiographic features suggest an intracavernous location of an aneurysm:

a) The aneurysm lies partly above and below the anterior clinoid process; this argues for a partly intradural and partly intracavernous location (Fig. 7.24)

b) The ophthalmic artery arises more proximally on the carotid trunk than the most

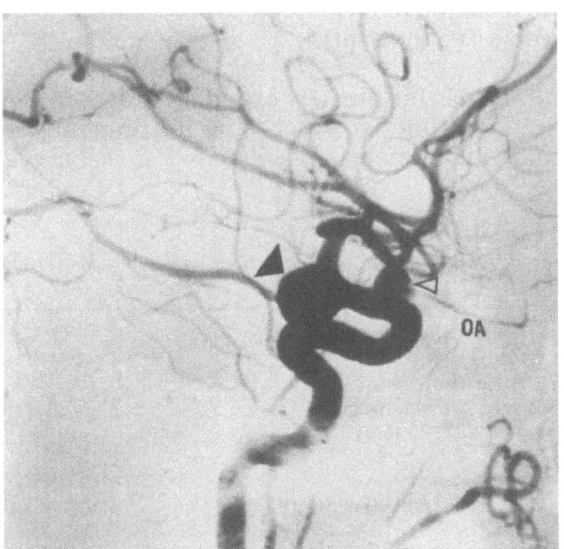

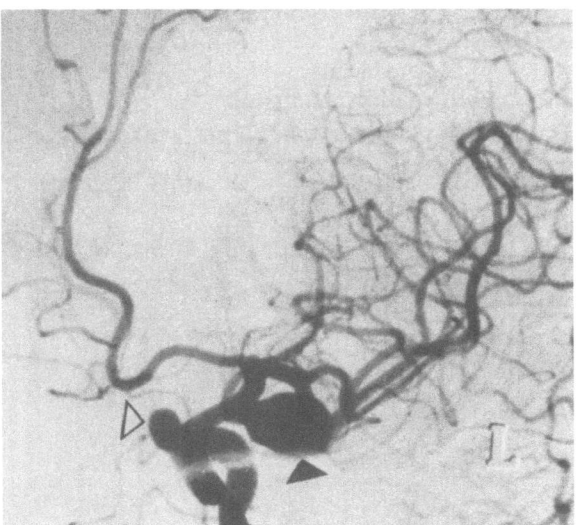

Fig. 7.23. a Lateral projection showing a small carotid ophthalmic artery (*OA*) aneurysm (*open arrowhead*) and a larger posterior communicating artery aneurysm (*black arrowhead*). **b** Townes oblique projection showing posterior communicating artery aneurysm (*black arrowhead*) projecting laterally and the carotid ophthalmic artery aneurysm (*open arrowhead*) projecting medially.

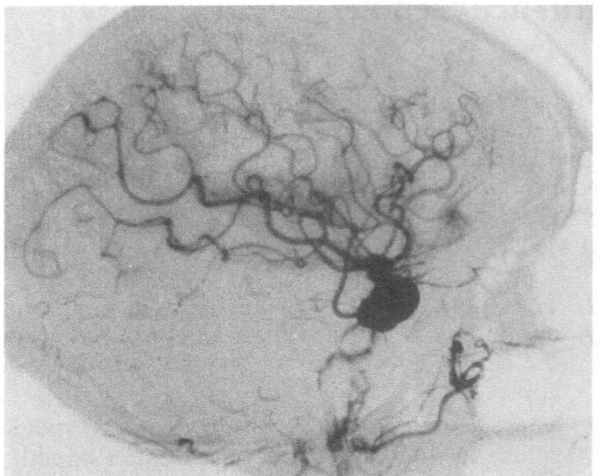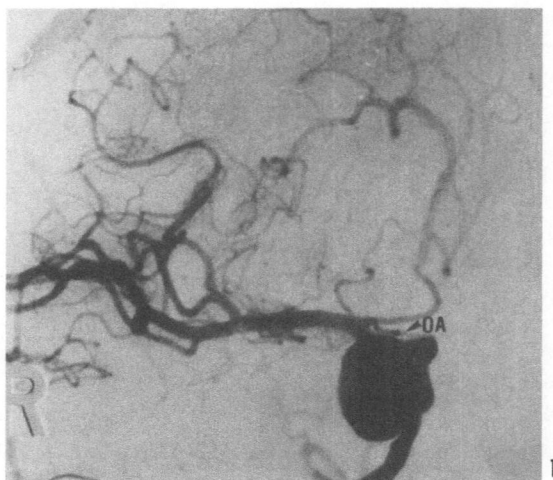

Fig. 7.24a, b. Intracavernous aneurysm. **a** Lateral projection. The fundus of the aneurysm lies mainly below the anterior clinoid process and is superimposed on the intracavernous carotid artery, indicating that the aneurysm is largely intracavernous in location. **b** Magnified oblique projection clearly shows that the aneurysm arises from the intracavernous portion of the internal carotid artery below the origin of the ophthalmic artery (*OA*).

proximal part of the aneurysm (Fig. 7.24)
c) In the lateral projections the fundus of an intracavernous aneurysm is superimposed on the intracavernous carotid artery (Fig. 7.24)

Vertebrobasilar Aneurysms

Vertebrobasilar aneurysms constitute between 5% and 10% of all aneurysms. They may be classified as:

1. Basilar bifurcation aneurysms
2. Basilar trunk aneurysms. These may be fur-

ther divided into:
a) Basilar and anterior inferior cerebellar artery junction aneurysms
b) Basilar and superior cerebellar artery junction aneurysms
c) Aneurysms in the region of union of the vertebral arteries
d) Posterior cerebral aneurysms which may arise either at the junction with the posterior communicating artery (P_1 segment) or at the first major branching on the side of the midbrain (P_2 segment).

Drake has the greatest experience, and in 1979 he reported on 546 cases. The distribution (excluding giant aneurysms) is shown in Table 7.2.

Table 7.2. Distribution of vertebrobasilar aneurysms (Drake 1979)

Basilar bifurcation aneurysms (12 mm)	*174*
Vertical	110
Posterior projection	41
Forward projection	23
Bulbous (12–25 mm)	59
Basilar trunk aneurysms	*123*
At superior cerebellar artery	72
At AICA	28
Region of union of vertebral arteries	23
Vertebral–PICA aneurysms	*65*
Posterior cerebral aneurysms	*18*

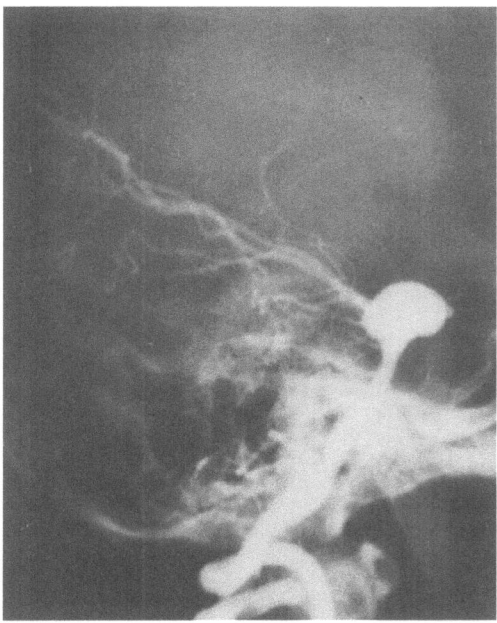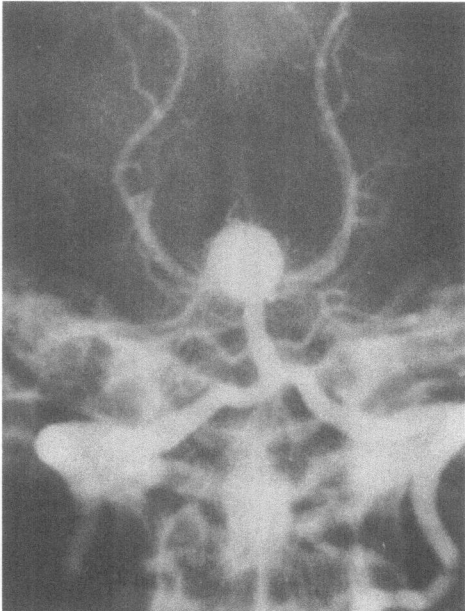

Fig. 7.25. Basilar bifurcation aneurysm projecting anteriorly.

Basilar Bifurcation Aneurysms

In basilar bifurcation aneurysms the lateral projection is important to assess whether the aneurysm projects directly upwards in line with the basilar artery, posteriorly into the interpeduncular cistern or anteriorly with the dome of the aneurysm above the dorsum sellae (Figs. 7.25, 7.26). Anteriorly projecting aneurysms will lie free of any perforating vessels and can be surgically obliterated. Posteriorly projecting aneurysms projecting into the interpeduncular fossa and posterior perforated substance will be intimately related to small perforating vessels so that direct clipping will be hazardous. Assessment of the height of the basilar bifurcation (in relationship to the dorsum sellae) is also important. A high bifurcation may necessitate greater retraction on the temporal lobe, while low bifurcation (base of dorsum sellae or lower down on the clivus) may mean that the tentorial edge hides the base of the aneurysm sac (Fig. 10.36). Angiography will allow evaluation of the relationship of the aneurysm to the posterior cerebral arteries and will define the angle at which the cerebral arteries originate from the basilar tip as well as demonstrate the course of the penduncular segment.

Basilar Trunk Aneurysms

Examples of aneurysms arising near the origin of the superior cerebellar artery and at the vertebrobasilar junction are shown in Figs. 7.27 and 7.28, respectively.

Posterior Inferior Cerebellar Artery (PICA) Aneurysms

These aneurysms usually arise at the PICA–vertebral artery junction but more rarely from distal PICA branching sites. They are often obscured on the lateral projection because of the dense petrous bone. Vertebral oblique projections making use of subtraction techniques are ideal to show the relationship of the neck of the aneurysm to the origin of the PICA, the level of origin of the PICA (e.g. high or low) as well as any vascular anomalies (e.g. vertebral artery ending as a PICA) (Figs. 7.29–7.31). Hirschfeld and Flamm (1981) reported a case of SAH from an aneurysm arising from an extracranial loop of the right posterior inferior cerebellar artery below the foramen magnum. They emphasised the need for a complete four-vessel study in evaluating patients with SAH.

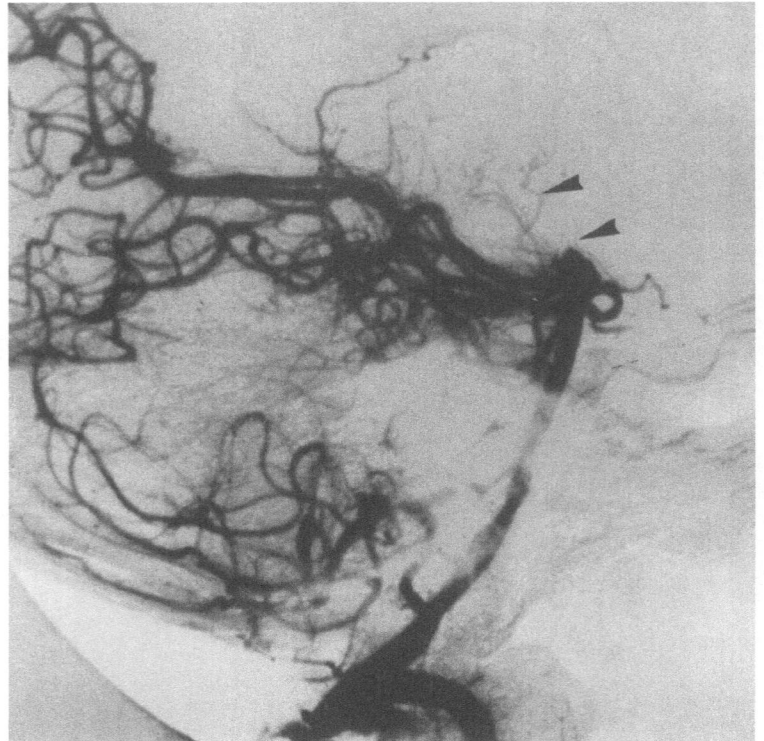

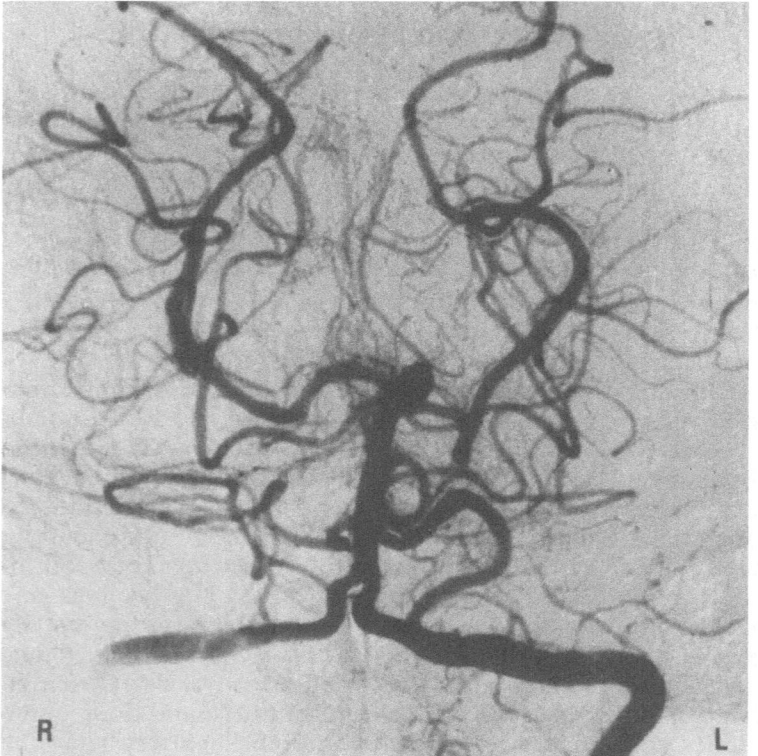

Fig. 7.26. a Basilar bifurcation aneurysm projecting posteriorly. Notice how the sac of the aneurysm is intimately related to numerous perforating vessels (*arrowheads*). **b** Townes projection shows the aneurysm projects to the left side.

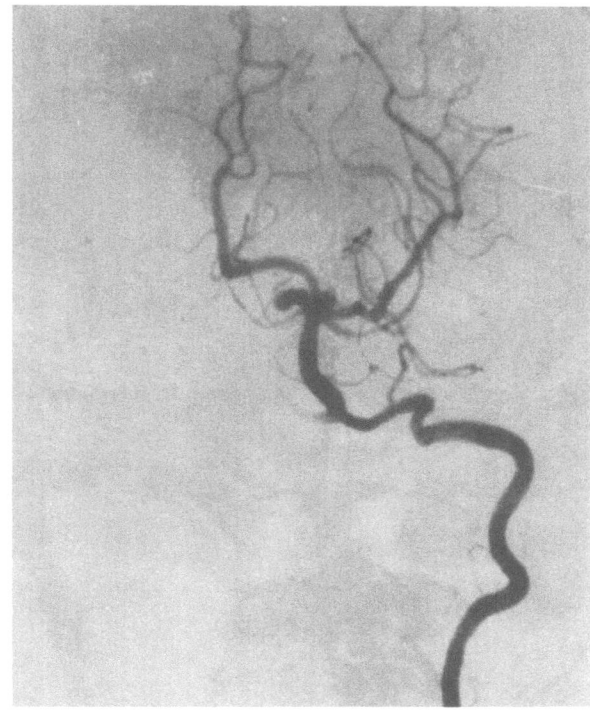

Fig. 7.27. Bilocular aneurysm arising at the junction of the basilar trunk and the superior cerebellar artery.

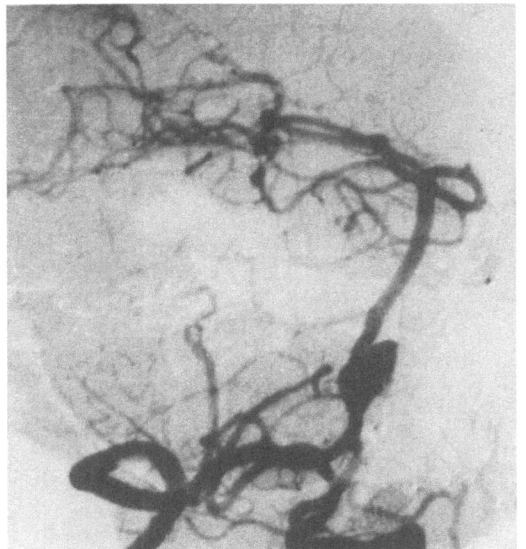 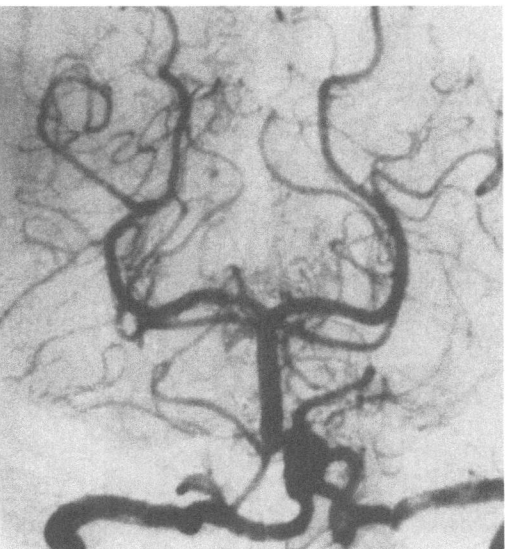

Fig. 7.28. Aneurysm arising at the vertebrobasilar junction.

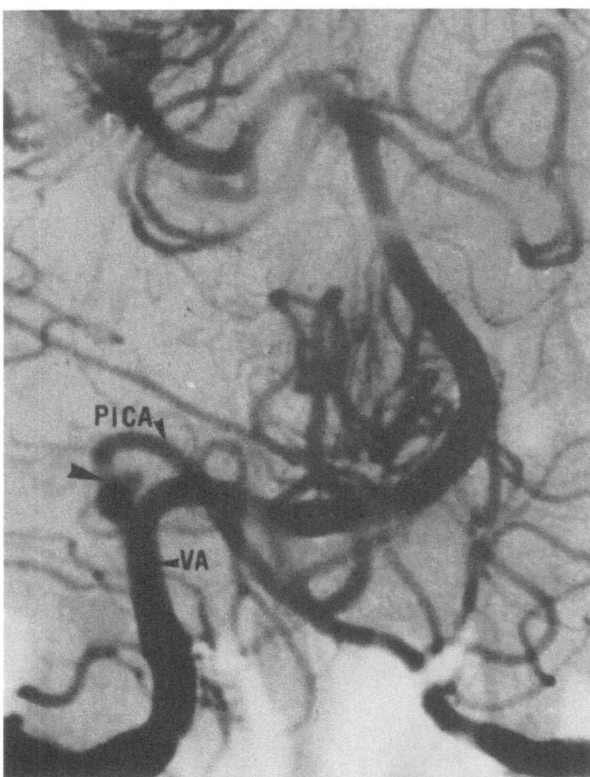

Fig. 7.29. Vertebral angiogram oblique projection showing aneurysm arising from the junction of the posterior/inferior cerebellar artery (*PICA*) and the vertebral artery (*VA*).

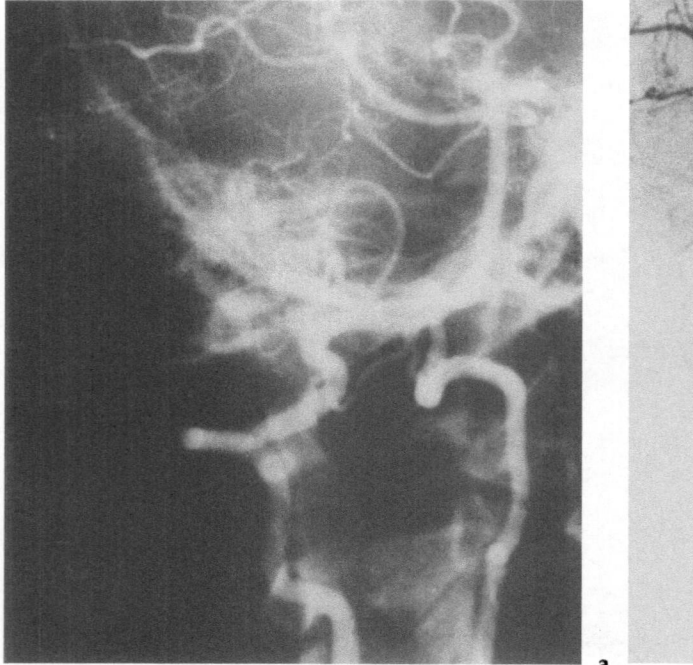 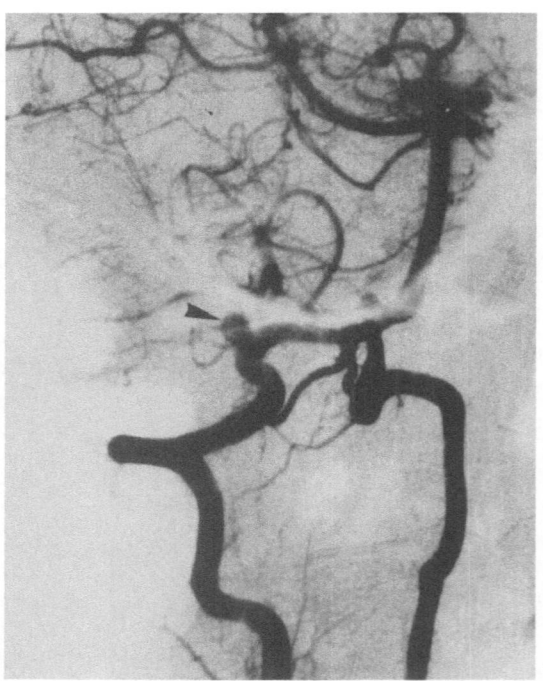

a   b

Fig. 7.30. a Unsubtracted vertebral oblique projection angiogram. **b** Subtracted vertebral oblique projection angiogram clearly shows a PICA aneurysm (*arrowhead*)

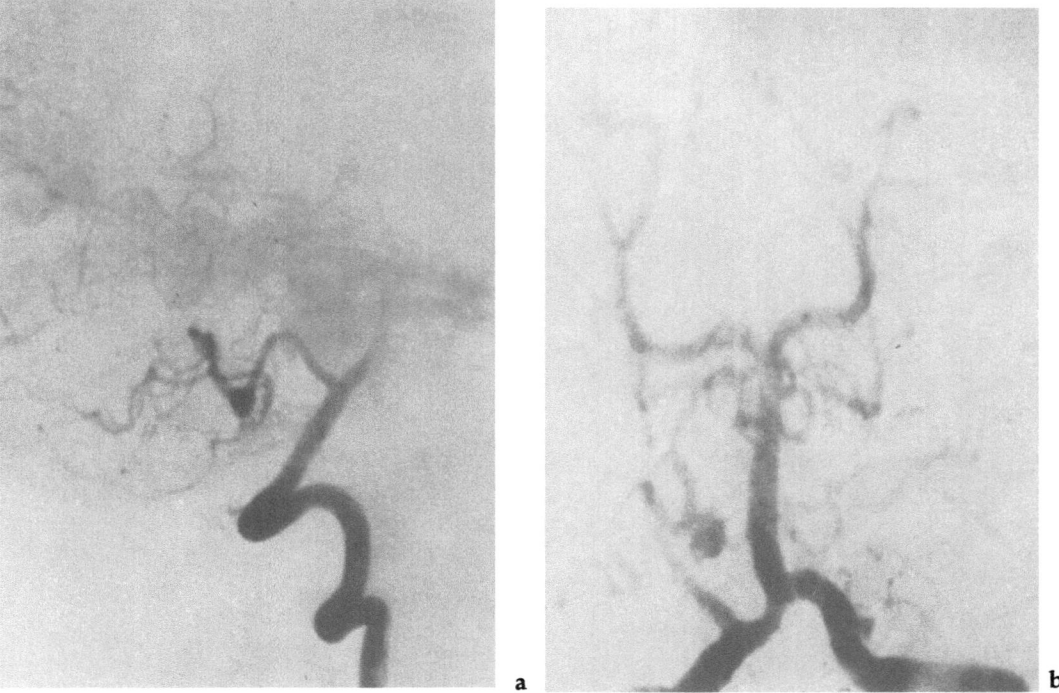

Fig. 7.31a, b. Peripheral PICA aneurysm. **a** Lateral and **b** Townes projections show the aneurysm arising about 3 cm from the origin of the PICA.

Congenital peripheral aneurysms are uncommon but occur more frequently on the vertebrobasilar arterial system. They mostly involve the PICA (Fig. 7.31) but can occur at other sites (Fig. 7.32). An example of a posterior cerebral artery aneurysm arising from the artery during its course on the side of the mid-brain is shown in Fig. 7.33. Hiscott and Crockard (1982) have reported a case of multiple aneurysms of the distal posterior inferior cerebellar artery.

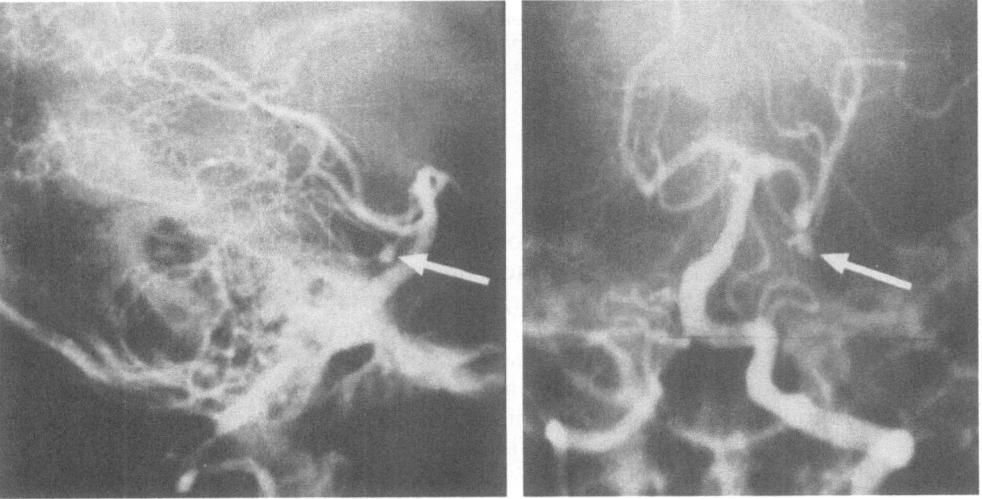

Fig. 7.32. Peripheral superior cerebellar artery aneurysm (*arrows*).

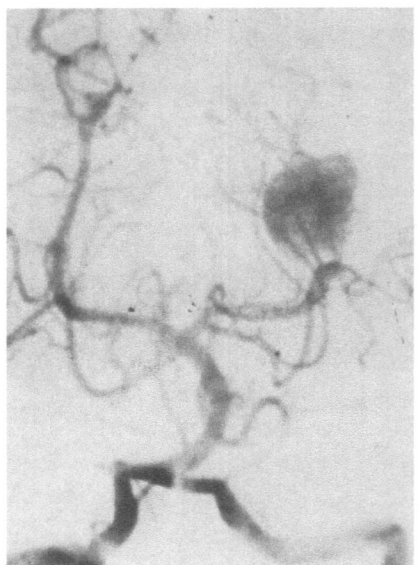
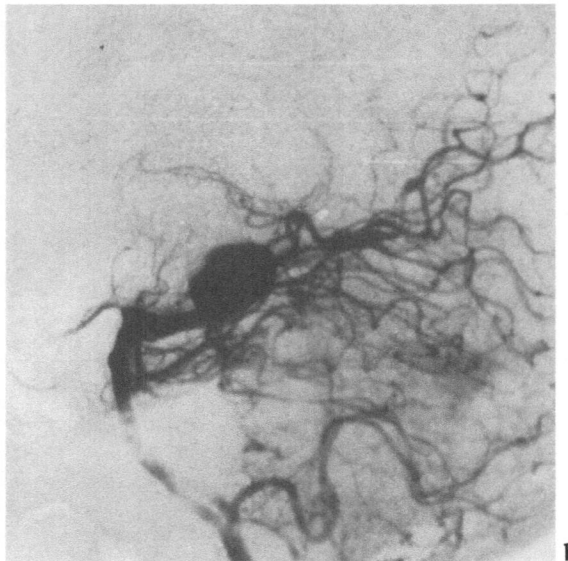

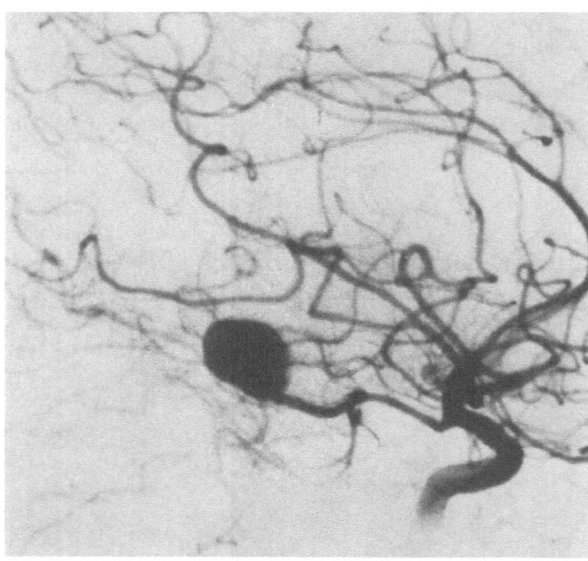

Fig. 7.33a–c. Posterior cerebral artery aneurysm arising on the side of the mid-brain. **a** Townes and **b** lateral projection angiogram; **c** lateral projection carotid angiogram

Angiotomography and Magnification Angiography

Agnoli et al. (1979) analysed the relative values of these techniques. Angiotomography and magnification angiography were most helpful in those cases in which routine angiography could not differentiate between an aneurysm and an arterial loop. Very small aneurysms may be more clearly demonstrated by these techniques. Identification of the exact origin and configuration of the neck of large aneurysms may also be facilitated. Agnoli et al. concluded that neither investigation should be used routinely because both are time consuming and require a large amount of contrast medium. On the whole, magnification angiography is more advantageous. It is our practice to take a magnification study of the projections which show the aneurysm anatomy to best advantage.

Angiographic Findings in Ruptured Aneurysms

Site of Rupture

Aneurysms nearly always rupture at or near the dome of the sac. Crompton (1966) found that 80% of aneurysms ruptured near the apex and 20% elsewhere. Irregularity or loculation of the aneurysm sac suggests recent rupture. Wood (1964) reported such loculation in 76% of aneurysms that had ruptured. du Boulay (1965) emphasised that in the presence of multiple aneurysms a loculated aneurysm is the one most likely to have bled (Fig. 7.34).

Vessel Spasm (Vasospasm)

It is postulated that following aneurysmal rupture blood fills the subarachnoid space and surrounds the arteries lying in the basal cisterns. The subarachnoid clot contains vasospasmogenic substances which, when activated, result in the arterial narrowing demonstrated at angiography and referred to as vasospasm.

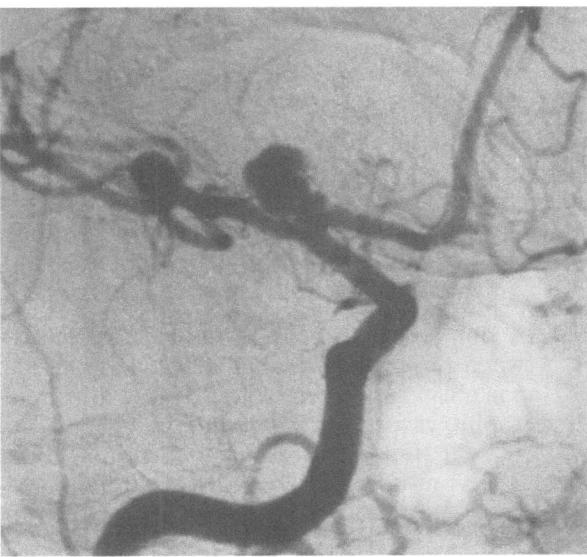

Fig. 7.34. Two aneurysms have been demonstrated—a smooth-walled aneurysm arising near the trifurcation of the right middle cerebral artery, and a larger, irregular (loculated) aneurysm arising near the bifurcation of the right internal carotid artery.

The nature of vasospasmogenic substances remains unclear; indeed, it is far from clear whether the arterial narrowing represents smooth muscle contraction or is related to structural changes which have been demonstrated in arterial walls in SAH (Hughes and Schianchi 1978; Hughes 1980).

The arterial narrowing results in increased vascular resistance, which, if of a sufficient degree, decreases perfusion pressure below the limits of autoregulation and results in reduced cerebral blood flow. This may cause ischaemia and, if severe, infarction. In patients with infarction the degree of vessel constriction is usually more than 60% (Schneck and Kricheff 1964).

Vasospasm can be classified as:

1. Local, when spasm is limited to one vessel (Fig. 7.35)
2. Segmental, when only a part of the artery is involved (Fig. 7.36)
3. Generalised, when there is a spasm in at least two major vessels (Fig. 7.37).

In our 500 operated aneurysm cases, pre-operative vasospasm occurred in 42.8% and consisted of localised spasm in 21.2%, segmental spasm in 5.2% and generalised spasm in 16.3%.

Vasospasm is probably a two-stage phenomenon (Brawley et al. 1968; Symon et al. 1972). The immediate stage corresponds with the traumatic rupture of the aneurysm and probably only lasts about half an hour, while the second stage occurs over the next few days and may persist for 2–3 weeks. Vasospasm is rarely seen in the first few days following SAH. It becomes evident on angiography 2–3 days following rupture and becomes more frequent with time, reaching a peak between the first and second weeks (Zervas 1979). Our experience of the timing of onset of vasospasm is very similar (Chap. 12).

Vessel narrowing due to vasospasm has to be differentiated from that due to atherosclerosis or an arteritic process. Differentiation between a hypoplastic A_1 segment and vasospasm is important but is not difficult in most cases. In hypoplasia there is usually a characteristic curvature of the internal carotid artery, and the contralateral A_1 segment artery tends to be large. Streaming of blood in the proximal part of the basilar artery may occasionally stimulate the appearance of spasm.

Pre-operative angiographic vasospasm in the 500 case series has been correlated with factors such as age, sex, neurological grade, aneurysm

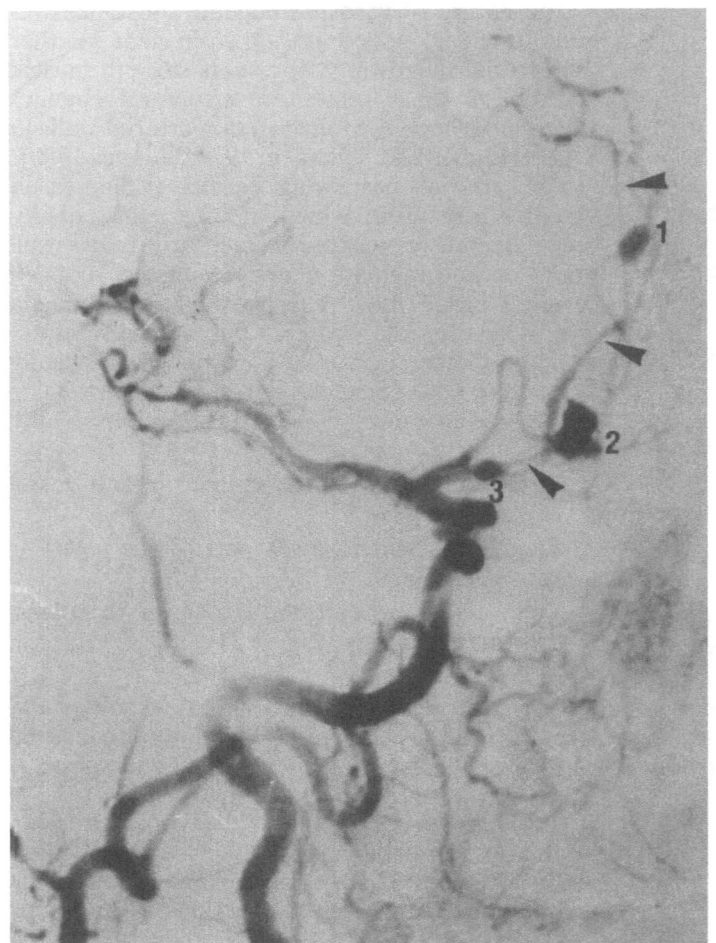

Fig. 7.35. Local spasm involving the A_1 and A_2 segments of the right anterior cerebral artery (*arrowheads*). Three aneurysms are demonstrated: *1* = pericallosal, *2* = anterior communicating, *3* = A_1 segment.

site, rebleeding, ischaemic complications, condition of the brain at surgery, mortality and hydrocephalus, and these are fully discussed in Chaps. 11 and 12. In summary:

1. There was no evidence that age had any influence on the incidence of vasospasm.
2. The incidence of vasospasm showed no sex predilection.
3. There was no real correlation between aneurysm site and the incidence of vasospasm except that it appeared to be more commonly seen in middle cerebral artery aneurysms ($P < 0.05$).
4. Pre-operative vasospasm is more common in those patients with haematoma ($P < 0.01$):

5. The brain at operation was abnormal in only 34% of patients with angiographic spasm compared to 47% with spasm ($P < 0.001$).
6. In our series there was no correlation between pre-operative angiographic spasm and mortality. However, some degree of angiographic vasospasm was noted in 34 (68%) of the 51 patients with ischaemic complications in the pre-operative period ($P < 0.001$).
7. Hydrocephalus is significantly more common in patients with pre-operative vasospasm ($P < 0.01$).
8. There was no correlation between the incidence of pre-operative vasospasm and postoperative vasospasm.

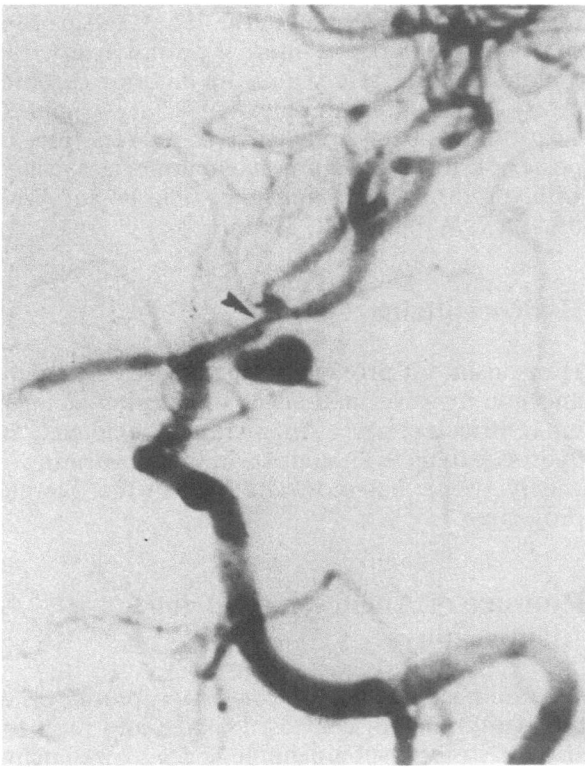

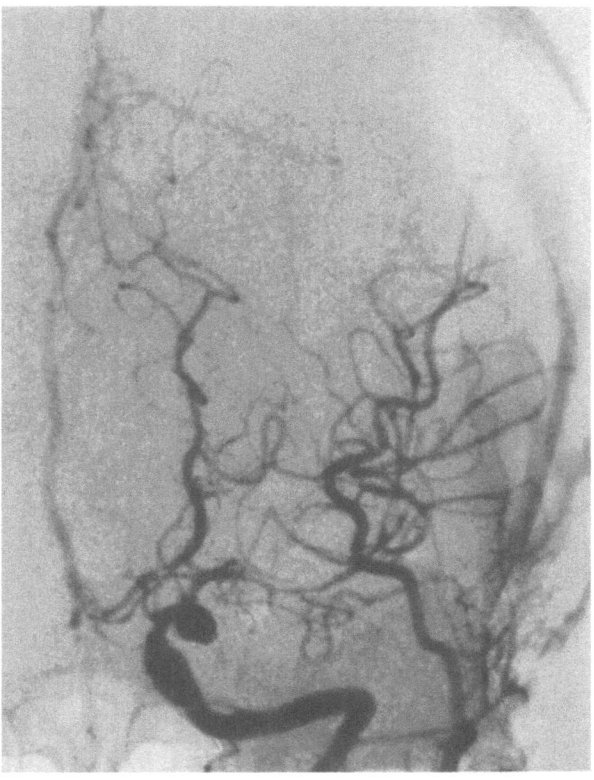

Fig. 7.36. Segmental spasm (*arrowhead*).

Fig. 7.37. Carotid angiogram showing generalised vasospasm.

9. The incidence of further SAH (rebleed) was not influenced by the presence of pre-operative vasospasm.

10. In a separate study of the complications following angiography in 440 patients we have shown that neurological complications are significantly more common in patients with severe generalised pre-operative vasospasm.

There has been a review of the radiologists' (du Boulay 1980) and neurosurgeons' (Mohan 1980) current views on vasospasm.

Intracranial Haematoma

Small haematomas are more accurately demonstrated by CT. Larger haematomas can be demonstrated by angiography, usually in patients in poor clinical grades in whom surgical evacuation of the clot is considered necessary. A detailed analysis of the patterns of haematoma produced by aneurysms at different anatomical sites is outlined in Chap. 6.

In intraventricular haematoma CT allows a precise diagnosis whereas at angiography the diagnosis may be impossible or at most only suggestive. Blood within the ventricular system may obstruct the CSF pathways at the foramen of Munro or the aqueduct or exit foramina of the fourth ventricle, leading to hydrocephalus which may be demonstrated at angiography.

Subdural Haematoma

Barton and Tudor (1982) in a review of the literature quote an incidence of 0.5%–7.9% of subdural haematomas in association with ruptured intracranial aneurysms. Many of these subdural collections were, however, only demonstrated at autopsy and were so small in size that they would be impossible to demonstrate angiographically or even at CT. In a review of 839 angiograms they reported 11 cases in which a subdural haematoma was demonstrated radiologically (incidence 1.3%).

The commonest aneurysm sites responsible for subdural haematoma were similar to those re-

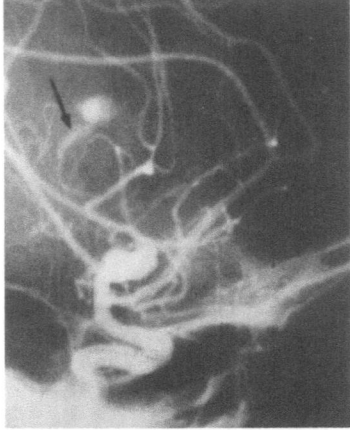

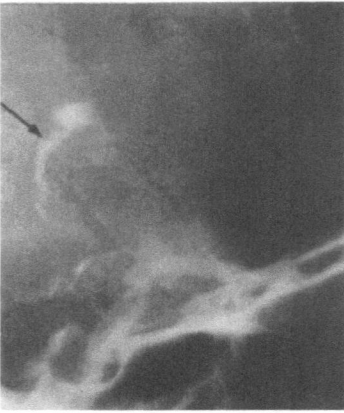

ported previously (Strange et al. 1951), and in order of frequency were the internal carotid artery, the middle cerebral artery and the anterior cerebral artery/anterior communicating artery complex. There have been only two cases reported of posterior fossa subdural haematoma associated with vertebrobasilar aneurysms (Clarke and Walton 1953; Wright et al. 1965).

Hydrocephalus

Here again, CT provides a much more convenient and non-invasive method of monitoring changes in ventricular size. Angiographic evidence of hydrocepahlus will consist in demonstrating a widely swept thalamostriate vein in the Townes projection.

Rupture of Aneurysms During Angiography

On rare occasions aneurysms may rupture during angiography, with contrast leakage into the ventricular system, subarachnoid space or parenchyma (Figs. 7.38, 7.39). It occurs most commonly in the supratentorial compartment (Waga et al.

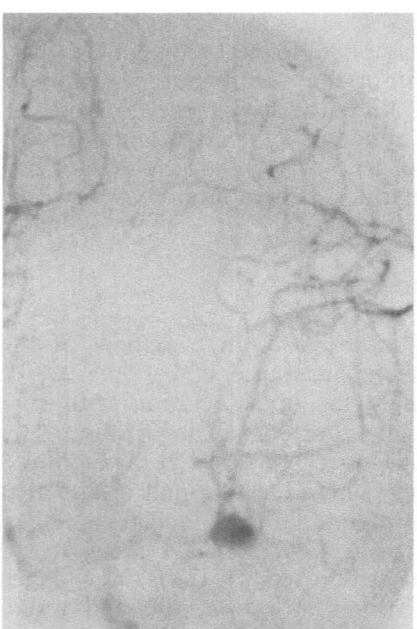

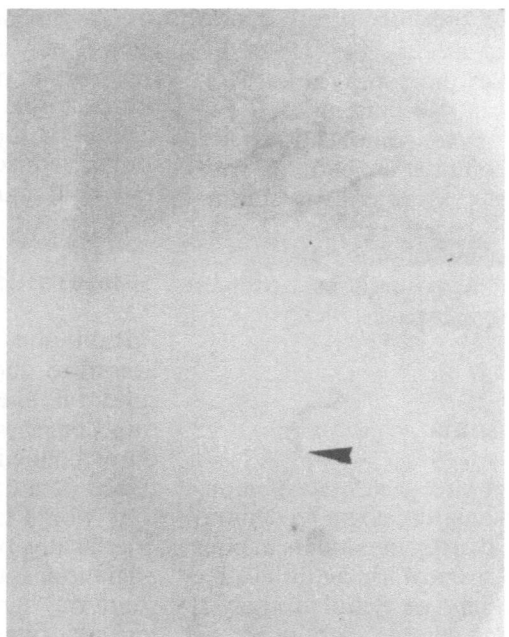

Fig. 7.38. a Lateral and **b** Townes projections showing leakage of contrast from a left middle cerebral artery aneurysm into the brain substance (*arrows and arrowhead*).

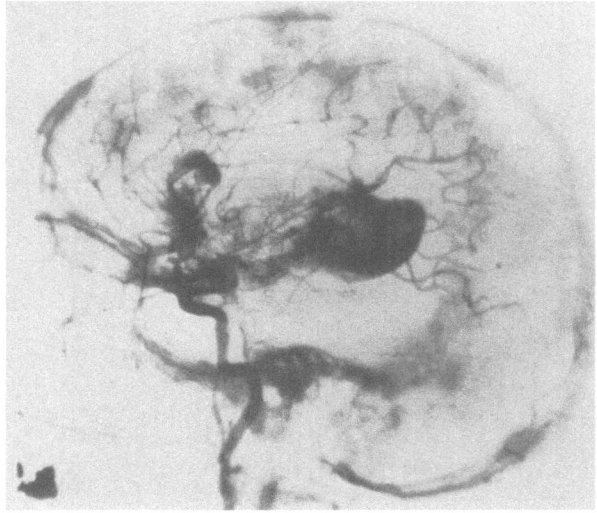

Fig. 7.39. A further case of intraparenchymal rupture of an aneurysm during angiography. (By courtesy of Dr. B Liliequist)

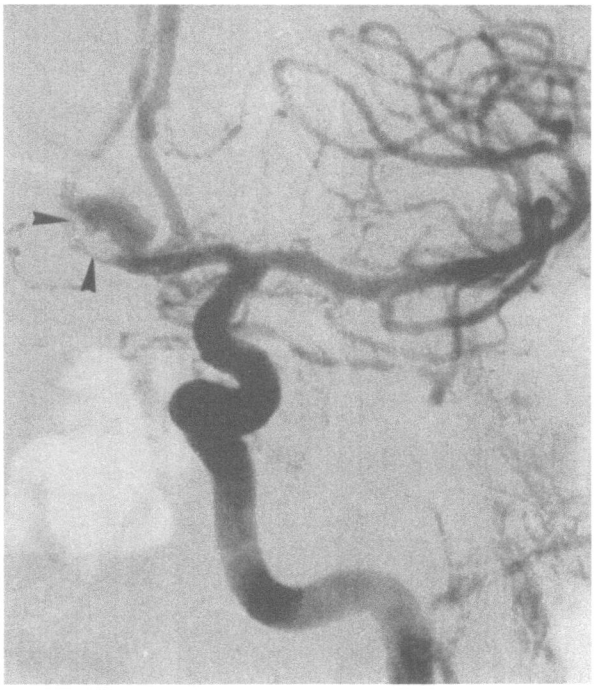

Fig. 7.40. Clot in an aneurysm sac (*arrowheads*).

1973), but it has been described in association with a posterior–inferior cerebellar artery aneurysm. The condition is extremely rare, occurring only once in 5484 patients investigated by Perret and Nishioka (1966a) for SAH. However, Allan and Whitcombe (1977) reported from their own patient material (about 6000 patients) a complication rate of 0.1%. The angiographic demonstration of extravasation of contrast medium from an aneurysm is an extremely grave sign, and the majority of these patients will die.

Multiple Aneurysms

Multiple aneurysms occur in 15%–25% of cases. In our series of 500 operated cases, 25% had multiple aneurysms. CT scanning, as discussed previously, will help localise the site of the bleed in the majority of cases. If, in the absence of localising clinical or CT findings, more than one aneurysm is found at angiography, certain angiographic features may be helpful in deciding which aneurysm has ruptured:

1. The largest aneurysm is most likely to have ruptured (Crompton 1966) (Fig. 7.34). It is rare for an aneurysm less than 5 mm in size to rupture.
2. Irregularity of outline or a multilocular appearance of the aneurysm (Fig. 7.34) usually indicates previous rupture (du Boulay 1965).

3. Localised spasm or adjacent mass effect due to haematoma or infarction indicates the site of the haemorrhage (Fig. 7.36).

Less common features indicating the offending aneurysm include:

4. Demonstration of clot in the aneurysm (Fig. 7.40)
5. Rapid enlargement of an aneurysm on serial angiography (Fig. 7.41).

Accuracy of Angiography

Perret and Bull in 1959 reported an 89% accuracy for angiography compared with necropsy findings in 210 patients. They indicated that other lesions were missed because of the presence of vessel spasm (2.5%), observer error (3%) or an inadequate angiographic examination (2%). In addition a ruptured aneurysm was missed in 2% after another aneurysm had been shown. They concluded that the potential accuracy of angiography is about 96%. It is likely that at the

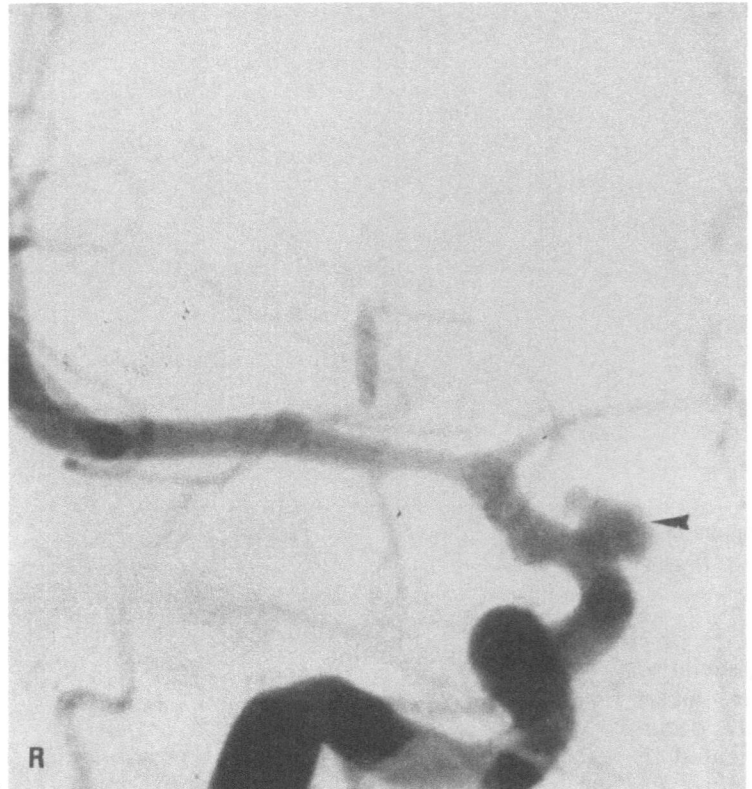

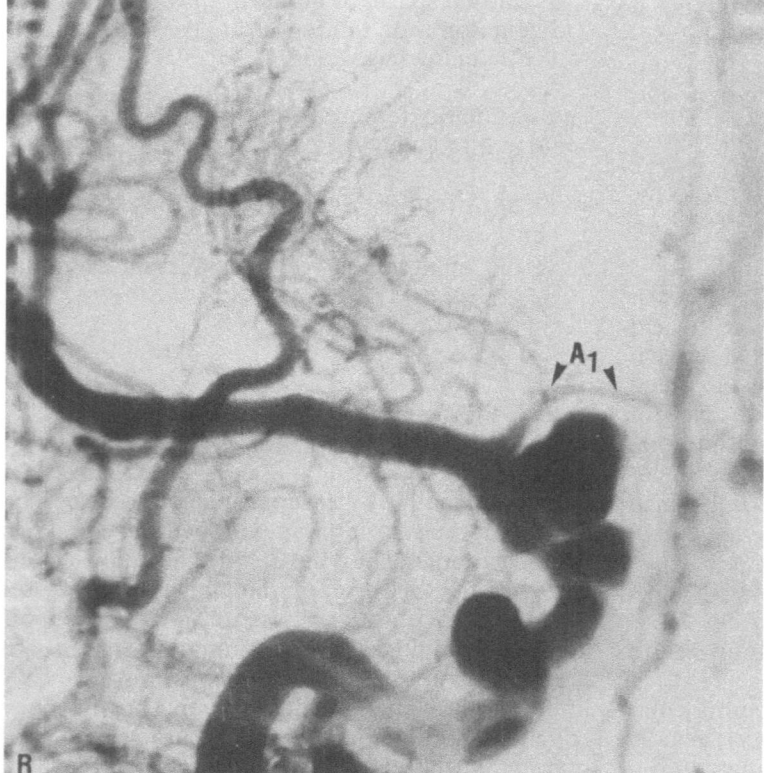

Fig. 7.41. **a** Right carotid angiogram showing a bilocular carotid ophthalmic aneurysm (*arrowhead*). **b** Repeat angiography 5 days later shows that there has been a considerable increase in the size of both loculi. Notice now that the A_1 segment of the right anterior cerebral artery appears elevated by the aneurysm sac (*arrowheads*).

present time with improved techniques such as magnification angiography, the accuracy of diagnosis is even higher.

A negative four vessel angiogram does not exclude an aneurysm or micro-angioma. In patients with a definite SAH but negative angiography one should consider a number of factors:

1. Is the angiogram of adequate quality and have adequate projections been taken to demonstrate a possible aneurysm?

2. Observer error can be eliminated by a careful reappraisal of the angiogram films.

3. In a few patients initial angiography may fail to demonstrate an aneurysm which is subsequently shown on repeat angiography. The failure of contrast to enter the aneurysm sac could be due to (a) the presence of severe spasm (though in our experience this is rare), (b) a clot in the aneurysm neck which later resolves, or (c) haemodynamic factors, e.g. a large aneurysm with a narrow neck in which too early films fail to demonstrate the aneurysm, or a combination of these factors.

4. In the remaining cases one should consider the possibility of spontaneous thrombosis of the aneurysm due to the clot which develops at the site of the bleed or the presence of a micro-aneurysm or microangioma too small to be visualised angiographically. Occlusion of an aneurysm due to clot may occasionally be demonstrated on follow-up angiography (Fig. 7.42). The subject of disappearing aneurysms on serial angiographic studies has been reviewed by Moritake (1981). The presence of vasospasm and a relatively narrow neck may play roles in spontaneous thrombosis, which tends to occur most commonly in larger

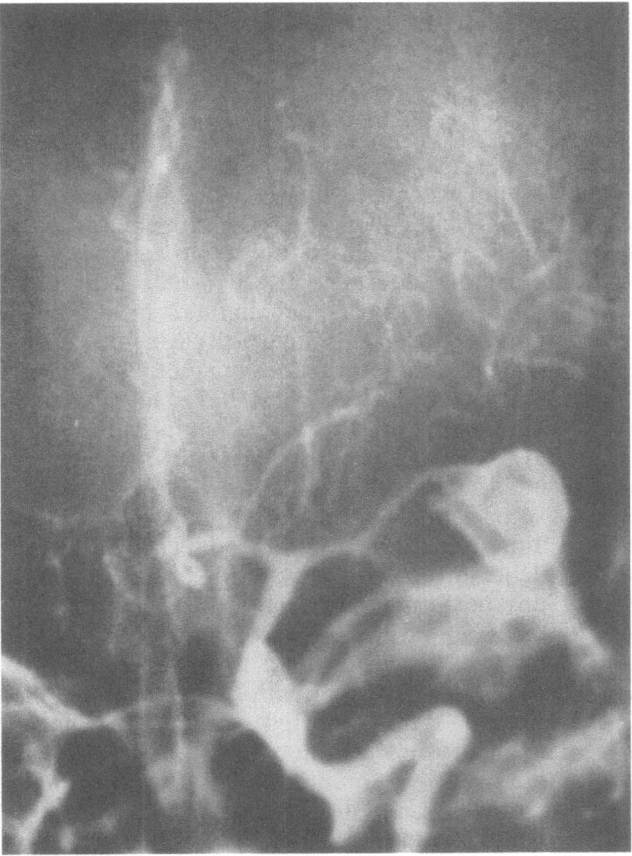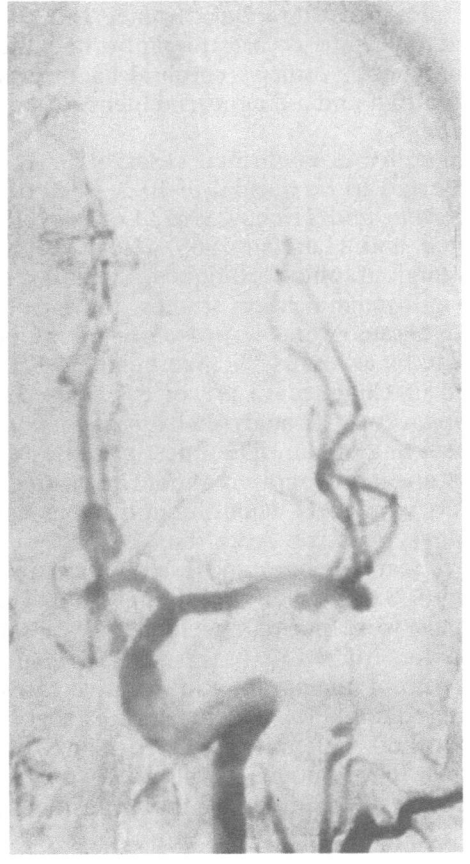

a   b

Fig. 7.42. **a** Left carotid angiogram showing a large middle cerebral artery aneurysm which contains clot. There is considerable spasm of the middle cerebral group of vessels, which also shows some upward displacement due to the presence of a temporal lobe haematoma. **b** Repeat carotid angiogram 15 days later shows that there has been considerable obliteration of the middle cerebral artery aneurysm, except for a portion of its neck. The middle cerebral artery displacement and spasm has now disappeared.

aneurysms. The disappearance and reappearance of an aneurysm on serial angiography has been well documented (Spetzler et al. 1974).

Thrombosis of ruptured aneurysms and of the middle cerebral artery contralateral to an aneurysm has been described in association with epsilon-aminocaproic acid (EACA) therapy (Edner et al. 1978; Sengupta et al. 1976; Scott and Garrido 1977). Intermittent angiographic appearance and disappearance of aneurysms on serial angiography has also been described in association with EACA therapy (Bohmfalk and Story 1980).

Magnification angiography can demonstrate microaneurysms up to 2 mm in diameter. Cole and Yates (1967) reported that multiple microaneurysms can be demonstrated at post-mortem angiography in up to 46% of hypertensive patients compared with only 9% of normal controls. Angiographic demonstration of such microaneurysms is certainly of theoretical interest but of little practical therapeutic value. Indeed, as discussed in Chap. 6, arteriography in patients with spontaneous primary cerebral haemorrhage is often normal and a diagnosis dependent on CT scan findings.

Angiography in confirmed cases of SAH has been reported to be normal in 10%–27% of patients (Sutton and Trickey 1962; Locksley 1966; Bjorkesten and Halonen 1965). However, with modern angiographic techniques, including subtraction and magnification studies, the incidence of negative angiograms in proven SAH has been reported to be as low as 7% (West et al. 1977). As discussed in Chap. 5, 13.1% of 547 consecutive cases of proven SAH analysed by us had a normal four vessel angiogram. The question arises as to whether repeat angiography should be carried out in patients with SAH when the initial four vessel angiogram is negative. According to Forster et al. (1978), repeat angiographic examination in patients with SAH when the initial four vessel angiograms were normal, yielded the causative factor in less than 3% of cases. The value of repeat cerebral angiography in negative cases is, therefore, debatable, unless severe spasm is present or there is definite evidence of an SAH on the CT scan. The remote possibility of a spinal SAH should be considered under such circumstances.

Peroperative Angiography

Some workers (Cummins et al. 1974) advocate the use of peroperative angiography to see if the aneurysm neck has been completely obliterated or if an adjacent vessel has been compressed or occluded. The surgeon may then, if necessary, make appropriate alterations to the position of the aneurysm clip. It is also useful in AVMs to confirm that the lesion has been completely obliterated and to show the exact location of any residual feeding vessels. The technique is carried out by retrograde catheterisation of the superficial temporal artery but can be carried out by catheterisation from the femoral route. We do not carry out peroperative angiography because it requires an indwelling catheter with its attendant problems and with the use of operating theatre radiographic equipment; the quality of X-rays is often suboptimal.

Postoperative Check Angiography

Postoperative angiography is not universally practised and will of course be dependent on one's neurosurgical colleague's commitment to further surgical intervention if the aneurysm sac is not completely obliterated. It will also be indicated in patients who have had limited pre-operative angiography if one's neurosurgical colleague is committed to operating on incidental aneurysms. Allcock and Drake (1963) have advocated the routine use of postoperative angiography. In an analysis of 70 cases they showed evidence of a residual aneurysm in 13 cases (18.64%); four of these patients subsequently died within a month of the operation from a re-bleed. There was evidence of vessel occlusion in six cases. Stevens (1966) performed postoperative angiography in 250 cases and found incomplete occlusion in 17.6% and occlusion of a main artery in 24%, some of which were intentional. Drake and Vanderlinden (1967) reported incomplete occlusion of an aneurysm in 43 out of 329 cases (13.1%) and emphasised the potential risks of rebleeding. In this series incomplete obliteration of an aneurysm occurred in 13.8% of cases. Non-filling of a vessel due to operative occlusion was seen in 3% of cases and due to vessel spasm in 4%. They believe, and we agree, that postoperative angiography is an integral part of the surgical management.

To avoid complications angiography is carried out 5–7 days after the operation under local anaesthesia using non-ionic contrast media; two or three injections in the optimal projection is in most cases all that is necessary. If postoperative angiography shows that a large proportion or the entire aneurysm has remained due to ineffective clipping of its neck, depending on the clinical condition of the patient early surgery is advocated to avoid the potential dangers of a rebleed (Drake and Vanderlinden 1967).

In those cases in which angiography shows that the aneurysm sac is not entirely obliterated, there is evidence from serial angiography that such residual aneurysms may disappear due to thrombosis (Bonnal and Stevenaert 1969) or may show enlargement. Under such circumstances repeat angiography after a period of 2–3 months should be considered.

There have been no serious permanent complications following 376 check angiograms carried out, and this includes a careful prospective study of the potential complications in 150 cases examined under local anaesthesia (J. W. Whitby, personal communication).

Complications

The comprehensive report by Perret and Nishioka (1966a) on the cooperative study of intracranial aneurysms and SAH showed an overall complication rate of 7.6%. They reported fatal complications showing a plausible relationship with angiography in 64 patients, representing a mortality of 1.17%. In this group a rebleed during angiography was reported to have occurred in seven cases but extravasated contrast media was demonstrated in only one case. Mani and Eisenberg (1978) analysed the complication rate in 5000 consecutive catheter cerebral arteriograms (including tumours, stroke and SAH cases). They found no statistically significant difference between the complication rate when the carotid artery alone was injected and that when the carotid artery was injected in combination with the vertebral artery. Complication rates were significantly higher when the procedure lasted more than 80 min, and when carried out in patients more than 40 years of age. These authors, as mentioned previously, emphasised that the complication rate for training hospitals was significantly higher than that for non-training hospitals.

The angiographic complications in 440 cases of SAH have been analysed in our unit. Any unexpected deterioration in a patient's condition within the first 24 hours after angiography was regarded as a complication of that procedure. Minor complications, such as small neck haematomas, subintimal injections or allergic skin reactions, were not included. Distinction between complications due to a rebleed which may be unrelated to angiography and can occur at any time, and neurological complications due to vasospasm, is difficult. A diagnosis of vasospasm was made in patients who awoke from anaesthesia unchanged and subsequently showed progressive neurological deterioration. More recently the CT scan has been used to confirm that there is a rebleed. The complications are outlined in Table 7.3 and compared with previous series in Table 7.4. The overall complication rate was 5.7% and excluding rebleeds 4.8%. There were no deaths. Reversible neurological complications occurred in 16 cases (3.6%) and permanent neurological complications in two cases (0.45%). Complications were more frequent in patients in the fifth to seventh decade (13/18 cases). In this series most neurological complications were associated with vasospasm 17/18 cases, and in 12/18 cases it was severe, although the patients were of grades 1–3. *Angiography should therefore be terminated if one finds severe spasm to be present.* There was no significant difference in

Table 7.3. Angiographic complications (440 cases)

Complication	No.
Non-neurological	
Haematoma (neck)	
Difficulty swallowing	1
Respiratory difficulties	1
(intubation required)	
?Septicaemia	1
Rebleed	4
Reversible neurological complications	
Hemiparesis	6
Hemiparesis and dysphasia	3
Dysphasia, worsened	2
Dysphasia	1
Monoparesis	1
Third nerve palsy	1
Weakness of both legs	1
Convergent squint and paresis of right lateral rectus muscle	1
Permanent neurological complications	
Dysphasia (mild)	1
Monoparesis (leg)	1

Table 7.4. Complications of angiography in SAH

Study	No. of cases	Type of angiography	Overall rate (%)	Permanent (%)	Deaths (%)
Field et al. (1962)	180	Direct puncture	3.3	0.6	1.1
Patterson et al. (1964)	76	Direct puncture	6.6	0	0
Perret and Nishioka (1966a)	5685	Direct puncture	5.5	0.5	0.6
Field et al. (1972)	152	Brachial	6.6	–	–
Miller et al. (1977)	171	Direct puncture	3.5	–	–
Mani and Eisenberg (1978)	461 (non-training)	Catheter femoral	1.3	0.4	0
	153 (training)		2.6	0	0
Authors' series	440	Direct puncture or catheter femoral	4.8	0.45	0

complications in patients undergoing a neck puncture or femoral catheter angiography.

Cortical blindness may follow vertebral angiography, but fortunately in the majority of cases it is not permanent. It is probably related to contrast medium toxicity rather than embolism. Prompt treatment with intravenous dextran 40 is beneficial.

Arteriovenous Malformations

Arteriovenous malformations occur with one-tenth of the frequency of intracranial aneurysm (Perret and Nishioka 1966b). In our experience AVMs were the cause of SAH in 6.4% of cases (Chap. 5). They are congenital lesions that arise at an early foetal stage (about 3 weeks) when there is division into primitive arteries, capillaries and veins. An arrest in development results in the formation of direct arterial to venous communications without an intervening capillary bed. The angiographic demonstration of an arteriovenous malformation was first made by Bergstrand Olivecrona and Tonnis in 1936.

Classification

Arteriovenous malformations may be classified as to their anatomical site and type of vascular supply, e.g. pial or dural.

In a review of 800 cases (Krayenbuhl and Yasargil 1958), their location was supratentorial in 85.7%, infratentorial in 6.2% and extradural in

Table 7.5. Anatomical location of AVMs (Perret and Nishioka 1966b)

Supratentorial	93%
Frontal region	22%
Temporal region	18%
Peri-ictal and porto-occipital	27%
Occipital	5%
Deep (intra- or paraventricular)	18%
Whole hemisphere	1%
Multiple locations	1%
Infratentorial	7%
Brain stem	2%
Cerebellar	5%

8.1%. Perret and Nishioka (1966b) analysed 549 confirmed AVMs, and their anatomical location is shown in Table 7.5.

Newton and Cronqvist (1969) studied the vascular supply in AVMs and showed that 73% had a purely pial, 15.5% a mixed pial and dural and 11.5% a purely dural supply. Posterior fossa AVMs have a dural blood supply in 50% of cases, compared with only 27% in the supratentorial compartment.

Technique

The arterial feeding vessels, as well as the draining veins, must be carefully demonstrated at angiography. This is best achieved by separate selective injection of the internal and external carotid arteries and the vertebral arteries when necessary. We have found the percutaneous femoral catheter technique particularly useful when multiple arteries need to be selectively examined. Rapid serial angiography is necessary to define adequately the origin of feeding arteries and the course of draining veins, especially in those AVMs with rapid blood flow. Magnification angiography may help define small arterial feed-ers. Subtraction techniques are routinely carried out and are especially valuable when vessel detail is obscured by bone. The value of selective angiographic studies is shown by the case illustrated in Fig. 7.43.

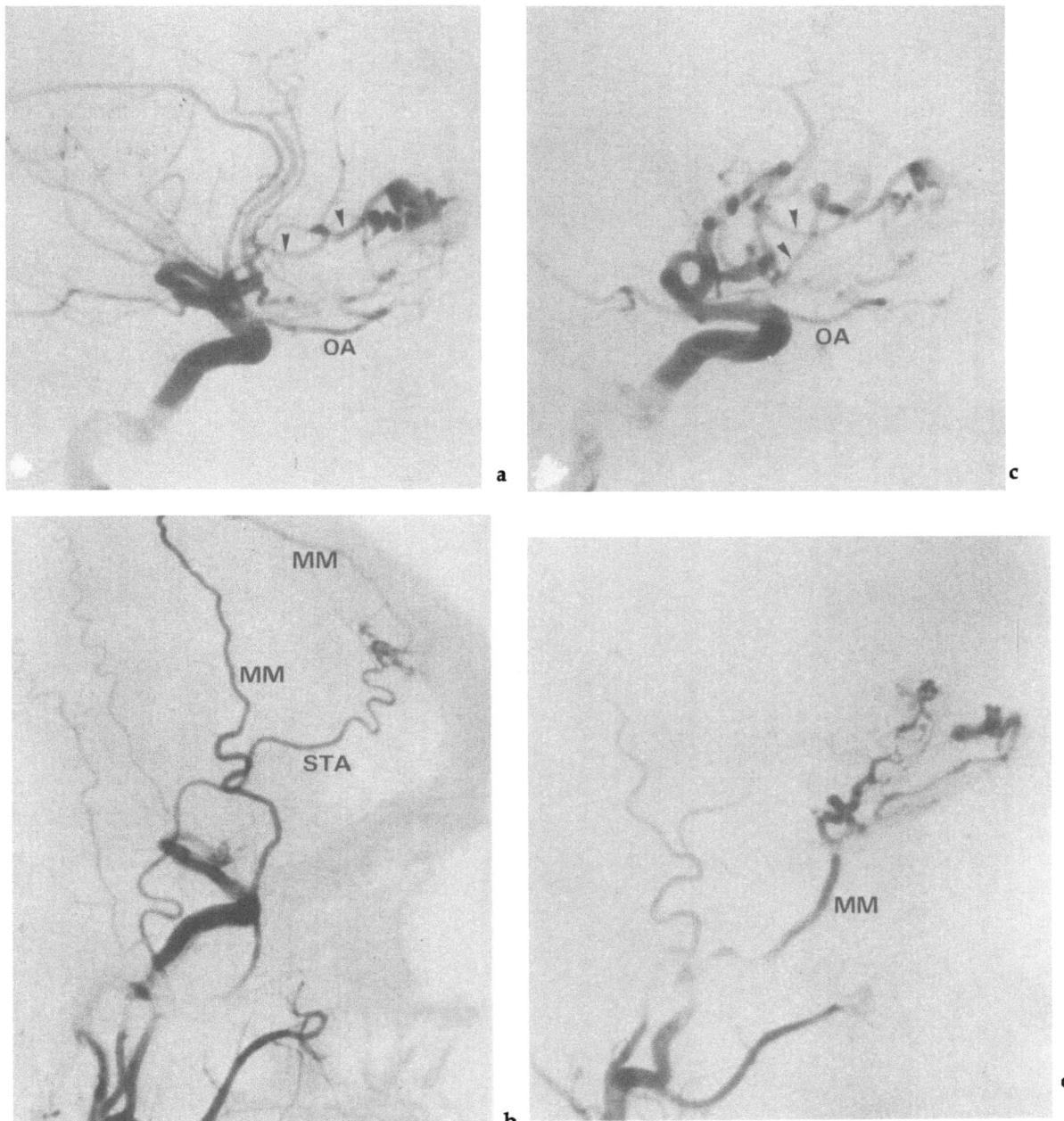

Fig. 7.43a–d. Patient with a large midline, frontal arteriovenous malformation. **a** Selective right internal carotid angiogram clearly shows the feeding vessels from the anterior cerebral artery (*arrowheads*) and also a feeding vessel from the ophthalmic artery (*OA*). **b** Selective right external carotid angiogram showing supply to the malformation from the middle meningeal artery (*MM*) and also from the superficial temporal artery (*STA*). **c** Selective left internal carotid angiogram shows a similar supply as is shown in **a**. **d** Selective left external carotid angiogram shows supply to the malformation from enlarged left middle meningeal artery (*MM*).

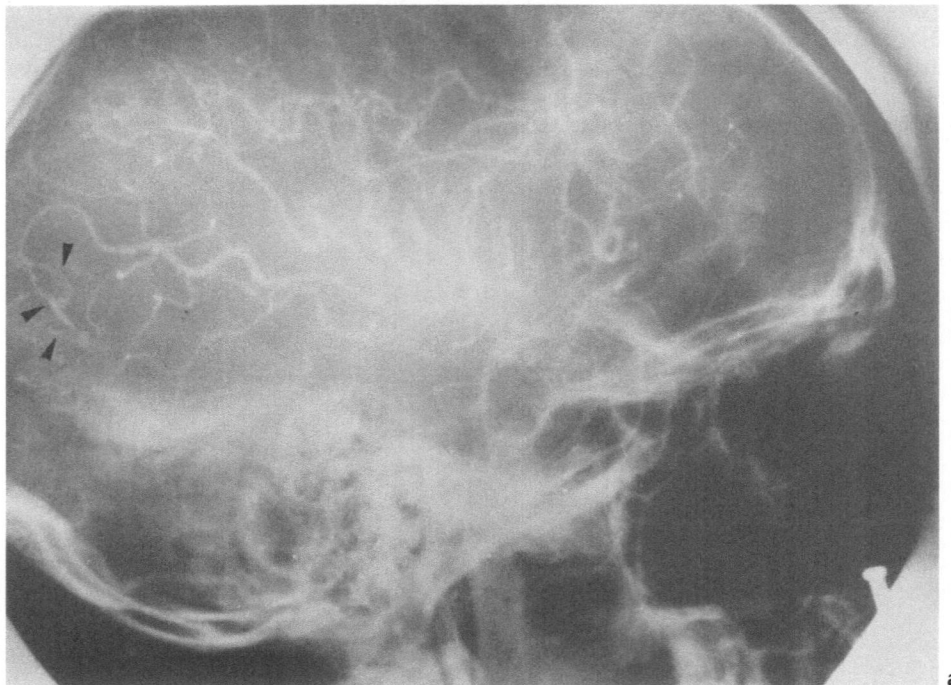

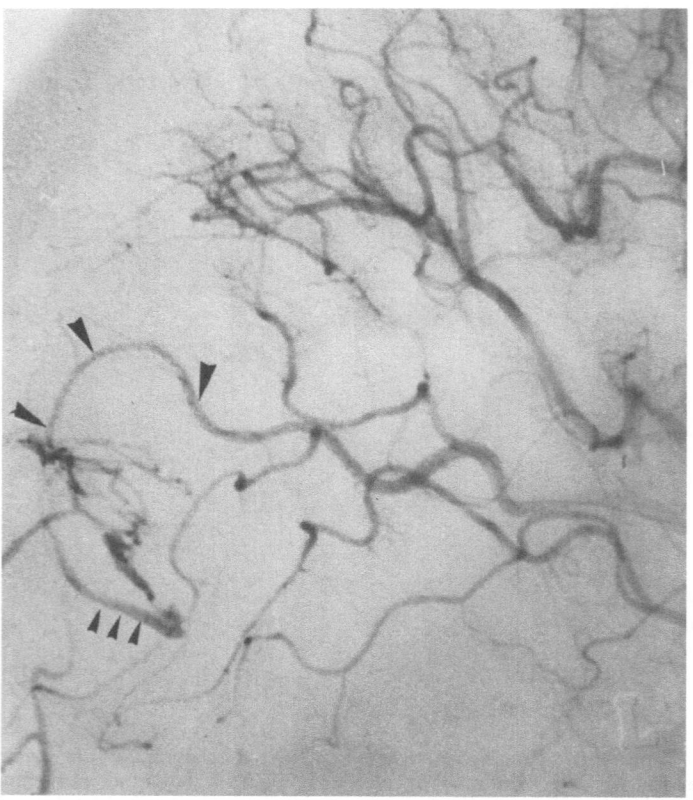

Fig. 7.44a, b. AVM with a single feeding artery and draining vein. **a** Left carotid angiogram shows a small posterior parietal AVM (*arrowheads*). **b** Magnification study shows the AVM has a single feeding artery (*large arrowheads*) and draining vein (*small arrowheads*).

Angiographic Features

Arteriovenous malformations characteristically show (a) large feeding arteries, (b) a central tangle of vessels, (c) arteriovenous shunting with enlarged tortuous draining veins and (d) a rapid circulation time. However, several different angiographic patterns may be seen:

1. An AVM with a single feeding artery and draining vein (Fig. 7.44).
2. An AVM consisting of a tangle of vessels with a draining vein but with no obvious enlarged arterial feeders (Fig. 7.45).

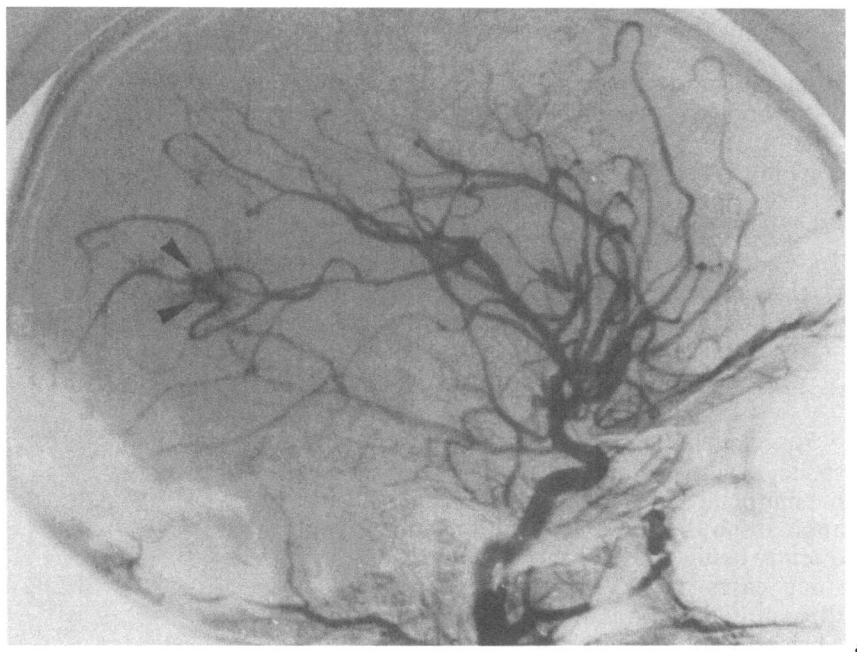

a

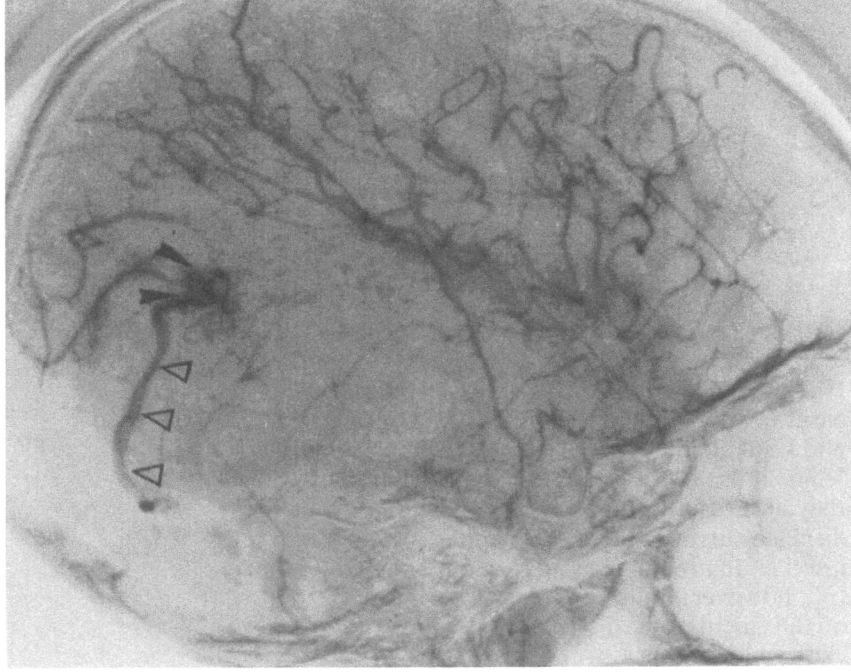

b

Fig. 7.45a, b. Small parietal AVM consisting of a small leash of vessels (*arrowheads*) with no obvious feeding artery, but with some prominent draining veins (*open arrowheads*).

3. An AVM with multiple feeding vessels and draining veins (Fig. 7.46). This is the commonest type.

4. AVMs with mixed pial and dural blood supply (Fig. 7.43).

5. Microangiomas where the angioma site is often only clearly demonstrated on magnification studies (Fig. 7.47).

6. Pure dural AVMs which are most commonly seen in the posterior fossa, the main feeding vessels coming from the occipital, middle meningeal or tentorial branch of the internal carotid, with venous drainage most commonly into the transverse or sigmoid sinuses (Fig. 7.48). Subarachnoid haemorrhage is a less common presenting feature of this type of AVM, however (see Chap. 13).

7. Predominantly intraventricular AVMs with their arterial feeders from the choroidal arteries and involvement of the choroid plexus of the lateral ventricle, the roof of the third ventricle or the fourth ventricle (Fig. 7.49).

Arteriovenous malformations are generally not space occupying unless there is an associated haematoma. They may not be demonstrated at angiography, however, the diagnosis subsequently being made at surgery or postmortem. In some cases an AVM may have spontaneously thrombosed or in rupturing destroyed itself. Thrombosed AVMs not detectable at angiography may be demonstrated at CT as a high density lesion with contrast enhancement (Kramer and Wing 1977).

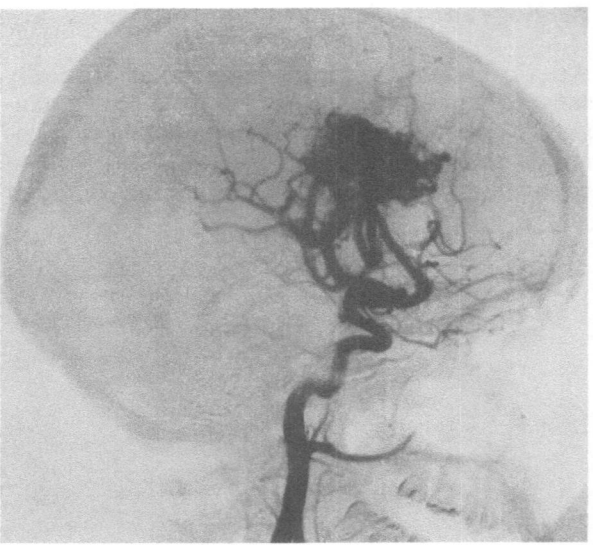

a

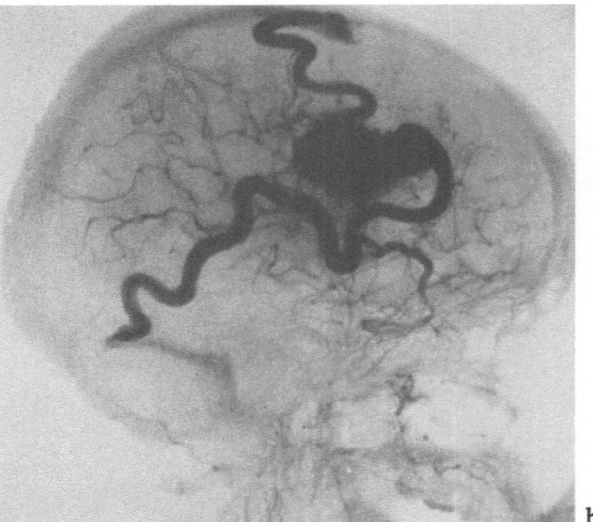

b

Fig. 7.46a, b. Large AVM with multiple feeding arteries and draining veins (**a** arterial; **b** venous).

Intracerebral Haematoma

Haemorrhage from AVMs occurs in 30%–50% of cases (Patterson and McKissock 1956; Olivecrona and Ladenheim 1957) and is usually intracerebral. When it occurs near the surface of the brain, SAH may also result. An intracerebral haematoma will displace surrounding vessels and is usually recognised as an area of avascularity on the angiogram. CT, however, will more clearly reveal the extent of the haematoma as well as demonstrate intraventricular extension.

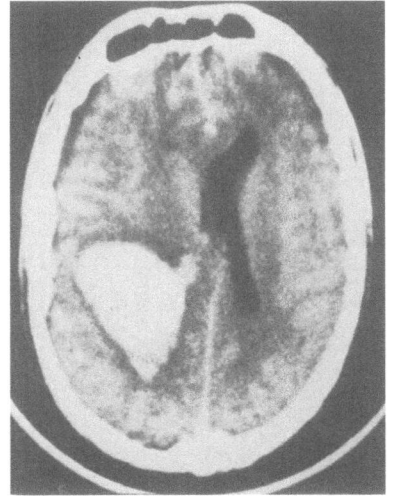

a

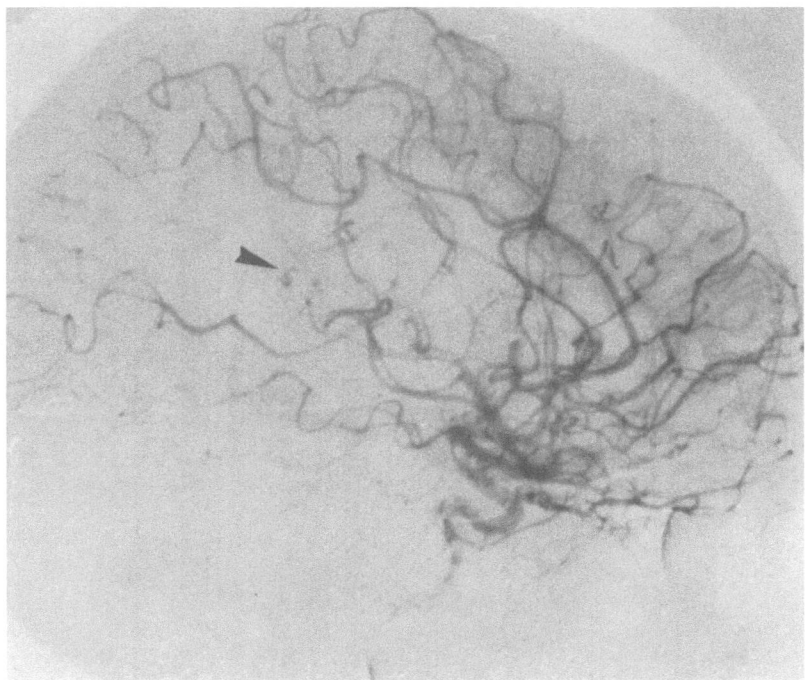

b

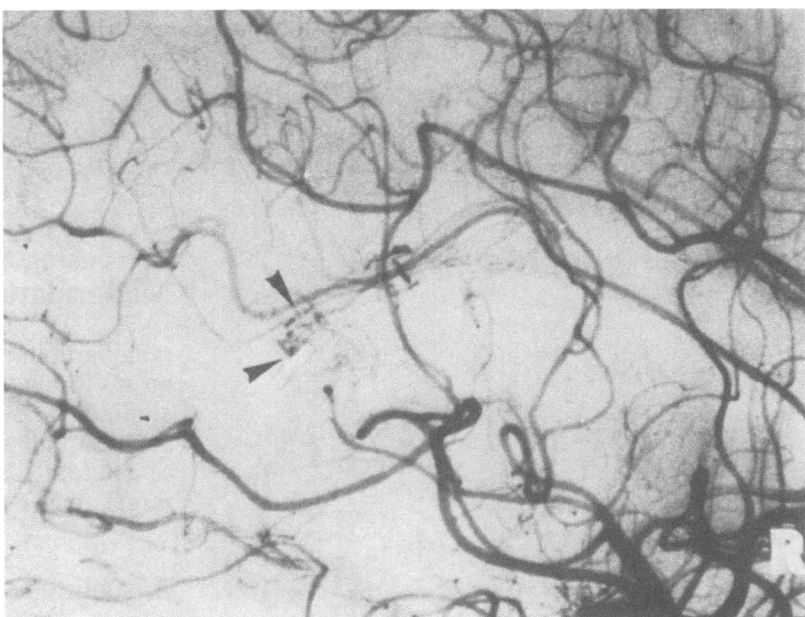

c

Fig. 7.47a–c. Microangioma. **a** CT scan showing a large haematoma deep in the left parietal lobe. At surgery, during evacuation of the haematoma, an abnormal leash of vessels, thought to be an AVM, was seen. **b** Left lateral carotid angiogram shows displacement of the vessels in the parietal region. In addition there was a suspicious area of abnormal circulation, thought to represent a possible small AVM (*arrowhead*). **c** Magnification studies confirm the presence of a small AVM (*arrowheads*).

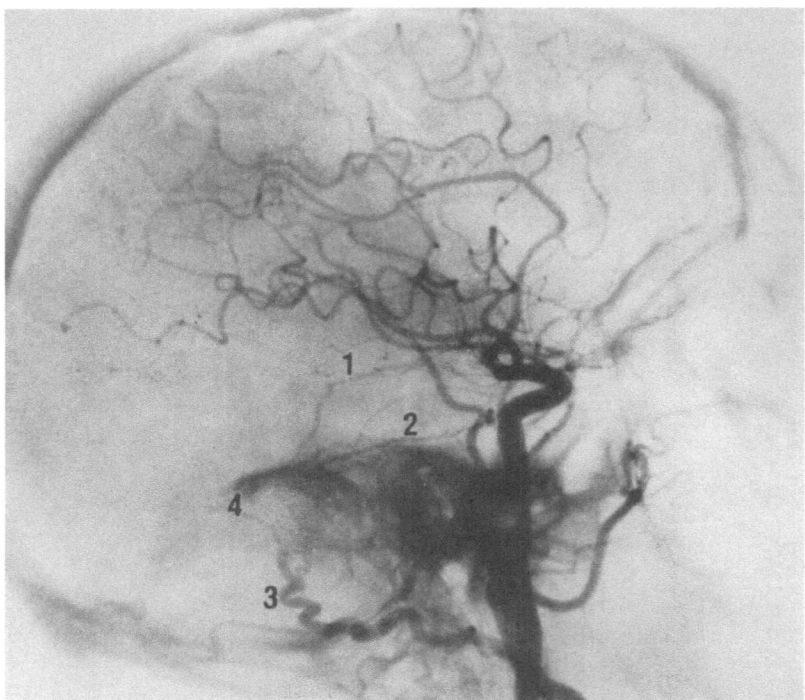

Fig. 7.48. Posterior fossa dural AVM supplied by (*1*) the posterior division of the middle meningeal artery, (*2*) the tentorial artery and (*3*) an enlarged occipital artery. There is early venous drainage into the sigmoid sinus (*4*).

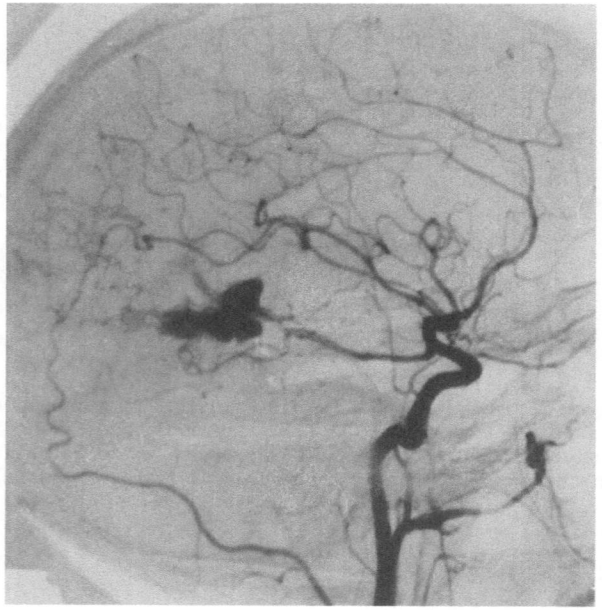

Fig. 7.49. Predominantly intraventricular AVM supplied by the posterior choroidal arteries.

Increasing Size of Arteriovenous Malformations

Angiographic documentation of increased size of an AVM may be seen (Fig. 7.50). Waltimo (1973) studied the size of AVMs and showed that the smallest had a tendency to increase in size, those of moderate size to remain unchanged and the larger ones even to decrease slightly in size.

Associated Aneurysms

Perret and Nishioka (1966b) showed a 7.6% incidence of aneurysms associated with AVMs, and Suzuki and Onuma (1979), a 6.4% incidence. The aneurysm may be located on the main arterial feeder of the AVM but may be anatomically unrelated to the AVM (Figs. 7.51, 7.52). Cronqvist and Troup (1966) reported that about 70% were on the main arterial feeders. It seems likely that their development is related to haemodynamics of increased flow. The report by

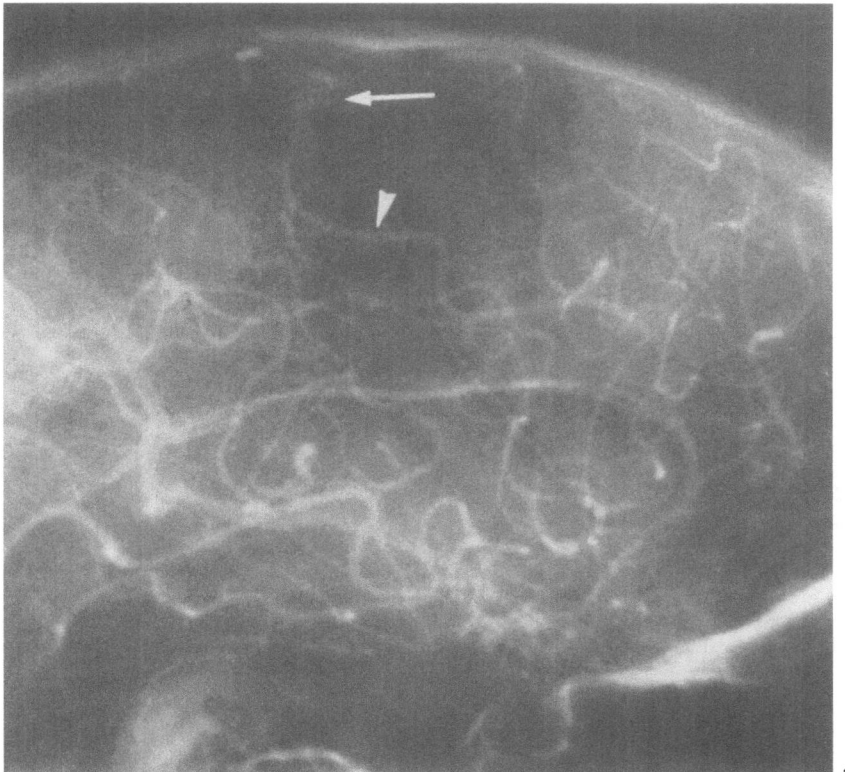

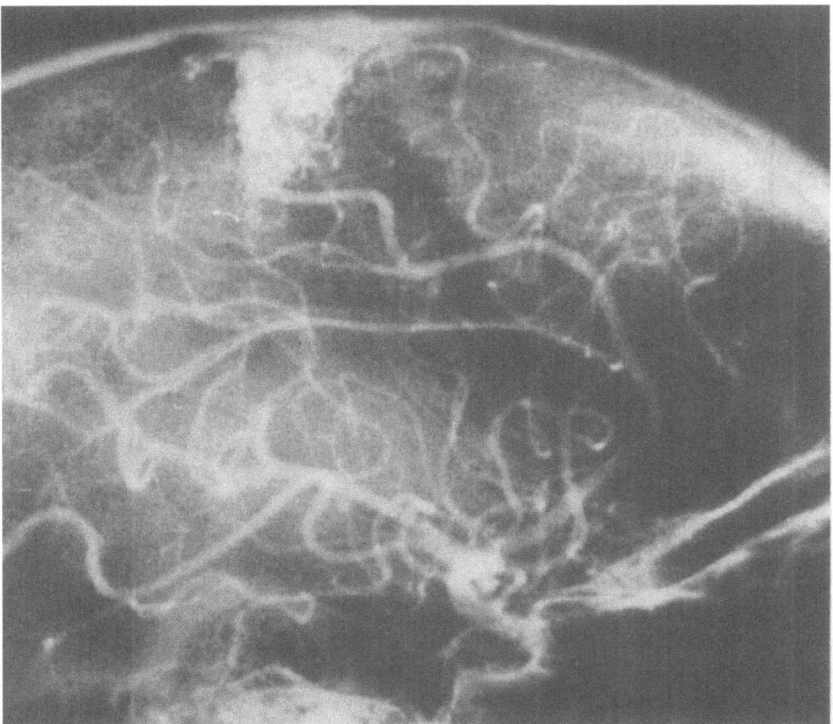

Fig. 7.50. a Angiogram on 6.5.1971 shows a small AVM (*arrow*) supplied by the callosomarginal artery (*arrowhead*). **b** A repeat angiogram on 7.8.1976 shows considerable enlargement of the AVM and its feeding vessels.

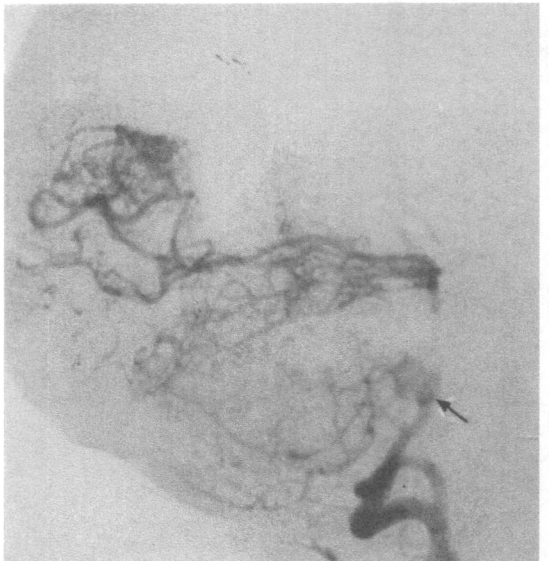 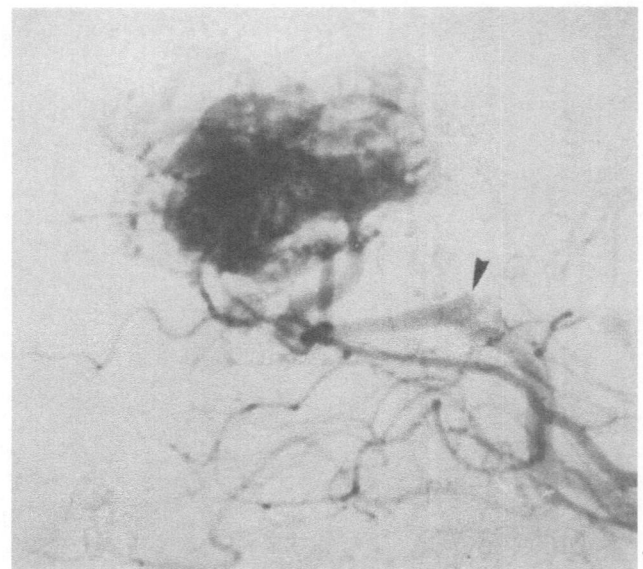

Fig. 7.51. a Aneurysm arising from the basilar trunk associated with an AVM supplied by the posterior cerebral artery. **b** Magnified lateral vertebral angiogram. There is an AVM supplied by an enlarged posterior cerebral artery with a small aneurysm (*arrowhead*) arising from this main feeding vessel.

Shenkin et al. (1971) of an aneurysm on the main feeder of an AVM which diminished in size due to thrombosis following excision of the AVM perhaps supports this hypothesis.

It may be very difficult to decide which has bled, but according to Perret and Nishioka (1966b) in an analysis of 29 patients, SAH was slightly more frequent from the AVM (nine cases bled from the AVM, seven cases from the aneurysm, and in 13 cases it was unclear). CT scanning is now an extremely accurate method of making this distinction (Chap. 7).

Vasospasm

Cerebral vasospasm associated with a ruptured AVM is relatively rare. Nishimura and Hawkins (1975) reviewed 52 cases of ruptured AVM and found vasospasm in six (12%) patients. The reason for this lower incidence of vasospasm compared with ruptured aneurysms is because AVMs, usually being parenchymal in location, are less likely to produce extensive haemorrhage into the subarachnoid space and therefore formation of clot around the arteries of the circle of Willis.

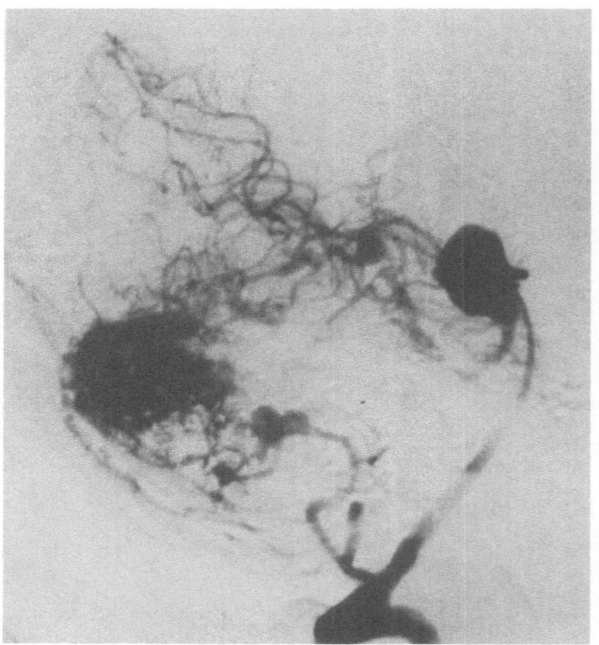

Fig. 7.52. Left vertebral angiogram carried out in 1966 showed a posterior fossa AVM fed by the superior cerebellar artery and the posterior inferior cerebellar artery (PICA). Vertebral angiogram in the same patient in 1980 now shows a large basilar tip aneurysm, a peripheral aneurysm on the superior cerebellar artery and multiple peripheral PICA aneurysms.

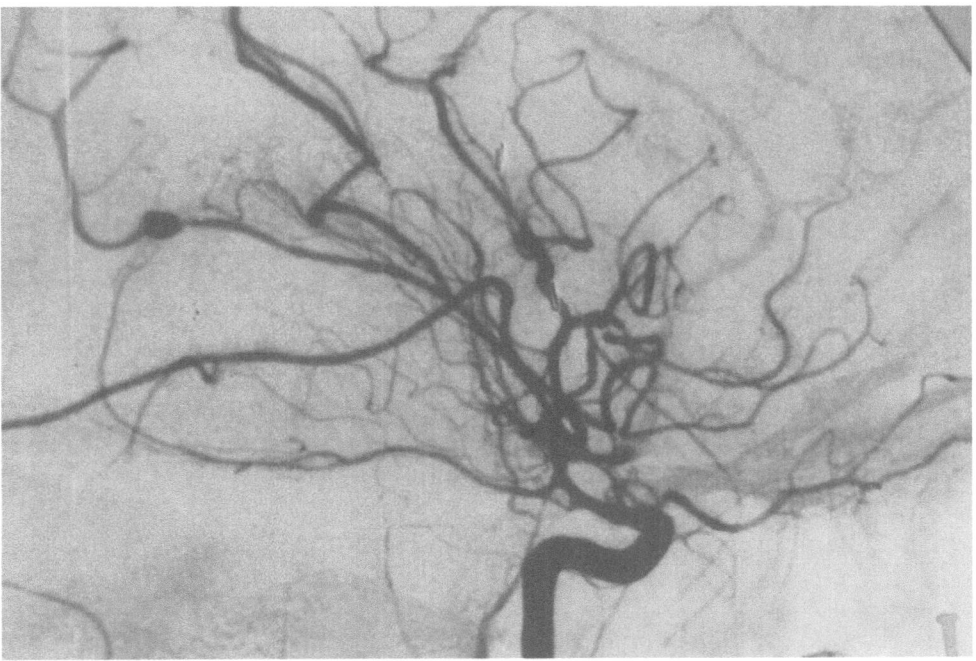

Fig. 7.53. Mycotic aneurysm arising from a peripheral branch of the middle cerebral artery. The aneurysm is spindle shaped and has no definable neck.

Angiographic Extravasation of Contrast Medium

Contrast extravasation from a ruptured AVM during angiography is extremely rare. Doi et al. (1980) reported one case and could find only two other cases reported in the literature, by McLennan et al. (1974) and Allan and Whitcombe (1977)

Mycotic Aneurysms

Mycotic aneurysms may be due to intravascular infection (most commonly bacterial endocarditis) or to extravascular infection such as meningitis (Heidelberger et al. 1968; Davis et al. 1970), cavernous sinus thrombosis and osteomyelitis (Suwanwella et al. 1972). Rupture is frequent and may be catastrophic. Bacterial mycotic aneurysms characteristically are found on peripheral arterial branches—most frequently the middle cerebral artery but also the anterior and internal carotid arteries. They are usually spindle or fusiform in shape and have no neck (Fig. 7.53). Angiography may occasionally demonstrate a false aneurysm sac in the parenchyma (Fig. 7.54). Multiple peripheral aneurysms may occur and this should point to an infective aetiology (Fig. 7.55).

Serial angiography may show rapid increase in aneurysm size (Sato et al. 1979), development of new aneurysms (Roach and Drake 1965) or disappearance of mycotic aneurysms due to thrombosis (Cantu et al. 1966) (Fig. 7.55). The reports of spontaneous complete regression of these aneurysms, especially multiple ones after antibiotic therapy, has favoured an approach aimed at adequate control of infection prior to considering surgical intervention (Valadares et al. 1979; Leipzig and Brown 1985).

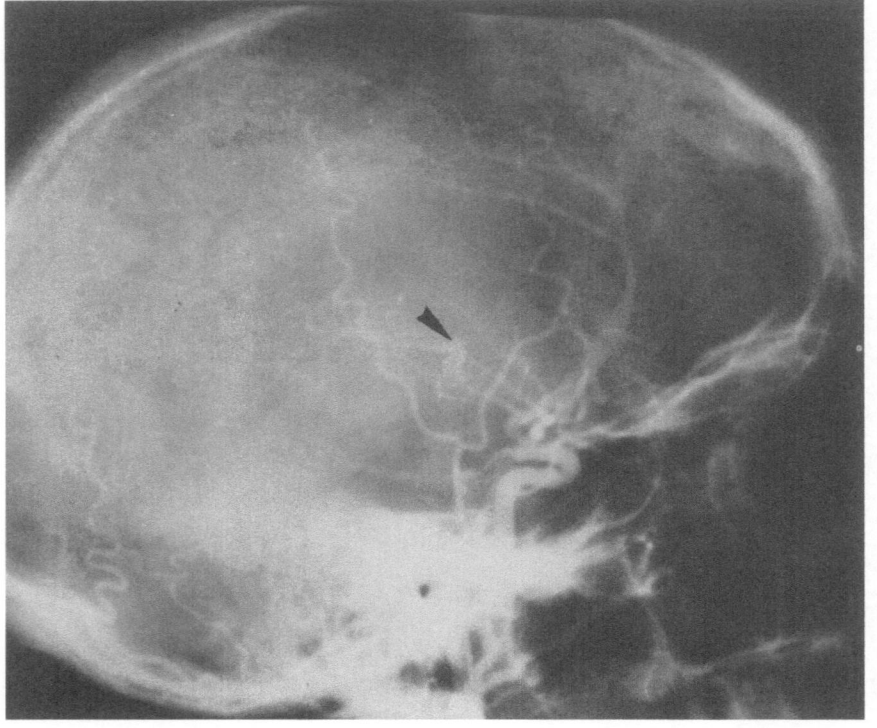

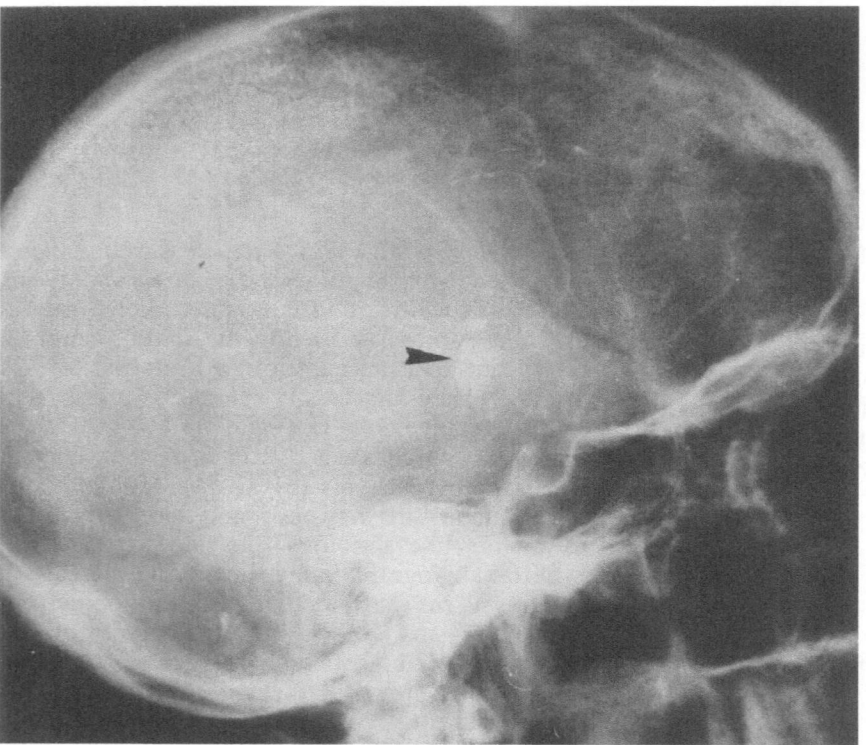

Fig. 7.54a, b. Ruptured mycotic middle cerebral artery aneurysm, which has produced a false aneurysm sac (*arrowheads*).

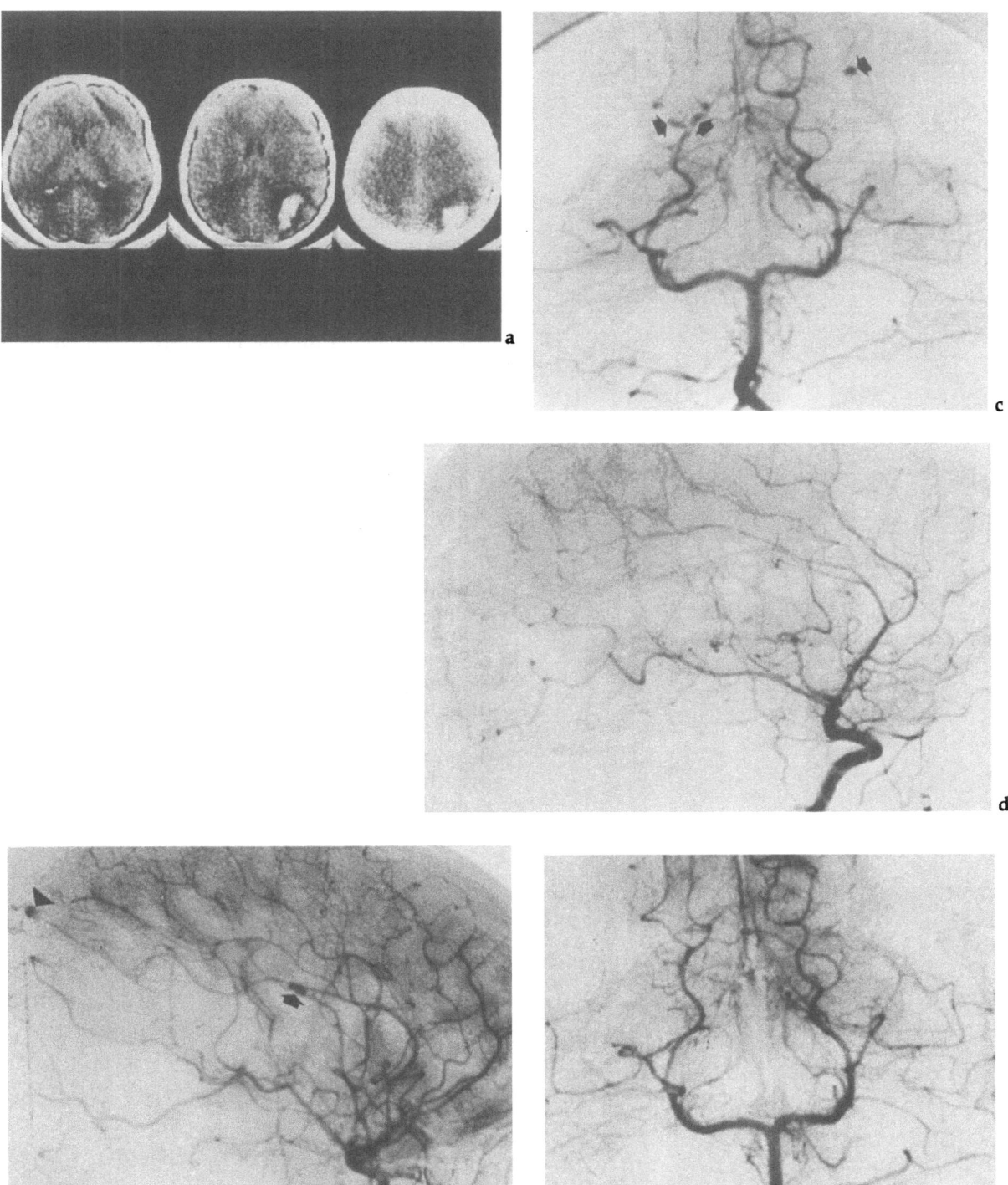

Fig. 7.55. a CT scan shows a right posterior parietal haematoma. The patient showed stigmata of an acute bacterial endocarditis.
b Right carotid and **c** vertebral angiograms show multiple peripheral mycotic aneurysms (*arrow*). The *arrowhead* points to the most likely source of the haemorrhage. A left carotid angiogram on this patient showed a few further aneurysms, including a peripheral middle cerebral and an anterior cerebral artery aneurysm. **d** Repeat right carotid and **e** vertebral angiography after antibiotic therapy shows complete disappearance of the aneurysms. (By courtesy of J. B. Valadares)

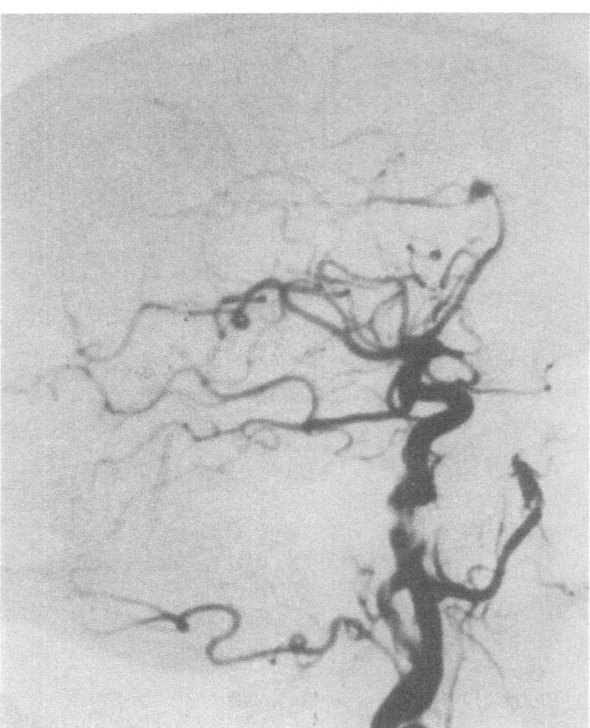

Fig. 7.56. Traumatic pericallosal artery aneurysm.

Traumatic Aneurysms

False and true aneurysms may occur after blunt and closed head injuries. They may also be iatrogenic in origin, arising after surgical operations (Lassman et al. 1974). A review of 73 cases of traumatic and iatrogenic aneurysms from the literature has been reported by Laun (1979).

Parkinson and West (1980) have reviewed the angiographic features differentiating traumatic from congenital saccular aneurysms. Traumatic aneurysms have no neck and are usually peripherally located on middle cerebral and anterior cerebral artery branches (Fig. 7.56). They may show delayed filling and emptying. The internal carotid artery and vertebrobasilar system are less common sites for traumatic aneurysms (Fig. 7.57).

The prognosis of traumatic aneurysms is poor owing to the fact that they are frequently associated with other severe brain injury. A review of the literature reveals that mortality from rupture exceeds 50% and in 50% of cases rupture occurs within 15 days after the injury.

Spontaneous disappearance of a traumatic aneurysm has been reported (Brenner 1962; Rumbaugh et al. 1970) but this is rare. One needs to be aware of this complication of head injury, but it is unlikely that traumatic aneurysms will be diagnosed prior to rupture now that CT has taken over from angiography the role of primary diagnostic procedure in head injury.

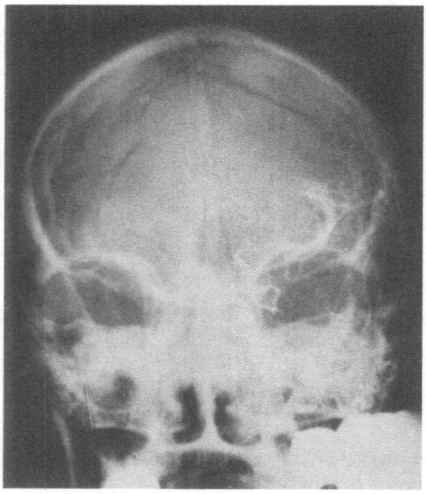
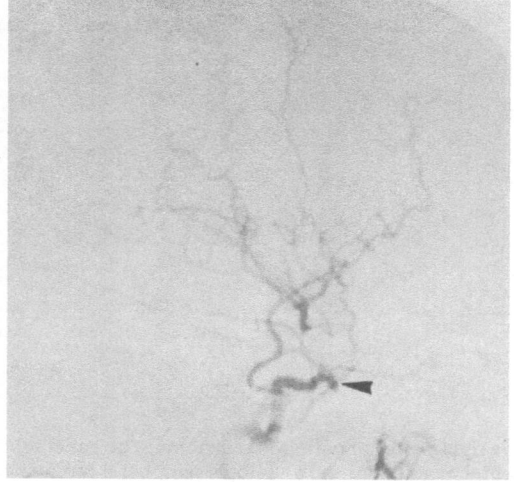

Fig. 7.57. a Patient who was involved in a road traffic accident, with a fracture of the anterior cranial fossa above the sella demonstrated on plain X-rays. **b** Left carotid angiogram shows a traumatic aneurysm of the left carotid siphon (*arrowhead*) together with evidence of severe spasm.

Neoplastic Aneurysms

Aneurysms from choriocarcinoma are peripherally located and fusiform (Montaut et al. 1971).

They resemble mycotic or traumatic rather than congenital berry aneurysms. New et al. (1970) have reviewed the literature concerning aneurysms resulting from embolic cardiac myxoma. The radiological abnormalities include irregular filling defects in cerebral vessels, occlusion of vessels and fusiform and saccular aneurysms.

Arterial Anomalies

Aneurysms may be associated with persistent embryonic vessels (caroticobasilar anastomoses). There are descriptions of a primitive trigeminal artery in combination with an aneurysm of almost every major trunk of the carotid and vertebrobasilar system (Lie 1972) (Fig. 7.58).

An aneurysm of the trigeminal artery has been described by Wolpert (1966) and a ruptured aneurysm of the hypoglossal artery has been reported by Udvarhelyi and Lai (1963). Aneurysms have been described in association with absence or hypoplasia of the internal carotid artery. It has already been pointed out that anomalies of the circle of Willis are frequently associated with aneurysm cases.

Fibromuscular Hyperplasia

Angiography shows the classic string of beads appearance (Fig. 7.59). Houser et al. (1972) in a study of 7000 angiograms found 42 patients with fibromuscular hyperplasia. In nine patients intracranial aneurysms were demonstrated and in six of these cases the aneurysm had ruptured. Palubinskas et al. (1966) showed a surprisingly high incidence (50%) of intracranial aneurysms in patients with fibromuscular hyperplasia of the renal arteries.

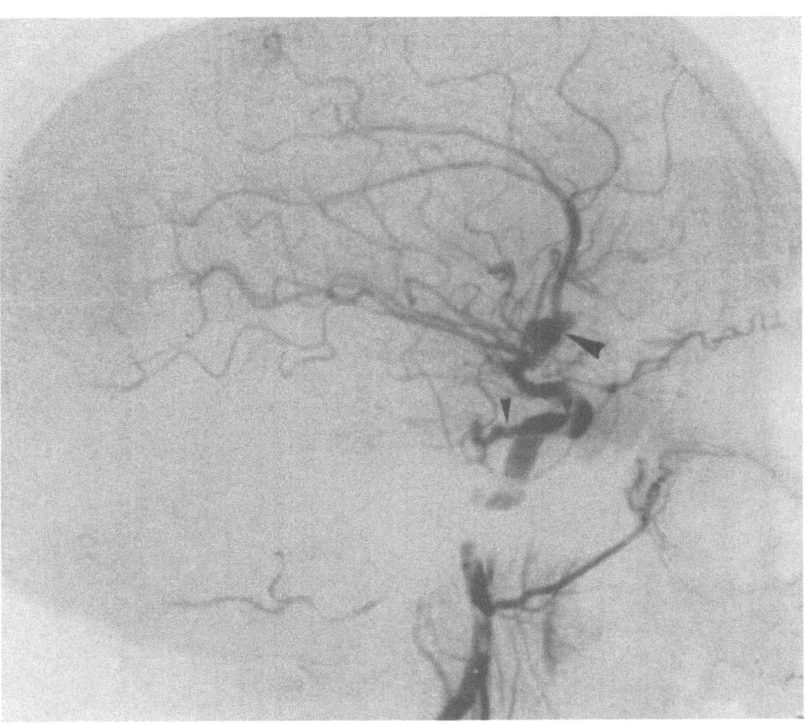

Fig. 7.58. Anterior communicating artery aneurysm (*large arrowhead*) associated with a persistent trigeminal artery (*small arrowhead*).

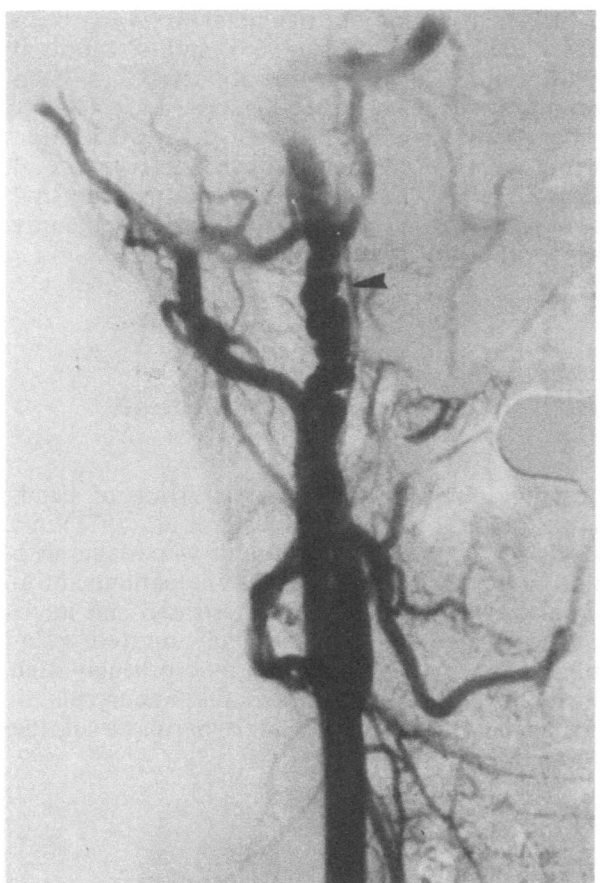

Moya Moya Syndrome

Subarachnoid, subdural or parenchymal haemorrhage may result from rupture of the characteristic dilated arterial channels or an associated aneurysm (Figs. 7.60, 15.8). Subarachnoid haemorrhage as a presenting feature is uncommon under 116 years of age (Nishimoto and Takeuchi 1972), though we have seen one case present at the age of 10 years. Nagamine et al. (1981) published a case of multiple aneurysms with Moya Moya disease and reviewed 22 other cases in which an aneurysm and Moya Moya were associated. Subarachnoid haemorrhage was the initial symptom in 84% of these cases. Aneurysms occurred most frequently in the vertebrobasilar system (43.3%). Kodama and Suzuki (1978) and Adams et al. (1979) postulate that the development of aneurysms might be induced by the

◀ **Fig. 7.59.** Fibromuscular hyperplasia of the internal carotid artery (*arrowhead*). This patient had an SAH from a ruptured anterior communicating artery aneurysm.

▼ **Fig. 7.60**

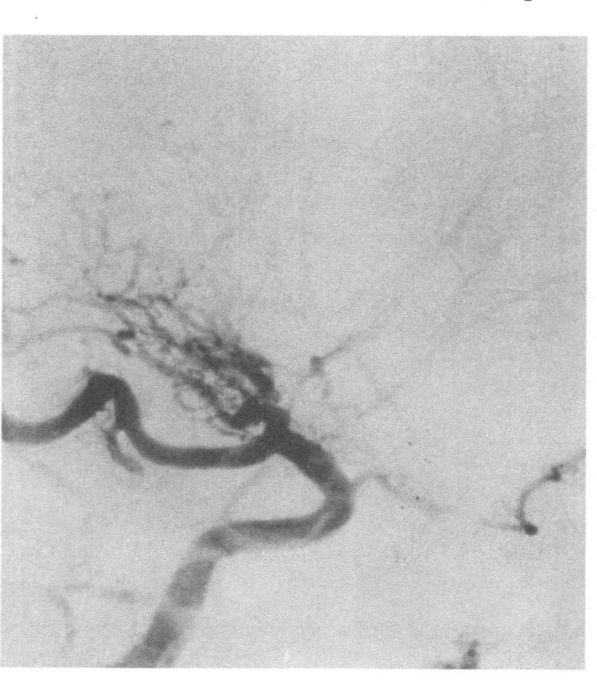

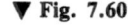

a

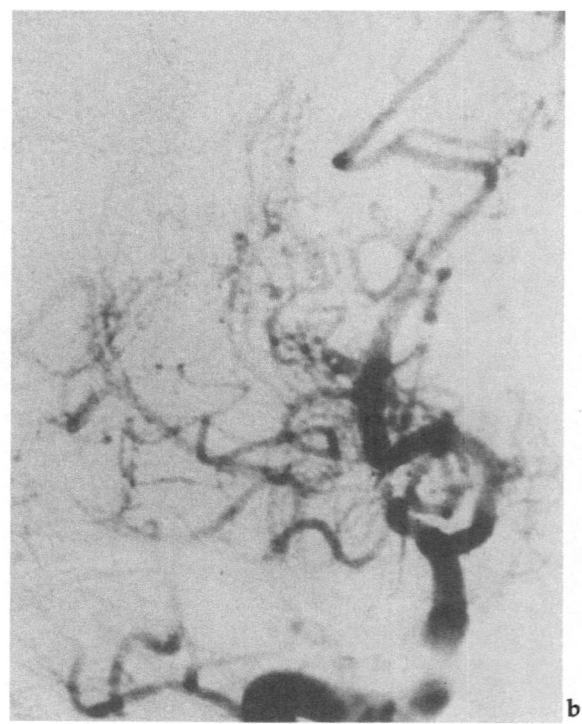

b

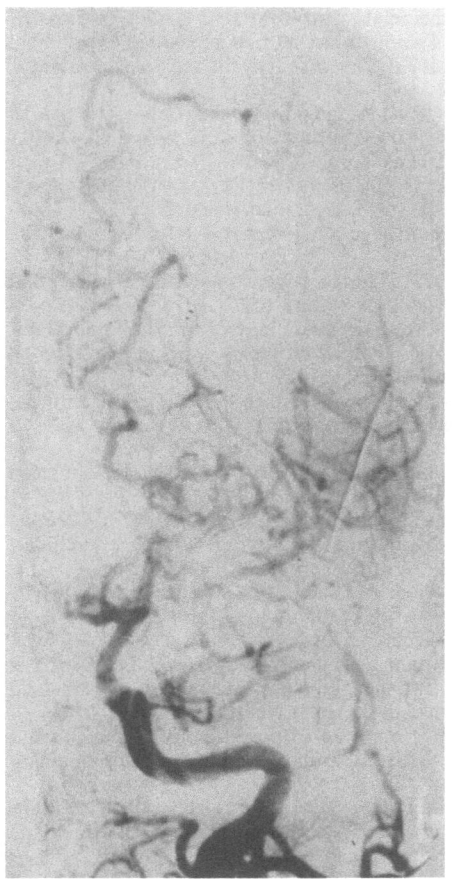
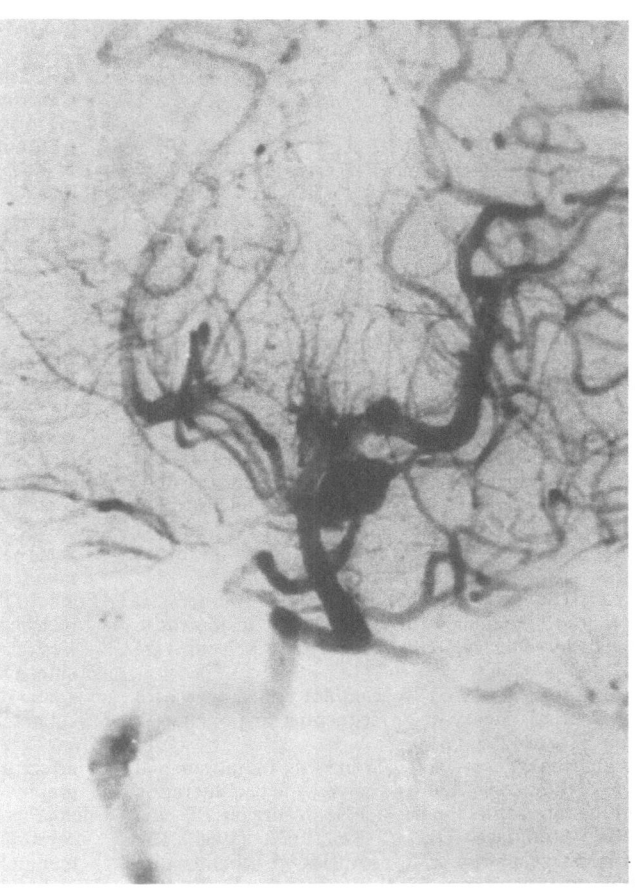

Fig. 7.60a–d. Adult female patient presenting with SAH. a, b Right carotid angiogram showing occlusion of the middle cerebral artery near the bifurcation. There are numerous collateral vessels typical of "moya moya". c Left carotid angiogram also shows occlusion of the horizontal segment of the middle cerebral artery, with numerous collateral vessels. d Vertebral angiography shows a small aneurysm arising from the left posterior cerebral artery and a larger, more irregular aneurysm arising from the basilar trunk, probably near the origin of the superior cerebellar artery.

increased blood flow in the posterior circulation as a result of decreased carotid circulation caused by stenosis or occlusion of the internal carotid arteries.

Cerebral Arteritis

Cerebral arteritis is a well recognised entity which most commonly occurs in patients with collagen vascular disease, a history of drug abuse (especially amphetamine) or intracranial infections. Parenchymal and subarachnoid haemorrhage are uncommon complications of intracranial arteritis, a subject which has been reviewed by Edwards (1977).

Angiographic demonstration of aneurysm formation has been described in periarteritis nodosa (Leonhardt et al. 1972) and lupus erythematosus (Ferris 1974).

Digital Subtraction Angiography

The potential impact of this new imaging technique in SAH is discussed in Chap. 7.

References

Adams HP Jr, Kassell NF, Wisoff HS et al. (1979) Intracranial saccular aneurysm and moya moya disease. Stroke.10:174–179

Agnoli AL, Pia HW, Zierski J (1979) Magnification and tomography In: Pia HW, Langmaid C, Zierski J (eds) Cerebral aneurysms. Advances in diagnosis and therapy. Springer, Berlin Heidelberg New York, pp 175–181

Allan DM, Whitcombe JB (1977) Intracranial extravasation of contrast medium during carotid angiography. Br J Radiol 50:404–411

Allcock JM, Drake CG (1963) Post-operative angiography in cases of ruptured intracranial aneurysms. J Neurosurg 20:752–759

Barton E, Tudor J (1982) Subdural haematoma in association with intracranial aneurysms. Neuroradiology 23:157–160

Bergstrand H, Olivecrona H, Tonnis W (1936) The history of cerebral angiography. In: Krayenbuhl HA, Yasargil MG (eds) Cerebral angiography, 2nd edn. Butterworth, London pp 1–3.

Björkesten G, Halonen V (1965) Incidence of intracranial vascular lesions in patients with subarachnoid haemorrhage investigated by four vessel angiography. J Neurosurg 23:29–32

Bohmfalk L, Story JL (1980) Intermittent appearance of a ruptured cerebral aneurysm on sequential angiograms. J Neurosurg 52:263–265

Bonnal J, Stevenaert A (1969) Thrombosis of intracranial aneurysms of the circle of Willis after incomplete obliteration by clip or ligature across the neck. J Neurosurg 30:158–165

Brawley BW, Strandness DE Jr, Kelly WA (1968) The biphasic response of cerebral vasospasm in subarachnoid haemorrhage. J Neurosurg 28:1–8

Brennen H (1962) Frontal Schadelsspaltung mit traumatischein Aneurysm der Arteria pericallosa. Acta Neurochir (Wien) 10:145–152

Cantu RC, Lemay M, Wilkinson HA (1966) The importance of repeated angiography in the treatment of mycotic intracranial aneurysms. J Neurosurg 25:189–193

Clark E, Walton JN (1953) Subdural haematoma and angioma. Brain 76:378–404

Cole FM, Yates P (1967) Intracerebral microaneurysms and cerebrovascular lesions. Brain 90:759–768

Crompton MR (1966) Mechanism of growth and rupture in cerebral aneurysms. Br Med. J I:1138–1142

Cronqvist S, Troupp H (1966) Intracranial arteriovenous malformation and arterial aneurysm in the same patient. Acta Neurol Scand 42:307–316

Cummins BH, Griffith HB, Thompson JLG (1974) Perioperative cerebral angiography. Br J Radiol 47:257–260

Davis DO, Dilenge D, Schlaephen W (1970) Arterial dilatation in purulent meningitis. J Neurosurg 32:112–115

Doi H, Kuwabana S, Sakoda K, Mori S, Shima T, Uozimi T, Okamoto S (1980) Angiographic extravasation of contrast medium in a case of ruptured arteriovenous malformation. Neuroradiology 20:83–85

Drake CG (1979) The treatment of aneurysms of the posterior circulation. Clin Neurosurg 26:96–144

Drake CG, Vanderlinden RG (1967) The late consequences of incomplete surgical treatment of cerebral aneurysms. J Neurosurg 27:226–238

Drake CG, Vanderlinden RG, Amacher AL (1968) Carotid ophthalmic aneurysms. J Neurosurg 29:24–31

du Boulay GH (1965) Some observations on the natural history of intracranial aneurysms. Br J Radiol 38:721–757

du Boulay GH, Symon L, Ackerman L, Dorsch D, Kendall BE, Shah S (1973) The reactivity of the spastic arteries. Neuroradiology 5:37–39

du Boulay GH (1980) Angiography—the radiologist's view. In: Boullin DJ (ed) Cerebral vasospasm. Wiley, Chichester New York Brisbane Toronto, pp 47–79

Edner G, Forster DMC, Steiner L, Bergvall U (1978) Spontaneous healing of intracranial aneurysms after subarachnoid haemorrhage. Case report. J Neurosurg 48:450–454

Edwards KR (1977) Haemorrhagic complications of cerebral arteritis. Arch Neurol 34:549–552

Ferris EJ (1974) Arteritis. Radiology of the skull and brain. In: Newton DH, Potts DG (eds) Angiography, vol 2. Mosby, St Louis, pp 2566–2597

Field JR, Robertson JT, DeSaussure RL Jr (1962) Complications of cerebral angiography in 2,000 consecutive cases. J Neurosurg 19:775–781

Field JR, Lee L, McBurney RF (1972) Complications of 1,000 brachial arteriograms. J Neurosurg 36:324–332

Fischer CM, Roberson GH, Ojemann RG (1977) Cerebral vasospasm with ruptured saccular aneurysms. The clinical manifestations. Neurosurgery 1:245–248

Forster DMC, Steiner L, Hakanson S, Bergvall U (1978) The malformations of the brain. A long term clinical study. J Neurosurgery 37:562–570

Forster DMC, Steiner L, Hakanson S, Bergvall U (1978) The value of repeat panangiography in cases of unexplained subarachnoid haemorrhage. J Neurosurg 48:712–716

Gerlock AJ (1975) Rupture of posterior inferior cerebellar artery aneurysm into the subarachnoid space during angiography. J Neurosurg 42:469–472

Heidelberger KP, Layton WM, Fisher RG (1968) Multiple cerebral mycotic aneurysms complicating post-traumatic meningitis. J Neurosurg 29:631–635

Hirschfeld A, Flamm ES (1981) Extracranial aneurysm arising from the posterior inferior cerebellar artery. Case report. J Neurosurg 54:537–539

Hiscott P, Crockard A (1982) Multiple aneurysms of the distal posterior inferior cerebellar artery. Neurosurgery 10:101–102

Houser OW, Bank HL Jr, Sandok BA, Holley KE (1972) Fibromuscular dysplasia of the cephalic arterial vessels. In: Vinken PJ, Bruyn GW (eds) Vascular diseases of the nervous system. Elsevier, New York, pp 366–385, (Handbook of clinical neurology, vol 11)

Hughes JT (1980) Pathological changes associated with cerebral vasospasm. In: Boullin DJ (ed) Cerebral vasospasm. Wiley, Chichester New York Brisbane Toronto, pp 171–206

Hughes JT, Schianchi PM (1978) Cerebral artery spasm. A histological study of necropsy of the blood vessels in cases of subarachnoid haemorrhage. J Neurosurg 48:515–525

Kendall BE, Lee BCP, Claveria E (1976) Computerised tomography and angiography in subarachnoid haemorrhage. Br J Radiol 49:483–501

Kodama N, Suzuki J (1978) Moya Moya disease associated with aneurysms. J Neurosurg 48:565–569

Kramer RA, Wing DS (1977) Computerised tomography of angiographically occult cerebral vascular malformations. Radiology 123:649–652

Krayenbuhl HA, Yasargil MG (1968) Cerebral angiography, 2nd edn. Butterworth, London

Lassman LP, Ramani PS, Sengupta RP (1974) Aneurysms of peripheral cerebral arteries due to surgical trauma. Vasc Surg 8:1–5

Laun A (1979) Traumatic aneurysm. In: Pia HW, Landmaid

C, Zierski J (eds) Cerebral aneurysms. Advances in diagnosis and therapy. Springer, Berlin Heidelberg New York, pp 364–375

Leipzig TJ, Brown FD (1985) Treatment of mycotic aneurysm. Surg Neurol 23:403–407

Leonhardt ETG, Jacobson H, Ringquist OTA (1972) Angiographic and clinio-physiologic investigation of a case of polyarteritis nodosa. Am J Med 53:242–256

Lie TA (1972) Congenital malformations of the carotid and vertebral arterial systems including the persistent anastomoses In: Vinken PJ, Bruyn GW (eds) Vascular diseases of the nervous system. Elsevier, New York, pp 289–339 (Handbook of clinical neurology, vol 12)

Locksley HB (1966) Report on the co-operative studies of intracranial aneurysms and subarachnoid haemorrhage. Section V, Part II, Natural history of subarachnoid haemorrhage, intracranial aneurysms and arterio-venous malformations based on 6368 cases in the co-operative studies. J Neurosurg 25:321–368

Loman J, Myerson A (1936) Visualization of cerebral vessels by direct intracarotid injection of thorium dioxide. Arch Neurol Psychiatry 36:912–915

Mani RL, Eisenberg RL (1978) Complications of catheter cerebral arteriography. Analysis of 5,000 procedures. Relation of complication rates to clinical and arteriographic diagnosis. AJR 131:867–869

McLennan JE, Rosenbaum AE, Hedley-Whyte ET, Rischler AS, Scott RM (1974) Angiographic visualisation of fatal haemorrhage from a cerebral arterio-venous malformation. J Neurosurg 41:622–626

Miller JDR, Grace MG, Russell DB, Zacks DJ (1977) Complications of cerebral angiography and pneumography. Radiology 124:741–744

Mohan J (1980) The neurosurgeon's view. In: Boullin DJ (ed) Cerebral vasospasm. Wiley, Chichester New York Brisbane Toronto, pp 15–35

Moniz E (1927) L'encephalographic arterielle son importance dans la localisation des tumeurs cerebrales. Rev Neuriol 2:72–90

Montaut J, Hepner H, Tridon P, Picaud L, Floquet J, Lepoire J (1971) Aspects pseudo vasculaires des metastases intracraniennes des chorio epitheliomes. Neurochirurgie 17:119–128

Moritake K, Halda H, Sukas OHT, Hashimoto N (1981) Vanishing cerebral aneurysm in serial angiography. Surg Neurol 16:36–40

Nagamine Y, Takalashi S, Sondie M (1981) Multiple intracranial aneurysms associated with Moya Moya disease. Case report. J Neurosurg 54:673–676

New PFJ, Price DL, Carter B (1970) Cerebral angiography in cardiac myxomas, correlation of angiographic and histopathological findings. Radiology 96:335–345

Newton TH, Cronqvist S (1969) Involvement of dural arteries in intracranial arterio-venous malformations. Radiology 93:1071–1078

Nishimoto A, Takeuchi S (1972) Moya Moya disease cerebrovascular network in the cerebral basal region. In: Vinken PJ, Bruyn GW (eds) Vascular diseases of the nervous system. Elsevier, New York, pp 352–383 (Handbook of clinical neurology, vol 12)

Nishimura K, Hawkins TD (1975) Cerebral vasospasm with subarachnoid haemorrhage from arteriovenous malformations of the brain. Neurol Radiol 8:201–207

Norlen G, Barnum AS (1953) Surgical treatment of aneurysms of the anterior communicating artery. J Neurosurg 10:634–650

Olivecrona H, Ladenheim J (1957) Congenital arterio-venous aneurysms of the carotid and vertebral arterial systems.

Springer, Berlin Heidelberg New York

Palubinskas AJ, Perloff D, Newton TH (1966) Fibromuscular hyperplasia: an arterial dysplasia of increasing clinical importance. AJR 98:907–913

Parkinson D, West M (1980) Traumatic intracerebral aneurysms. J Neurosurg 52:11–20

Patterson JH, McKissock W (1956) A clinical survey of intracranial angiomas with special reference to the mode of progression and surgical treatment: a report of 110 cases. Brain 79:233–266

Patterson RH, Goodell H, Dunning HS (1964) Complications of carotid arteriography. Arch Neurol 10:513–520

Perret LV, Bull JWD (1959). Some aspects of subarachnoid haemorrhage, Section 4. Cerebral angiography: An analysis in demonstrating ruptured intracranial aneurysms. Br J Radiol 32:85–92

Perret E, Nishioka H (1966a) Report on the co-operative studies of intracerebral aneurysms and subarachnoid haemorrhage, Section 4. Cerebral angiography: An analysis of the diagnostic value and complications of carotid and vertebral angiography in 5,484 patients. J Neurosurg 25:98–114

Perret E, Nishioka H (1966b) Report on the co-operative study of intracranial aneurysms and subarachnoid haemorrhage, Section 6. Arterio-venous malformations: an analysis of 545 cases of craniocerebral malformations and fistulae reported to the co-operative study. J Neurosurg 25:467–490

Pia HW (1979) Aneurysms of the anterior cerebral artery. In: Pia HW, Langmaid C, Zierski J (eds) Cerebral aneurysms. Advances in diagnosis and therapy. Springer Berlin Heidelberg New York, pp 109–115

Rhoton AL Jr, Saeki N, Perlmutter D, Zeal A (1979) Microsurgical anatomy of common aneurysm sites. Clin Neurosurg 26:248–306

Roach MR, Drake CG (1965) Ruptured cerebral aneurysms caused by micro-organisms. N Engl J Med 1273:240–244

Rumbaugh CL, Bergeron RT, Talalla A, Kurtze T (1970) Traumatic aneurysms of the cortical cerebral arteries—radiographic aspects. Radiology 96:49–54

Sato T, Sakuta Y, Takaku A, Suzuki J (1979) Successful surgical treatment of intracranial mycotic aneurysms with brain abscess In: Suzuki J (ed) Cerebral aneurysms. Neuron, Tokyo, pp 683–689

Schneck SA, Kricheff II (1964) Intracranial aneurysm rupture, vasospasm and infarction. Arch Neurol 11:691–702

Scott RM, Garrido E (1977) Spontaneous thrombosis of an intracranial aneurysm during treatment with epsilon aminocaproic acid. Surg Neurol 7:21–23

Seldinger SI (1953) Catheter replacement of the needle in percutaneous arteriography. A new technique. Acta Radiol 39:368

Sengupta RP (1975) Anatomical variations in the origin of the posterior cerebral artery demonstrated by carotid angiography and their significance in the direct surgical treatment of posterior communicating aneurysms. Neurochirurgia 18:33–42

Sengupta RP, Sing CS, Villarejo-Ortega FJ (1976) Use of epsilon aminocaproic acid (EACA) in the pre-operative management of ruptured intracranial aneurysms. J Neurosurg 44:479–484

Sengupta RP, Lassman LP, Hankinson J (1978) Scope of surgery for intracranial aneurysm in the elderly: A preliminary report, Br Med J II:246–247

Shenkin HA, Jenkins F, Kim K (1971) Arterio-venous anomalies of the brain associated with cerebal aneurysm. J Neurosurg 34:225–228

Shimidzu K (1937) Beitrage zur Arteriographie des Gehirns—einfache perkutane Methode. Arch Klin Chir 188:295–316

Spetzler RF, Winestock D, Newton HT, Boldrey EB (1974) Disappearance and reappearance of cerebral aneurysm in serial arteriograms. J Neurosurg 41:508–510

Stevens JL (1966) Post-operative angiography in the treatment of intracranial aneurysms. Acta Radiol 55:536–547

Strang RR, Tovi D, Hugosson R (1951) Subdural haematomas resulting from the rupture of intracranial arterial aneurysms. Acta Chir Scand 121:345–350

Sutton, D, Trickey SE (1962) Subarachnoid haemorrhage and total cerebral angiography. Clin Radiol 13:297–303

Suwanwella C, Suwanwella N, Charuchinda S, Hongsapraphas S (1972) Intracranial mycotic aneurysms of extravascular origin. J Neurosurg 36; 552–559

Suzuki J, Onuma T (1979) Intracranial aneurysms associated with arteriovenous malformations. J. Neurosurg 50:742–746

Symon L, du Boulay GH, Ackerman RH, Dorsch NMC, Shah SH (1972) The time course of blood induced spasm of cerebral arteries in baboons. Neuroradiology 5:40–42

Udvarhelyi GB, Lai M (1963) Subarachnoid haemorrhage due to rupture of an aneurysm on a persistent left hypoglossal artery. Br J Radiol 36:843–847

Valadares JB, De Souza MTK, Hankinson J, Hall K, Sengupta RP (1979) Multiplos aneurysmus micoticos intracranianos

Regist. de um caso. Arq Neuropsiquiatr 37:311–318

Waga S, Kondo A, Moritake K, Handa H (1973) Rupture of intracranial aneurysm during angiography. Neuroradiology 5:169–173

Waga S, Morooka Y, Kojima T (1981) Aneurysm on a persistent hypoglossal artery. Acta Neurochir 59:71–78

Waltimo O (1973) The change in size of intracranial arteriovenous malformations. J Neurol Sci 19:21–27.

West HH, Mani RL, Eisenberg RL, Tuenk K, Stucken TB (1977) Normal cerebral arteriography in patients with spontaneous subarachnoid haemorrhage. Neurology 27:592–594

Wolpert SM (1966) The trigeminal artery and associated aneurysms. Neurology 16:610–614

Wood EH (1964) Angiographic identification of the ruptured lesion in patients with multiple cerebral aneurysms. J Neurosurg 21:182–198

Wright JR, Slavin RE, Wagner JA (1965) Intracranial aneurysm as a cause of subdural haematoma of the posterior fossa. J Neurosurg 22:86–89

Zervas NT (1979) Vasospasm: an update. Clin Neurosurg 26:643–656

Ziedses des Plantes BG (1963) Application of the roentgenographic subtraction method in neuroradiology. Acta Radiol [Diag] 1:961

8 Management of Subarachnoid Haemorrhage

Management of patients with SAH involves a co-ordinated medical and surgical approach. Medical management is very important in the pre- and postoperative period, and, furthermore, in some conditions the treatment remains purely non-surgical.

The aims of treatment in SAH are:

1. To allow the brain to recover from the initial insult of the SAH.
2. To minimise or prevent the risk of rebleeding before definitive surgical treatment can be undertaken.
3. To detect early and to treat complications such as cerebral vasospasm, ischaemia and hydrocephalus before irreversible damage occurs.
4. To prevent the general complications that may result from a disturbance of consciousness.

This chapter largely deals with the role of medical therapy in the management of SAH, particularly from ruptured aneurysm. Where relevant, however, the role of surgery is briefly mentioned.

In patients in whom surgery is contraindicated, medical management plays an important role in reducing the mortality and morbidity. The following groups of patients usually fall into this category.

1. Patients in clinical grade 4 or worse, unless the condition is due to a haematoma
2. Patients who have generalised atherosclerosis and severe extracranial arterial disease
3. Patients with serious systemic illness, such as uncontrolled hypertension or renal disease
4. Patients who have crippling, chronic cardiac and respiratory disease
5. Patients with inoperable intracranial vascular lesions
6. Patients above 70 years of age in general, unless they are exceedingly fit
7. Patients with no angiographically demonstrable lesion

Management at the Receiving Hospital

Once the diagnosis is established, subsequent management depends upon the clinical condition of the patient. If the patient is in clinical grade 4 or more, mannitol 500 ml of a 15% solution and/or frusemide (Lasix) should be given. If the patient improves, then he should be referred to a neurosurgical centre immediately. If, however, the patient remains comatose from the outset, neurosurgery has little role to play.

In the less severely affected patients, sedation should be given, taking particular care not to use drugs that will interfere with the pupils, respiration or blood pressure. Codeine phosphate or chlormethiazole (Heminevrin) are suitable for this purpose. Antifibrinolytic therapy should be commenced as soon as possible; the dose and mode of administration are outlined later in the chapter. Meanwhile, arrangements should be made for the patient to be transferred to the nearest neurosurgical centre. Patients with a mild to moderate uncomplicated SAH should be allowed to settle prior to being transferred, as harm can result from the anxiety and stress produced by urgent transfer.

One point that requires particular emphasis is the question of management of hypertension at the receiving hospital. If the patient is on anti-hypertensive therapy this should be continued. When evidence of longstanding untreated hypertension is present (i.e. hypertensive cardiac or retinal disease), gentle lowering of the blood pressure is indicated. (The role of antihypertensive therapy in the management will be discussed further.)

General Measures

Bed-rest

The value of bed-rest in the treatment of SAH cannot be over-emphasised. Before surgical therapy was available in the management of SAH, bed-rest was the mainstay of treatment (Richardson and Hyland 1941). Even today, with the greater emphasis on early definitive surgical intervention, this time-honoured measure should not be overlooked. Absolute bed-rest in a quiet and darkened room is essential. The duration of bed-rest should be at least 3 weeks, or longer, if necessary, in a conservatively treated patient. A darkened room is also helpful to relieve photophobia.

The head should be moderately elevated to promote venous drainage and lessen cerebral oedema. When the conscious state is severely impaired, the patient should be turned every 1–2 h to prevent bed sores. Development of deep venous thrombosis in patients with prolonged bed-rest should be borne in mind.

Nursing Care

From the moment a patient with SAH is admitted to hospital, he should be kept under constant observation for the first few days, ideally in an intensive care unit with the facilities for monitoring vital signs. This, however, is not always practicable, and not essential for a large number of patients with an uncomplicated SAH. Frequent observation and assessment by skilled and trained nurses in the management of neurological problems are adequate.

Recording of Vital Functions

Every neurological department has its own system of recording vital functions, and we use a chart for recording the vital signs, such as the conscious level, blood pressure, pulse, temperature, respiration, pupillary size and reaction and limb movements, which is based on the Glasgow Coma Scale. Four-hourly observations are adequate in a patient with an uncomplicated SAH, but half-hourly observations are necessary in patients with a more severe SAH. Careful recording of fluid balance is necessary, especially in the unconscious patient. Serum electrolytes, urea, haemoglobin and haematocrit should be checked daily. In special circumstances, estimation of serum osmolality may be necessary.

Headache and Neck Pain

These are very common symptoms after SAH. Morphine, once used extensively, should not be given, as it depresses both respiration and the conscious level, and furthermore interferes with the assessment of the pupillary reaction to light. The phenothiazine group of drugs is also not recommended because of their propensity to produce hypotension. In the majority of cases codeine phosphate 60 mg given intramuscularly at regular intervals is sufficient. Oxycodone (Prolodone) suppositories are also useful, and, although this is a narcotic, it has little effect on the pupils, blood pressure or respiration. The dosage is usually 30 mg three times per day. When analgesics fail to relieve headache the patient should be investigated (CT scan) for evidence of developing hydrocephalus.

Sedation

This is necessary if a patient is restless, and we use amylobarbitone sodium or chlormethiazole to ensure rest and sleep. Sedation may also be required to avoid stress during transfer to the neurosurgical unit.

Laxatives

Meadows (1951) stressed the importance of the judicial use of laxatives to avoid strain at stool, and we use lactulose (Duphalac) 30 mg at bedtime routinely to soften the stool during the pre-operative period.

Nutrition and Fluid Requirements

Provision of adequate food and nourishment is necessary, and the fluid and electrolyte balance needs to be carefully monitored. Overhydration can easily lead to cerebral oedema, and dehydration may cause haemoconcentration and consequent poor cerebral perfusion. Fluid replacement should be 2 litres per day, and we recommend alternating normal saline with 4% dextrose in a fifth normal saline. Adequate nourishment is afforded by a diet of 1300–1400 calories per day. In severely ill patients a nasogastric tube may be required for feeding. Intravenous nutrition is rarely necessary.

Lowering the Intracranial Pressure

Raised intracranial pressure invariably follows SAH, but usually settles rapidly in uncomplicated cases. Clinically raised intracranial pressure is manifest by intense headache, drowsiness and lethargy. When the CT scan has excluded a space-occupying lesion, the raised pressure may be lowered gradually by lumbar puncture or external ventricular drainage, and this will, in addition to alleviating headache, often improve the level of consciousness. Care should be taken to avoid stress during the lumbar puncture to prevent rebleed. Diazepam 5 mg half an hour before the lumbar puncture may be given for this purpose. It is also important to emphasise that the intracranial pressure should not be lowered below 200–250 mm water. Dexamethasone, although often used in these circumstances, has a doubtful role in reducing raised intracranial pressure due to SAH.

Prevention of Seizures

The role of anticonvulsant therapy in the management of SAH remains to be clearly defined. Epilepsy after SAH has been reported to occur in 10%–22% of patients (Rose and Sarner 1965; Storey 1967; Cabral et al. 1976; Winn et al. 1978; Richardson and Uttley 1980), and is 20 times greater than in the general population (Rose and Sarner 1965). Interestingly, there is no difference in the incidence between the operated and the conservatively treated groups (Storey 1967). Epilepsy is more common with middle cerebral artery aneurysmal rupture than with other aneurysms (Rose and Sarner 1965; Storey 1967; Cabral et al. 1976; Richardson and Uttley 1980). There is no relationship between the type of seizure and the site of the aneurysm (Rose and Sarner 1965). The chances of epilepsy developing after intracranial aneurysmal rupture are not increased by the occurrence of a single fit at the time of haemorrhage in our experience, or in that of Rose and Sarner (1965). However, cerebral oedema and cortical damage (Carbral et al. 1976), as well as an intracerebral haematoma (Rose and Sarner 1965; Storey 1967; Cabral et al. 1976; Richardson and Uttley 1980) are significantly correlated with a greater incidence of epilepsy. Seizures are usually well controlled by anticonvulsant medication (Rose and Sarner 1965; Storey 1967; Cabral et al. 1976; North et al. 1980). Prophylactic anticonvulsant therapy has been recommended in all patients with SAH (Cabral et al. 1976; Richardson and Uttley 1980; North et al. 1980). In the author's series of 500 patients with aneurysmal SAH 6% had epilepsy at the onset of SAH. The incidence of epilepsy was 9% at the time of discharge from hospital. Epilepsy was more commonly seen with middle cerebral artery aneurysms. We recommend prophylactic anticonvulsants in all patients with SAH undergoing craniotomy. In our opinion, the development of grand mal epilepsy in the early postoperative period is best avoided, as it may lead to further cerebral damage, with higher mortality and morbidity (see Chap. 11). We use phenytoin 300 mg per day, with a loading dose of 1–1.5 g in the 24 h immediately prior to surgery. This daily dose may need adjustment, depending upon the serum levels. We have not used anticonvulsant therapy in conservatively treated patients. However, a prospective controlled study is being carried out in our department to evaluate the role of prophylactic anticonvulsant therapy in aneurysmal SAH.

Treatment of Hypertension

Patients with SAH often show transient hypertension. This is regarded as part of Cushing's reflex, where secondary hypertension occurs in order to maintain cerebral perfusion in the presence of an elevated intracranial pressure. As mentioned before, the blood pressure often comes down to the normal level with improvement of the clinical condition of the patient, and, therefore, hypotensive therapy is not required. Patients with pre-existing hypertension on a drug regime should continue their previous therapy. If, in spite of general measures, the blood pressure remains high, this may indicate raised intracranial pressure and attempts should be directed to finding the cause and instituting appropriate therapy, rather than placing the patient on hypotensive medication.

Management of the Comatose Patient

Coma in a patient with SAH is usually due to a complication (such as intracerebral haemorrhage, hydrocephalus or cerebral oedema), and here surgery may have a role to play in management. General measures should, however, not be omitted. Protection of the airway is essential in such patients to prevent aspiration pneumonia, as vomiting is common.

Patients who have severe haemorrhage are likely to die without regaining consciousness. Fifty per cent of the patients dying after SAH do so within the first 48 h, and half of these within the first 24 h (Dandy 1944). Walton (1956), in an analysis of 312 patients, noted 113 patients to be in coma lasting more than 12 h, and only 27 of them recovered. This does not include those patients who died at home or who were admitted to peripheral hospitals in a moribund state and thus considered unsuitable for transfer. McKissock and his colleagues (1962) found that the results of medical treatment of unconscious patients were no different to those of surgical treatment. The Co-operative Study (Sah 1966) provides similar evidence regarding the lack of efficacy of surgical treatment in moribund patients. Such evidence has led to the conclusion that patients in coma cannot be helped. Before the advent of CT scanning, the pathological process could

only be revealed in life by various invasive investigations, including angiography or ventriculography, which in themselves carried the risk of aggravating the situation. The CT scan now reveals the pathology of SAH and it can identify those patients who may be retrieved without compromising their chance of recovery by invasive investigation. Advances in neuroanaesthesia and in the management of intracranial pressure and cerebral oedema have improved the chances of recovery of these patients. Active treatment, including emergency surgery, is now sometimes rewarding. It is obvious that a large proportion of comatose patients will die, irrespective of the form of therapy, but treatment at the earliest opportunity may prevent others from developing irreversible brain damage. The management of comatose patients following SAH depends upon the underlying intracranial pathology. Whatever is the pathological process which results in coma, irreversible brain damage will occur from rapidly rising intracranial pressure. The rapid infusion of 500 ml of 15% mannitol will reduce the pressure temporarily, gaining time to re-assess the clinical status and to detect the underlying cause by CT scan. Coma is usually due to one of the following:

1. Massive SAH
2. Intracerebral haematoma
3. Subdural haematoma
4. Acute hydrocephalus
5. Diffuse brain swelling

In the presence of massive SAH, little can be done. We would advocate draining intraventricular blood if it is obstructing the CSF pathway, causing acute hydrocephalus.

If there is improvement following mannitol and/or frusemide therapy, any further deterioration in a patient with a space-occupying intracerebral haematoma will be due to the combined result of secondary oedema and the mass effect of the haematoma itself. Evacuation of the haematoma will reduce the intracranial pressure, but before embarking on surgery to this end, the nature of the vascular lesion responsible should be identified by angiography. This is necessary in case the vascular lesion itself requires surgical treatment during the emergency evacuation. Subdural haematoma, causing significant shift, should be evacuated.

As a temporary measure, acute hydrocephalus is best dealt with by an external ventricular drain inserted under local anaesthesia. A ventriculoperitoneal shunt may be required later.

Diffuse cerebral oedema is treated with fluid restriction. The role of dexamethasone in these circumstances is controversial. We use dexamethasone 5 mg 6-hourly for its doubtful beneficial value.

Mannitol, conventionally used in a dose of 1–1.5 g/kg body weight, effectively reduces the intracranial pressure. When used as a long-term measure to control intracranial pressure, it is found to cause disturbances in serum osmolarity and electrolytes, as well as a rebound elevation of intracranial pressure. Smaller doses of mannitol, repeated at 4- to 6-hourly intervals, are recommended when it is being used for long-term control of ICP (Marsh et al. 1977).

McGraw et al. (1978) analysed the intracranial pressure (ICP) monitoring records of 150 patients receiving 20% mannitol infusions to evaluate its effectiveness in relation to dose. Initial ICP, ICP after various doses of mannitol and the time interval between its administration and the pressure recording were considered. They concluded that smaller doses of mannitol were as effective as larger doses, without having the latter's problems, such as disturbance of osmolarity and rebound elevation of ICP. They recommended 50–100 ml of 20% mannitol as a bolus dose with ICP monitoring in patients with raised ICP.

Prevention of Recurrent Haemorrhage

One of the most important problems in the management of SAH is rebleeding, which occurs in approximately 20%–30% of patients, with a mortality of 20% within the first 2 weeks. To minimise the risk of rebleeding in the pre-operative period, hypotensive therapy and antifibrinolytic agents have been recommended.

Induced Hypotension

The role of hypotension in the management of patients with aneurysmal SAH has been, and remains, the subject of considerable controversy. Holmes (1958) found some apparent benefit, but the results were not spectacular. Slosberg (1960) analysed 15 cases treated with hypotension alone, and found that there were no deaths in the 12 patients who received hypotensive therapy within 48 h after the onset of SAH. He stressed that it is

most important to induce hypotension during the early stages (i.e. within 48 h) after SAH. Meyer and Bauer (1962) also thought that hypotension had a place in the management of SAH. In the Co-operative Study (Sahs 1966) hypotension was used in 109 patients. In reasonable risk cases there was a suggestion that the incidence of rebleeding and subsequent death was diminished; there was, however, no definite evidence that drug-induced hypotension had a beneficial role. In the small number of patients in whom hypotension and hypothermia were combined, there were no survivors. All these patients fell into the poor surgical risk category or the aneurysms were inoperable. Mullan (1975) found hypotensive therapy in moribund patients to be dangerous, as it further reduced the cerebral perfusion. It is worth remembering the experimental work of Ralston et al. (1955), in which the effect of induced hypotension in 16 monkeys who underwent middle cerebral artery occlusion was compared with that in five normotensive animals. Blood letting-induced hypotension caused marked infarction, and similarly, hypotension due to the drug methylhexitone resulted in slight but additional infarction when compared to the control group. *We do not use, nor recommend, hypotensive therapy in the pre-operative management of patients with SAH.*

Antifibrinolytic Therapy

The factors responsible for the spontaneous arrest of haemorrhage after rupture of intracranial aneurysms are still not clearly defined. It is assumed that clot formation in and around the sac occurs, and is responsible for the cessation of haemorrhage. As the clot becomes organised, fibrosis and endothelial overgrowth take place, and thus the rent in the aneurysm is repaired. In spite of this physiological response, rebleeding is more common in the first 3 weeks after SAH, and it is reasonable to assume that the fibrinolytic mechanism may be counteracting this clotting process. On this assumption, antifibrinolytic agents have been used in the management of aneurysmal SAH. These substances act by competitive inhibition of the activator that converts plasminogen into plasmin. The two drugs currently available are epsilon amino-caproic acid (EACA) 24–36 g/day and tranexamic acid (AMCA) 4–6 g/day. The rationale behind the treatment of patients with SAH by means of antifibrinolytic therapy is to delay or prevent the dissolution of the clot at the site of the aneurysm. Sengupta et al. (1976) and Chowdhary et al. (1979) found that EACA had a beneficial role in the prevention of recurrent haemorrhage in the pre-operative management of patients with SAH. Similar results were also reported by Ransohoff et al. (1972) and Post et al. (1977). Mullan (1975) had noticed a shift of the rebleeding curve to the right with EACA at a dose of 24 g/day, whilst Shucart et al. (1980) were unable to demonstrate any benefit from the use of EACA. Chandra (1978) in a double-blind trial in 39 patients found a significant reduction of rebleeding with 6 g AMCA daily. Fodstad et al. (1980) noted AMCA to be effective for the first 10–12 days only, and after that the rebleed rate was equal to that of the control group. Van Rossum et al. (1977) and Kaste and Ramsay (1979) in a double-blind trial did not find any beneficial effects from the use of tranexamic acid. AMCA has a beta-sympathomimetic action (Norman 1975) and hence it should not be used in combination with chlorpromazine, as this may lead to hypotension (Fodstad et al. 1981). Alvarez Garijo et al. (1980) suggested monitoring the CSF fibrinolytic activity, and adjusting the dosage of the antifibrinolytic therapy. Schisano (1978) used AMCA with the kallikrein inhibitor Trasylol in a small study of 20 patients. He found that the dose of AMCA could be reduced to 0.5 g daily with the addition of 100 000 units of Trasylol twice daily. Trasylol has an inhibitory action on the transformation of plasminogen into plasmin, and a direct inhibitory affect on the already formed plasmin.

Ameen and Illingworth (1981) and Fodstad et al. (1981) found fewer episodes of rebleeding but a greater incidence of cerebral infarction in patients treated with antifibrinolytic drugs, and an overall greater mortality in the treated group, although this was not statistically significant. Fodstad et al. (1981) further cautioned against the use of such drugs in elderly patients because of their propensity to cause ischaemic complications. Sonntag and Stein (1974) noted angiographic intracranial vascular changes 5–14 days after commencing EACA; these were widespread, and affected the internal carotid artery and its branches, with punctate arterial narrowing involving a few millimetres of the vessels. Chowdhary et al. (1979) reported diarrhoea, deep vein thrombosis and pulmonary embolism as complications of EACA. Adams (1982) noted prolonged bleeding times and qualitative platelet function defects in some patients who had been given EACA.

Delayed myopathy after EACA therapy in patients with SAH has been reported (Korsan-Bengsten et al. 1969; Frank et al. 1972; Mackay et al. 1978; Brown et al. 1982). The myopathy is insidious in onset, and progresses as long as the patient is receiving EACA. The course of the myopathy is benign, and the symptoms resolve with the return of muscle enzyme levels to normal, once the EACA therapy is stopped. There is no correlation between the serum levels of the antifibrinolytic drug and the occurrence of myopathy. It involves the skeletal muscles preferentially. Most of the patients have pigmented urine (Brodkin 1980). The females are more prone and the initial symptoms are myalgia, muscle tenderness and weakness of proximal muscles (Brown et al. 1982). Histological examination of the muscles shows no inflammatory infiltrates. The myopathy is necrotising in type, with random distribution of regenerating and degenerating myofibrils. The remarkable feature is the reversal of the histological features after recovery. Intravascular thrombosis (Korsan-Bengsten et al. 1969) and disruption of sarcolemmal integrity (Frank et al. 1972) are some of the features responsible for myopathy. Hydrocephalus is seen more often in patients on antifibrinolytic therapy (Knibestol et al. 1976; Park 1979).

We recommend EACA to be commenced immediately after confirming the diagnosis of SAH, as the great majority of patients with SAH will have an aneurysm as the underlying cause. Furthermore, early surgery in the management of SAH means that the duration of therapy with antifibrinolytic drugs will be short and, therefore, the incidence of side-effects minimal. We do not use antifibrinolytics as an alternative to surgery, as they have been shown only to delay rather than prevent recurrent haemorrhage. Currently we use a dose of 3 g EACA syrup 3-hourly or 1.5 g AMCA 6-hourly.

Therapy in Bleeding Disorders

Subarachnoid haemorrhage due to thrombocytopenia is best treated with platelet transfusions, and, in patients with a bleeding diathesis due to a low prothrombin, replacement with PPF (plasma protein fraction) and the administration of vitamin K may be useful. The use of barbiturates is contraindicated in such patients, as it may further reduce the prothrombin content of the blood.

Treatment of Complications

Vasospasm

The aetiology and management of vasospasm will be discussed in Chap. 12. However, brief principles in the management of patients with vasospasm will be outlined here.

1. Whole blood or colloid (haemocell or PPF) is effective in increasing the circulating blood volume. Central venous pressure should be maintained at between 8 and 12 cm H_2O.
2. We use isoprenaline and lignocaine infusions with the aim of achieving cerebral vasodilatation and improving cerebral perfusion.
3. When vasospasm develops postoperatively, we use dopamine infusions to induce hypertension when isoprenaline fails to improve the patient's condition.

Haematoma

More cases of intracerebral haematoma following aneurysmal rupture are being recognised with the advent of CT scan. The incidence of intracerebral haematoma is reported to be between 4% (Sano 1979) and 17% (Pia 1979) following ruptured aneurysms. The incidence of intracerebral haematomas in our series is 10%. In spite of early diagnosis afforded by CT scan, and the availability of intensive care facilities, the mortality and morbidity due to intracerebral haematomas from ruptured aneurysms remain high. Most haematomas occur following rupture of anterior cerebral and middle cerebral lesions. They are commonly seen in the subfrontal, temporal, and interhemispheric regions.

Energetic management of these patients is essential. Steroids, mannitol, and, if necessary, elective ventilation, form the main modes of treatment. The question of surgical intervention and its timing remains controversial. Richardson (1976) suggested that only those patients with mild deficits, showing late neurological deterioration, and not responding to medical management, benefit from surgery. Tindall and Odom (1972) advocated immediate evacuation of the clot with definitive treatment of the offending aneurysm. Wheelock et al. (1983) reviewed 132 cases collected from 11 centres, and concluded that early surgery offers marginal benefit. They found morbidity and mortality following acute intracerebral

haematoma to be worse in patients with high blood pressure, signs of herniation, poor neurological grades, associated vasospasm and ischaemic deficits, and a haematoma in the parietal lobe. The mortality was higher in those who had evacuation alone than in those who had their aneurysms clipped at the time of evacuation of haematoma. Lougheed and Marshall (1973) were against clipping of the aneurym at the time of evacuation of the haematoma.

Our approach to this problem depends on the patient's condition at the time of admission. We find that it is futile to operate on a patient with irreversible brain damage. However, if a patient presents with signs of progressive secondary deterioration, we evacuate the haematoma. No attempt is made to clip the aneurysm at the same time, but occasionally this is required when the aneurysm becomes exposed after evacuation of haematoma.

Hydrocephalus

Hydrocephalus is common following aneurysmal SAH, its incidence varying from 10% to 35%. It can occur immediately after SAH or later. The insidious onset of impaired mentation and memory, sometimes associated with gait disturbance, should make one suspect the gradual development of hydrocephalus (Yasargil et al. 1973). In some cases, the dilated ventricles may by asymptomatic and need no special treatment.

Galera and Greitz (1970) calculated the ventriculocranial index in 100 patients with SAH. Only 19% were symptomatic, although 34% showed enlarged ventricles. Vassilouthis and Richardson (1979) expressed ventricular size as a ratio of the width of the lateral ventricles at the level of the foramen of Munro, immediately behind the caudate nucleus, and the transverse inner diameter of the skull at the same level. The normal ratio is 1:6.4. The enlargement is considered moderate if the ratio is between 1:4 and 1:5, and minimal if it is between 1:5 and 1:6.4. A value of more than 1:4 represents marked dilatation. On CT scan, periventricular lucencies (Mori et al. 1977), rounding of the frontal horns and obliteration of the cerebral sulci (Gunasekara and Richardson 1977), in addition to ventricular size, help in making a diagnosis.

We have classified hydrocephalus into preoperative and postoperative groups, depending upon the time of diagnosis. In our series (Kolluri and Sengupta 1984) symptomatic hydrocephalus was seen in 82 (16.4%) patients. The hydrocephalus was seen either pre- or postoperatively in only 7% and 6.6% respectively. In 2.8% of these patients, it was seen both pre- and postoperatively. In seven patients, emergency external ventricular drainage was done before definite surgery for the offending aneurysm. Most patients responded to repeated lumbar punctures and CSF drainage. Great care should be taken to avoid sudden reduction of the pressure, which should be maintained above 200–250 mm H_2O.

Sixty-four per cent of the patients with preoperative hydrocephalus had some degree of vasospasm. Hydrocephalus is also more common in patients receiving antifibrinolytic therapy (Knibestol et al. 1976; Park 1979). Immediate drainage of CSF in patients with acute hydrocephalus removes haemorrhagic fluid and reduces cerebral oedema (Raimondi and Torres 1973), and improves the neurological condition (Kusske et al. 1973) and the cerebral blood flow (Hartmann et al. 1977). In experimental animals, parenteral steroids have significantly reduced the incidence of hydrocephalus after SAH (Wilkinson et al. 1974).

Hydrocephalus after aneurysmal SAH is self-limiting in most cases. Although 16.4% of the 500 patients seen by us had symptomatic hydrocephalus, definitive CSF drainage procedures were required in only 5.8% of the patients (Kolluri and Sengupta 1984).

Metabolic, Electrolyte and Haematological Changes

After SAH there is sympathetic overactivity due to the normal stress reaction and hypothalamic dysfunction. The hypothalamic dysfunction is due to disturbances in the arterial supply to the hypothalamic nuclei (Jenkins et al. 1969). Transitory hyperglycaemia, eosinopenia (Thurlin and Rais 1958), elevated haematocrit (Bruch and de Pasquale 1965) and leukocytosis (Neil-Dwyer et al. 1974) are also regarded as non-specific responses to stress.

Elevated circulating catecholamines (Neil-Dwyer et al. 1974; Peerless and Griffiths 1972; Benedict and Loach 1978) and diurnal variations in cortisol secretion (Jenkins et al. 1969) are noted following SAH. There is also good evidence relating autonomic dysfunction in patients with SAH to functional and morphological changes in the heart (Greenhoot and Reichen-

back 1969; Cruickshank et al. 1974; Weintraub and McHenry 1974). The CSF lactate/pyruvate ratio is increased due to a combination of red cell metabolism of sugar in the subarachnoid space (Forman et al. 1967; Sambrook et al. 1973; Sugi and Fugishima 1975), hyperventilation (Sambrook et al. 1973) and brain tissue hypoxia (Sugi and Fujishima 1975). The mortality is directly proportional to the decrease in CSF pH (Sambrook et al. 1973). The neurological state of a patient who has suffered an SAH may result from disturbance in cerebral energy metabolism due to lactic acidosis promoted by systemic hyperglycaemia.

Water and electrolyte disturbances occur due to disturbances of various hypothalamic nuclei Disturbance of water and electrolyte metabolism is common after rupture of anterior communicating artery aneurysms (Joynt et al. 1965; Landolt 1972; Takaku et al. 1979; Mather et al. 1981; Doczi et al. 1981). The mortality in patients with hyponatraemia is comparatively low (15%) when compared with that in patients with hypernatraemia (42%) (Takaku et al. 1979). Massive haemorrhage in the hypothalamic region is common in patients with hypo- or hypernatraemia (Joynt et al. 1965; Landolt 1972; Takaku et al. 1979). Hypothalamic lesions may isolate supraoptic nuclei, resulting in inappropriate and excessive ADH release (Joynt et al. 1965).

Diabetes insipidus is usually monophasic, but may also be multiphasic (Landolt 1972). The diagnosis is established by first excluding iatrogenic diabetes insipidus due to excessive fluid administration or renal dysfunction. Urinary output of more than 1000 ml per 4 h should be viewed with suspicion, and specific gravity and serum osmolality examined. When a patient is conscious, i.v. fluids should be discontinued and the patient encouraged to take oral fluids (either plain water or glucose water). A strict fluid balance chart should be maintained on an hourly basis. If not controlled, DDAVP (desmopressin) should be given. It is advisable to give the initial dose intramuscularly, followed by nasal spray. Shucart and Jackson (1976) recently reviewed the management of diabetes insipidus in neurosurgical patients.

Inappropriate ADH Secretion

Schwartz et al. first described the syndrome of inappropriate ADH secretion in 1957. It is called inappropriate because ADH secretion is no longer regulated by the osmotic and volume changes

(Joynt et al. 1965). The classical features of the syndrome are:

1. Low serum sodium (less than 125 mEq/1)
2. High urinary sodium (more than 25 mEq/1)
3. Low serum osmolality (less than 280 mosmol/kg)
4. Urinary osmolality more than plasma osmolality

One should exclude other causes, such as increased fluid intake, excessive diuretic therapy, inadequate salt intake, kidney disease and cardiac failure, before making a final diagnosis. The pathogenesis is the failure of the kidney to conserve sodium in the face of low serum sodium concentration due to depression of the reabsorptive capacity of the proximal tubules. It does not respond to the hypertonic salines. In fact, hypertonic sodium and diuretics will aggravate the condition due to the decreased aldosterone secretion (Doczi et al. 1981). The restriction of crystalloid and colloid replacement in the form of packed cells or plasma is useful (Nelson et al. 1979). The patients with SIADH (syndrome of inappropriate ADH secretion) have decreased blood volume (Nelson 1981) and resemble those with the cerebral salt-wasting syndrome (Peters et al. 1950). Both SIADH and cerebral salt wasting may be contributing to the electrolyte disturbances noticed in these patients following aneurysmal SAH (Nelson 1981). Significantly higher levels of ADH are found in patients with SAH (Nelson et al. 1977) compared to those with unruptured aneurysms. The levels are increased more often in patients with rupture of the anterior communicating aneurysm (Mather et al. 1981). The incidence of SIADH varies from 9% to 29% in patients with SAH (Fox et al. 1971; Doczi et al. 1981). It is important to realise that not all cases of hyponatraemia are due to SIADH; excessive fluid administration during operation and in the postoperative period also results in hyponatraemia (Shenkin et al. 1976).

Elevated packed cell volume, ESR (Buckell) 1966), and leucocytosis (Neil-Dwyer et al. 1974) are found to have a prognostic significance after SAH.

In addition to the vasoregulatory mechanisms, cerebral blood flow is affected by haematological factors—the whole blood viscosity, the viscosity of blood sub faces and the properties of the formed elements. The whole blood viscosity is in turn influenced by haematocrit, plasma viscosity, red cell aggregation and deformability. Thomas et al. (1977) found an increase in cerebral blood flow at lower haematocrit levels. Haemoconcentration and reduction in circulating blood volume are potential risks, especially in patients with a poor level of consciousness. Buckell (1966) found increased packed cell volume in 35% of patients who were comatose, but in only 13% of patients who were alert. Increased intravascular aggregation may be exacerbated by increased platelet stickiness and haemoconcentration, which may be a normal reaction to stress (Bruch and de Pasquale 1965).

In view of the above-mentioned stress reactions following aneurysmal SAH, a prospective study was undertaken in our department (Kolluri 1982) to correlate the biochemical and haematolgical changes to progressive neurological deterioration. Over an 18-month period, 99 patients were studied.

Whole Blood Viscosity. In 61% of the patients, the whole blood viscosity was in the upper limits of the normal range. The mean blood viscosity during days 5–8 of SAH was significantly higher in patients with neurological deterioration than in those without such deterioration. Viscosity was measured by capillary viscometer.

Packed Cell Volume. The packed cell volume was within the upper limits of normal in the majority of the patients. It was above the normal value of 45% in 24% of the patients who had neurological deterioration, compared to 10% in those without such deterioration. This difference was not significant.

White Blood Cells. The white cell count was more than 10×10^9 per litre in 69% of the patients in the immediate post-bleed period (within 8 days). It could not be used as an indicator of prognosis as suggested by Neil-Dwyer et al. (1974).

ESR. The ESR was not high on admission. A steady increase in the mean values was noted, probably due to physiological response to surgery.

Blood Sugar. The mean fasting blood sugar values were around and above the upper limits of the normal range until day 14 after SAH. There was a significant increase in the incidence of raised fasting blood sugar values in patients who had progressive neurological deterioration.

Urinary Catecholamines. Urinary catecholamines were significantly raised in patients with angiographic cerebral vasospasm ($P < 0.05$). The elevation was also significantly less frequent in patients without spasm or neurological deterioration than in the remainder of the patients ($P < 0.01$).

In this study systemic metabolic and rheological variables, together with the pre-operative neurological status of the patient, were found to be related to the development of neurological deterioration from SAH due to ruptured aneurysms.

In conclusion, the management of SAH involves consideration of the effects of the acute bleed on the brain. Careful evaluation of neurological, biochemical and rheological disturbances helps assessment of the condition of the brain while deciding upon the surgical treatment. Early detection and treatment of complications such as hydrocephalus, haematoma, ischaemia and infarction prevent further injury to the brain. The medical treatment of the patient remains an important part of the overall management of SAH.

References

Adams HP Jr (1982) Current concepts of cerebrovascular disease. Stroke 13:256–259

Alvarez Garijo JA, Vilches JJ, Aznar JA (1980) Pre-operative treatment of ruptured intracranial aneurysms with tranexamic acid and monitoring of fibrinolytic activity. J Neurosurg 52:453–455

Ameen AA, Illingworth R (1981) Antifibrinolytic treatment in the pre-operative management of subarachnoid haemorrhage caused by ruptured intracranial aneurysms. J Neurol Neurosurg Psychiatry 44:220–226

Benedict CR, Loach AB (1978) Clinical significance of plasma adrenaline and nor-adrenaline concentrations in patients with subarachnoid haemorrhage. J Neurol Neurosurg Psychiatry 41:113–117

Brodkin HM (1980) Myoglobinuria following epsilon amino-caproic acid (EACA) therapy. J Neurosurg 53:690–692

Brown TA, Woltzman RL, Mullan S (1982) Myopathy induced by epsilon amino-caproic acid—A case report. J Neurosurg 56:130–134

Bruch GE, de Pasquale NB (1965) Haematocrit viscosity and coronary blood flow. Dis Chest 48:225–232

Buckell M (1966) Biochemical changes after spontaneous subarachnoid haemorrhage. J Neurol Neurosurg Psychiatry 29:291–298

Cabral RJ, King TT, Scott DF (1976) Epilepsy after two different neurosurgical approaches to the treatment of ruptured intracranial aneurysm. J Neurol Neurosurg Psychiatry 39:1052–1056

Chandra B (1978) Treatment of subarachnoid haemorrhage from ruptured intracranial aneurysm with tranexamic acid: A double blind clinical trial. Ann Neurol 3:502–504

Chowdhary UM, Carey PC, Hussien MM (1979) Prevention of early recurrence of spontaneous subarachnoid haemorrhage by epsilon amino-caproic acid. Lancet I:741–743

Cruickshank JM, Neil-Dwyer G, Brice J (1974) ECG changes and their prognostic significance in SAH. J Neurol Neurosurg Psychiatry 37:755–759

Dandy WE (1944) Intracranial arterial aneurysms. Comstock Ithaca, New York, Quoted by Norlen G, Olivecrona E (1953) The treatment of aneurysms of the circle of Willis. J Neurosurg 10:404–415

Doczi T, Bende J, Huszka E, Kiss J (1981) The syndrome of inappropriate secretion of ADH after subarachnoid haemorrhage. Neurosurgery 9:394–397

Fodstad H, Kok P, Algers G (1980) Fibrinolytic activity (FA) of cerebral tissue after experimental subarachnoid haemorrhage, effect of tranexamic acid (AMCA). Presented at the 5th international conference on synthetic fibrinolytic thrombolytic agents, progress in fibrinolysis. Malmo, Sweden, June 17–20. (Abstr)

Fodstad H, Forssell A, Liliequist B, Schannong M (1981) Antifibrinolysis with tranexamic acid in aneurysmal subarachnoid haemorrhage. A consecutive controlled clinical trial. Neurosurgery 8:158–165

Fox JL, Falik JL, Shalhoub RJ (1971) Neurosurgical hyponatraemia. The role of inappropriate antidiuresis. J Neurosurgery 34:506–514

Frank MM, Serjent JS, Kane MA et al. (1972) Epsilon amino-caproic acid therapy in hereditary angioneurotic oedema. N Engl J Med 286:808–812

Galera RG, Greitz T (1970) Hydrocephalus in the adult secondary to the rupture of intracranial artery aneurysms. J Neurosurg 32:634–641

Greenhoot JH, Reichenback DD (1969) Cardiac injury and SAH—A clinical, pathological and physiological correlation. J Neurosurg 30:521–531

Gunasekara L, Richardson AE (1977) Computerised axial tomography in idiopathic hydrocephalus. Brain 100:748–754

Hartmann A, Alberti E, Lange D (1977) Effects of CSF drainage on CBF and CBV in subarachnoid haemorrhage and communicating hydrocephalus. Acta Neurol Scand [Suppl] 56:336–337

Holmes JMD (1958) The medical management of subarachnoid haemorrhage. Br Med J I:788–790

Jenkins AS, Bucchal AM, Barham E et al. (1969) Hypothalamic pituitary adrenaline function after subarachnoid haemorrhage. Br Med J 4:707–709

Joynt RJ, Afifi A, Harrison J (1965) Hyponatraemia in subarachnoid haemorrhage. Arch Neurol 13:633–638

Kaste M, Ramsay M (1979) Tranexamic acid in subarachnoid haemorrhage. A double-blind study. Stroke 10:519–522

Knibestol M, Karadayi A, Tovi D (1976) Echo encephalographic study of ventricular dilatation after subarachnoid haemorrhage with special reference to antifibrinolytic treatment. Acta Neurol Scand 54:57–70

Kolluri VRS (1982) Biochemical and haematological changes in aneurysmal subarachnoid haemorrhage. M.Sc. Thesis, University of Newcastle upon Tyne

Kolluri VRS, Sengupta RP (1984) Symptomatic hydrocephalus following aneurysmal subarachnoid haemorrhage. Surg Neurol 21:402–404

Korsan-Bengsten K, Ysander L, Blohme G et al. (1969) Extensive muscle necrosis after long-term treatment with amino-caproic acid—EACA, in a case of hereditary periodic oedema. Acta Med Scand 185:341–346

Kusske JA, Turner PT, Ojemann GA, Haris AB (1973) Ventriculostomy for the treatment of acute subarachnoid haemorrhage. J Neurosurg 38:591–595

Landolt AM, Yasargil MG, Krayenbuhl E (1972) Disturbance of the serum electrolytes after surgery of intracranial arterial aneurysms. J Neurosurg 37:210–218

Lougheed WT, Marshall BM (1973) Management of aneurysms of the anterior circulation by intracranial procedures: In Youmans JR (ed) Neurological surgery, vol 2. WB Saunders, London Philadelphia Toronto, pp 731–767

Mackay AR, Sane UH, Weinstein PR (978) Myopathy associated with epsilon-amino-caproic acid (EACA) therapy. Report of two cases. J Neurosurg 49:597–601

Marsh ML, Marshall LF, Shapiro HM (1977) Neurosurgical intensive care. Anaesthesiology 17:149–163

Mather HM, Ang V, Jenkins JS (1981) Vasopressin in plasma and CSF of patients with subarachnoid haemorrhage. J Neurol Neurosurg Psychiatry 44:216–219

McGraw CP, Alexander E, Howard G (1978) Effect of dose and dose schedule on the response of ICP to mannitol. Surg Neurol 10:127–130

McKissock W, Richardson A, Walsh L (1962) Middle cerebral aneurysms. Further results in the controlled trial of conservative and surgical treatment of ruptured intracranial aneurysms. Lancet II:417–421

Meadows SP (1951) Intracranial aneurysms. In: Feiling A (ed) Modern trends in neurology. Butterworth, London, pp 391–405

Meyer JS, Bauer RB (1962) Medical treatment of spontaneous intracranial haemorrhage by the use of hypotensive drugs. Neurology 12:36–47

Mori K, Murata T, Nakano Y, Handa H (1977) Periventricular lucency in hydrocephalus on computer tomography. Surg Neurol 8:337–340

Mullan S (1975) Conservative management of the recently ruptured aneurysm. Surg Neurol 3:27–32

Nelson PB, Seir SM, Robinson AG et al. (1977) Increased secretion of antidiuretic hormone in patients with intracranial aneurysms. Stroke 8:13. Abstract, 2nd Joint Meeting on Stroke and Cerebral Circulation, Florida, February 1977

Nelson PB, Seir SM, Maroon JL, Robinson AG (1979) Hyponatraemia in patients with subarachnoid haemorrhage. A study of vasopressin and blood volume, Part B. In: Wilkins RH (ed) Cerebral vasospasm. Williams and Wilkins, Baltimore, pp 654–658

Nelson P (1981) Comments: Doczi T, Bende J, Huszka E, Kiss J. SIADH after SAH. Neurosurgery 9:394–397

Neil-Dwyer G, Cruickshank J, Scott A et al. (1974) Urinary catecholamines and plasma cortisol levels in patients with subarachnoid haemorrhage. J Neurol Sci 22:375–382

North JP, Hanich A, Challen RC et al. (1980) Post-operative epilepsy. A double-blind trial of phenytoin after craniotomy. Lancet I:384–386

Norman SR (1975) The sympathomimetic actions of trans-4-amino methyl cyclo hexane carboxylic acid–AMCA–cyclocapron in anaesthetised cats—Data on file. AB–KABI. Stockholm, Sweden. Quoted by Fodstad et al. 1981

Park BE (1979) Spontaneous subarachnoid haemorrhage complicated by communicating hydrocephalus: Epsilon aminocaproic acid as a possible predisposing factor. Surg Neurol 11:73–80

Peerless SJ, Griffiths JC (1972) Plasma catecholamines following subarachnoid haemorrhage. Ann R Coll Phys Surg Can 5:48–49

Peters JP, Welt LG, Seins EAH, Orloff J, Needham J (1950) Salt wasting syndrome associated with cerebral disease. Trans Assoc Am Phys 63:57–64

Pia HW (1979) Intracerebral haematomas. In: Pia HW, Langmaid C, Zierski J (eds) Cerebral aneurysms. Advances in diagnosis and therapy. Springer, Berlin Heidelberg New York, p 407

Post KD, Flanım ES, Goodgold A, Ransohoff J (1977) Ruptured intracranial aneurysms. Case morbidity and mortality. J Neurosurg 46:290–295

Raimondi AJ, Torres H (1973) Acute hydrocephalus as a complication of subarachnoid haemorrhage. Surg Neurol 1:23–26

Ralston B, Rasmussen T, Kennedy T (1955) Occlusion of middle cerebral artery under normotension and chemically induced hypotension. J Neurosurg 12:26–33

Ransohoff J, Goodgold A, Benjamin MV (1972) Pre-operative management of patients with ruptured intracranial aneurysms. J Neurosurg 36:525–530

Richardson JC, Hyland HH (1941) Intracranial aneurysm. A clinical and pathological study of subarachnoid and intracerebral haemorrhage caused by berry aneurysms. Medicine 20:1–88

Richardson AE (1976) Spontaneous intracerebral and cerebellar haemorrhage. In: Russel RWR (ed) Cerebral arterial disease. Churchill Livingstone, Edinburgh, pp 210–230

Richardson AE, Uttley D (1980) Prevention of post-operative epilepsy (letter). Lancet I:650

Rose FC, Sarner M (1965) Epilepsy after ruptured intracranial aneurysm. Br Med J I:18–21

Sahs AL (1966) Hypotension and hypothermia in the treatment of intracranial aneurysms. In Sahs, AL, Perret GE, Locksley HB, Nishioka H (eds) Intracranial aneurysms and subarachnoid haemorrhage—a co-operative study. Lippincott, Philadelphia Toronto, pp 143–149

Sambrook MA, Hudgson EC, Amber GM (1973) Metabolic studies in subarachnoid haemorrhage and stroke. Part 1. Serial changes in acid base values in blood and CSF. Brain 19:171–190

Sano K (1979) Intracerebral haematomas. In: Pia HW, Langmaid C, Zierski J (eds) Cerebral aneurysms. Advances in diagnosis and therapy. Springer, Berlin Heidelberg New York, pp 402–407

Schisano G (1978) The use of antifibrinolytic drugs in aneurysmal subarachnoid haemorrhage. Surg Neurol 10:217–222

Sengupta RP, So SC, Villarejo-Ortega FJ (1976) Use of epsilon aminocaproic acid (EACA) in the pre-operative management of ruptured intracranial aneurysm. J Neurosurg 44:479–484

Shenkin HA, Bezier HS, Bouzrht WF, Debu F (1976) Restricted fluid intake: Rational management of the neurosurgical patient. J Neurosurg 45:432–436

Schucart WA, Jackson I (1976) Management of diabetes insipidus in neurological patients. J Neurosurg 44:65–71

Shucart WA, Hussain SK, Cooper PR (1980) Epsilon aminocaproic acid and recurrent subarachnoid haemorrhage. A clinical trial. J. Neurosurg 42:28–31

Slosberg PS (1960) Medical treatment of intracranial aneurysms: An analysis of 15 cases. Neurology 10:1085–1089

Sonntag VKH, Stein BM (1974) Arteriopathic complications during treatment of subarachnoid haemorrhage with epsilon amino-caproic acid. J Neurosurg 40:480–485

Storey PB (1967) Psychiatric sequelae of subarachnoid haemorrhage. Br Med J I:261–266

Sugi D, Fujishima M (1975) Lactate and pyruvate concentrations and acid base balance of CSF in experimentally induced intracerebral and subarachnoid haemorrhage in dogs. Stroke 6:715–719

Takaku A, Shindo K, Tanaka S et al. (1979) Fluid and electrolyte disturbances in patients with intracranial aneurysms. Surg Neurol 1:349–356

Thomas DJ, Marshall J, Russell RW et al. (1977) Effect of haematocrit on cerebral blood flow in man. Lancet II:941–945

Thurlin C, Rais O (1958) Metabolic response to acute closed cranio-cerebral injuries of different degrees of severity. Glycaemia and blood eosinophil count in 28 cases. Acta Chir Scand 115:332–342

Tindall GT, Odom GL (1972) Saccular aneurysms of brain—surgical treatment. In: Vinken PJ, Bruyn GW (eds) Handbook of clinical neurology, vol 12. North Holland, Amsterdam New York, pp 205–226

Van Rossum J, Wintzen AR, Endtz LJ et al. (1977) Effects of tranexamic acid on rebleeding after subarachnoid haemorrhage. Double-blind controlled clinical trial. Ann Neurol 2:242–245

Vassilouthis J, Richardson AE (1979) Ventricular dilatation and communicating hydrocephalus following spontaneous subarachnoid haemorrhage. J Neurosurg 51:341–351

Walton JN (1956) Subarachnoid haemorrhage. E and S Livingstone, Edinburgh London

Weintraub BM, McHenry LC Jr (1974) Cardiac abnormalities in subarachnoid haemorrhage. A resume. Stroke 5:384–392

Wheelock B, Weir B, Watts R et al. (1983) Timing of surgery for intracerebral haematomas due to aneurysm rupture. J Neurosurg 58:476–481

Wilkinson HA, Wilson RB, Patel PP, Esmaili M (1974) Corticosteroid therapy of experimental hydrocephalus after intraventricular subarachnoid haemorrhage. J Neurol Neurosurg Psychiatry 37:224–229

Winn HR, Richardson AE, O'Brien W, Jane JA (1978) The long-term prognosis in untreated cerebral aneurysms. II. Late morbidity and mortality. Ann Neurol 4:418–426

Yasargil MG, Yonekawa Y, Zumstein B, Stahl HJ (1973) Hydrocephalus following subarachnoid haemorrhage. Clinical features and treatment. J Neurosurg 39:474–479

9 Anaesthesia

J. D. Whitby

Historical Background

The anaesthetic techniques used for intracranial operations on cerebral aneurysms have undergone many changes during the last 40 years. Between 1940 and 1950 the intravenous barbiturates began to supplant rectal bromethol for the induction of anaesthesia in patients being subjected to craniotomy (Hewer 1948). During this period most anaesthetists were maintaining anaesthesia with nitrous oxide and oxygen and allowing their patients to breathe spontaneously, often through an open circuit with an Ayre's T-piece (Ayre 1937). Maintenance was made easier when trichloroethylene was introduced (Hewer 1941).

During the next decade, deliberate hypotension was introduced, mainly to reduce the severity of the bleeding if the aneurysm should rupture. The first technique used was Gardner's method of inducing haemorrhagic hypotension by arteriotomy (Gardner 1946; Hale 1948; Bilsland 1951), but this was soon superseded by the simpler and safer pharmacological method of using ganglion blocking agents (Aserman 1953; Anderson and McKissock 1953).

The introduction of halothane into clinical practice in 1956 gave neurosurgical anaesthetists a more powerful non-inflammable inhalation agent than trichloroethylene without the toxic disadvantages of chloroform (Johnstone 1956).

The next new method to be tried out was the induction of deliberate hypothermia (Vandewater et al. 1955; Burrows et al. 1956). It was hoped that this would improve operating conditions, allow the temporary clipping of vital arteries and improve the safety of hypotensive techniques. Starting with moderate hypothermia produced by surface cooling, a few units went on to induce still lower temperatures by using more elaborate techniques of direct blood cooling through an extracorporeal circulation in order to produce a temporary cardiac arrest while the aneurysm was being clipped (Uihlein et al. 1962; Drake et al. 1964; Michenfelder et al. 1964; Campkin 1965). The early hopes that hypothermia would reduce operative mortality have not been realised (Hamby 1963; Drake 1966) and it has been suspected of causing cerebrovascular spasm (Drake 1968a, b). Its use, therefore, has gradually declined and most neurosurgical units have now abandoned it (McDowall 1971; Brophy 1974).

The most notable advance during this decade was the introduction of controlled ventilation. There is no doubt that by preventing respiratory depression and cerebral congestion, controlled ventilation has made it much easier for the anaesthetist to provide good operating conditions for the neurosurgeon (Furness 1957; Mortimer 1957).

From 1960 onwards, the use of hypotension had been declining, but it was revived again towards the end of the decade when it was realised that a low arterial blood pressure would decrease the tension in the aneurysmal sac and reduce the likelihood of its rupturing during surgical dissection and manipulation (Drake 1966).

During the last 15 years the experimental work done on the adverse effects of volatile inhalation agents on the intracranial pressure (Wollman et al. 1964; McDowall et al. 1966; Fitch and McDowall 1971) led many anaesthetists to replace them with the newly discovered neuroleptic drugs (Brophy 1974; Nilsson and Janssen 1961; Brown et al. 1963). Some continued to use the older methods without any apparent ill-effects and found halothane useful as a sensitiser to the action of hypotensive agents (Editorial, Br J Anaesth 1969; Gordon 1975; Johnstone 1969; Foster et al. 1969; Christensen et al. 1969; Adams et al. 1972; Taylor et al. 1970; Hart and Willats 1975). The introduction and popularity of sodium nitroprusside has given this effect of halothane some significance as it allows the dosage of nitroprusside to be reduced and so decreases the chances of an inadvertent and fatal overdosage (Siegel et al. 1971; Griffiths et al. 1974; Drake and Aitken 1974; Clark 1976; Greenbaum 1976).

Introduction

Every neurosurgical unit will tend to develop its own anaesthetic technique for operations on intracranial aneurysms. In describing our present methods, no claim is made that they are superior to those being used elsewhere. The safety of any technique depends less on the agents used than on the experience of the anaesthetist and the surgeon. The practical success of any method is more important than paying undue attention to any particular facet of the large amount of experimental work that has been done on intracranial pressure and the cerebral blood flow. Excessive attempts to avoid one possible theoretical risk may subject the patient to some other potential and more practical danger.

Pre-operative Management

All patients are seen and examined by the anaesthetist concerned. The usual routine pre-operative investigations are done, including an electrocardiogram, which is often abnormal in cases of subarachnoid haemorrhage (SAH) (Koskelo et al. 1964; Hoffbrand and Morgan 1965; Greenhoot and Reichenbach 1969; Brice et al. 1973; Neil-Dwyer et al. 1978).

Particular attention is paid to the respiratory system. Bronchospasm and obstructive airway disease can lead to high inflation pressures being required during controlled ventilation. High inflation pressures can increase the cerebral venous pressure and result in difficult operating conditions for the surgeon. Patients with audible wheezing sounds in the chest or a history of asthma are put on oral promethazine, 25 mg 8-hourly, for 24 h before operation.

Hypertension is common as a partial cause or as a result of SAH and some patients will be receiving an antihypertensive drug such as methyldopa. It is our policy to avoid giving these drugs within 8 h of the induction of anaesthesia. Whether they are resumed after the aneurysm has been dealt with will depend on the behaviour of the patient's blood pressure.

The patient's condition and the proposed operation are discussed with the surgeon before any craniotomy is undertaken.

Anaesthesia for Angiography

Angiography should not be treated lightly. It can lead to a hemiplegia or a deterioration in conscious level. Vertebral angiography may be accompanied by bradycardia, cardiac arrythmias and a fall in blood pressure and can produce a cortical blindness. Fortunately most of the neurological deficits that occur are temporary. Anaemia, dehydration or a fall in blood pressure may play a part in producing these complications.

Although it is possible to carry out angiography under local analgesia, with or without sedation, we prefer to use general anaesthesia for pre-operative investigations and have done since 1952 (Brophy 1974; Kay et al. 1970). The possibility of the patient moving during the injection is abolished and this makes for better definition on the films taken (Chap. 7).

It has been said that controlled ventilation with some degree of hyperventilation and a low arterial PCO_2 will give a better picture of a cerebral aneurysm than spontaneous ventilation with a normal or slightly raised arterial PCO_2 (Edmonds-Seal et al. 1967). The opposite has also been claimed (Cane 1973). We have followed the preference of the radiologist concerned over the years and at present controlled ventilation is the method of choice. The degree of cerebral vasoconstriction produced does not appear to interfere with the radiological diagnosis of local vascular spasm, and even respiratory movement can be temporarily abolished while the films are being taken if so desired. There has been no obvious difference between the two methods in the incidence of complications. As always, the experience and the ability of the anaesthetist and the radiologist concerned are probably more important than the technique that is chosen.

It is our custom to premedicate the patient with atropine. Induction is with a small dose of fentanyl, usually 50 mg, followed by methohexitone and suxamethonium. After intubation the patient is mechnically ventilated with a minute volume of 8–10 litres a minute and maintained on nitrous oxide and 0.1%–0.3% trichloroethylene. Pancuronium, 3–4 mg, is usually given to keep control of the ventilation and is reversed with neostigmine and atropine at the end of the procedure in the usual manner.

We prefer to avoid using halothane for angiography and to reserve it for craniotomy because of the possibility of jaundice occurring after repeated exposure to this agent (Inman and Mushin 1978). Using a little trichloroethylene instead of a larger dose of fentanyl reduces the possibility of any postoperative respiratory depression (Becker et al. 1976; Adams and Pybus 1978; McQuay et al. 1979; Stoeckel et al. 1979).

Both blood pressure and pulse rate must be monitored. Hypotension must be avoided and injections of contrast are not allowed if the systolic pressure is below 100 mm Hg. Very occasionally small doses of vasopressor have been required to raise the systolic pressure above this level, but these agents must be used cautiously as hypertension is also undesirable. Changes in pulse rate or a cardiac arrythmia can occur while the vertebral arteries are being catheterised and injected with dye.

Check angiography after craniotomy is usually done under local lignocaine infiltration, supplemented by intravenous diazepam and pentazocine sedation. The procedure is a short one and definition on the films is not as critical as in the pre-operative investigation. Doses of 4–10 mg diazepam and 30–60 mg pentazocine are usually quite sufficient. By balancing the two agents, any discomfort caused by the contrast injection can be made minimal, even if meglumine iothalamate is used. With iopamidol or iohexol there need be no discomfort other than that caused by the local injection of the lignocaine.

Anaesthesia for Craniotomy

Premedication is light. Pethidine, 25–50 mg, and atropine, 0.2–0.4 mg, are given intramuscularly, the dose depending on the build and general condition of the patient. If the conscious level is low, only atropine is given. Patients with chronic bronchitis, asthma or severe allergies of any kind also receive promethazine, 20–25 mg.

Anaesthesia is induced with a barbiturate, usually methohexitone, followed by suxamethonium for intubation. The patient is then immediately connected to a ventilator. Anaesthesia is maintained with nitrous oxide, oxygen and 0.1%–0.3% trichloroethylene; relaxation with either pancuronium or tubocurarine.

Two intravenous cannulae, gauge 14 or 16, are inserted, usually into the feet as they are a little more accessible than the arms during the course of a craniotomy.

A 20 gauge Teflon catheter is inserted percutaneously into a radial artery. This size is adequate and there is some evidence that larger sizes may increase the incidence of a subsequent thrombosis (Bedford 1977). A smaller gauge may be used in the case of a child, but SAH is rare before puberty. Occasionally, if cannulation of a radial artery is difficult, a brachial artery is used instead.

The patient is covered with two blankets under either a metal foil surfaced reflecting space blanket or a large polythene sheet. It is well known that patients can become hypothermic during a long operation, even if the ambient temperature is maintained at over 20°C (Morris and Wilkey 1970; Morris 1971). Working in a cool theatre, it was not uncommon in the past to record a lower oesophageal temperature of less than 35°C at the end of a craniotomy. Temperature falls can still occur, but they have been reduced considerably by using adequate covering. To eliminate them completely, a heating mattress would be required (Radford and Thurlow 1979). It is not the mild reduction of body temperature during operation that matters, but the shivering that it may cause later during recovery.

In the theatre the patient is tilted into an 8–10° head-up position, partly to produce a slight decrease in the intracranial cerebrospinal fluid and cerebral venous pressures and partly to facilitate the induction of hypotension later on in the operation.

Halothane, in concentrations of up to 0.5%, is added before the surgeon injects the skin flap with lignocaine and adrenaline, unless there has been a marked fall of blood pressure after the induction of anaesthesia. It is not given until the radial artery has been cannulated as this procedure is easier if the blood pressure is maintained at normal or near normal levels. Also it has been stated that halothane produces little increase in the intracranial pressure if it is not given until after 10–20 min of hyperventilation (McDowall et al. 1966; Adams et al. 1972).

The local injection of lignocaine and adrenaline, the skin incision and the turning of the osteoplastic flap all tend to cause an increase in the blood pressure. Our aim has been to prevent the systolic pressure, which has often fallen a little with induction, from rising above its original level. Apart from the obvious danger of an aneurysm rupturing if the blood pressure rises above normal levels, there is also the possibility that the upper level of autoregulation may be exceeded (Alexander and Lassen 1970; Shapiro et al. 1972; Strandgaard et al. 1973). β-Adrenergic blockade has been suggested as a method of prevention (Greenbaum 1976) and we have frequently used labetalol at this stage. Often a small dose of fentanyl is given as well, particularly if the patient has only had atropine as premedication or if the pulse rate is slow. The total dosage for the operation does not normally exceed 100 μg.

When a patient has multiple aneurysms, aggressive surgical treatment may result in two or more craniotomies over a period of time; in these cases halothane is never used twice. For any subsequent operations either enflurane or trichloroethylene supplemented by fentanyl is used instead.

When the dura mater has been opened, the blood pressure usually falls a little, but it may rise again when the surgeon starts to retract the brain.

The trichloroethylene is normally discontinued either soon after the incision or when the flap has been turned. The halothane is reduced when the aneurysm has been clipped and is discontinued during closure. The patient should be answering and obeying commands before leaving the theatre.

Monitoring

Three parameters are monitored electronically: the arterial blood pressure, the electrocardiogram and the expired carbon dioxide. These are displayed on a large screen oscilloscope and also on the tracing of a direct writer.

The arterial blood pressure recording is calibrated to measure the pressure at the level of the site of the aneurysm. When mechanical ventilation with a large tidal volume is being used, there is no single level of blood pressure as both systolic and diastolic pressures can vary by as much as 10 mmHg during the different phases of the respiratory cycle. Even the mean arterial pressure may vary by up to 5 mmHg.

The intra-arterial cannula is removed at the end of the operation. There is evidence that the incidence of complications is related to the length of time that a catheter remains in an artery (Bedford and Wollman 1973), and regular recording of the blood pressure at 15-min intervals using a cuff and auscultation of the Korotkoff sounds is considered to be adequate in the ward.

Controlled Ventilation

The patient is mechanically ventilated with a tidal volume of 800–1000 ml and a minute volume of 8–11 litres. This seems to produce the optimum operating conditions. No improvement will be achieved by a more vigorous hyperventilation, possibly because it can only be obtained by a considerable increase in the mean intrathoracic pressure (Shettini et al. 1967). We commonly use a negative phase of 5–8 cm H_2O as we feel that this may confer a marginal advantage (Ressel 1958), though it is usually omitted during deliberate hypotension.

Doubts have been raised as to the safety of using hyperventilation for neurosurgery (Clutton-Brock 1957; Sugioka and Davis 1960; Allen and Morris 1962; Geffin 1967; Wollman and Orkin 1968). Any lowering of intracranial pressure and vascularity that it produces will be due to a cerebrovascular constriction and a consequent decrease in the cerebral blood flow (Kety and Schmidt 1946; Rosamoff 1963; Ueyama and Loehning 1963; Wollman et al. 1965). It is said that it is safe as long as the arterial PCO_2 is not allowed to fall below a level of 20 mmHg (0.27 kPa) (Wollman and Orkin 1968; Wollman and Cohen 1971) and that at this level the reduction of the cerebral blood flow is 40%. It has also been claimed that if the PCO_2 does fall below this level, there will be a compensatory cerebral vasodilation, though this does not necessarily imply safety as it may be an anoxic reaction (Wasserman and Patterson 1961; Harper 1965; Kitahata et al. 1971; Harp and Wollman 1973; Lassen and Christensen 1976).

Another view is that maximal cerebral vasoconstriction occurs when the arterial PCO_2 is 30 mmHg (4 kPa) and that the cerebral arteries are no narrower at a PCO_2 of 25 mmHg (3.3 kPa) than they are at one of 35 mmHg (4.6 kPa) (du Boulay and Symon 1971; du Boulay et al. 1972).

Whatever the safe level may be, there is some experimental evidence to suggest that hyperventilation can confer a partial immunity against cerebral infarction when the blood supply to an area of brain tissue is compromised (Soloway et al. 1968). Perhaps the total cerebral blood flow is less important than the local flow through any vessels in spasm, and increasing the total flow could result in the cerebral steal phenomenon (Cohen 1968), though the increase caused by halothane (McDowall 1967) is said to apply as much to ischaemic areas of the brain as to those with an intact blood supply (Smith et al. 1973).

We normally try to keep the PCO_2 between 3 and 4 kPa. Cerebral vasoconstriction does not appear to be excessive. The vasoconstrictive effects of the hyperventilation may well be mitigated by the vasodilatory effect of the halothane, and vice versa (Wollman et al. 1964; McDowall 1967; Harp and Wollman 1973; du Boulay et al. 1972).

Because of the hyperventilation, the total dose of relaxant used does not normally exceed 6–8 mg pancuronium or 20–30 mg tubocurarine. Nevertheless, we always reverse it at the end with 2.5 mg neostigmine and either 1.2 mg atropine or 0.5 mg glycopyrrolate, even when the measure seems superfluous.

Intracranial Pressure

Dehydrating agents such as mannitol are not used routinely; nor is continuous spinal drainage. The surgeon is concerned more with brain volume, retractability and vascular congestion than with intracranial pressure. Many of these patients will have an internal hydrocephalus, and tapping and draining the ventricles will provide the surgeon with all the room that he requires. If there is increased intracranial pressure due to the presence of a haematoma, it will be relieved by the removal of the clot.

If the brain is pale, swollen and difficult to retract, this is an indication of cerebral anoxia. The ventricles will probably be small and the intracranial pressure normal or nearly normal. If the swelling is considerable, it is questionable whether the surgeon should proceed with the operation and even more questionable whether a hypotensive technique should be used. If the surgeon does continue, the oedema is likely to

worsen during the postoperative period. Fortunately this is a rare occurrence. It is unlikely to be connected with anaesthesia. Faults in the anaesthetic technique would tend to produce a vascular congestion rather than a pallid ischaemic oedema. Hyperventilation will not correct this type of brain swelling (Rosamoff 1963; Ueyama and Loehning 1963). Mannitol will have some effect, but will not remove the underlying cause.

One possible indication for using mannitol regularly is when temporary clipping of the artery feeding the aneurysm has been planned. It has been claimed that the prior administration of 500–1000 ml of 20% mannitol is as effective as hypothermia in prolonging the time for which the temporary clips can be applied and that it produces fewer complications. This effect is said to last up to 2 h, and it is advised that the mannitol should be given in two doses, one before the dura mater has been opened and one just before the application of the temporary clip (Watanabe et al. 1979; Suzuki and Yoshimoto 1979). It is difficult to see why mannitol should have this specific effect, though if it is injected rapidly it will produce a temporary increase in the cerebral blood flow (Wilkins et al. 1972) and a decrease in brain volume may offer some protection against retractor anaemia.

Controlled Hypotension

There are two main reasons for using controlled hypotension during surgery on intracranial aneurysms. The first is that it will decrease the tension in the aneurysmal sac, making it softer and less liable to rupture during surgical manipulation (Drake 1966, 1968a, b). The second is that if the sac should still rupture, the resulting haemorrhage will be less catastrophic and the achievement of haemostasis will be made both easier and safer. Additional advantages such as less oozing from small vessels and a reduction in the total operative blood loss are of less importance.

Hypotension is not undertaken lightly. One does not know the exact level of blood pressure at which cerebral autoregulation will begin to fail in any particular patient, unless one has the facilities for measuring cerebral blood flows during the course of the operation (Johnson and Harper 1973; Pickard et al. 1980; Nornes 1975). The cerebral function monitor (Patel 1981) is probably not sensitive enough to be a useful indicator of the point at which either focal or general cerebral blood flows become inadequate.

It is said that autoregulation will start to be impaired at about 65% of the normal mean arterial pressure when the hypotension is induced by haemorrhage and at about 40% of normal when it is induced by halothane, trimetaphan or sodium nitroprusside (Drake and Aitken 1974; Fitch et al. 1976). Other figures quoted have been at a mean pressure of 60 mmHg or two-thirds of the normal pressure (Strandgaard et al. 1973; Harp and Wollman 1973; Strunin 1975). Experiments on monkeys have suggested that the mean pressure has to be held at a level of one-third normal for 30 min in order to produce conditions leading to a reactive cerebral oedema (Gamache et al. 1976).

These figures only apply to normal animals or humans with an intact autoregulation system. The lower limit is raised in hypertensive individuals (Strandgaard et al. 1973). Patients with SAH may have a higher than normal level of blood pressure because of an increased output of catecholamines (Brice et al. 1973). It is not always possible to know whether their hypertension has been caused by the bleed.

In addition, SAH impairs autoregulation and this effect may still be present a week after the event (Boïsvert et al. 1979). The degree of impairment correlates with the neurological state of the patient, being greater in cases graded 3 on the Botterell scale than in cases graded 1–2 (Nornes et al. 1977). It has also been shown that the cerebral blood flow decreases progressively during the first week after a bleed and remains subnormal for at least a further fortnight (Meyer et al. 1982).

Lowering the blood pressure by using vasodilating hypotensive agents may produce an initial increase in the cerebral blood flow. As the blood pressure continues to fall, a point will be reached when the cerebral blood flow begins to decrease below the starting level. Pickard found when taking intra-operative cerebral blood flow measurements that 15 out of 20 patients showed an increased cerebral blood flow when the mean arterial pressure was reduced by an average of 39%, but that the other five showed a decrease. The latter group had a higher incidence of late postoperative neurological defects. Halothane was the main hypotensive agent used during these operations (Pickard et al. 1980).

Our aim in fit young adults is to reduce the systolic pressure at head level to between 60 and 75 mmHg, with a mean pressure of 50–60 mmHg while the surgeon is working in the vicinity of the aneurysm. Occasionally with giant or exceptionally difficult aneurysms, a slightly lower level may be desirable for a short period. With older patients, particularly those over 60 years of age, or patients having some other relevant concomitant disease, a higher level is chosen. In some cases hypotension may be contraindicated and the aim then is to prevent any inadvertent fall of the blood pressure during anaesthesia. Examples are patients being treated for severe cerebral vasospasm in which the risks of a rebleed are thought to outweigh the risks of operation and patients aged 70 years or more.

Hypotension is not induced until after the dura mater has been opened. If the brain looks pale, oedematous and anoxic, hypotension is either not attempted or only a mild drop in blood pressure is induced, even if the patient is otherwise healthy and has shown no clinical evidence of vasospasm or of raised intracranial pressure. The blood pressure is lowered slowly as this is said to reduce the risk of interfering with cerebral autoregulation (Harper 1965; Turner et al. 1977; Cope and Crawford 1979).

The usual agent employed is trimetaphan, given in a concentration of 1 mg/ml in an intravenous dextro-saline infusion. With hyperventilation and the administration of 0.5% halothane, many of the older patients require very little trimetaphan. Occasionally this concentration of halothane will produce more than the required effect on its own.

The pulse rate is controlled, if necessary, with a β-adrenergic blocker, usually labetalol, 2–40 mg in intermittent 1–2 mg doses. Provided the patient has not already got a bradycardia, there is much to be said for giving a β-adrenergic blocker before the trimetaphan and preventing any marked rise in the pulse rate rather than attempting to treat one that has already occurred. Labetalol tends to potentiate the hypotensive effect of halothane (Cope and Crawford 1979) and in some cases the addition of trimetaphan has been unnecessary, especially when only a mild degree of hypotension has been desired.

A few patients have been given pentolinium, particularly when the surgeon has requested two stages of hypotension. A mild first stage after the dura mater has been opened has been achieved with the pentolinium and a second, deeper stage while the aneurysm has been dissected out and clipped, with trimetaphan (Nornes 1975). The first stage can usually be produced equally well with labetalol, and we have not used pentolinium recently. If a patient's blood pressure is particularly resistant to ganglionic blockade, we are prepared to settle for a systolic pressure of 80–90 mmHg rather than push any single agent to its limit (Drake and Aitken 1974). If a lower pressure is, for a short while, deemed essential by the surgeon, switching off the negative phase of the ventilator and increasing the concentration of halothane should achieve the objective.

When the aneurysm has been clipped, or otherwise dealt with, the blood pressure is allowed to rise slowly to at least 100 mmHg systolic before the dura mater is closed. If it should start to rise excessively during closure of the flap, it is controlled with a further but reduced dosage of trimetaphan.

We have not felt any need for sodium nitroprusside. Experimental work has indicated that it may preserve cerebral autoregulation and blood flow better than trimetaphan does at low levels of arterial pressure (Griffiths et al. 1974, Ishikawa and McDowall 1979). This would be an advantage, but other work suggests the opposite (Brown et al. 1978) and also that when hypotension reaches a level at which autoregulation is lost, nitroprusside produces an increase in cerebral oxygen utilisation whereas trimetaphan does not (Grubb and Raichle 1982).

Although nitroprusside, unlike trimetaphan, causes an initial increase in intracranial pressure, this is probably of no clinical significance during operation (Miller et al. 1977). Its tendency to activate the release of renin is a disadvantage, but can be mitigated by giving propranolol (Ishikawa and McDowall 1979; Miller et al. 1977). It is also said to reduce the arterial PO_2 (Griffiths et al. 1974; Khambatta 1979; Wildsmith et al. 1975), but its main danger is that it is possible to give a fatal dose without the appearance of any warning signs, except possibly a systemic acidosis (Wildsmith et al. 1975; Macrae and Owen 1974; McDowall et al. 1974). This is particularly liable to occur if the drug is pushed in an attempt to overcome a resistant patient. In this situation the rate of administration should not be increased; either any attempt to lower the blood pressure further should be abandoned or an adjuvant, such as halothane, should be added (Annotation, Br Med J 1975; Ishikawa and McDowall 1979; Vesey et al. 1975).

It is said that nitroprusside is safe provided that the dose is limited to 1.5 mg/kg body weight, though the rate of administration may be as important as the total dose given (Greenbaum 1976; Simpson et al. 1979; Cole 1978; Wildsmith et al. 1979). It is certainly widely used for aneurysm surgery. Nevertheless, it does seem potentially more dangerous than trimetaphan and

halothane. Even its claimed advantage when extreme levels of hypotension are required is questionable.

Nitroglycerin has been recently introduced as a hypotensive agent for intracranial operations (Fahmy 1978; Chestnut et al. 1978). It is said to be controllable, non-toxic and free from any rebound phenomenon. Opinions vary as to whether it has any effect on intracranial pressure (Fahmy 1978; Cottrell et al. 1980).

Transfusion

Blood loss during intracranial operations is always difficult to estimate. Normal methods, such as weighing the swabs and drapes used, are not applicable as the wound is frequently flooded with saline solution. Also some blood always finds its way to the theatre floor. When there has been extensive haemorrhage, the use of a haemoglobinometer will give a rough indication of the amount of blood contained in the suction bottles. There is no doubt that most cases can be managed without a blood transfusion, provided the aneurysm does not rupture, but it is probable that all patients lose at least 500 ml of blood when the postoperative loss from under surgical flap is added to the operative loss.

When the aneurysm does rupture during surgery, rapid transfusion will be required. If there is any difficulty in obtaining an adequate rate of transfusion through the two intravenous cannulae, the indwelling radial catheter is available as an additional route. Blood can be injected rapidly through it by means of a two-way tap and a syringe. There is evidence that keeping the blood volume and its osmolality high will give some protection against the effects of postoperative vasospasm and oedema (Kosnik and Hunt 1976; Sundt et al. 1977; Fleischer and Tindall 1980). It can be argued that dextran or other plasma substitutes are the best way of doing this because they will lower the viscosity of the blood that has to pass through the narrowed vessels (Burke et al. 1979; Thomas et al. 1977). However, 15 years ago it was the practice here to give all aneurysm patients at least 500 ml of dextran 40 daily for the first 3 postoperative days, and this regime was abandoned because it appeared to have no effect on either mortality or morbidity.

A moderate dilution of the blood may increase capillary blood flow and effective oxygenation (Biro 1980), but dilution of the blood with saline will also increase its coagulability (Janvrin et al.

1980). The relative importance of the blood pressure and the osmolality and viscosity of the blood is still uncertain.

We therefore replace blood loss with blood, though plasma and plasma substitutes may also be used during an emergency and we tend to err on the side of generosity. Some patients do have a period of relative hypertension during the first 24 h after operation, but this does not appear to increase the incidence of reactionary haemorrhage and is less dangerous than a period of hypotension.

Techniques for Special Aneurysms

Carotid Ophthalmic Aneurysms

For some carotid ophthalmic aneurysms a trapping operation is used. The first stage consists in exposing the internal carotid artery in the neck. The second stage is the turning of an osteoplastic cranial flap and the forming of an anastamosis between a branch of the external carotid artery, usually the superficial temporal, and a cortical branch of the middle cerebral artery. In the third stage, the aneurysm is trapped by occluding the internal carotid artery in two places, in the neck and intracranially distal to the aneurysm.

The anaesthetic technique is therefore modified and the patient's blood pressure is maintained at normal or slightly above normal levels during the anastamosis and trapping. Trichloroethylene, with or without small doses of fentanyl, is the main anaesthetic agent. Halothane is either not used or is used sparingly, the concentration usually not exceeding 0.3%.

Cerebellar Aneurysms

Cerebellar aneurysms are operated on with the patient in the semi-sitting position. The legs are encased in elastic stockings while the patient is horizontal and the sitting up is done in stages to prevent any undue postural hypotension. Halothane is not given until the blood pressure has been stabilised with the patient in the operating position. If the blood pressure shows any sensitivity to this agent, trichloroethylene and small doses of fentanyl are used instead.

If any degree of hypotension is required later by the surgeon, it is induced carefully, but only if the patient has a healthy cardiovascular system and is not elderly. No attempt is made to lower the systolic pressure below 90–100 mmHg at atrial level, and the reduction is maintained only for as long as it is strictly necessary.

As with any operation done with the patient in the sitting or semi-sitting position, there is always the possibility of air embolism occurring. In addition to the usual monitoring of the blood pressure, electrocardiogram and end-tidal carbon dioxide, we also use an oesophageal stethoscope. As a further precaution, the neck veins are compressed frequently by the anaesthetist during the surgical approach.

Undoubtedly the Doppler device is a highly sensitive detector of small amounts of air in the heart (Edmonds-Seal and Maroon 1969; Chang et al. 1980), but it is not quantitative and we found it too sensitive for clinical use (Michenfelder et al. 1972). It was impossible to get any valid information from it when the diathermy was being used. More recent models may be less subject to electrical interference.

We do not catheterise the right atrium. This procedure will offer the advantage of enabling air to be aspirated once it has entered the heart (Michenfelder et al. 1966), but the efficiency of the aspiration will depend on the type of catheter used and the site of its tip. A catheter with a single terminal opening placed at the mid-atrial level may allow only 5% of the air in the atrium to be removed (Albin et al. 1981). The procedure is invasive and is not without its complications (Csànky-Treels 1978; Hunter and Sebel 1979; Jones 1979). Nor do we measure pulmonary artery pressures (Chang et al. 1980; Munson et al. 1976; Brechner and Bethune 1971). The insertion of a Swan-Ganz catheter is again an invasive procedure. It is relatively ineffective for the removal of air and can cause cardiac arrhythmia (Chang et al. 1980; Shaw 1979). Less common but more serious complications include perforation of the carotid and pulmonary arteries, pneumothorax and damage to the tricuspid valve (Lowenstein and Teplick 1980; Brown and Horton 1966).

Basilar Aneurysms

These are the most difficult and dangerous of all the cerebral aneurysms because of their proximity to the brain stem and the danger of compromising its blood supply, particularly if they should happen to rupture during operation. The risks of taking the blood pressure to lower levels than usual for a short period may therefore be considered justifiable (Drake 1968a, b).

In most cases the hypotensive method used has been our standard one. In a few cases the surgeon has requested a deeper level of hypotension. To achieve this we have used a pacemaker technique. Several have been described in the past (Brown and Horton 1966; Small et al. 1966; Rovitt 1971) and the one that we employ is a modification of Rovitt's. The basic difference is that a β-adrenergic blocker, usually labetalol, is given so that the required level of hypotension can be attained with only a moderate degree of tachycardia. This method is only used in patients under the age of 50 and with normal cardiovascular systems.

These patients are always examined by a cardiologist before operation. Before the incision, the cardiologist inserts the pacemaker into the left ventricle by means of a catheter passed up through the brachial or the femoral vein under radiological control. Labetalol is started after the incision, and when the surgeon is approaching the aneurysm the systolic pressure is lowered to between 60 and 70 mmHg with trimetaphan, further labetalol being given if there is any tendency for the pulse rate to rise. For the actual clipping a tachycardia is induced with the pacemaker and the systolic pressure is lowered to between 35 and 50 mmHg. This level of hypotension should be reached with a pulse rate of 108–120 a minute. Its duration should be kept as short as possible and should never exceed 5 min. The inspired oxygen is raised to at least 60% for this period.

The advantage of the pacemaker is that it gives a much more precise control of the blood pressure than any pharmacological control. Its danger is the possibility of myocardial damage or ventricular fibrillation. The latter is particularly likely to occur if the heart rate is allowed to rise above 160 a minute. Our aim is to achieve the desired degree of hypotension without allowing the heart rate to exceed 120 beats a minute.

Postoperative Management

All patients are given additional oxygen through a small nasopharyngeal catheter or a B.L.B. face mask for at least 4 h after the operation. This is to counteract any hypoxia produced by pulmonary shunting during the postanaesthetic period (Sulli-

van and Patterson 1968; Conway and Payne 1964; Conway and Payne 1963; Bay et al. 1968).

Nursing attention is on an intensive care basis for the first 3 days, or as long as may prove necessary. An intravenous fluid drip is usually kept going for this period. The blood electrolytes are checked daily. Either hypernatraemia or hyponatraemia can occur after surgery (Landolt et al. 1972; Collins 1976; Takaku et al. 1979). A low blood pressure is more dangerous than a high one. Some recent experiments on cats have suggested that SAH protects the blood–brain barrier against damage caused by hypertension (Peterson and Cardoso 1983). Only very occasionally will some postoperative antihypertensive therapy be necessary in patients who were known hypertensives and on antihypertensive therapy before their SAH. Care is needed to prevent an overswing with treatment and a reduced dosage will usually produce an adequate result.

If cerebral vasospasm occurs, it is usually treated by intravenous drip infusion of isoprenaline and lignocaine (Sundt 1975). The blood volume may also be increased by giving blood, plasma or plasma substitutes. It has recently been suggested that the circulating red cell volume may be more important than the circulating fluid volume, though in the cases quoted the haemoglobin was on the low side of normal (Kudo et al. 1981). It has also been claimed that naloxone will reverse the clinical effects of cerebral ischaemia provided that infarction has not already occurred (Baskin and Hosobuchi 1981), but we have not had sufficient experience with this agent to judge whether it has any effect. Cerebral oedema is treated with dexamethasone. If it is severe, mannitol is also given.

Arteriovenous Malformations

Arteriovenous malformations differ from aneurysms in that haemorrhage from them during operation has a venous element, though the veins concerned are arterialised as well as being dilated. The haemorrhage does tend to be less immediately catastrophic than that produced by a ruptured aneurysm, but with the larger AVMs it can be both severe and prolonged because of the size and the number of abnormal vessels involved.

Our basic anaesthetic technique is similar to that adopted for aneurysms, but only a moderate degree of hypotension, with a systolic pressure of

80–90 mmHg, is used. This is because of the greater length of time for which it may be required.

References

Adams AP, Pybus DA (1978) Delayed depression after use of fentanyl during anaesthesia. Br Med J I:278–279.

Adams RW, Gronert GA, Sundt TM, Michenfelder JD (1972) Halothane, hypocapnia and cerebrospinal fluid pressure in neurosurgery. Anesthesiology 37:510–517.

Albin MS, Bunegin L, Babinski M, Smith RB (1981) Venous air embolism—where should the catheter be placed for maximal aspiration. Br J Anaesth 53:315

Alexander SC, Lassen NA (1970) Cerebral circulatory response to acute brain disease: implications for anaesthetic practice. Anesthesiology 32:60–68

Allen GD, Morris LE (1962) Central nervous system effects of hyperventilation during anaesthesia. Br J Anaesth 34:296–305

Anderson S, McKissock W (1953) Controlled hypotension with Arfonad in neurosurgery. Lancet II:754–757

Annotation (1975) Sodium nitroprusside in anaesthesia. Br Med J I:524–525

Aserman D (1953) Controlled hypotension in neurosurgery with hexamethonium and procaine amide. Br Med J I:961–964

Ayre P (1937) Anaesthesia for intracranial operation. Lancet I:561–562

Baskin DS, Hosobuchi Y (1981) Naloxone reversal of ischaemic neurological effects in man. Lancet II:272–276

Bay J, Nunn JF, Prys-Roberts C (1968) Factors influencing arterial PO_2 during recovery from anaesthesia. Br J Anaesth 40:398–407

Becker LD, Paulson BA, Miller RD, Severinghaus JW (1976) Biphasic respiratory depression after fentanyl-droperidol or fentanyl alone used to supplement nitrous oxide anaesthesia. Anesthesiology 44:291–296

Bedford RF (1977) Radial arterial function following percutaneous cannulation with 18 and 20 gauge catheters. Anesthesiology 47:37–39

Bedford RF, Wollman H (1973) Complications of percutaneous radial-artery cannulation: an objective prospective study in man. Anesthesiology 38:228–236

Bilsland WL (1951) Controlled hypotension by arteriotomy in intracranial surgery. Anesthesia 6:20–25

Biro GP (1980) Anaemia and haemodilution. In: Pryce-Roberts C (ed) The circulation in anaesthesia. Blackwell, Oxford, pp 327–350

Boisvert DPJ, Pickard JD, Graham DI, Fitch W (1979) Delayed effects of subarachnoid haemorrhage on cerebral metabolism and cerebrovascular response to hypocapnia in the primate. J Neurol Neurosurg Psychiatry 42:892–898

Brechner VL, Bethune RWM (1971) Recent advances in monitoring pulmonary air embolism. Curr Res Anesth Analg 50:255–261

Brice J, Dwyer G, Cruikshank G, Stott B (1973) Metabolic response to subarachnoid bleeding. J Neurol Neurosurg Psychiatry 36:885

Brophy T (1974) Anaesthesia for intracranial vascular surgery. Aust NZ J Surg 44:232–240

Brown AS, Horton JM (1966) Elective hypotension with intracardiac pacemaking in the operative management of

intracranial aneurysms. Acta Anaesthesiol Scand 23:665–669

Brown AS, Horton JM, Macrae WR (1963) Anaesthesia for neurosurgery. Anaesthesia 18:143–150

Brown FD, Crockard HA, Johns LM, Mullan S (1978) The effects of sodium nitroprusside and trimetaphan camsylate on cerebral blood flow in rhesus monkeys. Neurosurgery 2:31–34

Burke AM, Chien S, McMurty JG, Quest DO (1979) Effects of low molecular weight dextran on blood viscosity after craniotomy for intracranial aneurysms. Surg Gynecol Obstet 148:9–15

Burrows M, Dundee JW, Francis IL, Lipton S, Sedzimir CB (1956) Hypothermia for neurosurgical operations. Anaesthesia 11:4–18

Campkin TV (1965) Moderate hypothermia and circulatory arrest for neurosurgical operations. Br J Anaesth 37:528–532

Cane RD (1973) Cerebral angiography: two anaesthetic techniques. South Afr Med J 47:777–780

Chang JL, Albin MS, Bunegin L, Hung T (1980) Analysis and comparison of venous air embolism detection methods. Neurosurgery 7:135–141

Chestnut JS, Albin MS, Gonzales-Abola E, Newfield P, Maroon JC (1978) Clinical evaluation of intravenous nitroglycerin for neurosurgery. J Neurosurg 48:704–711

Christensen MS, Ellis DB, Freeman J, Michenfelder JD (1969) Halothane and neurosurgery. Br J Anaesth 41:906

Clark K (1976) Complications of aneurysm surgery. Clin Neurosurg 23:342–356

Clutton-Brock J (1957) The cerebral effects of overventilation. Br J Anaesth 29:111–113

Cohen PJ (1968) Things are seldom what they seem. Anesthesiology 29:865–866

Cole P (1978) The safe use of sodium nitroprusside. Anaesthesia 33:473–477

Collins WF (1976) Hyponatremia following neurosurgery. Clin Neurosurg 23:418–423

Conway CM, Payne JP (1963) Post-operative hypoxaemia and oxygen therapy. Br Med J I:844–845

Conway CM, Payne JP (1964) Hypoxaemia associated with anaesthesia and controlled respiration. Lancet I:12–14

Cope DHP, Crawford MC (1979) Labetalol in controlled hypotension. Br J Anaesth 51:359–365

Cottrell JE, Gupta B, Rappaport H, Turndorf H, Ransohoff J, Flamm ES (1980) Intracranial pressure during nitroglycerin-induced hypotension. J Neurosurg 53:309–311

Csànky-Treels JC (1978) Hazards of central venous pressure monitoring. Anaesthesia 33:172–177

Drake CG (1966) On the surgical treatment of ruptured intracranial aneurysms. Clin Neurosurg 13:122–155

Drake CG (1968a) Further experience with surgical treatment of aneurysms of the basilar artery. J Neurosurg 29:372–379

Drake CH (1968b) The surgical treatment of vertebral-basilar aneurysms. Clin Neurosurg 16:114–169

Drake CG, Aitken RR (1974) Technique of anaesthesia with induced hypotension for surgical correction of intracranial aneurysms. Clin Neurosurg 21:107–114

Drake CG, Barr HWK, Coles JC, Gergely NF (1964) The use of extracorporeal circulation and profound hypothermia in the treatment of ruptured intracranial aneurysms. J Neurosurg 21:575–581

du Boulay G, Symon L (1971) The anaesthetist's effects on the cerebral arteries. Proc R Soc Med 64:77–81

du Boulay G, Symon L, Shah S, Dorsch N, Ackerman R (1972) Cerebral arterial reactivity and spasm after subarachnoid haemorrhage. Proc R Soc Med 65:80–82

Editorial (1969) Halothane and neurosurgery. Br J Anaesth

41:277–278

Edmonds-Seal H, Maroon JC (1969) Air embolism diagnosed with ultrasound. Anaesthesia 24:438–440

Edmonds-Seal J, du Boulay G, Bostick T (1967) The effect of intermittent positive pressure ventilation on cerebral angiography with special reference to the quality of the films. Br J Radiol 40:957–958

Fahmy NR (1978) Nitroglycerin as a hypotensive drug during general anesthesia. Anesthesiology 49:17–20

Fitch W, McDowall DG (1971) Effect of halothane on intracranial pressure gradients in the presence of intracranial space-occupying lesions. Br J Anaesth 43:904–912

Fitch W, Ferguson GG, Sengupta D, Garibi J, Harper AM (1976) Autoregulation of cerebral blood flow during controlled hypotension in baboons. J Neurol Neurosurg Psychiatry 39:1014–1022

Fleischer AS, Tindall GT (1980) Cerebral vasospasm following aneurysm rupture: a protocol for therapy and prophylaxis. J Neurosurg 52:149–152

Foster B, Jones WK, Keen RI (1969) Halothane and neurosurgery. Br J Anaesth 41:561

Furness DN (1957) Controlled respiration in neurosurgery. Br J Anaesth 29:415–418

Gamache FW, Myers RE, Monell E (1976) Changes in local cerebral blood flow during profound systemic hypotension. J Neurosurg 44:215–225

Gardner WJ (1946) The control of bleeding during operation by induced hypotension JAMA 132:572–574

Geffin B (1967) Spinal fluid and hyperventilation during anesthesia in man. Anesthesiology 28:251–252

Gordon E (1975) Anaesthesia for neurosurgery. In: Gordon E (ed) A basis and practice of neuro-anaesthesia. Excerpta Medica, Amsterdam Oxford New York, pp 175–182 (Monographs in anaesthesiology)

Greenbaum R (1976) General anaesthesia for neurosurgery. Br J Anaesth 48:773–781

Greenhoot JH, Reichenbach DD (1969) Cardiac injury and subarachnoid haemorrhage. J Neurosurg 30:521–531

Griffiths DPG, Cummins BH, Greenbaum R, Griffith HB, Staddon G, Wilkins DG, Zorab JSM (1974) Cerebral blood flow and metabolism during hypotension induced with sodium nitroprusside. Br J Anaesth 46:671–679

Grubb RL, Raichle ME (1982) Effects of hemorrhagic and pharmacologic hypotension on cerebral oxygen utilization and cerebral blood flow. Anesthesiology 56:3–8

Hale DE (1948) Controlled hypotension by arterial bleeding during operation and anesthesia. Anesthesiology 9:498–505

Hamby WB (1963) Intracranial surgery for aneurysms. The effects of hypothermia on survival. J Neurosurg 20:41–45

Harp TR, Wollman H (1973) Cerebral metabolic effects of hyperventilation and deliberate hypotension. Br J Anaesth 45:256–262

Harper AM (1965) Physiology of cerebral blood flow. Br J Anaesth 37:225–235

Hart W, Willats S (1975) An anaesthetic technique for intracranial aneurysms. Anaesthesia 30:233–234

Hewer CL (1941) Trichloroethylene as an inhalation anaesthetic. Br Med J I:924–927

Hewer CL (1948) Recent advances in anaesthesia and analgesia, 6th edn. Churchill, London, pp 246–247

Hoffbrand BI, Morgan BDG (1965) Functional significance of electrocardiographic changes associated with subarachnoid haemorrhage. Lancet I:844–845

Hunter D, Sebel PS (1979) Detection of venous air embolism. Anaesthesia 34:578–582

Inman WHW, Mushin WW (1978) Jaundice after repeated halothane: a further analysis of reports to the Committee on Safety of Medicines. Br Med J II:1455–1456

Ishikawa T, McDowall DG (1979) Differences in cerebral blood flow and cortical electrical activity during hypotension induced by trimetaphan and nitroprusside in the cat. Br J Anaesth 51:566

Janvrin SB, Davies G, Greenhalgh RM (1980) Post-operative deep vein thrombosis caused by intravenous fluids during surgery. Br J Surg 67:690–693

Johnson IH, Harper AM (1973) The effect of mannitol on cerebral blood flow. An experimental study. J Neurosurg 38:461–471

Johnstone M (1956) The human cardiovascular response to Fluothane anaesthesia. Br J Anaesth 28:392–410

Johnstone M (1969) Halothane and neurosurgery Br J Anaesthesia 41:561

Jones DF (1979) Central venous catheterisation. Hosp Update 5:484–496

Kay B, Keaney JPD, Taylor GJ (1970) Neuroleptanalgesia: a double-blind comparison of pentazocine and phenoperidine for neuroradiological investigations. Br J Anaesth 42:329–334

Kety SS, Schmidt CF (1946) The effects of active and passive ventilation on cerebral blood flow and on cerebral oxygen consumption, cardiac output and blood pressure of normal young men. J Clin Invest 25:107–119

Khambatta RJ, Stone JG, Khan E (1979) Propranolol abates nitroprusside-induced renin release. Anaesthesiology Abstr Suppl 51:S74

Kitahata LM, Galicich JF, Sato I (1971) The effect of passive hyperventilation on intraventricular pressure in the dog. J Neurosurg 34:185–193

Koskelo P, Punsar S, Sipila W (1964) Subendocardial haemorrhages and ECT changes in intracranial bleeding. Br Med J I:1479–1480

Kosnik EJ, Hunt WE (1976) Post-operative hypertension in the management of patients with intracranial arterial aneurysms. J Neurosurg 45:148–154

Kudo T, Suzuki S, Iwabuchi T (1981) Importance of monitoring the circulating blood volume in patients with cerebral vasospasm after subarachnoid haemorrhage. Neurosurgery 9:515–520

Landolt AM, Yasargil MG, Krayenbühl H (1972) Disturbance of the serum electrolytes after surgery of intracranial aneurysms. J Neurosurg 37:210–218

Lassen NA, Christensen MS (1976) Physiology of cerebral blood flow. Br J Anaesth 48:719–734

Lowenstein E, Teplick R (1980) To (PA) catheterise or not to (PA) catheterise. Anesthesiology 53:361–363 (editorial)

Macrae WR, Owen M (1974) Severe metabolic acidosis following hypotension induced with sodium nitroprusside. Br J Anaesth 46:795–797

McDowall DG (1967) The effects of clinical concentrations of halothane on the blood flow and oxygen uptake of the cerebral cortex. Br J Anaesth 39:186–196

McDowall DG (1971) The current usage of hypothermia in British neurosurgery. Br J Anaesth 43:1084–1087

McDowall DG, Barker J, Jennett WB (1966) Cerebrospinal fluid pressure measurements during anaesthesia. Anaesthesia 21:98–99

McDowall DG, Keaney NP, Turner JM, Lane JR, Okuda Y (1974) The toxicity of sodium nitroprusside. Br J Anaesth 46:327–332

McQuay HJ, Moore RA, Paterson GMC, Adams AP (1979) Plasma fentanyl concentrations and clinical observations during and after operation. Br J Anaesth 51:543–550

Meyer CHA, Lowe W, Meyer M, Richardson PL, Neil-Dwyer G (1982) Subarachnoid haemorrhage: older patients have low cerebral blood flow. Br Med J 285:1149–1153

Michenfelder JD, MacCarty CS, Theye RA (1964) Physiologic studies following closed-chest technique of profound hypothermia. Anesthesiology 25:131–136

Michenfelder JD, Terry HR, Daw EF, Miller RH (1966) Air embolism during neurosurgery: a new method of treatment. Curr Res Anesth Analg 45:390–391

Michenfelder JD, Miller RH, Gronert GA (1972) Evaluation of an ultrasonic device (Doppler) for the diagnosis of venous air embolism. Anesthesiology 36:164–167

Miller ED, Ackerly JA, Vaughan ED, Peach MJ, Epstein RM (1977) The renin-angiotensin system, during controlled hypotension with sodium nitroprusside. Anesthesiology 47:257–262

Morris RH (1971) Operating room temperature and the anaesthetised paralysed patient. Arch Surg 102:95–97

Morris RH, Wilkey BR (1970) The effects of ambient temperature during surgery not involving body cavities. Anesthesiology 32:102–107

Mortimer PLF (1957) Controlled respiration in neurosurgery. Br J Anaesth 29:528–530

Munson ES, Paul WC, Perry JC, De Padua CB, Rhoton AL (1976) Early detection of venous air embolism using a Swan-Ganz catheter. Anesthesiology 42:223–226

Neil-Dwyer G, Walter P, Cruickshank JM, Doshi B, O'Gorman P (1978) Effect of propranolol and phentolamine on myocardial necrosis after subarachnoid haemorrhage. Br Med J II:990–992

Nilsson E, Janssen P (1961) Neurolept-analgesia, an alternative to general anaesthesia. Acta Anaesth Scand 5:73–84

Nornes H (1975) Monitoring of patients with intracranial aneurysms. Clin Neurosurg 22:321–331

Nornes H, Knutzen HB, Wikeby P (1977) Cerebral arterial blood flow and aneurysm surgery. J Neurosurg 47:819–827

Patel H (1981) Experience with cerebral function monitor during deliberate hypotension. Br J Anaesth 53:639–645

Peterson EW, Cardoso ER (1983) The blood–brain barrier following experimental subarachnoid haemorrhage. J Neurosurg 58:338–344

Pickard JD, Matheson M, Patterson J, Wyper D (1980) Prediction of late ischaemic complications after cerebral aneurysm surgery by the intraoperative measurement of cerebral blood flow. J Neurosurg 53:305–309

Radford P, Thurlow AC (1979) Metallised plastic sheeting in the prevention of hypothermia during neurosurgery. Br J Anaesth 51:237–239

Ressel G (1958) Beatmung and intrakranieller Druck. Anaesthetist 7:33

Rosamoff HL (1963) Distribution of intracranial contents with controlled ventilation: Implications for neuroanaesthesia. Anesthesiology 24:640–645

Rovitt RL (1971) Operative hypotension for intracranial vascular surgery using pacemaker-induced tachycardia. J Neurosurg 31:51–58

Shapiro H, Wyle SR, Harris AB, Galindo A (1972) Acute interoperative hypertension in neurosurgical patients. Mechanical and pharmacological factors. Anesthesiology 37:399–405

Shaw TJI (1979) The Swan-Ganz pulmonary artery catheter. The incidence of complications with particular reference to ventricular dysrhythmias and their prevention. Anaesthesia 34:651–656

Shettini A, Cook AW, Owre ES (1967) Hyperventilation in craniotomy for brain tumour. Anesthesiology 28:363–371

Siegel P, Moraca PP, Green JR (1971) Sodium nitroprusside in the surgical treatment of cerebral aneurysms and arteriovenous malformations. Br J Anaesth 43:790–795

Simpson PJ, Adams L, Vesey CJ, Cole P (1979) Some physiological and metabolic effects of sodium nitroprusside and cyanide in the dog. Br J Anaesth 51:81–87

Small JM, Stephenson SCF, Campkin TV, Davison PH, McIlveen DJS (1966) Elective circulatory arrest by artificial pacemaker. Lancet I:570–572

Smith A, Larson CP, Hoff JT (1973) Effects of halothane on regional cerebral blood flow in experimental focal ischaemia. Anesthesiology 39:377–381

Soloway M, Nadel W, Albin MS, White RJ (1968) The effect of hyperventilation on subsequent cerebral infarction. Anesthesiology 29:975–980

Stoeckel H, Hengstmann JH, Schüttler J (1979) Pharmacokinetics of fentanyl as a possible explanation for the recurrence of respiratory depression. Br J Anaesth 51:741–745

Strandgaard S, Oleson J, Skinhøj E, Lassen NA (1973) Autoregulation of brain circulation in severe arterial hypertension. Br Med J I:507–510

Strunin L (1975) Organ perfusion during controlled hypotension. Br J Anaesth 47:793–798

Sugioka K, Davis DA (1960) Hyperventilation with oxygen— a possible cause of cerebral hypoxia. Anesthesiology 21:135–143

Sullivan SF, Patterson RW (1968) Post-ventilation hypoxia: theoretical considerations in man. Anesthesiology 29:981–986

Sundt TM (1975) Management of ischemic complications after subarachnoid haemorrhage. J Neurosurg 43:418–425

Sundt TM, Szurzewski J, Sharbrough FW (1977) Physiological considerations important for the management of vasospasm. Surg Neurol 7:259–267

Suzuki J, Yoshimoto T (1979) The effect of mannitol in prolongation of permissible occulsion time of cerebral arteries. In: Suzuki J (ed) Cerebral aneurysms. Neuron, Tokyo, pp 330–337

Takaku A, Shindo K, Tanaka S, Mori T, Suzuki J (1979) Fluid and electrolyte disturbances in patients with intracranial aneurysms. Surg Neurol 11:349–356

Taylor TT, Styles M, Lamming AJ (1970) Sodium nitroprusside as a hypotensive agent in general anaesthesia. Br J Anaesth 42:859–864

Thomas DJ, Marshall J, Russell RWR, Wetherby-mein G, du Boulay GH, Pearson TC, Symon L, Zilkha E (1977) Effect of haematocrit on cerebral blood flow in man. Lancet II:941–945

Turner JM, Powell D, Gibson RM, McDowall DG (1977) Intracranial pressure changes in neurosurgical patients during hypotension induced with sodium nitroprusside or trimetaphan. Br J Anaesth 49:419–425

Ueyama H, Loehning RW (1963) Effect of hyperventilation on cerebrospinal fluid pressure and brain volume. Curr Res Anesth Analg 42:581–587

Uihlein A, Terry HR, Payne WS, Kirklin JW (1962) Operations on intracranial aneurysms with induced hypothermia below 15° and total circulatory arrest. J Neurosurg 19:237–239

Vandewater SL, Botterell H, Lougheed WM (1955) A method of anaesthesia and hypothermia in cerebral vascular surgery. Can Anaesth Soc J 2:319–326

Vesey CJ, Cole P, Simpson P (1975) Sodium nitroprusside in anaesthesia. Br Med J II:229

Wasserman AJ, Patterson JL (1961) The cerebral vascular response to reduction in arterial carbon dioxide tension. J Clin Invest 40:1297–1303

Watanabe T, Yoshimoto T, Suzuki J (1979) The effect of mannitol in preventing the development of cerebral infarction. In: Suzuki J (ed) Cerebral aneurysms. Neuron, Tokyo, pp 359–365

Wildsmith FAW, Drummond GB, Macrae WR (1975) Blood-gas changes during induced hypotension with sodium nitroprusside. Br J Anaesth 47:1205–1211

Wildsmith FAW, Drummond GB, Macrae WB (1979) Metabolic effects of induced hypotension with trimetaphan and sodium nitroprusside. Br J Anaesth 51:875–879

Wilkins DG, Griffith HB, Cummins BH, Greenbaum R, Zorab JSM (1972) Repeated measurements of cerebral blood-flow during intracranial surgery. Lancet II:402–403

Wollman H, Cohen PJ (1971) Hyperventilation and cerebral oxygenation. In: Gray TC, Nunn JF (eds) General anaesthesia, 3rd edn, vol 1. Butterworth, London, pp 291–298

Wollman SB, Orkin LR (1968) Post-operative human reaction time and hypocarbia during anaesthesia. Br J Anaesth 40:920–926

Wollman H, Alexander SC, Cohen PJ, Chase PE, Melman E, Behar MG (1964) Cerebral circulation of man during halothane anaesthesia. Anesthesiology 25:180–184

Wollman H, Alexander SC, Cohen PH, Smith TC, Chase PE, Van de Molen RA (1965) Cerebral circulation during general anesthesia and hyperventilation in man. Anesthesiology 26:329–334

10 Basic Principles of Surgical Treatment of Intracranial Aneurysms

The role of surgery for intracranial aneurysms is usually preventive. From the natural history of ruptured aneurysms, it is well recognised that life or neurological function may be further threatened by a recurrent haemorrhage from the aneurysm. The risk of rebleeding is most frequent in the first 2 weeks after the initial bleed, but remains for the rest of the patient's life to a variable degree. Surgical obliteration of the aneurysm after the first haemorrhage is the best way to prevent a recurrent bleed. However, the surgical treatment of an intracranial aneurysm is a formidable measure, with a potential risk of mortality and morbidity. When the brain has already been injured by the SAH, the risk of complication from surgical intervention is proportionately high. The role of aneurysm surgery must, therefore, be considered in terms of its effectiveness, its complications and the natural history of the aneurysm.

Selection of Patients

Selection of patients for surgical treatment is the most important decision for the neurosurgeon. All of the factors discussed below should be taken into account, as each of them may influence the outcome. They also influence the timing of surgical treatment, which will be discussed later.

Severity of Subarachnoid Haemorrhage

Clinical evaluation of the condition of the patient may show a variable degree of consciousness, meningeal signs and neurological deficit. These are usually expressed in various grades (see Chap. 4). In a patient who is dying from the effect of SAH itself, there is no indication for surgical obliteration of the aneurysm. In patients with an adverse clinical condition due to a haematoma or hydrocephalus, surgical treatment should be confined to treating these complications only. In practice, therefore, patients in grades 4 and 5 are excluded from aneurysm surgery, unless they improve to a higher grade. It should also be recognised that the clinical condition of the patient may fluctuate. For example, a patient admitted in grade 1 or 2 may deteriorate to grade 3 or worse. The opposite can also happen. A patient who is showing progressive deterioration, however slowly, should not be subjected to surgery until the neurological condition is stable or improving. In essence, manipulation of the brain or its blood supply in a patient severely affected by SAH will only add insult to injury, and surgery will not help him. Our views about the timing and extent of angiography have been discussed in Chap. 7.

Age of the Patient

Ruptured intracranial aneurysms usually occur between the ages of 40 and 60. With increasing longevity and improved geriatric care, patients in the seventh or eight decade may be referred for neurosurgical evaluation. There is no doubt that with advancing age the cardiovascular and respiratory reserves diminish and a formidable surgical undertaking and prolonged anaesthesia impose greater risks. The benefit of surgery in such patients should be balanced against not only the natural history of the aneurysm but also the increased probability of death from an unrelated illness.

After careful analysis of the outcome, Martindale and Garfield (1978) questioned the value of any further investigation for patients above the age of 59. On the other hand, successful treatment with a good quality of life in older patients has been reported (Sengupta et al. 1978). It is well known that the chronological age of the patient does not always reflect his physiological status. Each patient should, therefore, be evaluated individually when considering surgical treatment. In practice, however, we have found that, up to the age of 65, the outcome of surgery is no different to that in a younger age group, and the result drops appreciably after 65 years of age (Sengupta et al. 1978). The selection of patients above this age limit should thus be strict.

Hypertension

Patients with chronic hypertension show morphological changes in the blood vessels. Manipulation of cerebral circulation by direct surgical treatment or by other alternative methods carries an unfavourable risk. These patients tolerate hypotensive anaesthesia badly, because of poor cerebral autoregulation. On the other hand, the risk of recurrent bleeding is significantly higher in hypertensive patients, and the need to treat their ruptured aneurysms is therefore all the greater. With careful pre-operative management and advanced anaesthetic techniques, the result of surgery is still considerably better than the natural history.

Associated Major Illness

In patients with associated chronic respiratory or myocardial disease, consideration of surgery is greatly influenced by the risk of anaesthesia. In patients with ischaemic heart disease, manipulation of blood pressure during surgery or an unintentional drop during anaesthesia is dangerous. In these patients, the expertise of the anaesthetist and the facilities available should be taken into account in the assessment. Recently, we have operated upon a patient under local anaesthesia for clipping of a posterior communicating aneurysm, through a frontotemporal craniotomy. He was an alcoholic and crippled with chronic respiratory disease. General anaesthesia was contraindicated. The whole operation, taking 2 h, was undertaken with intravenous sedation and injection of local anaesthetic for craniotomy. The condition of the brain was ideal, and clipping of the aneurysm was performed without difficulty. During his hospital stay it was possible to withdraw his alcohol addiction. This case reminded us of those great surgeons of the past who carried out major intracranial surgery under local anaesthesia, before general anaesthesia became safe for neurosurgery.

Location, Size and Shape of the Aneurysm

The location of an aneurysm has a considerable bearing on the technical aspects of surgery. Aneurysms on the anterior carotid circulation can be more easily obliterated than those on the vertebrobasilar system. Low basilar bifurcation aneurysms and those at the vertebrobasilar junction are notorious for their difficult access and poor surgical outcome. On the basis of the location of the aneurysm alone, surgical treatment may be considered unsafe if the previously mentioned adverse factors are present. The size and shape of the aneurysm are not contraindications to surgical treatment, although they may determine the suitability of a particular method.

Multiple Aneurysms

At least one in five patients with ruptured aneurysm will have more than one aneurysm, and the surgical outcome in such patients is worse than in those with single aneurysm (Paterson and Bond 1973). Poor outcome is often due to failure of identification and treatment of the symptomatic lesion, or the over-enthusiastic application of surgical treatment to all of the aneurysms. With advances in neuroradiology (see Chap. 7) and clinical methods (Sengupta and Lassman 1974), it has become possible to determine the offending

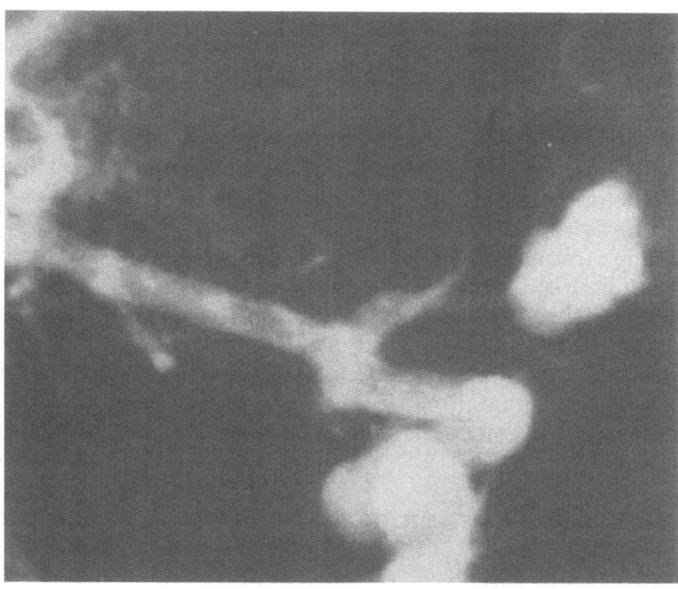

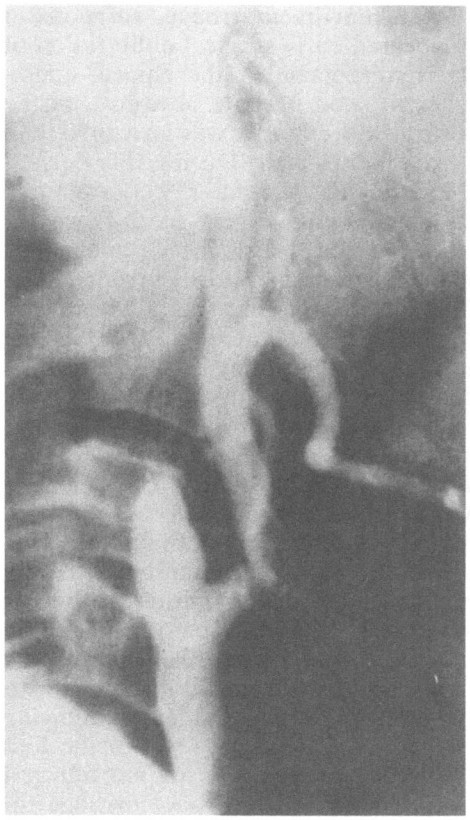

Fig. 10.1a, b. Bilateral carotid angiograms of a 50-year-old man who presented with subarachnoid haemorrhage in 1980. **a** Right carotid angiogram showing the ligated internal carotid artery, which was carried out for ruptured posterior communicating artery aneurysm in 1956. No other aneurysm was demonstrated at that time. **b** Left carotid angiogram showing a large anterior communicating artery aneurysm and an unruptured posterior communicating artery aneurysm.

lesion accurately, and to obliterate it by direct surgery. If there is any doubt as to the source of the SAH, it is unwise to treat an operable aneurysm only, as the risk of recurrent bleeding from the offending unobliterated aneurysm is increased considerably during the postoperative period. It should be recognised that proximal occlusion of the parent artery, as opposed to direct obliteration, which will be discussed later, may lead to formation, growth and rupture of asymptomatic aneurysms due to a change in the haemodynamics of cerebral circulation (Fig. 10.1).

Whether surgery is indicated for unruptured aneurysms is debatable, since their natural history is poorly understood. Some authors (Bailey and Loeser 1971; Paterson and Bond 1973) suggest that surgical treatment is not indicated. However, Mount and Brisman (1974) believe that all intracranial aneurysms should be treated to prevent possible rupture in the future. The risk of rupture

of an intact aneurysm is 1% per year (Winn et al. 1983). In our view, clipping of an unruptured aneurysm, even in the same territory as the offending lesion, adds an unnecessary hazard in a patient with recent SAH. Our practice is to treat such aneurysms later, when the risk is minimal.

Association of Aneurysm and Arteriovenous Malformation

On rare occasions, an aneurysm may be associated with an arteriovenous malformation, either in the same or a remote vascular territory. In such a situation, identification of the bleeding source may be difficult. In six of our patients with a coexistent arteriovenous malformation and aneurysm, the CT scan and/or operative findings indicated that an aneurysm was responsible for the haemorrhage in three cases (see Chaps. 5, 7).

Anomaly of the Circle of Willis

Anomalies of the circle of Willis are more common with intracranial aneurysms (see Chap. 2). These anomalies alter the area of supply of the major cerebral arteries and the collateral circulation is compromised. As the surgical result is significantly affected in patients with vascular anomalies (Sengupta 1975), they should be carefully studied on the angiograms pre-operatively. Timing of surgery and the method of surgical treatment are also influenced by the anomalies (*vide infra*). Asymptomatic occlusion of an intracranial or extracranial major vessel by atheromatous disease will impose a similar hazard.

Angiographic Vasospasm

Vasospasm following SAH or intracranial surgery is an ill-understood phenomenon. This will be discussed in Chap. 12. There is no correlation between the clinical condition of the patient and vasospasm seen at angiography. If vasospasm causes a reduction in cerebral perfusion, resulting in ischaemia, the clinical condition is affected. Otherwise, it can be assumed that the area of the brain related to the spastic vessels has received sufficient collateral circulation to maintain its function. Surgery on a patient who is clinically in a favourable condition is not contraindicated on the basis of angiographic vasospasm alone.

Consent for Operation

The surgical treatment of ruptured aneurysms is a prophylactic measure to prevent recurrent haemorrhage. Relatives, and the patient to a certain extent, must be made to understand the natural history of the aneurysm, the purpose of surgery and the risks involved. There is nothing more frustrating to a surgeon than a relative or patient who wonders whether consent for surgery was the right decision when the patient was getting over the effects of haemorrhage so well before operation.

Timing of Surgery

Timing of surgical treatment for a ruptured aneurysm is the most important consideration a neurosurgeon has to make in his surgical practice.

To prevent recurrent haemorrhage, surgeons in the fifties advocated early surgical obliteration of the aneurysm irrespective of the clinical condition. However, it soon became obvious that the outcome of surgical treatment was far worse than no surgical treatment at all. During this period, however, Norlen and Barnum (1953) obtained good results by delaying surgery for 2–3 weeks. As the natural history of intracranial aneurysms in relation to their tendency to recurrent bleeding became apparent, surgery was advocated in the second week, before the period of highest rebleeding. Delay in the timing of surgery allows the condition of the brain to improve, and, along with other advances in the surgical management, makes it possible to obtain an extremely low surgical mortality and morbidity. The delaying policy, however, does not take into account two important considerations. First, although the surgical result improves concomitantly with the improvement in the clinical condition of the patient that occurs with the passage of time, some patients continue to deteriorate from the effects of the initial haemorrhage and do not come to surgery any more. The other problem in delaying surgery is the recurrent bleeding within the first week or 10 days in patients who are not affected by the initial bleed. Recurrent haemorrhage increases the risk of death and disablement, and may contraindicate surgical treatment altogether.

Recently there has been some renewed enthusiasm for early surgery. Some surgeons (Hori and Suzuki 1979) advocate surgery within the first few hours if possible, and certainly within the first 3 days. They believe that the development of vasospasm may be prevented by removing blood clots from the subarachnoid cisterns and around the major vessels at operation. Surgical treatment between the fifth and eighth days of the haemorrhage has been reported to produce a poor result (Sano and Saito 1978). Because of the controversy on the timing of surgery, a multinational cooperative study (including the Newcastle Regional Neurological Centre) has recently been completed by the University of Iowa. There was no significant difference as regards mortality and morbidity in the early surgery (0–3 days) and late surgery (7–14 days) groups (see Chap. 17). This study, however, includes only the practice of an individual surgeon on his timing of surgery and the surgical outcome. It does not answer the question of the role of overall management in relation to the natural history of the disease. Hunt and Miller (1977) approached the problem of timing of surgery by regarding the clinical condition of the patient as the dominant factor. They advocate surgery as soon as the patient's neurological condition becomes stable or is improving. Our practice during the last 15 years has been similar to that of Hunt and Miller. We believe that in an ideal situation, the surgical treatment should be carried out at the earliest opportunity. In practice, we rarely receive patients on day 1 or 2, and therefore most of our good-risk patients are operated on towards the latter half of the first week. The factors which affect the outcome of surgery, as discussed before, should be taken into account in planning the timing of surgery. In our view, by carefully considering various circumstances in an individual patient, postoperative vasospasm no longer causes an irremediable problem. The timing of surgery and its outcome in Newcastle is given in Chap. 11.

Methods of Surgical Treatment

Obliteration of the aneurysm from the cerebral circulation by ligation at its neck is the ideal method of treatment (Fig. 10.2). With experience and modern technical aids (*vide infra*) the majority of aneurysms can be treated in this manner. However, in some aneurysms, particularly the larger ones, with difficult morphological features, it may prove difficult to achieve this goal. These cases may require alternative surgical procedures. The available methods of surgical treatment for intracranial aneurysms are considered below.

Parent Artery Occlusion

Principle

In this technique the artery is ligated proximal to the site of the aneurysm in order to reduce the blood flow through the aneurysm. The collateral circulation nourishes the part deprived of direct flow. John Hunter introduced the technique more than 200 years ago for the treatment of large popliteal aneurysm. Ligation of the carotid artery in the neck has been practised for over 100 years. Proximal artery occlusion was also carried out for anterior communicating aneurysms by ligating the origin of one of the anterior cerebral arteries (Logue 1956) and for vertebrobasilar aneurysms by ligating the vertebral artery intracranially (Drake 1975). The method of cervical carotid

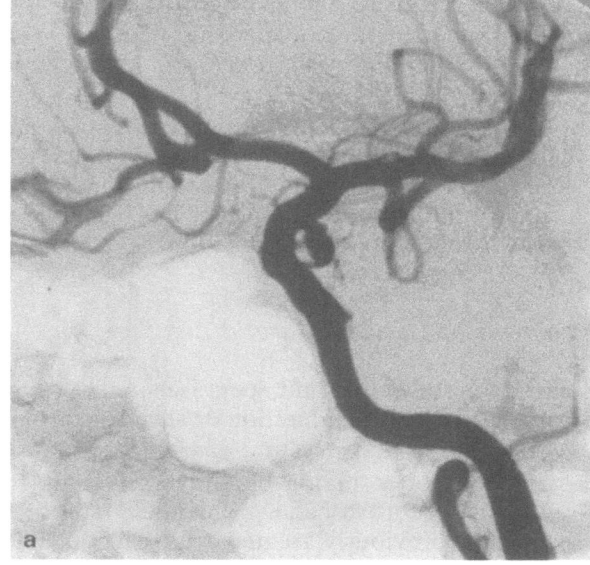

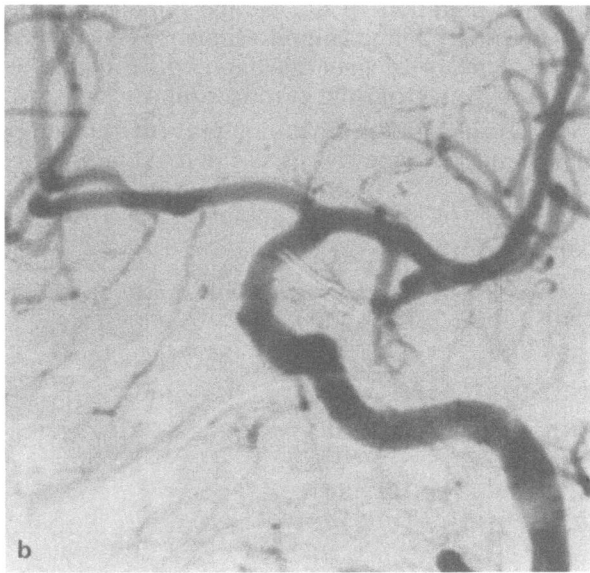

Fig. 10.2. a Pre- and b postoperative angiograms of a patient with ruptured posterior communicating artery aneurysm showing successful clipping of aneurysm.

ligation still remains a useful procedure for certain aneurysms.

Advantages of Cervical Carotid Ligation

1. It is technically a simple procedure.
2. An intracranial exploration is not required, and dissection of the aneurysm is avoided.

3. The method is effective in preventing re-bleeding in certain aneurysms, such as posterior communicating or carotid ophthalmic aneurysms.

4. It can remove the compression effects of some of the larger aneurysms on the cranial nerves. For example, trigeminal neuralgia due to an aneurysm of the carotid artery has been effectively treated by carotid ligation.

Problems of Cervical Carotid Ligation

1. It is unpredictable and acute ischaemia, causing fatal cerebral infarction or severe neurological deficit, may occcur.

2. The loss of a major blood vessel leads to various cerebrovascular problems in later life. Patients previously treated with carotid ligation develop hypertension more frequently than members of the normal population. Delayed ischaemic complications may also occur as a result of haemodynamic disturbances or embolism from the carotid stump.

3. Carotid ligation does not prevent rebleeding from those aneurysms situated at the internal carotid bifurcation or beyond, as the flow to the aneurysm is not effectively reduced.

4. Increased blood flow through the remaining carotid artery may lead to further aneurysm formation in later years.

Methods to Reduce Ischaemic Complications from Carotid Ligation

1. Ligation of the common carotid artery rather than the internal carotid provides increased collateral circulation via the external carotid artery.

2. Gradual obliteration of the artery is considered to be safer than acute ligation. Furthermore, it is thought to encourage increased flow through the collateral supply.

3. Peroperative carotid blood flow or stump pressure studies may indicate the tolerance of carotid ligation.

4. Simultaneous internal carotid occlusion and extracranial–intracranial arterial bypass shunt (Spetzler et al. 1980; Sengupta 1982b) (Fig. 10.3). A new collateral system is created by anastomosing a branch of the external

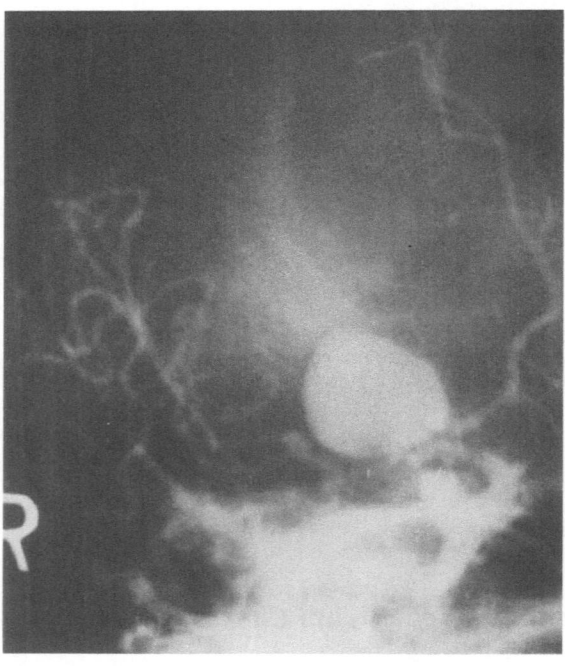
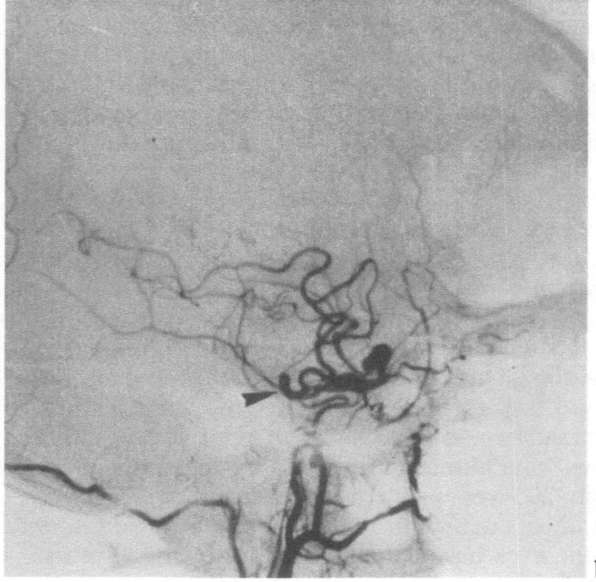

Fig. 10.3. a Left carotid angiogram showing a large carotid ophthalmic aneurysm which was found to be inoperable at direct surgery—internal carotid ligation with EC/IC anastomosis was carried out. **b** Postoperative carotid angiogram (lateral views) showing superficial temporal artery (*arrowhead*) and site of anastomosis. *Note*: a small residual filling of the aneurysm is seen.

carotid, usually the superficial temporal artery, to a cortical branch of the middle cerebral artery. It should be pointed out that the carotid ligation should be performed acutely, after performing the bypass shunt, as, in the presence of a normal carotid flow, the shunt tends to lose patency. If there is any doubt about the adequacy of the flow through the shunt, the internal carotid should be clamped with a reversible Selverstone clamp acutely, with provision for later release if necessary.

Intravascular Balloon Occlusion

Serbinenko (1974) introduced the technique of detachable balloon occlusion of the intracranial vessels though the cervical carotid route, and it has since been successfully used for carotid–cavernous fistulae and intracranial aneurysm (Debrun et al. 1978; Romodanov and Shcheglov 1979). In this method, the neck of the aneurysm is occluded by inflating a detachable balloon within the sac of the aneurysm without compromising the patency of the parent artery (Fig. 10.4). The

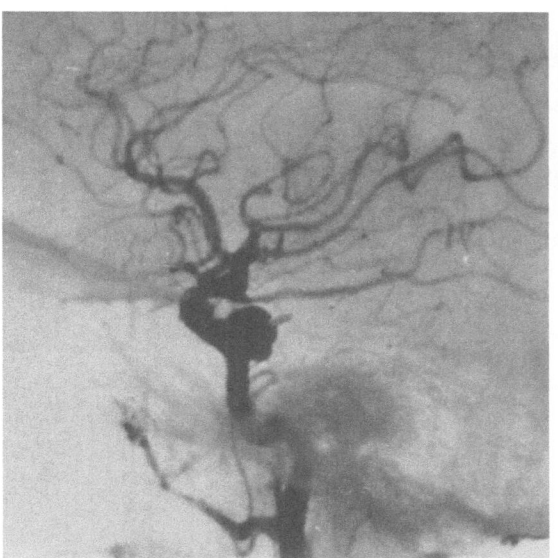
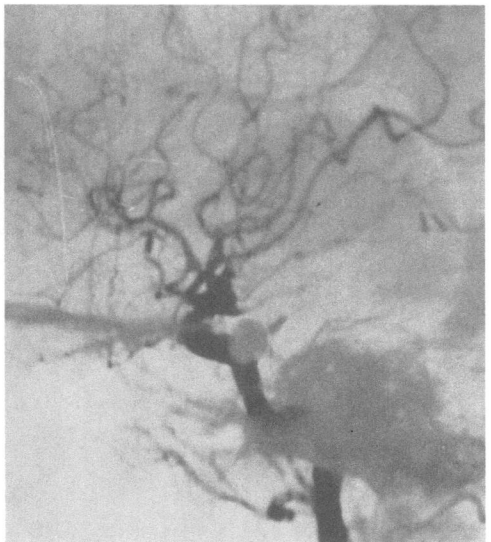
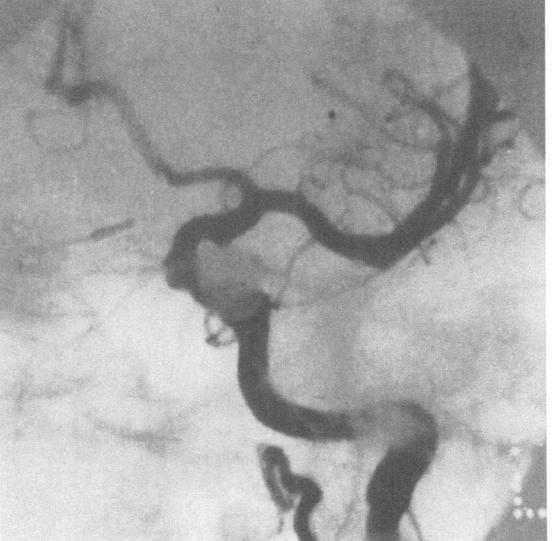

Fig. 10.4. a Lateral and **b** Townes oblique projection showing balloon occlusion of an aneurysm arising from the cavernous part of the right internal carotid artery with a patent parent artery. (Courtesy of Dr. Desmond Hawkins)

results of balloon occlusion are excellent in carotid–cavernous fistulae, but the treatment of aneurysms by this method is difficult and dangerous, with the risk of rupture of the aneurysm during balloon inflation.

Reinforcement of Aneurysmal Sac (Wrapping)

The first aneurysm ever to be treated by direct surgery was a carotid bifurcation aneurysm, which was wrapped by Dott (1933) with muscle. Gillingham (1975) used this technique for middle

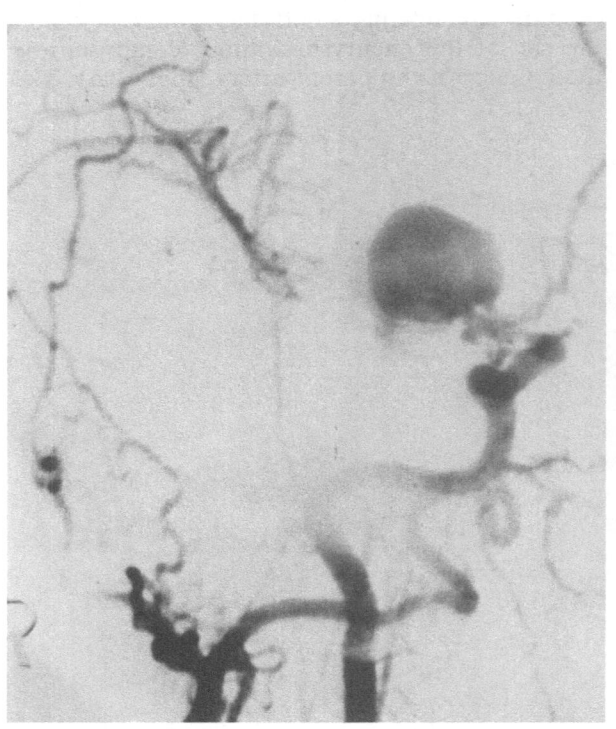

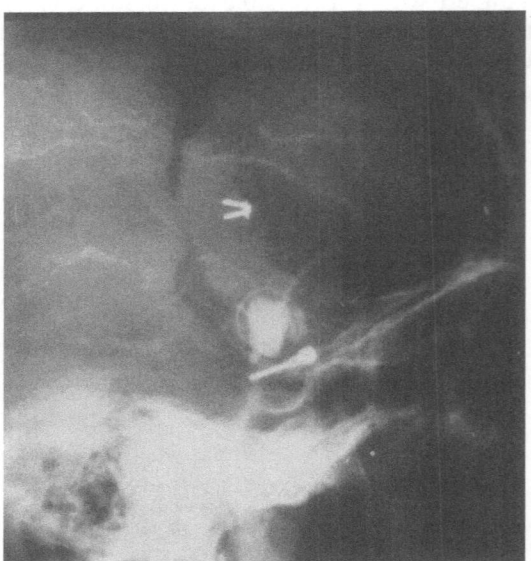

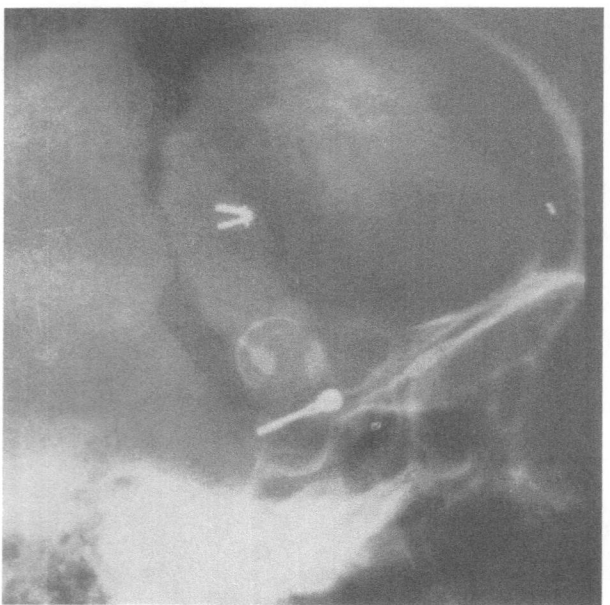

Fig. 10.5. a Patient with a large internal carotid artery bifurcation aneurysm, in which **b** intraluminal thrombosis using copper wire has been carried out (*arrow*). **c** Postoperative angiogram showing incomplete occlusion of the aneurysm. The clip shown was for occlusion of a posterior communicating artery aneurysm done previously.

cerebral aneurysms for many years with remarkable success. The wall of the aneurysm is reinforced with muslin or glue, without the risk of compromising the parent artery or its branches. The technique is not, however, generally favoured since it requires excessive dissection around the base of the aneurysm, and there is a risk of early rebleeding before fibrosis around the aneurysmal wall has taken place.

Intraluminal Thrombosis

Induced thrombosis of the sac with hair, glue or copper wire is an attractive method of treating intracranial aneurysms, as there is no dissection involved. However, the extent of thrombosis often cannot be controlled, either leading to thrombosis of the parent vessel or leaving part of the aneurysm unoccluded (Fig. 10.5). Although Mullan et al. (1965) have obtained excellent results with this technique, we found it extremely tedious and difficult in practice.

Trapping of the Aneurysmal Neck

Trapping of the aneurysmal neck is a very effective technique where neck occlusion is not possible. It is a method of choice for giant aneurysms, where a considerable part of the parent artery is involved in the aneurysmal neck formation. Simultaneous extracranial–intracranial bypass surgery can overcome the problem of collateral circulation, as part of the parent artery is necessarily occluded in this procedure.

Neck Occlusion

Obliteration of the aneurysmal neck is the ideal method of treatment, as there is no compromise of any vessel and it removes the threat of recurrent haemorrhage permanently.

Technical Points During Neck Occlusion

1. It should be remembered that more aneurysms may be clippable than would appear to be the case on angiograms, or even during operation at initial examination (Fig. 10.6)
2. Sac obliteration with multiple clips, leaving a few millimetres at the neck, is preferable if there is any danger of arterial kinking.

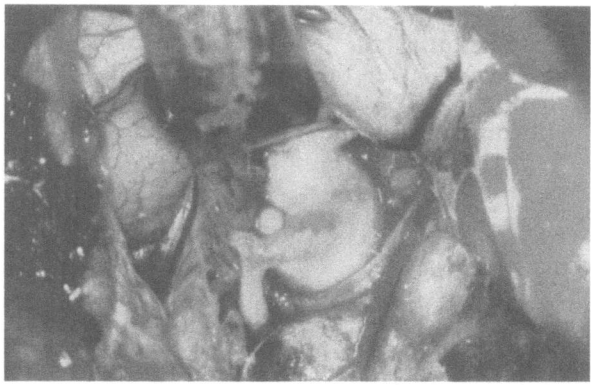

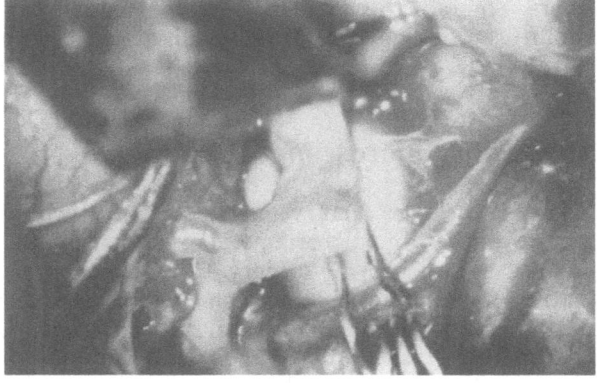

Fig. 10.6a, b. Operative photographs of right middle cerebral aneurysm. **a** On initial examination aneurysm appears to be a blow-out of the middle cerebral artery without an apparent neck. **b** The same aneurysm satisfactorily clipped after further dissection.

3. A large aneurysm can rarely be shrunken by bipolar coagulation because of atheroma and calcification.
4. On a large or giant aneurysm the application of a clip must be done when it is slack, otherwise there is a risk of a tear or kinking at the neck (Sengupta 1982b).

Methods to Reduce Operative Rupture

1. Induced hypotension to a level of up to 60% of the patient's blood pressure during dissection.
2. Temporary occlusion of the parent vessel shortly before application of a clip to the neck.
3. Cardiac pacing to provide extreme hypotension if proximal occlusion is not possible, as in the case of giant basilar bifurcation aneurysms. The pacemaker is inserted intravenously, and placed in the right atrium by radiological control (see Chap. 8). It gives a

highly controllable and sensitive method of manipulating the blood pressure. Mannitol infusion is given during the period of extreme hypotension to reduce cerebral ischaemia (Suzuki and Yashimoto 1979).

Technical Aids for Intracranial Surgery

There have been considerable advances in the facilities available for aneurysm surgery in recent years. Some of the ancillary measures and equipment used during operation are discussed briefly here.

Operating Microscope

Dissection of the aneurysmal neck, with the use of the operating microscope, has improved the results of aneurysm surgery in recent years. Although it is possible to achieve a successful clipping without magnification, the anatomy in the region of the aneurysm is better identified through the microscope. Furthermore, it provides excellent illumination of the operating field. Significantly, the microtechnique requires extremely gentle dissection and only minimal brain retraction, which, understandably, improves the outcome.

Micro-instruments

For microvascular technique, it is necessary to have various micro-instruments which are of adequate length and quality (Fig. 10.7).

Bipolar Coagulation

Bleeding points during dissection can be stopped with less trauma using bipolar coagulation than with unipolar diathermy. Occasionally, the neck of an aneurysm can be narrowed by using bipolar coagulation before applying a clip. Special care should be taken to avoid the forceps becoming adherent to the tissues. This may be achieved by holding the tissue intermittently rather than continuously during coagulation. The tips of the forceps should be cleaned often, by scraping with a moist gauze. Working in a wet field is also helpful in this respect.

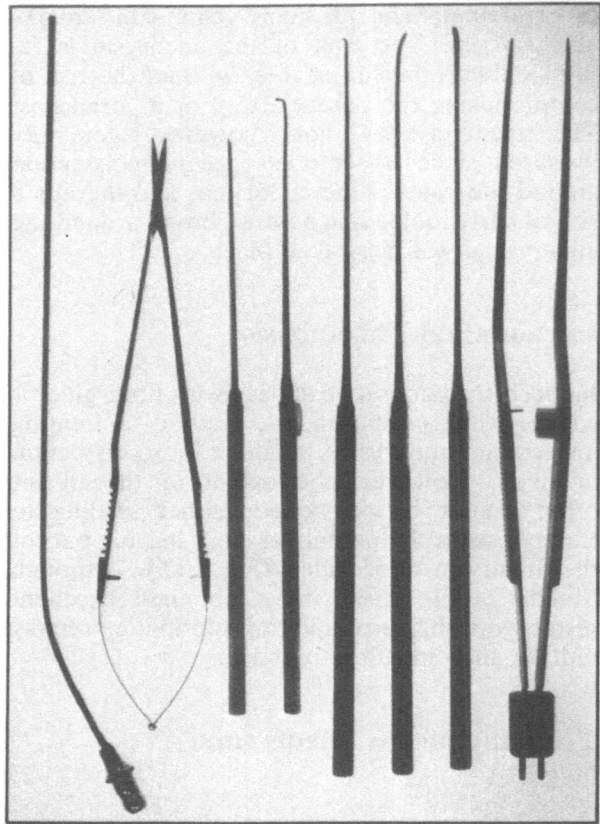

Fig. 10.7. Some of the micro-instruments used in aneurysmal surgery.

Self-retaining Brain Retractors

The use of self-retaining retractors is as beneficial as the operating microscope in the prevention of operative trauma to the brain tissue. During a long operation the retractor should be released from time to time to avoid constant compression on a particular area of the brain. Of the various types available, the self-retaining retractor designed by Yasargil and made by Aesculap of West Germany is the most versatile and easy to apply.

Suction Apparatus

Special care is needed in respect of the suction facilities during aneurysm surgery. The pressure of suction tubes during dissection should not be more than 4 lb/in.^{2} as powerful suction disturbs the tissue and may precipitate premature rupture. However, in the event of an untimely rupture,

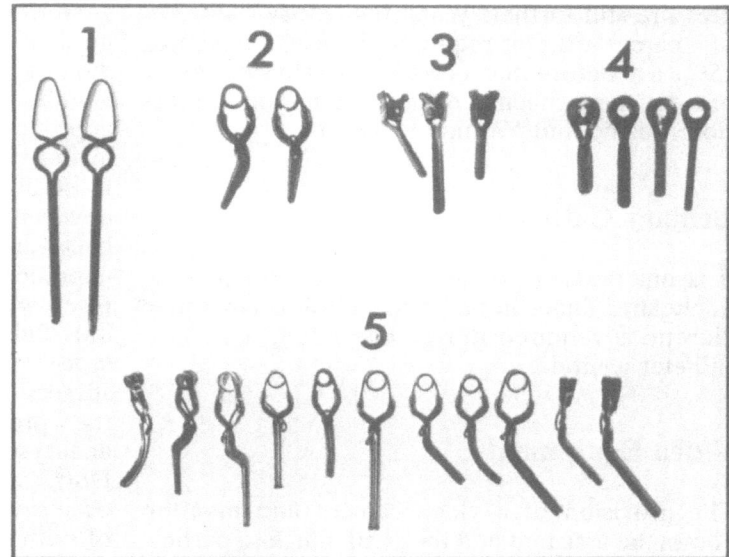

Fig. 10.8. Some of the clips used for occlusion of aneurysm in our practice. *1*, Drake; *2*, Yasargil; *3*, Heifitz; *4*, Scoville, *5*, Sugita.

rapid suction of the blood from the operating field may be necessary. It is, therefore, useful to have two suction facilities with different pressures.

Aneurysm Clips

Spring clips of various size and shape are now designed for aneurysm surgery (Fox 1978), and these should be readily available during operation. It is useful to remember that the strength of a clip varies with the need for permanent or temporary occlusion. We have found that the clips designed by Sugita are applicable for most of the aneurysms. Some of the clips used in our centre are shown in Fig. 10.8.

Reinforcing Agents

On rare occasions, when clipping is not possible, the wall of the aneurysm may be wrapped. Muslin and histoacryl glue, made by Braun Melsunge of West Germany, are easy to apply, and no less effective than other similar agents advocated for this purpose.

Spasmolytic Agent

Papaverine 2.5% solution is very effective to reverse spasm of vessels induced during dissection. Some surgeons prefer phentolamine for a longer lasting effect.

Hypotensive Anaesthesia

The technique of anaesthesia used in aneurysm surgery has been described in Chap. 8. It is essential, however, to appreciate that tension within the aneurysm drops considerably during induced hypotension. With a pliable sac, dissection and obliteration of the neck can be performed with less risk of rupture. Pharmacologically induced hypotension to a systolic pressure of 60 mmHg can be achieved for a short period of time without inflicting neurological damage. If the surgeon has wide experience, the need for hypotension to such a low level may be less frequent. We have commonly used ganglion blocking agents. It is useful to remember that a sudden fall in blood pressure may lead to breakdown of cerebral autoregulation, with a consequent reduction in the cerebral perfusion, leading to ischaemic damage. A similar reduction may result if low blood pressure is allowed to persist during bleeding from rupture of the aneurysm. We hasten to add that elevation of blood pressure to a normal level should also be gradual, to avoid sudden strain on the clip.

Dehydrating Agents

With careful timing of surgery and ideal anaesthetic conditions, reduction of intracranial pressure with a dehydrating agent is not necessary and is counterproductive. Aspiration of CSF from the subarachnoid cistern or the ventricle reduces the pressure still further. When temporary occlusion of a parent artery is required, the use of mannitol 15% 1 h before the occlusion is considered to prevent the ischaemic effect of temporary occlusion (Suzuki and Yashimoto 1979).

Urinary Catheter

It is our practice to catheterise the patient routinely after anaesthesia. If mannitol or any other diuretic is required during operation, a urinary catheter is vital.

Video Equipment

The provision of a video camera and monitor allows the assistant and the scrub nurse to participate in the surgical procedure in a more helpful manner. It also allows teaching of the trainee, and further improvement of operative technique.

Aneurysms in Various Sites

There are many operative surgery textbooks which give excellent descriptions of the operative stages (Kempe 1968; Symon 1980; Schmidek and Sweet 1982). The main purpose here is to present the personal philosophy of the authors in approaching an intracranial aneurysm.

Anterior Communicating Artery Aneurysms

Direct surgical treatment of anterior communicating artery aneurysms is considered to be hazardous, because of their close proximity to the anterior hypothalamus and optic chiasma. Lying buried between the frontal lobes, they are often enclosed and obscured by the parent trunks of the anterior cerebral arteries. The practice of surgical treatment, in terms of access and mode of therapy, has been revised due to these problems.

Historical Note on the Evolution of Surgical Treatment

Tonnis (1936) was the first to operate on an anterior communicating artery aneurysm directly; he did so through the midline, by splitting the genu of the corpus callosum. This extensive surgical destruction of an important area of the brain did not find general acceptance. Falconer (1951), Hamby (1952) and others used the subfrontal approach to gain access to these aneurysms. Following the observation of Falconer (1951) that most of these aneurysms project forwards and downwards, and the remainder upwards and backwards, Norlen and Barnum (1953) approached the former type subfrontally, and reserved a midline approach along the falx without dividing the corpus callosum for the latter type. However, the outcome following direct surgery remained generally poor. To overcome the problem of premature rupture of the aneurysm at operation, Logue (1956) popularised Dott's method of proximal anterior cerebral occlusion. Hamby (1952) recommended exposure of both carotid arteries in the neck so that they could be temporarily occluded to avoid premature rupture. Pool (1961) popularised the technique of a midline approach with temporary occlusion of both anterior cerebral arteries, and this gained universal acceptance. Kempe (1968), in his excellent monograph, recommends an approach to these aneurysms based on their projection. In his technique, a non-dominant subfrontal exposure is used. The region of the anterior communicating artery is approached by dissecting the internal carotid to the bifurcation and then proceeding along the anterior cerebral artery. Subsequent steps follow, according to the projection of the aneurysm. For those projecting upwards and backwards, the aneurysms are approached from below through the longitudinal fissure, while for those projecting downwards and forwards, access to the aneurysm is gained from above, by removing a small area of the gyrus rectus. The principle of this approach is to avoid exposing the fundus of the aneurysm, which is the commonest area of rupture, before exposing the neck of the aneurysm (Fig. 10.9).

Anatomical and Physiological Considerations

In the authors' experience, most of the aneurysms in this region can be obliterated more successfully with careful study of the angiograms, which will provide useful information, as outlined below.

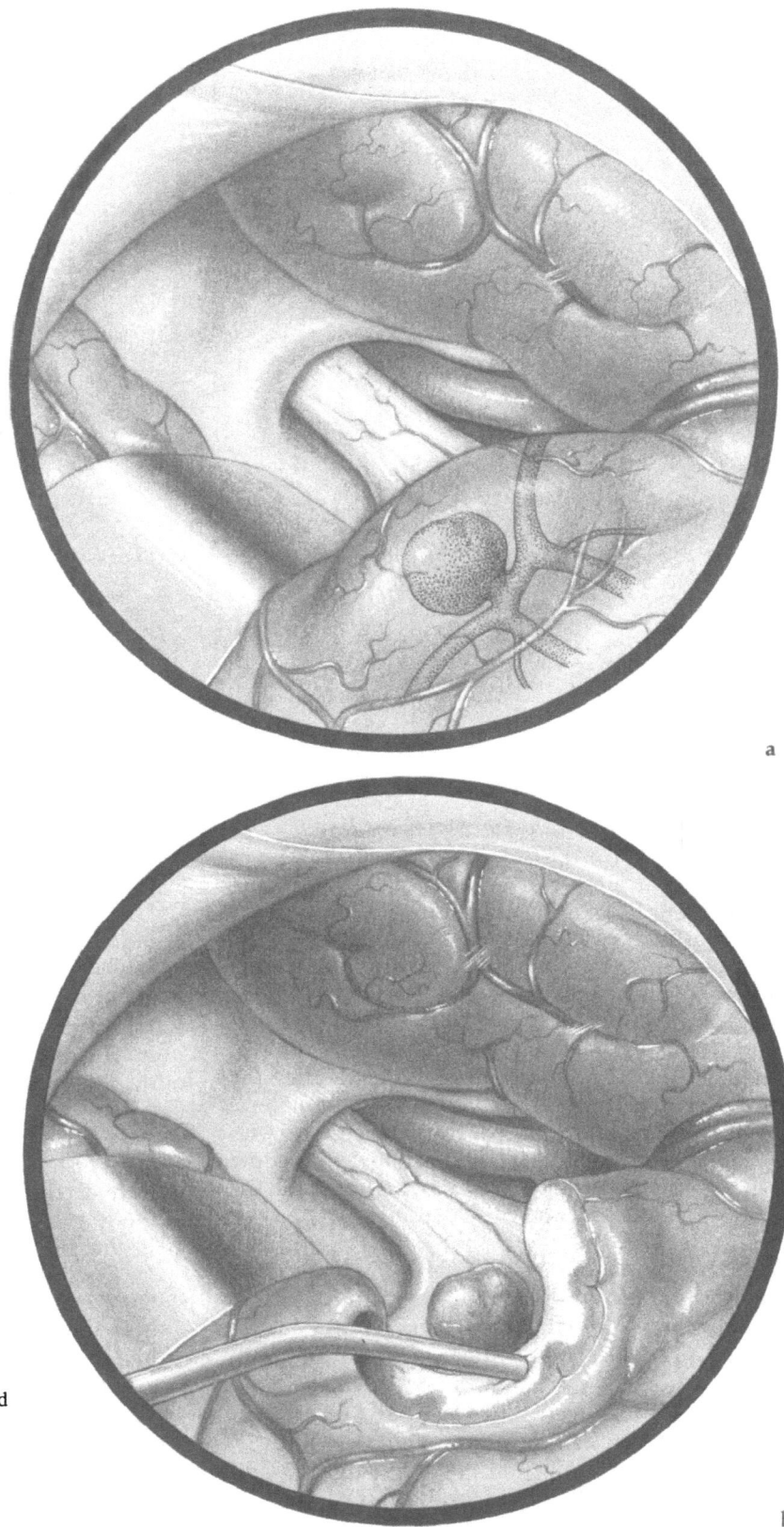

a

b

Fig. 10.9. a Illustration of an anterior communicating artery aneurysm projecting anteriorly and inferiorly and its relation to major vessels. **b** Gyrus rectus approach to aneurysm as in **a**. **c** Anterior communicating artery aneurysm with clip in situ.

Fig. 10.9c *overleaf*

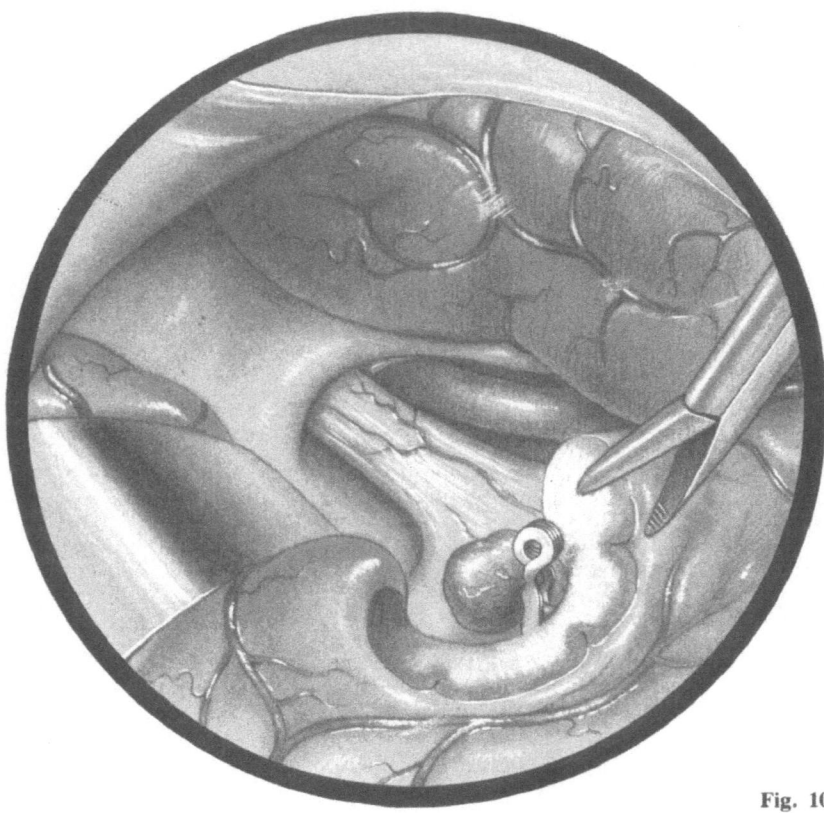

Fig. 10.9c

Circulation Through the Anterior Part of the Circle of Willis

Norlen and Barnum (1953) drew attention to the different patterns of circulation through the anterior part of the circle of Willis in patients with anterior communicating artery aneurysms, stressing their importance for the various surgical procedures. Knowledge of different types of circulation is also important in understanding the effects of vasospasm, as the available collateral supply differs. In an analysis of 100 patients with anterior communicating aneurysms, Sengupta (1977) noted four types of circulation, and the aneurysms were classified accordingly:

Type 1 (Ipsilateral)—66%. In this type, the aneurysm and the distal anterior cerebral artery filled from one proximal anterior cerebral artery.

1. Right anterior cerebral–anterior communicating artery aneurysms. The pattern of circulation in these aneurysms may be as follows (Fig. 10.10a):
a) Right carotid injection fills the aneurysm and both distal anterior cerebral arteries.
b) Right carotid injection fills the aneurysm and right distal anterior cerebral artery.
c) Left carotid injection fills the left distal anterior cerebral artery only.
d) Left carotid injection with right carotid compression fills both distal anterior cerebral arteries but not the aneurysm.
e) As in d), but the aneurysm fills.

2. Left anterior cerebral–anterior communicating artery aneurysms. In these aneurysms the following patterns of circulation are possible (Fig. 10.10b):
a) Left carotid injection fills the aneurysm and both distal anterior cerebral arteries.
b) Left carotid injection fills the aneurysm and the left distal anterior cerebral artery.
c) Right carotid injection fills the right distal anterior cerebral artery only.
d) Right carotid injection with left carotid compression fills both distal anterior cerebral arteries but not the aneurysm.
e) As in d), but the aneurysm fills.

Type 2 (Bilateral)—14%. In this type, the aneurysm and both anterior cerebral arteries fill from both carotid injections (Fig. 10.11a). This pattern of circulation is often associated with

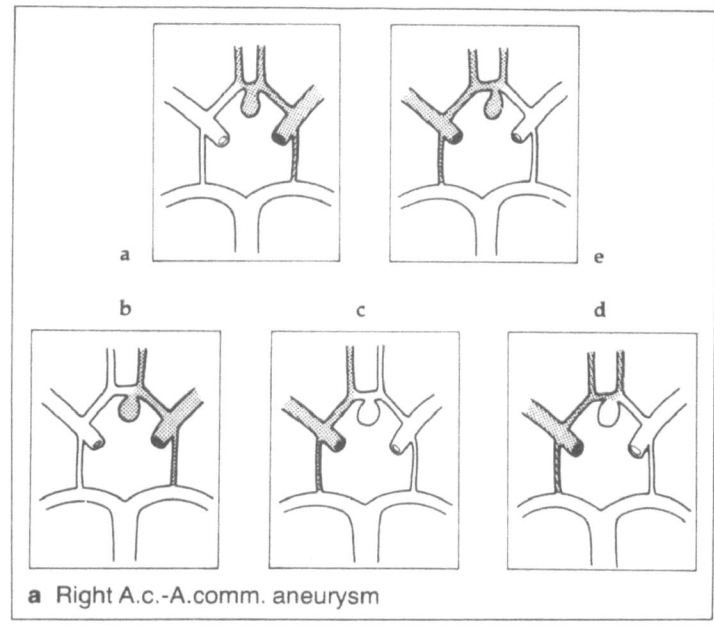

a Right A.c.-A.comm. aneurysm

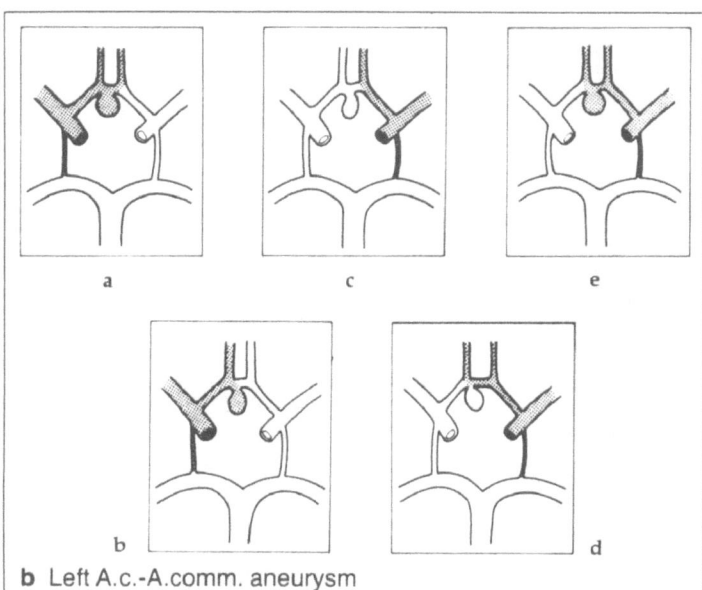

b Left A.c.-A.comm. aneurysm

Fig. 10.10a, b. Anterior communicating artery aneurysm. Type I (ipsilateral): **a** right; **b** left.

rudimentary anterior communicating arteries. In fact, both anterior cerebral arteries may be fused to each other (Fig. 10.11b). On the other hand, the anterior communicating artery may be seen as a prominent structure on the angiograms (Fig. 10.11c). The significance of this analysis is that in this type of circulation the region of the anterior communicating artery receives good collateral supply, and the effect of vasospasm is minimal. In cases of rudimentary anterior communicating arteries, however, application of a clip may lead to kinking of both anterior cerebral arteries, leading to severe ischaemic problems, as discussed later

Type 3 (Dominant Anterior Cerebral Artery)—12%. In this type, the aneurysm arises from the axilla of the two distal anterior cerebral arteries, both of which are divisions of the dominant anterior cerebral artery, and the contralateral artery is hypoplastic (Fig. 10.12).

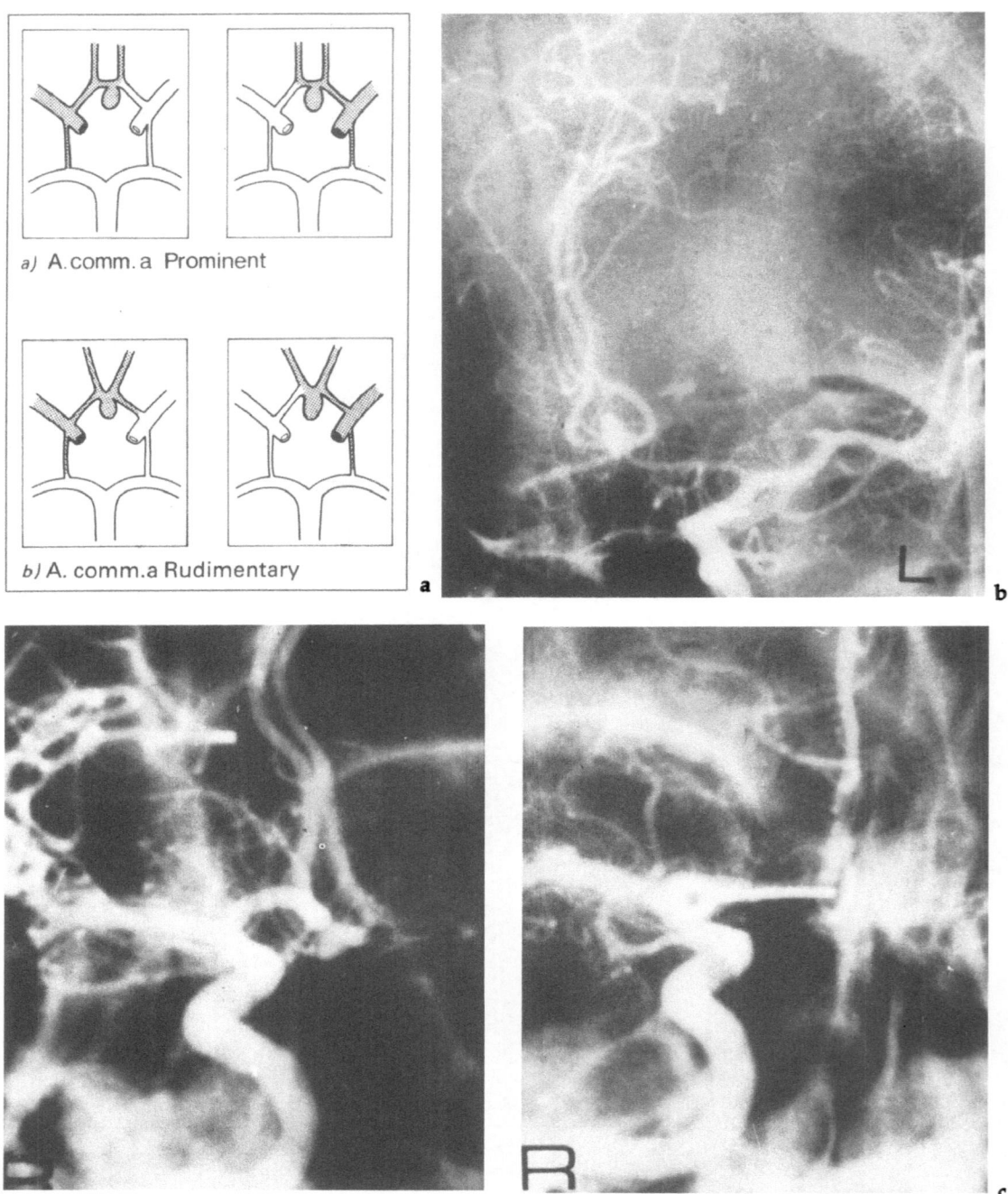

Fig. 10.11. a Anterior communicating artery aneurysm. Type II (bilateral). **b** Left carotid angiogram showing anterior communicating artery aneurysm with fused anterior cerebral arteries. Anterior communicating artery is almost nonexistent. **c** Right carotid angiogram showing anterior communicating artery aneurysm with a prominent anterior communicating artery. Figure on the *right* shows postoperative angiogram of the same patient after clipping the aneurysm.

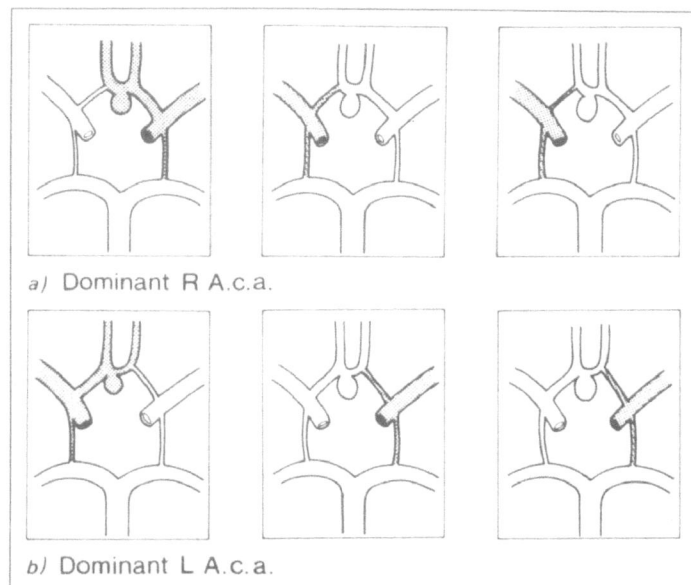

Fig. 10.12. Anterior communicating artery aneurysm. Type III (dominant ACA).

Type 4 (Dominant Anterior Cerebral Artery with Foetal Posterior Cerebral Artery)—8%. In this type, the circulatory patterns are like those in type 3, but there are other associated anomalies in the circle (Fig. 10.13).

In types 3 and 4 the effects of postoperative vasospasm are considerable.

Location of the Neck

These aneurysms rarely arise from the anterior communicating artery itself; rather their exact site of origin is usually close to its junction with one of the anterior cerebral arteries. From the angiograms, the position of the neck of the aneurysm

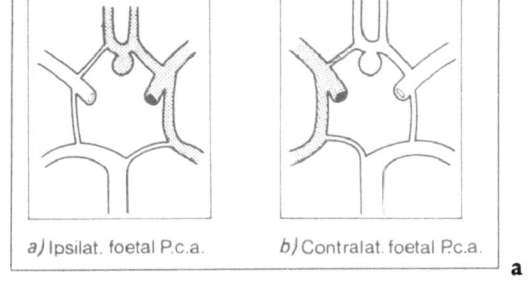

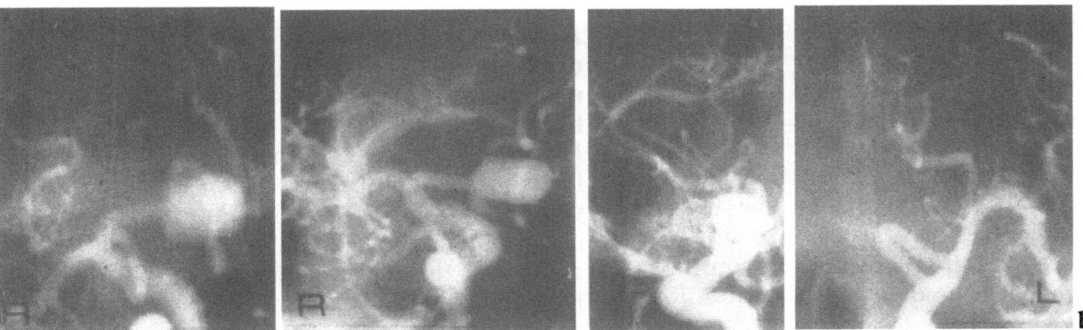

Fig. 10.13. a Anterior communicating artery aneurysm. Type IV (dominant ACA with foetal PCA). **b** Right carotid angiogram showing anterior communicating artery aneurysm arising from a dominant anterior cerebral artery. Left carotid angiogram showing hypoplastic anterior cerebral artery and a foetal posterior cerebral artery.

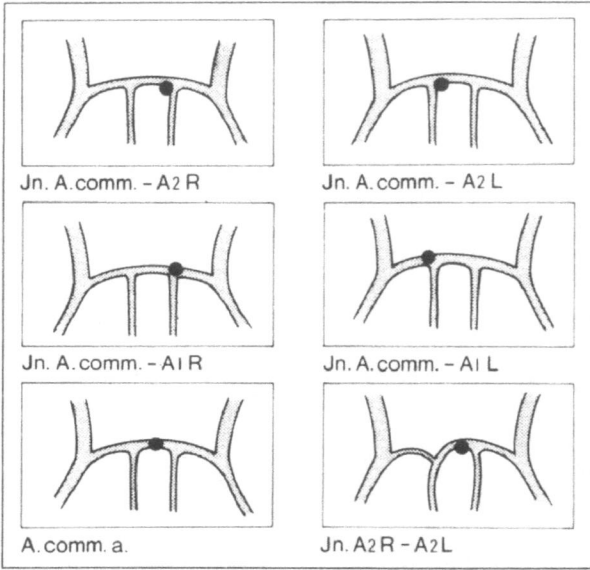

Fig. 10.14. Variations in the location of the neck.

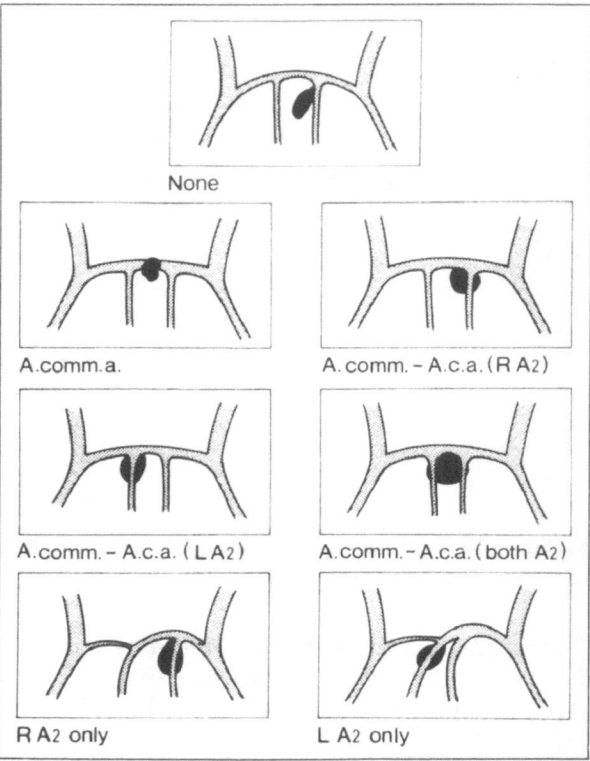

Fig. 10.15. Anatomical relationship of the sac to the major vessels.

can be ascertained to a certain extent. It may be pointed out that occasionally angiographic evidence is misleading, and the aneurysm may appear to have no clippable neck. The following variations in the location of the neck have been noted (Fig. 10.14; Table 10.1) (Sengupta 1977).

1. Junction of the anterior communicating artery and right distal anterior cerebral artery
2. Junction of the anterior communicating artery and left distal anterior cerebral artery
3. Junction of the anterior communicating artery and proximal right anterior cerebral artery
4. Junction of the anterior communicating artery and proximal left anterior cerebral artery
5. Junction of the right and left distal anterior cerebral arteries in type 3 and 4 circulation, as described before
6. Anterior communicating artery alone

Relationship of the Aneurysmal Sac to Major Vessels

It is useful to know the precise relationship of the major vessels to the aneurysmal sac to avoid trauma to these vessels during dissection. In a study of 100 cases, the following relationships of the sac to the major vessels were found (Fig. 10.15; Table 10.2) (Sengupta 1977).

1. No relation to any major vessel
2. Anterior communicating artery alone

3. Anterior communicating and right distal anterior cerebral artery.
4. Anterior communicating and left distal anterior cerebral artery.
5. Anterior communicating and both distal anterior cerebral arteries
6. Right distal anterior cerebral artery
7. Left distal anterior cerebral artery

Placement of the Clip

Application of a clip to the neck is the goal of direct surgery. Yasargil (1969) has shown that it is possible to occlude these aneurysms even with a broad neck, with the use of bipolar coagulation. However, we believe that excessive dissection leads to harmful vasospasm. On the other hand, with the appropriate circulatory pattern, the anterior communicating artery can be obliterated, along with the aneurysm if necessary, without any harmful effect. Considerable opinion has been expressed in recent years about the dangers of damaging small perforating vessels arising from the anterior communicating artery. From anatomical studies we have found that a maximum of

Table 10.1. Circulation via circle of Willis vs location of the neck

Location of the neck	Circulation				
	Type I	Type II	Type III	Type IV	Total
Junc. of ant. comm. a. and right a_2	19	3	1	–	23
Junc. of ant. comm. a. and left a_2	15	1	–	–	16
Junc. of ant. comm. a. and right a_1	13	1	–	1	15
Junc. of ant. comm. a. and left a_1	7	1	–	–	8
Junc. of right a_2 and left a_2	1	–	11	7	19
Ant. comm. a. only	11	8	–	–	19
Total	66	14	12	8	100

Abbreviations: ant. comm. a., anterior communicating artery; a_1, proximal anterior cerebral artery; a_2, distal anterior cerebral artery

Table 10.2. Circulation via circle of Willis vs relation of aneurysmal sac to major vessel

Relation of sac	Circulation				
	Type I	Type II	Type III	Type IV	Total
Ant. comm. a. only	32	7	–	–	39
Ant. comm. a. and right a_2	14	3	–	–	17
Ant. comm. a. and left a_2	6	–	–	–	6
Ant. comm. a. and both a_2	2	2	2	3	9
Right a_2 only	2	–	8	3	13
Left a_2 only	1	1	1	1	4
None	9	1	1	1	12
Total	66	14	12	8	100

Abbreviations: See Table 10.1

three perforating vessels arise from the anterior communicating artery. Moreover, embryological studies suggest that the purpose of the anterior communicating artery is primarily as a conduit for collateral channels rather than for nourishment of any particular area of the brain. When the artery is occluded, the perforating vessels may still receive blood from the opposite anterior cerebral artery. The possible effects of clipping this artery in various types of aneurysm with different circulatory patterns are shown in Fig. 10.16, which shows that although a clip on the neck is ideal, occlusion of the anterior communicating artery along with the clip is harmless in some and lethal in others (Sengupta 1977).

Side of Craniotomy

It is generally accepted that anterior communicating artery aneurysms should be approached through the right non-dominant side, with the exception of a left frontal lobe haematoma, or a dominant left anterior cerebral artery. We plan our approach on the basis of the position of the neck, relation of the sac, and the occasional need to expose the dominant anterior cerebral artery in large difficult aneurysms. Figure 10.17 clarifies the circumstances which decide the side of craniotomy for these aneurysms. If the neck is located at the left, a_1–ant. comm. a. junction, as in diagram (a), or if the sac is related to the left a_2 segment, as in diagrams (b) and (c), the approach should be left sided. In a situation as in diagram (d), with a large aneurysm, the approach should be bilateral at different stages. In diagram (e), although the dominant artery is on the left side, the approach is from the right, since the sac is intimately related to the right a_2 segment.

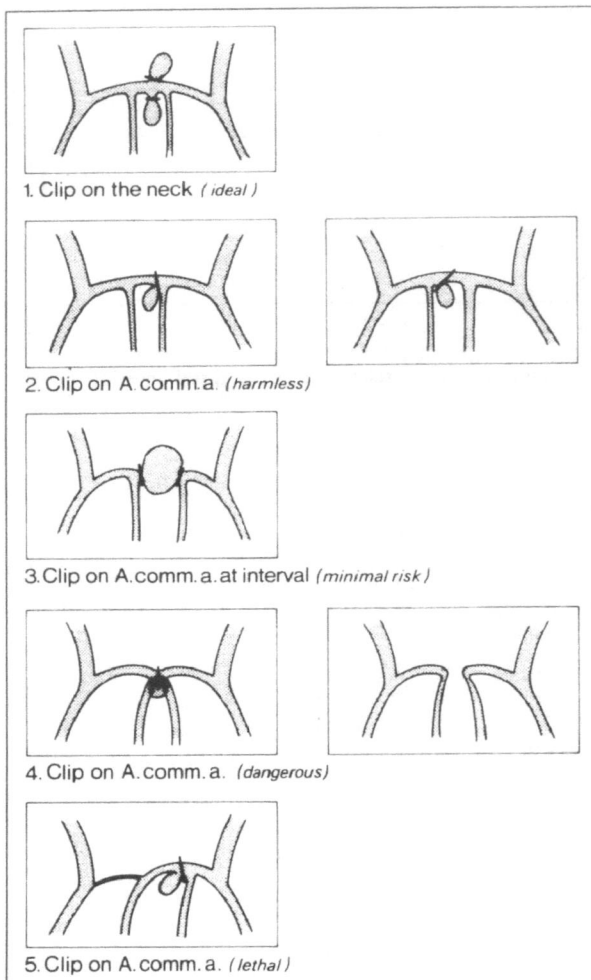

Fig. 10.16. Possible effects of clipping of the aneurysm in different circulatory patterns.

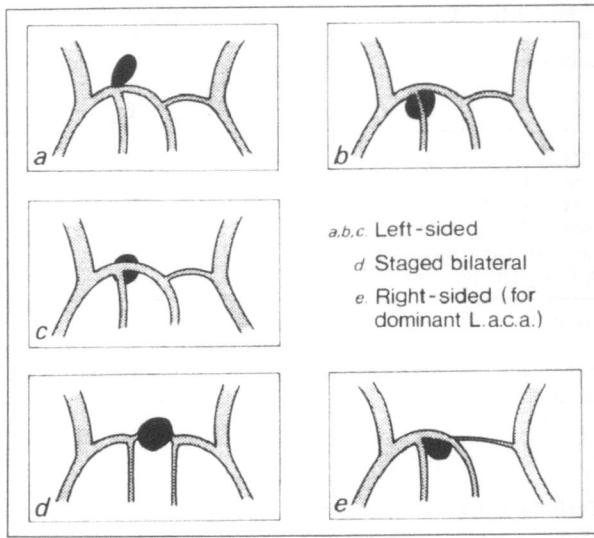

Fig. 10.17. Principles determining the surgical approach.

ries, including Heubner's artery, to the basal ganglia and the hypothalamus. (Fig. 2.10). Dissection of this artery can therefore produce harmful effects from vasospasm. With the use of hypotensive anaesthesia there is hardly ever any need for temporary occlusion of the proximal artery.

In this approach, the distal anterior cerebral artery in the longitudinal fissure is exposed through the gyrus rectus and further dissection is continued proximally until the anterior communicating artery is reached (Fig. 10.18b).

Results of Treatment

In our series of 500 patients, aneurysms of the anterior communicating artery were present in 164. There were 86 males and 78 females (Table 10.3). The age ranged from the second to the eighth decade, with the majority (55%) being in the fifth and sixth decades (Table 10.4).

At the time of operation 43 patients were in grade 1, 82 in grade 2, 34 in grade 3 and 5 in grade 4 (Table 10.5). Ninety-five patients (57%) were operated on before the 12th day of the last haemorrhage (Table 10.6). It should be pointed out that the patients in grade 4 or 5 with these or other aneurysms were operated on because of life-threatening haematoma.

Twenty patients (12%) had postoperative ischaemic neurological complication. One hundred and thirty-one patients (78%) had a good outcome. Twenty-three patients (14%) were in

A Modified Approach for Dissection of the Aneurysm Without Exposing the Proximal Anterior Cerebral Artery

This approach is based on two considerations:

1. The course of the anterior cerebral artery is such that from the point of origin it passes forwards and slightly upwards, until it meets its fellow from the opposite side in the longitudinal fissure. Therefore, to expose an aneurysm of the anterior communicating region, it is not necessary to dissect the carotid bifurcation, which is the deepest part of the circle (Fig. 10.18a).

2. The proximal anterior cerebral artery is the most important source of vital perforating arte-

fair condition, five patients (3%) had a poor outcome and five died (Table 10.7).

Table 10.3. Anterior cerebral artery (ACA) aneurysms: sex incidence

	Ant. comm. a.	Prox. ACA	Total
Male	85	1	86
Female	75	3	78
	160	4	164

Table 10.4. Anterior cerebral artery aneurysms: age incidence

Age (years)	Ant. comm. a.	Prox. ACA	Total
10–19	3	–	3
20–29	19	–	19
30–39	26	–	26
40–49	30	3	33
50–59	56	1	57
60–69	25	–	25
70–79	1	–	1
	160	4	164

Table 10.5. Anterior cerebral artery aneurysms: neurological grade at operation (Hunt and Hess)

Grade	Ant. comm. a.	Prox. ACA	Total
I	43	–	43
II	80	2	82
III	32	2	34
IV	5	–	5
V	–	–	–
	160	4	164

Table 10.6. Anterior cerebral artery aneurysm: timing of surgery

Days from last SAH	Ant. comm. a.	Prox. ACA	Total
0– 4	14	–	14
5– 7	33	1	34
8–11	45	2	47
12–14	24	–	24
15–18	12	–	12
19–21	12	–	12
>21	20	1	21
	160	4	164

Peripheral Anterior Cerebral Aneurysms (Pericallosal Aneurysms)

Peripheral anterior cerebral aneurysms are relatively rare and pose considerable difficulty in their management.

Table 10.7. Anterior cerebral artery aneurysms: outcome at discharge

Outcome	Ant. comm. a.	Prox. ACA	Total
Good	127	4	131
Fair	23	–	23
Poor	5	–	5
Dead	5	–	5
	160	4	164

Anatomical and Physiological Considerations

The anterior cerebral artery divides into pericallosal and callosomarginal arteries in the region of the genu of the corpus callosum. Aneurysms usually arise from the junction of these two arteries and are often termed pericallosal aneurysms. The point of division of the anterior

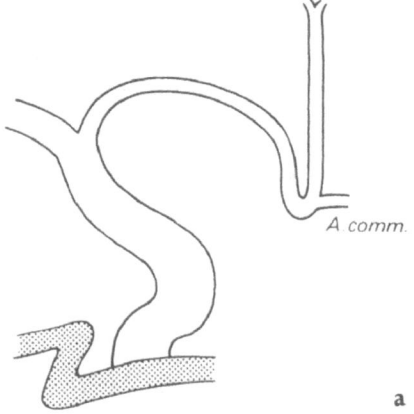

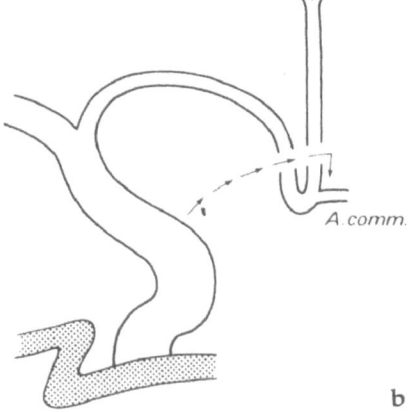

Fig. 10.18. a Schematic representation of the course of the anterior cerebral artery. **b** Surgical approach to the anterior communicating artery aneurysm. *Note*: Dissection has continued from internal carotid artery to the a_2 segment of the anterior cerebral artery through the gyrus rectus (*broken line*).

cerebral artery is, however, variable, and aneurysms arising from this area are difficult to locate at operation. Occasionally, the distal portions of both anterior cerebral arteries are fused into a common trunk, and the aneurysm arises from the origin of its first major branch (Fig. 10.19a). When associated with other intracranial aneurysms, pericallosal aneurysms are usually the offending lesions. They usually project along the course of the callosomarginal artery, and separation of the aneurysm may damage this vessel. As the two anterior cerebral arteries lie side by side in the interhemispheric fissure, the effect of SAH or surgical manipulation may involve the area of supply of both these arteries (Fig. 10.19b). Collateral circulation over the corpus callosum becomes ineffective in SAH because of involvement of the collaterals in the vasospastic process.

Method of Identification at Operation (Fig. 10.20)

The approach to aneurysms of the pericallosal artery is made along the falx through a frontal bone flap anterior to the coronal suture.

Identification of the aneurysm at operation may at times prove difficult. Certain guidelines while planning the scalp and bone flap and during the approach to the aneurysm will help keep the dissection to a mimimum and locate the aneurysm. A line is drawn on the lateral view of the angiogram from the nasion to the aneurysm. From the end of this line a perpendicular is drawn to meet the vault of the skull. The point where the second line joins the vault should be in the middle of the medial limb of the bone flap in the midline. Search for the aneurysm should be made along this imaginary perpendicular line.

Results of Treatment

Ten patients with pericallosal artery aneurysms have been operated on in this series. Nine patients were in the fifth and sixth decades (Table 10.8). One patient was male and the rest were female (Table 10.9). At the time of operation, one patient was in grade 1, six in grade 2, two in grade 3 and one in grade 4 (Table 10.10). Seven patients were operated on before the 12th day of the last haemorrhage (Table 10.11).

Of the ten patients, three had postoperative neurological complications. Three patients died, and the remaining seven had a good outcome (Table 10.12).

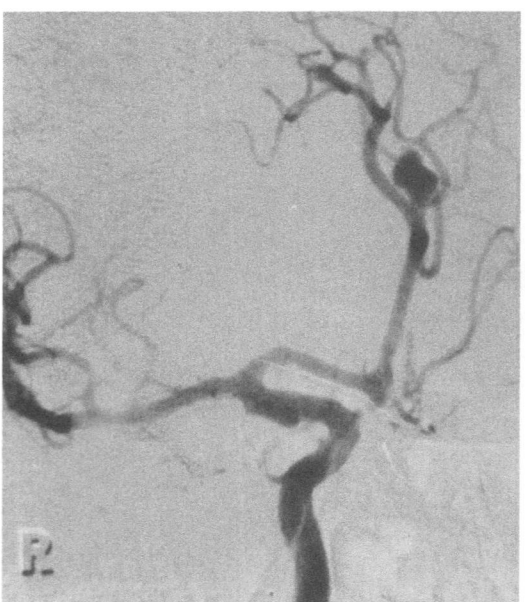

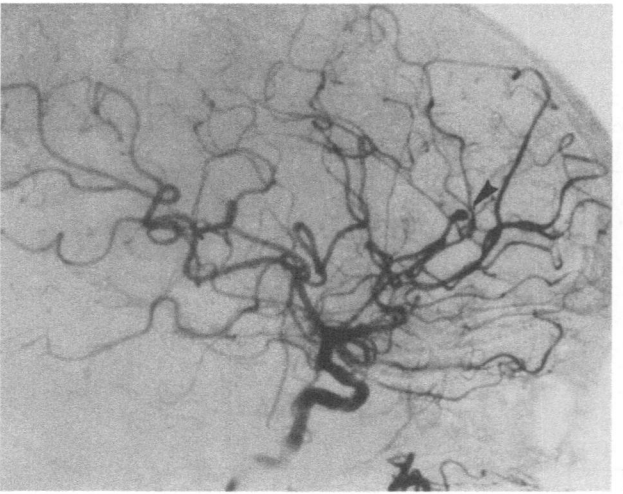

b

a

Fig. 10.19. a Right carotid angiogram showing fused common trunk of anterior cerebral artery (azygous anterior cerebral artery). Pericallosal artery aneurysm arises from the origin of the first major branch. **b** Right carotid angiogram showing a small pericallosal artery aneurysm (*arrowhead*). There is marked spasm of the adjacent anterior cerebral artery.

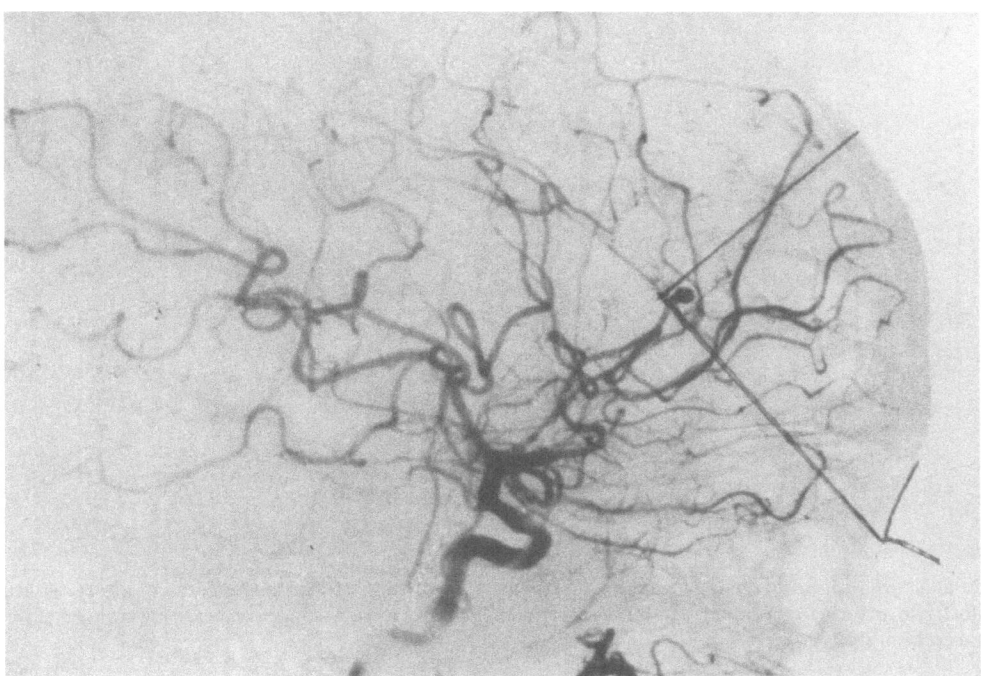

Fig. 10.20. Lateral carotid angiogram showing a pericallosal artery anerurysm with lines drawn to help identification of the aneurysm at surgery (see text).

Table 10.8. Pericallosal artery aneurysm: age incidence

Age (years)	10–19	20–29	30–39	40–49	50–59	Total
	1	–	–	4	5	10

Table 10.9. Pericallosal artery aneurysms: sex incidence

Male	1 (10%)
Female	9 (90%)
Total	10

Table 10.10. Pericallosal artery aneurysms: neurological grade at operation

Grade (Hunt and Hess)	I	II	III	IV	V	Total
	1	6	2	1	–	10

Table 10.11. Pericallosal artery aneurysms: timing of surgery

Days since last SAH	0–4	5–7	8–11	12–14	15–18	19–21	> 21
	2	3	2	1	–	1	1

Table 10.12. Pericallosal artery aneurysms: outcome at discharge

Outcome	Good	Fair	Poor	Dead
	7	–	–	3

Middle Cerebral Artery Aneurysms

Anatomical and Physiological Considerations

Middle cerebral artery aneurysms usually arise from the artery at its first major division. The main trunk of the middle cerebral artery varies in length and gives rise to important perforating branches along its course. An aneurysm arising from the main trunk, or at an early bifurcation or trifurcation, is often surrounded by these fine vessels (Fig. 10..21) and its fundus is buried within the frontal lobe. Branches of the middle cerebral artery invest an aneurysm at the primary division like a candelabra, and the sac is cushioned between the frontal and temporal

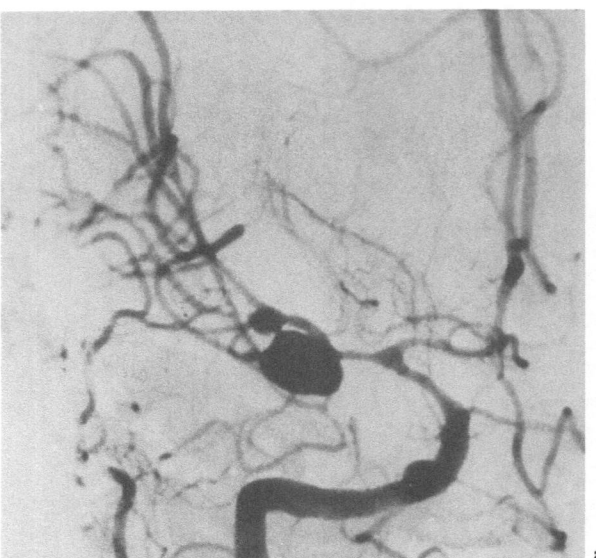 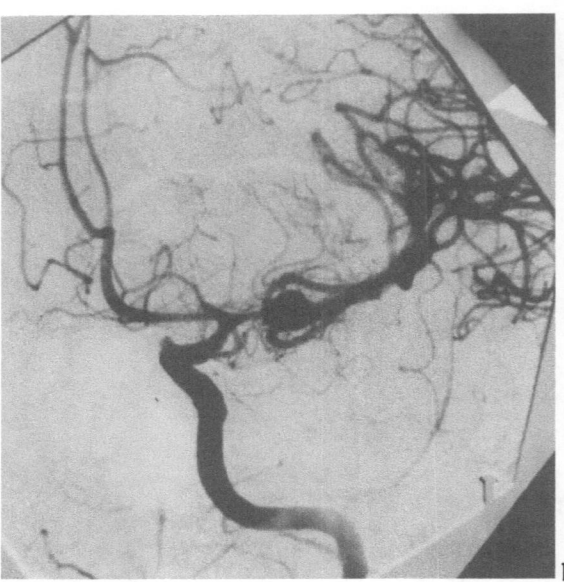

Fig. 10.21. a Right carotid angiogram showing an aneurysm arising from the main trunk of the middle cerebral artery. *Note*: Close proximity of lenticulostriate arteries to the aneurysm. **b** Left carotid angiogram showing an aneurysm arising from an early bifurcation of the middle cerebral artery.

lobes. Because of this confined space, temporal lobe haematomas are classically associated with these aneurysms, especially as the sac often projects laterally. An angiographically recognisable haematoma is usually associated with destruction of part of the temporal lobe (Fig. 10.22).

The configuration of the neck and the size of a large and multilocular sac require careful study before planning a direct surgical approach. Surrounding vessels grip the aneurysm as it grows in size, passing at times in between the loculations. With superimposition of radiopaque shadows in the angiogram, some of these vessels may seem to arise from the sac of the aneurysm itself. In addition to this, with further enlargement of the aneurysm the neck continues to widen until it encroaches upon the origin of one or more of the major branches. Pre-operative angiographic study or initial examination at operation may not distinguish between these two phenomena, and the aneurysm mistakenly be considered unclippable.

It is useful to remember that when these aneurysms bleed during dissection, the flow is not forceful because of their peripheral location in the carotid tree; if hypotensive anaesthesia is used, the bleeding is no more than a trickle. The speech centre lies alongside the sylvian fissure in the dominant left hemisphere.

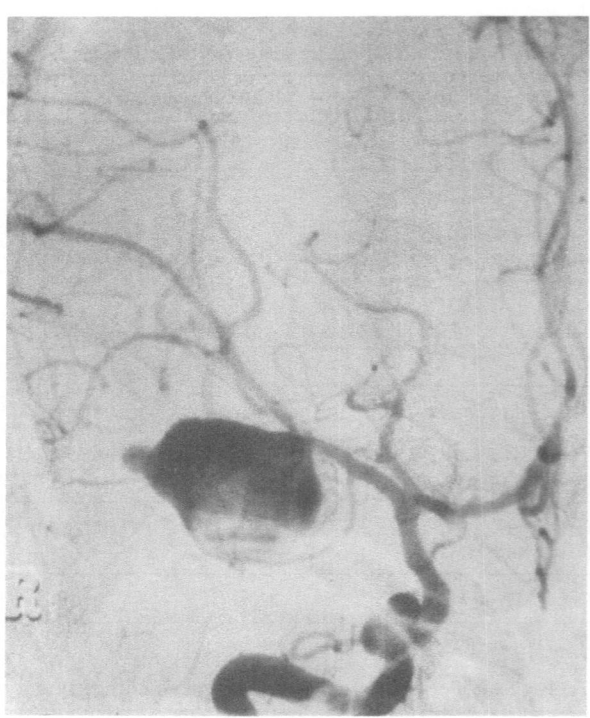

Fig. 10.22. Right carotid angiogram showing a large middle cerebral artery aneurysm. There is elevation of the horizontal part of the middle cerebral artery due to a temporal lobe haematoma.

Approaches to Middle Cerebral Artery Aneurysms

The main considerations in selecting an approach are that the aneurysm should be reached by the shortest route and with the least neuronal damage. Depending upon the circumstances, a middle cerebral artery aneurysm may be approached by one of three routes—(a) subfrontal, (b) sylvian fissure or (c) transtemporal. If the aneurysm arises from the main trunk or from the primary division, with a short proximal segment (M_1), particularly in the dominant side of the brain, the subfrontal route (Fig. 10.23a) is preferred. In most other instances, middle cerebral artery aneurysms are approached through the sylvian fissure (Fig. 10.23b, c). The sylvian fissure approach is particularly suitable if the middle cerebral artery takes a more anterior course, with the aneurysm projecting anteriorly. The transtemporal approach is ideal in the presence of a haematoma or when the aneurysm is situated peripherally. A careful study of the angiogram will afford some guidance.

Results of Treatment

Ninety-nine patients with middle cerebral artery aneurysms have been operated on in this series of 500 cases. Three aneurysms were on the proximal (M_1) section of the middle cerebral artery. There were 49 males and 50 females (Table 10.13). Their ages ranged from the second to the seventh decade, the majority being in the fifth and sixth decades (68%) (Table 10.14). Sixty-four patients were in grades 1 and 2, 27 in grade 3, and 8 in grade 4 at the time of operation (Table 10.15). Forty-nine patients were operated on before the 12th day of the last haemorrhage (Table 10.16).

Of the 99 patients, 17 had postoperative neurological complications. At the time of discharge, 71 patients had a good outcome and six had died (Table 10.17).

Table 10.13. Middle cerebral artery (MCA) aneurysms: sex incidence

	MCA trifurcation	Prox. MCA	Total
Male	48	1	49
Female	48	2	50
	96	3	99

Table 10.14. Middle cerebral artery aneurysms: age incidence

Age (years)	MCA trifurcation	Prox. MCA	Total
10–19	2	–	2
20–29	5	–	5
30–39	21	1	22
40–49	30	1	31
50–59	36	1	37
60–69	2	–	2
	96	3	99

Table 10.15. Middle cerebral artery aneurysms: neurological grade at operation (Hunt and Hess)

Grade	MCA trifurcation	Prox. MCA	Total
I	23	1	24
II	38	2	40
III	27	–	27
IV	8	–	8
V	–	–	–
	96	3	99

Table 10.16. Middle cerebral artery aneurysms: timing of surgery

Days since last SAH	MCA trifurcation	Prox. MCA	Total
0– 4	6	–	6
5– 7	23	1	24
8–11	19	–	19
12–14	15	–	15
15–18	10	1	11
19–21	7	–	7
> 21	16	1	17
	96	3	99

Table 10.17. Middle cerebral artery aneurysms: outcome at discharge

Outcome	MCA trifurcation	Prox. MCA	Total
Good	68	3	71
Fair	21	–	21
Poor	1	–	1
Dead	6	–	6
	96	3	99

Internal Carotid Artery Aneurysms (Posterior Communicating and Anterior Choroidal Aneurysms)

Most of the aneurysms of the internal carotid artery are situated in its supraclinoid part, distal to the origin of the ophthalmic artery. Aneurysms

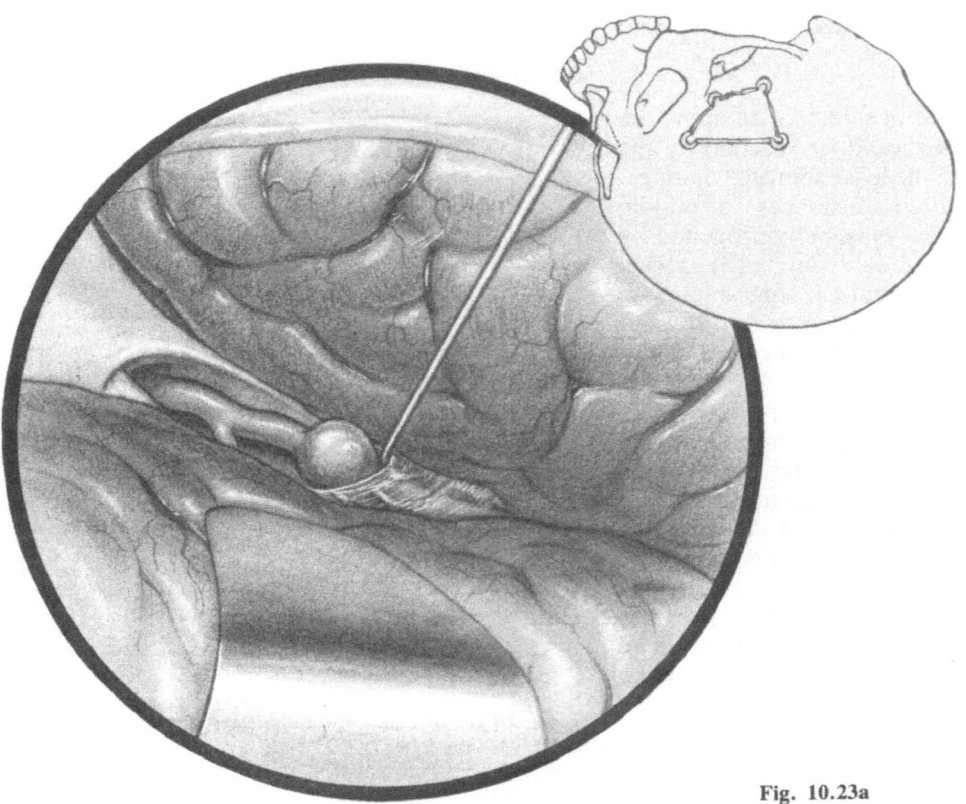

Fig. 10.23a

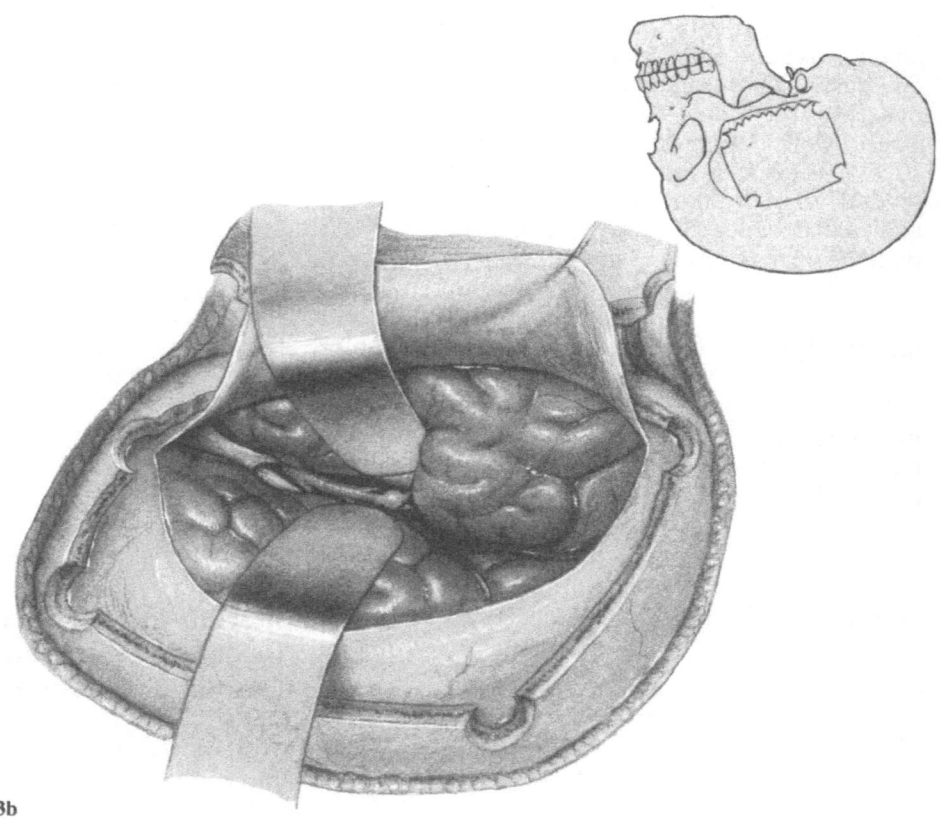

Fig. 10.23b

Fig. 10.23c

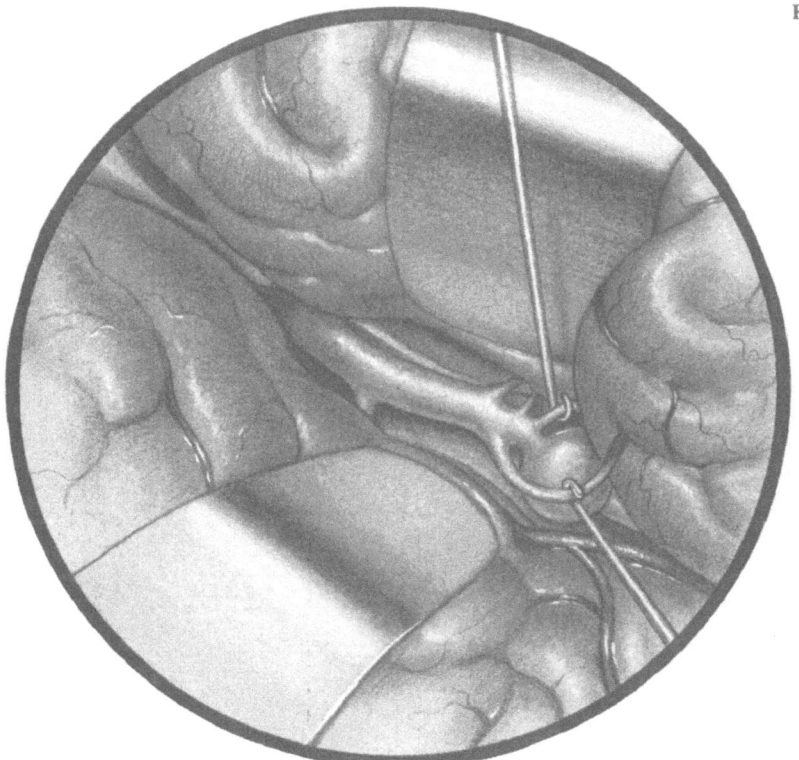

Fig. 10.23. a Middle cerebral artery aneurysm—subfrontal approach to the aneurysm following the internal carotid artery and opening the proximal part of the sylvian fissure. **b** Middle cerebral artery aneurysm in the sylvian fissure after the dissection of the arachnoid. *Note*: With microsurgical approach, total exposure of the sac is usually unnecessary. **c** Dissection of middle cerebral artery aneurysm from surrounding vessels.

in the internal carotid–posterior communicating region account for over 30% of all intracranial aneurysms, whereas the internal carotid–anterior choroidal aneurysms account for no more than 4%. However, there are a few other aneurysms which arise from this part of the internal carotid artery, without having a close relationship with any of its branches. On rare occasions, an aneurysm has been found to arise from the origin of an aberrant middle cerebral artery. The principles of surgical treatment in all these aneurysms are essentially similar, and will be described together (Fig. 10.24).

Anatomical and Physiological Considerations

These aneurysms are considered to be technically easy to obliterate by direct surgery. Yet postoperative cerebral infarction and death following a smooth, short operation, without any difficulty or encroachment of a major vessel, have occurred from time to time. Surgical occlusion of the posterior communicating artery or the anterior

choroidal artery is considered by some to be responsible, yet we have seen a similar problem even when the arteries were carefully protected. It has been previously mentioned that patients with an anomalous origin of the posterior cerebral artery are particularly vulnerable to the generally recognised adverse factors.

Embryological studies of the circle of Willis show that a large posterior communicating artery continues to depend on the internal carotid artery for its blood supply. Kirgis et al. (1960) have shown that an inverse relationship consistently exists between the posterior branch of the internal carotid artery (posterior communicating artery) in the circle of Willis and the adjacent posterior cerebral segment (proximal posterior cerebral artery) of the circle. When a primitive posterior cerebral artery showing as a large posterior communicating artery is demonstrated by carotid angiography, it can be found that the divisional branch of the basilar artery is hypoplastic (Fig. 10.25). When such a primitive posterior cerebral artery is occluded, the whole territory supplied by a normal posterior cerebral artery will

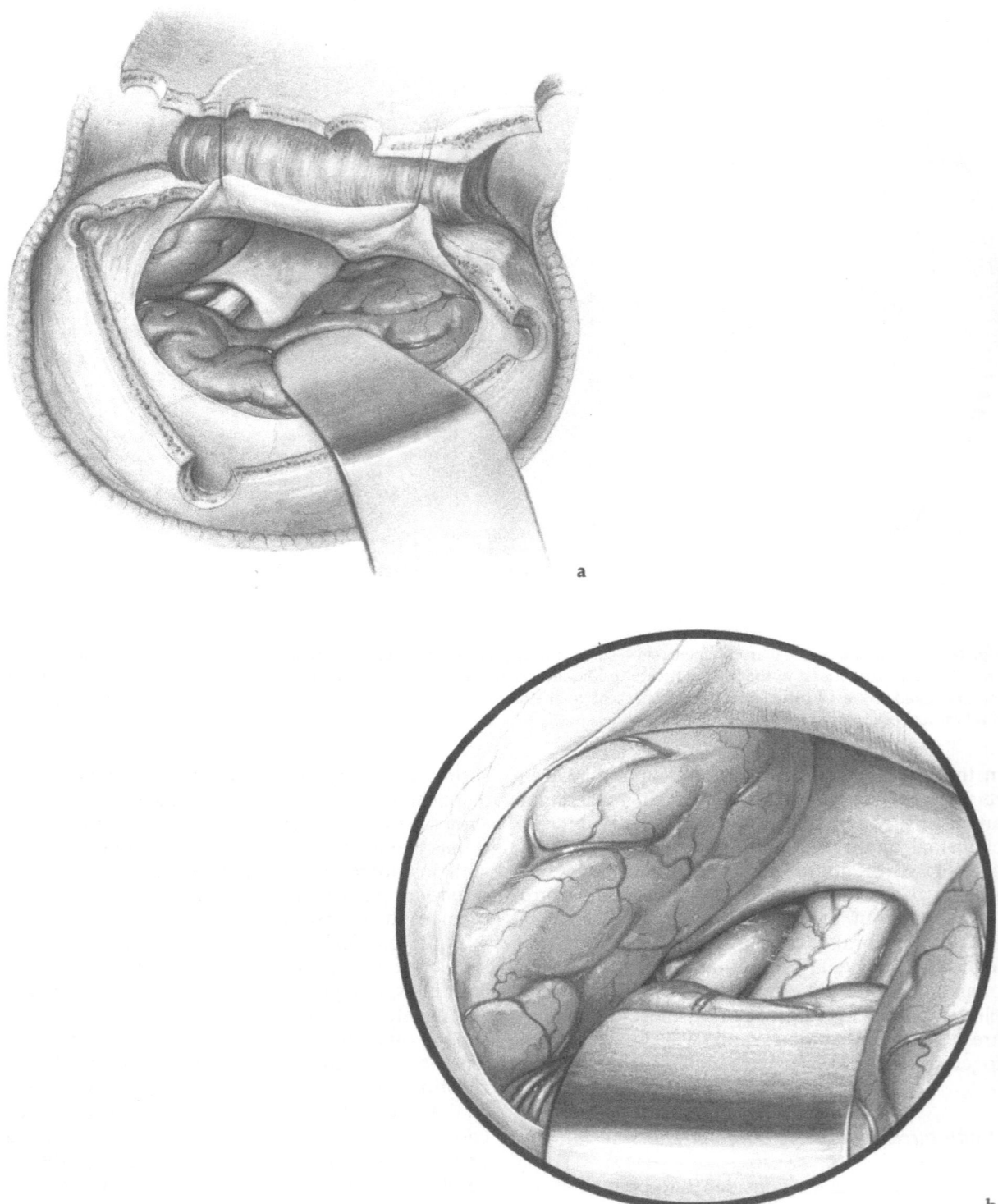

a

b

Fig. 10.24. a Subfrontal approach to aneurysm of the left internal carotid artery. Optic nerve and the internal carotid are exposed. In this illustration there is far greater retraction and exposure of the brain than is normally required in microsurgery. **b** Exposure as seen through the operating microscope. **c** Exposure of internal carotid artery showing the posterior communicating artery aneurysm. The arachnoid is demonstrated with a hook (in practice the arachnoid is divided with micro-scissors). **d** The aneurysm occluded with a spring clip.

Fig. 10.24c

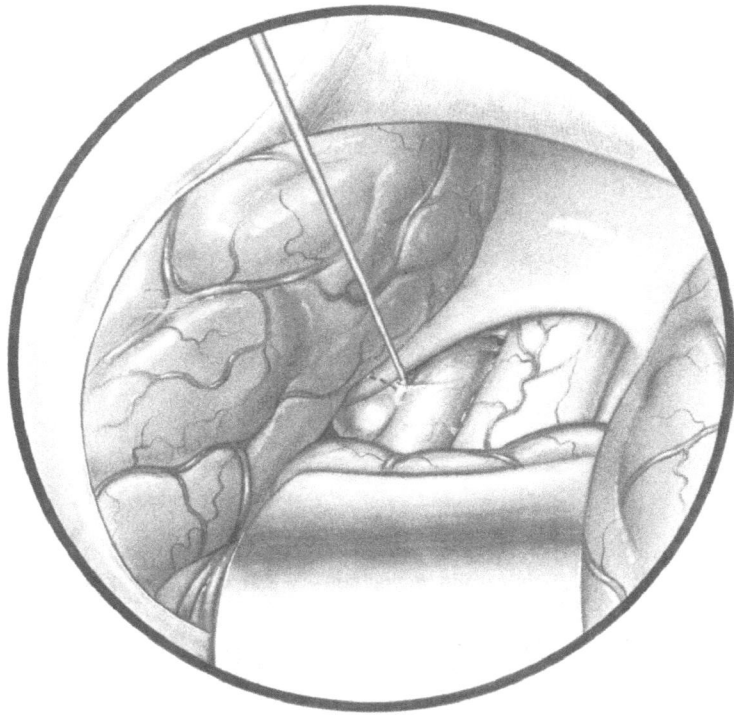

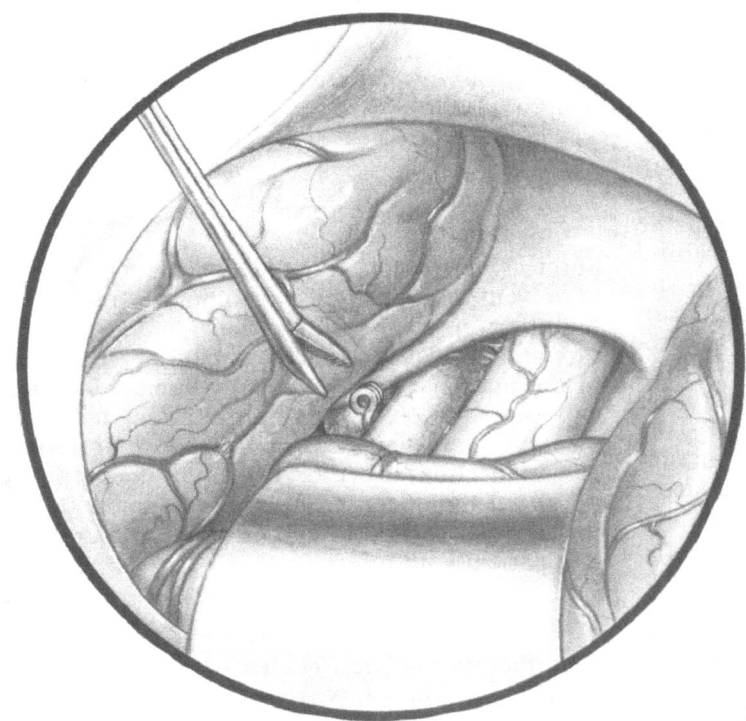

Fig. 10.24d

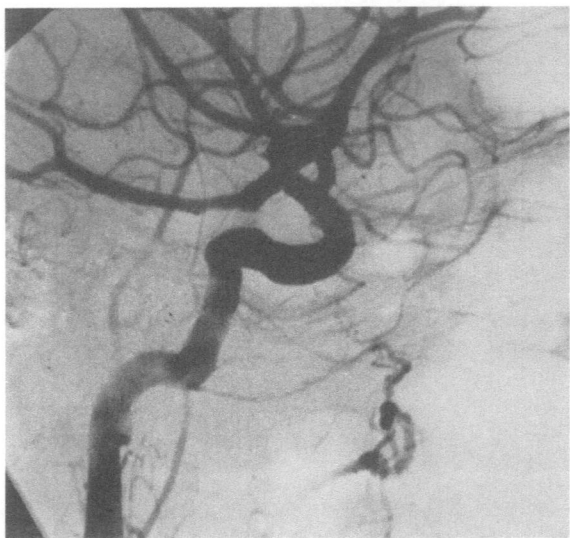 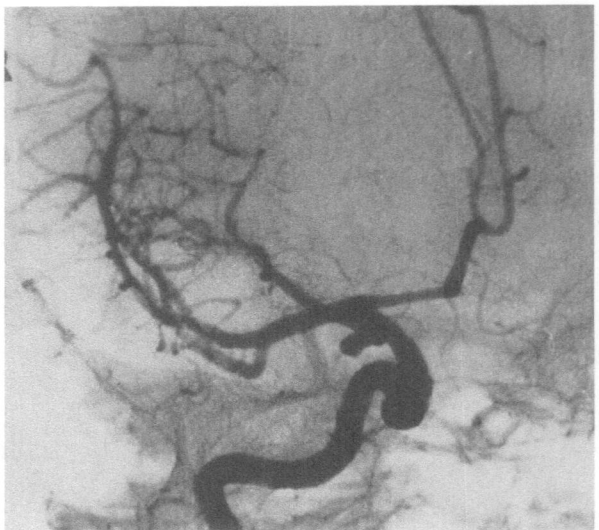

Fig. 10.25. a, b. Right carotid angiogram—lateral and Townes oblique projections showing a posterior communicating artery aneurysm and a foetal posterior cerebral artery.

be affected. However, in the case of a tiny normal posterior communicating artery, its territory will still be nourished by the blood from the posterior circulation, through the posterior cerebral artery. The presence of a primitive posterior cerebral artery in patients with generalised vasospasm creates a more complicated situation. When the internal carotid artery and its branches go into spasm, the ipsilateral cerebral hemisphere tries to maintain its essential blood supply through the collateral circulation from the opposite carotid system by the anterior communicating artery and the vertebrobasilar system via the cortical anastomosis between the branches of the middle cerebral and posterior cerebral arteries. When the primitive posterior cerebral artery goes into spasm along with the internal carotid artery, the collateral circulation through the cortical anastomosis from the vertebrobasilar system is reduced. Associated spasm or hypoplasia of the proximal part of the anterior cerebral artery will isolate the hemisphere from the opposite carotid system as well. If the flow across the anterior communicating artery is defective, due to a congenital anomaly, the consequences will be similar. The two cases illustrated in Figs. 10.26 and 10.27 show the significance of severe vasospasm in patients with normal and foetal posterior cerebral arteries.

There is a constant anastomosis of the anterior choroidal artery with the posterior choroidal artery at the level of the lateral geniculate ganglion. In a patient with a normal circle, occlusion

of the anterior choroidal artery with the aneurysmal neck produces a less deleterious effect. Occasionally, there may be an anomalous or accessory middle cerebral artery from this region which gives its blood supply to the anterior part of the temporal lobe.

Principles of the Surgical Approach

Surgical approach to these aneurysms should aim at prevention of vasospasm by minimal trauma to the artery, prevention of an intra-operative rupture and avoidance of encroachment of the lumen of the internal carotid artery by kinking or by a clip. A foetal posterior cerebral artery must be preserved. A diligent search for a small posterior communicating artery or the anterior choroidal artery, at the expense of undue manipulation of the internal carotid artery, is counterproductive in a patient with a recent SAH.

Identification of the Problems Which May Be Encountered at Surgery

From careful examination of the pre-operative angiograms, a surgical strategy should be devised; for this purpose, a Townes and a lateral view of the angiogram will give the following information.

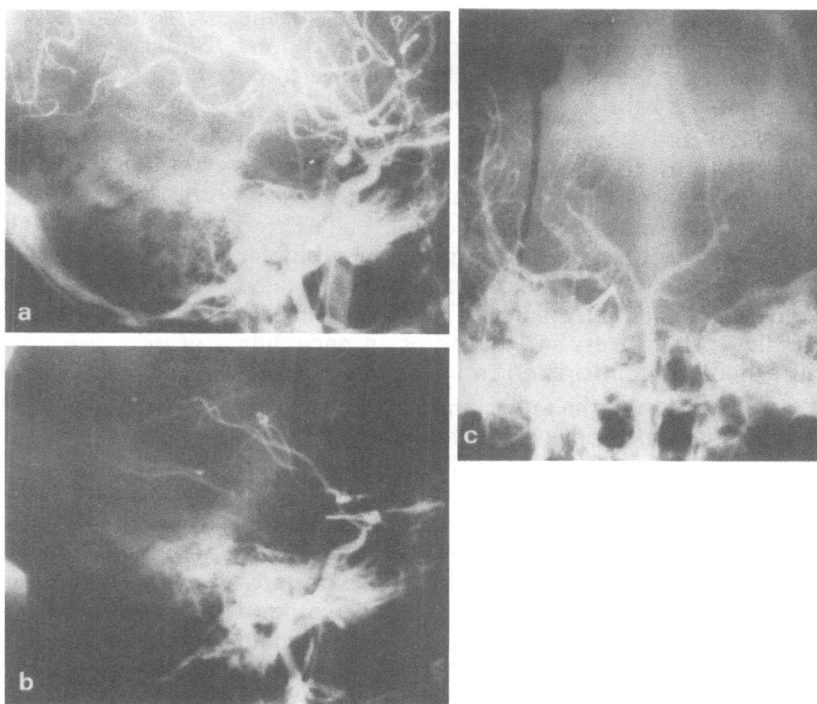

Fig. 10.26. a Right lateral carotid angiogram (pre-operative) in a 27-year-old housewife showing a posterior communicating artery aneurysm. Note absence of foetal circulation from internal carotid artery. **b** Right lateral carotid angiogram (postoperative) showing satisfactory occlusion of the aneurysm. There is marked spasm of the vessels and the posterior communicating artery is faintly outlined. **c** Carotid angiogram AP projection showing severe spasm of the carotid artery. Retrograde filling of the basilar and both posterior cerebral arteries can also be seen in this angiogram. In spite of severe spasm this patient showed no neuroligical deficit.

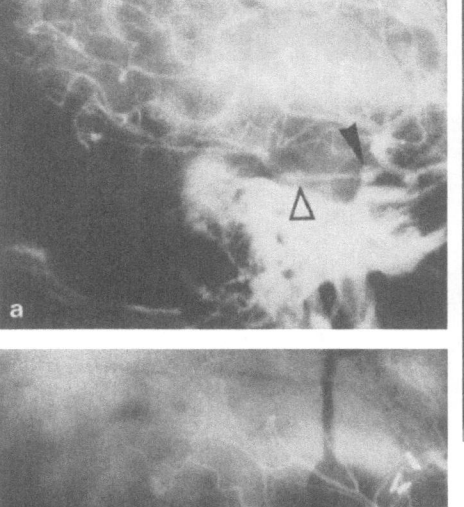

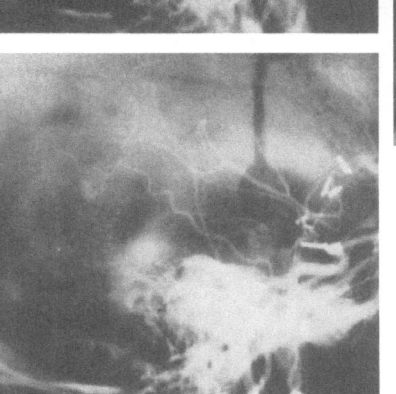

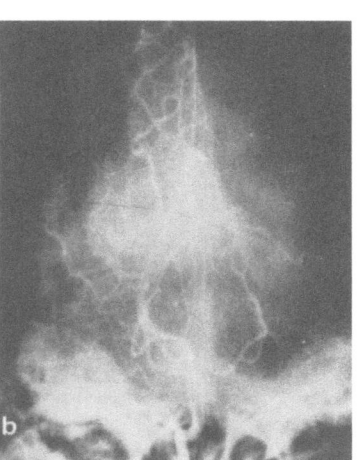

Fig. 10.27. a Lateral carotid angiogram (pre-operative) in a 40-year-old housewife showing posterior communicating artery aneurysm (*black arrowhead*) with a foetal posterior cerebral artery (*open arrowhead*). **b** Vertebral angiogram (pre-operative) showing non-filling of the posterior cerebral artery due to hypoplasia. **c** Lateral carotid angiogram (postoperative) showing occlusion of the aneurysm, but there is severe spasm of the vessels, including the foetal posterior cerebral artery. The patent died of massive infarction, confirmed at autopsy.

1. When the aneurysm is very close to the anterior clinoid process, removal of this bony obstacle from the path of the clip will have to be undertaken by the use of a dental drill.

2. Size and shape of the aneurysm: Small aneurysms in this region are notoriously thin walled, and even gentle manipulation may cause a tear with fearsome haemorrhage. A broad necked aneurysm can rarely be made smaller by bipolar coagulation without the risk of rupture. The need for obliteration of an aneurysm by placing the clip parallel to the artery, or by use of an encircling clip, should be anticipated from the angiograms.

3. Projection of the aneurysm: If the aneurysm is projecting posteriorly, its shadow will be completely overlapped by that of the internal carotid artery in the Townes view. With this projection, the aneurysm lies beneath the edge of the tentorium, and usually free from the temporal lobe. Most of the aneurysms, however, project postero-laterally, and may be adherent to the temporal lobe and/or the tentorium (Fig. 10.28). When an aneurysm projects medially or upwards, it may become adherent to the frontal lobe or the optic nerve, and retraction of the frontal lobe at the commencement of the exploration may cause premature rupture of the aneurysm.

4. Course of the internal carotid artery: In elderly or hypertensive patients, the internal carotid artery takes an unusually lateral course. The approach to the aneurysms arising from such an artery is difficult, and retraction of the temporal lobe is necessary.

5. Presence of foetal posterior cerebral artery (Fig. 10.29): The presence of a foetal posterior cerebral artery increases the risk of surgery, and preservation of the artery is essential. When the posterior communicating and anterior choroidal arteries are not visualised in the angiogram, excessive dissection to identify them is not necessary, as discussed previously.

Results of Treatment

One hundred and thirty-eight patients with internal carotid artery aneurysms were operated on in this series. One hundred and sixteen had aneurysms on the posterior communicating artery, ten had aneurysms on the anterior choroidal artery, and in 12, the aneurysms were classified as non-specific. Their ages varied from the second to the eighth decade, the majority being in the fifth and sixth decades (61%) (Table

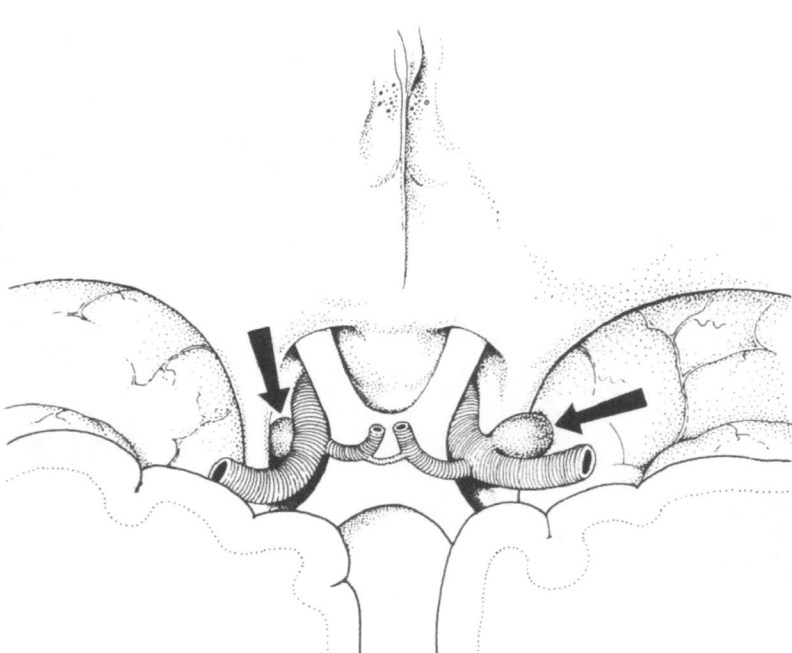

Fig. 10.28. Projections of the posterior communicating artery aneurysm. On the right, the aneurysm is above the tentorium, and adherent to the temporal lobe. On the left, the aneurysm lies medial to the tentorium and free from the temporal lobe.

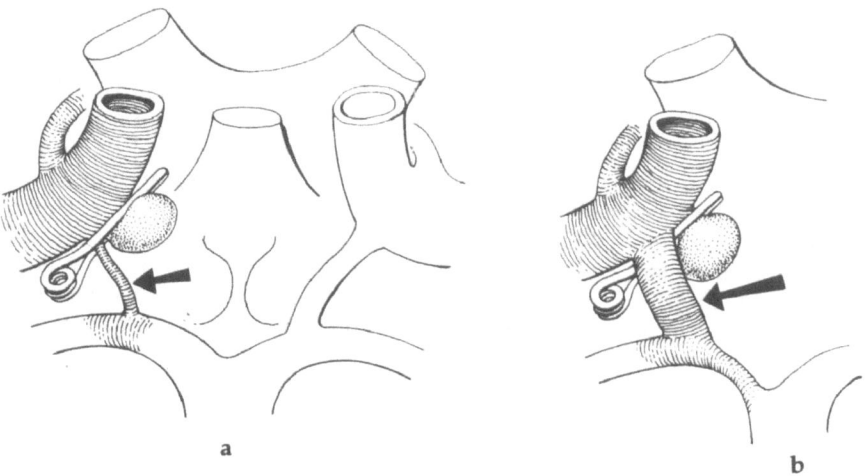

a   b

Fig. 10.29. a Small posterior communicating artery may be occluded along with the neck of the aneurysm if necessary. **b** A large posterior communicating artery (foetal posterior cerebral artery) must be preserved.

10.18). There were 38 males and 100 females. (Table 10.19). Forty-four patients were in grade 1, 66 in grade 2, 26 in grade 3, and 2 in grade 4 (Table 10.20). Eighty-four patients were operated on before the 12th day of the last haemorrhage (Table 10.21).

Of the 138 patients, 36 (26%) had postoperative neurological complications. One hundred and three patients had a good outcome and 11 patients (8%) died (Table 10.22).

Table 10.18. Internal carotid artery aneurysms: age incidence

Age (years)	Post. comm. a.	Ant. choroidal	Non-specific	Total
10–19	1	–	–	1
20–29	13	1	1	15
30–39	10	2	3	15
40–49	25	5	5	35
50–59	46	2	2	50
60–69	18	–	1	19
70–79	3	–	–	3
	116	10	12	138

Table 10.19. Internal carotid artery aneurysms: sex incidence

	Post. comm. a	Ant. choroidal	Non-specific	Total
Male	29	6	3	38
Female	87	4	9	100
	116	10	12	138

Table 10.20. Internal carotid artery aneurysms: neurological condition at operation (Hunt and Hess)

Grade	Post. comm. a.	Ant. choroidal	Non-specific	Total
I	39	1	4	44
II	58	5	3	66
III	17	4	5	26
IV	2	–	–	2
V	–	–	–	–
	116	10	12	138

Table 10.21. Internal carotid artery aneurysms: timing of surgery

Days since last SAH	Post. comm. a.	Ant. choroidal	Non-specific	Total
0– 4	16	–	3	19
5– 7	29	4	1	34
8–11	24	1	6	31
12–14	19	–	1	20
15–18	7	2	1	10
19–21	5	–	–	5
> 21	16	3	–	19
	116	10	12	138

Table 10.22. Internal carotid artery aneurysms: outcome at discharge

Outcome	Post. comm. a.	Ant. choroidal	Non-specific	Total
Good	86	8	9	103
Fair	17	–	2	19
Poor	5	–	–	5
Dead	8	2	1	11
	116	10	12	138

Internal Carotid Bifurcation Aneurysms

Anatomical and Physiological Considerations

Aneurysms in the region of the internal carotid bifurcation rarely arise from the tip of the bifurcation itself. Usually the neck involves one of the divisions of the internal carotid artery, and the sac is often closely adherent to either the anterior cerebral or the middle cerebral artery. Occasionally, the attachment of the neck is linear to the major vessel involved. Because of this, obliteration of the aneurysm without encroaching on the lumen of the parent artery is difficult. Although pre-operative angiography does not always define the neck clearly, it will often indicate the vessel which is contributing most to the formation of the neck (Fig. 10.30). Without this information, a search for the neck may lead to inadvertent rupture of the sac. Although there are no perforating vessels at the bifurcation itself, they may arise from the proximal part of the anterior cerebral or the middle cerebral artery, and supply the basal ganglia and other deep structures. These arteries often invest the sac of the aneurysm, and some of them may remain hidden from the surgeon's view behind the aneurysm.

It is essential to appreciate that the bifurcation point of the internal carotid artery is the deepest part of the anterior half of the circle of Willis. Surgical exposures of the aneurysm may, therefore, require considerable retraction of the brain.

Unlike aneurysms at the posterior communicating or anterior communicating regions, aneurysms at the carotid bifurcation are rarely associated with anomalies of the circle of Willis. Due to a good cross circulation between the hemispheres, development of postoperative ischaemia is unusual after satisfactory surgical obliteration.

Results of Treatment

Thirty-two patients with internal carotid bifurcation aneurysms were operated on in this series. Their ages varied from the second to the eighth decade (Table 10.23). There were 11 males and 21 females (Table 10.24). Nine patients were in grade 1, 17 in grade 2 and six in grade 3 at the

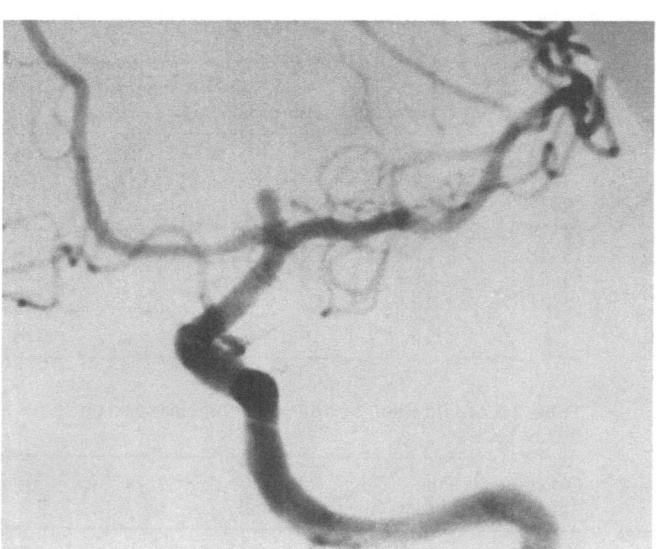
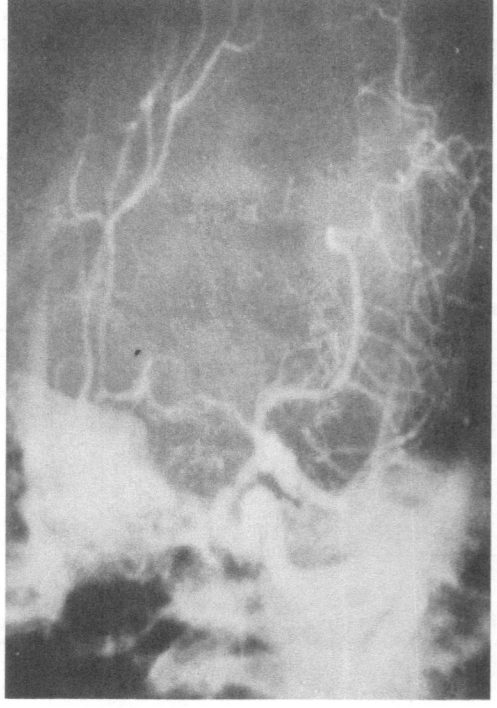

Fig. 10.30. a Carotid angiogram AP projection showing an internal carotid artery bifurcation aneurysm, in which the neck arises at the junction of the internal carotid and the anterior cerebral artery. b Carotid angiogram AP projection showing the internal carotid artery bifurcation aneurysm in which the neck arises at the junction of the internal carotid artery and the middle cerebral artery.

Table 10.23. Internal carotid bifurcation aneurysms: age incidence

Age (years)	10–19	20–29	30–39	40–49	50–59	60–69	70–79	Total
	5	2	3	9	9	3	1	32

Table 10.24. Internal carotid bifurcation aneurysms: sex incidence

Male	11 (34%)
Female	21 (66%)
	32

Table 10.25. Internal carotid bifurcation aneurysms: neurological grade at operation (Hunt and Hess)

I	II	III	IV	V	Total
9	17	6	–	–	32

Table 10.26. Internal carotid bifurcation aneurysms: timing of surgery

Days since last SAH	0–4	5–7	8–11	12–14	15–18	19–21	> 21
	7	7	7	1	3	1	6

Table 10.27. Internal carotid bifurcation aneurysms: outcome at discharge

Outcome	Good	Fair	Poor	Dead	Total
	25	5	1	1	32

time of operation (Table 10.25). Twenty-one patients (65%) were operated on before the 12th day of the last haemorrhage (Table 10.26).

Of the 32 patients, six (19%) developed postoperative ischaemic neurological complications. Twenty-five patients (78%) had a good outcome and one patient died (Table 10.27).

Carotid Ophthalmic Aneurysms

Aneurysms in the region of the ophthalmic artery require special attention for their surgical treatment. Arising from the most proximal part of the intracranial internal carotid artery, they are in close relation to the cavernous sinus, the optic nerve and the anterior clinoid process. Direct surgical obliteration of these aneurysms produces problems which can only be avoided by the experience and skill of the surgeon, and more significantly, by adapting the most pragmatic line of treatment to obtain maximum benefit from surgery with minimum neurological and visual deficit. These aneurysms have an unusual natural history and morphological features, which influence the surgical treatment considerably.

Natural History

Intracranial aneurysms, at all locations, are grouped together as one entity as far as the natural history is concerned. However, carotid ophthalmic aneurysms differ from the rest in a significant way, and the unusual features of these aneurysms should be recognised when considering surgery. All patients with carotid ophthalmic aneurysms admitted under the care of one of the authors between 1970 and 1982 were analysed in a separate study; this included the 24 cases which formed part of the 500 cases analysed in detail. The cases included both symptomatic and incidental aneurysms. Forty-nine patients were found to have one or more carotid ophthalmic aneurysms, making a total of 62. There were 22 patients with a single symptomatic carotid ophthalmic aneurysm only. In the other 27 patients, there were 40 carotid ophthalmic aneurysms and 36 other aneurysms, making a total of 98 aneurysms (Table 10.28). We have also noted a significant number of bilateral carotid ophthalmic aneurysms.

Multiplicity. From the management viewpoint, this factor is very important. It is generally recognised that the incidence of multiple aneurysms is

Table 10.28 Carotid ophthalmic aneurysms: multiplicity

No. of aneurysms	No. of patients	C. ophthalmic aneurysms	Others	Total
One	22	22	0	22
Two	13	18	8	26
Three	9	13	14	27
Four	2	3	5	8
Five	3	6	9	15
	49	62	36	98

about 20%. With carotid ophthalmic aneurysms, however, we have found it to be as high as 55% (Table 10.29).

Table 10.29. Carotid ophthalmic aneurysms: single versus multiple

	No. of patients
Single aneurysm	22 (45%)
Multiple aneurysms	27 (55%)

Lack of Tendency to Rupture. Although SAH can occur from carotid ophthalmic aneurysms, a considerable number of these aneurysms are discovered incidentally. Of 40 carotid ophthalmic aneurysms in the multiple aneurysm group, shown in Table 10.30, only ten caused SAH, whereas aneurysms in other regions, particularly in the posterior circulation, were more frequently responsible for SAH. In other words, in the presence of multiple aneurysms, carotid ophthalmic aneurysms are often incidental, and the offending lesion may be missed if it is not carefully searched for.

Table 10.30. Carotid ophthalmic aneurysms: lack of tendency to rupture when associated with other aneurysms

	No. of aneurysms	SAH	%
C. ophth.	40	10	25
MCA	14	3	21
Ant. comm. a.	8	2	25
Post. comm. a.	7	1	14
Basilar tip	2	2	100
PICA	2	2	100
ICA tip	2	2[a]	100
Perical	1	1	100

[a] One patient had an SAH 25 years previously.

Left-Sided Occurrence. It is of some significance that these aneurysms arise predominantly from the left internal carotid artery. Surgical therapy must ensure protection of the dominant side of the brain.

Sex Preponderance. It is a common experience that in women some aneurysms are more prevalent than others. It is fascinating that our experience reveals carotid ophthalmic aneurysms to be six times more common in women than in men (Table 10.31). Analysis of the data from the co-operative study (Locksley 1966) reveals the interesting but generally unrecognised fact that the female preponderance grows progressively as the aneurysmal origin is traced proximally towards the heart (Fig. 10.31).

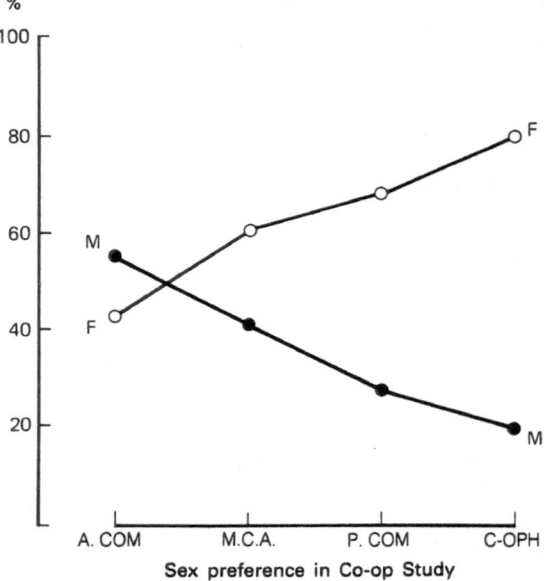

Fig. 10.31. Graph adopted from the figures from the Co-operative Study, illustrating the different incidence in the site of aneurysms in male and female.

Table 10.31. Carotid ophthalmic aneurysms: sex incidence

Male	7 (14%)
Female	42 (86%)
	49

Morphological Characteristics

The morphological features of carotid ophthalmic aneurysms explain the hazards of direct surgery. Because of its unique location, a carotid ophthalmic aneurysm shows specific features in its neck, wall of the sac and lumen. These features should be well understood to avoid serious problems during surgery.

Neck. A neat, pear-shaped aneurysm with a narrow neck is uncommon in this region. The aneurysm is attached to the carotid artery by a broad origin, and constriction produced by the radiolucent clinoid process gives a false impression of a neck. The neck may be hidden by the optic nerve and the clinoid process. In some cases, a part of the neck may be within the cavernous sinus. Furthermore, the aneurysm may be a blow-out of the carotid artery, without having a neck (Fig. 10.32).

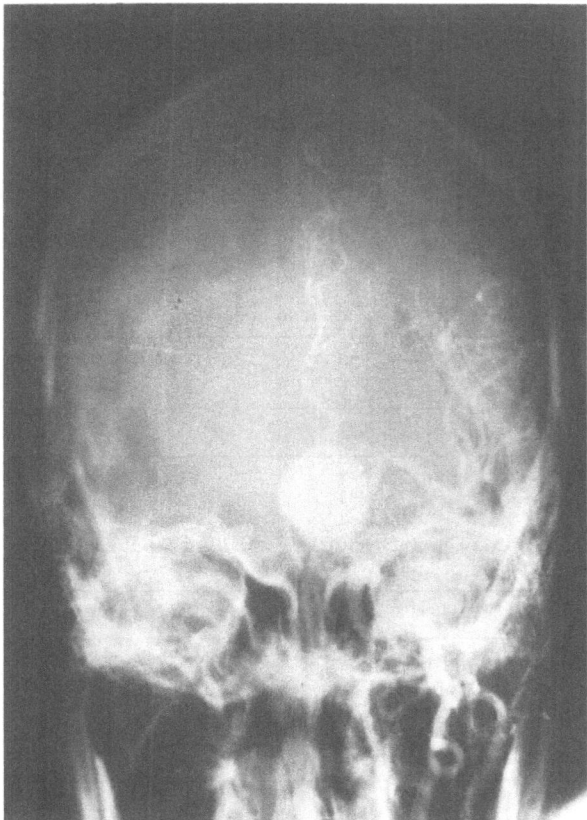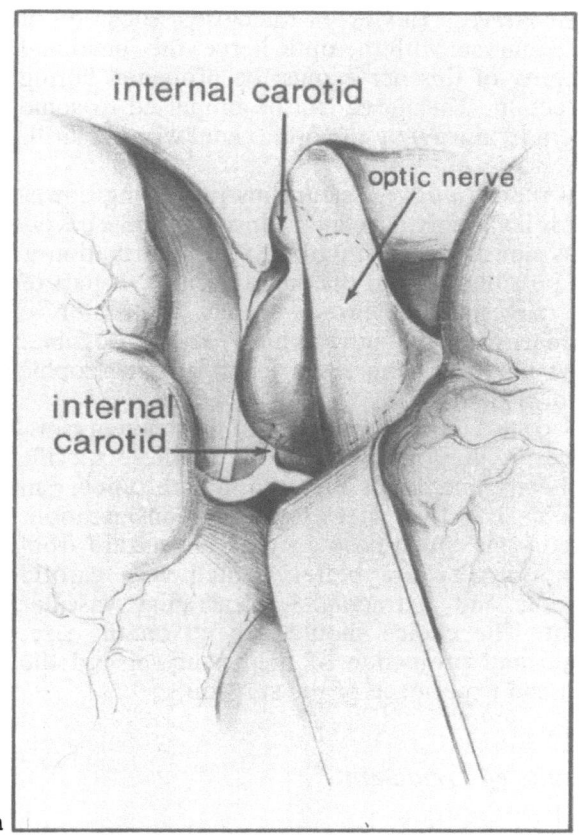

Fig. 10.32. a Left carotid angiogram showing a large carotid ophthalmic aneurysm. **b** Operative diagram of the same, indicating that the aneurysm is a blow-out of the carotid artery.

Wall of the Sac. The wall of the sac of a carotid ophthalmic aneurysms is extremely variable. It is often extremely thin and at some places thick with atheroma. In a large aneurysm, it is often anchored to the surrounding dura with fibrous strands, and devoid of elastic tissue. It cannot be shrunk by bipolar coagulation and is often prone to rupture during application of a clip. The ophthalmic artery may be closely adherent to the wall of the sac.

Lumen. Blood pressure within the lumen is very close to that in the carotid artery itself; hence intraluminal thrombus does not usually form, even in a large aneurysm in this location, as it occurs in middle cerebral artery aneurysms. Because of this flow phenomenon, bleeding from the aneurysm is extremely severe.

Problems Encountered at Direct Surgery

Torrential Bleeding. Bleeding is profuse if these aneurysms rupture during dissection, and, since one has no access to the carotid proximal to the aneurysm, it is difficult to control. The sac of an aneurysm projecting upwards may remain adherent to the frontal lobe and may give way during retraction of the lobe at the commencement of the exploration. In spite of temporary occlusion of the internal carotid artery in the neck, the aneurysm fills through the ophthalmic artery from the external carotid circulation. The external carotid artery should also be included for temporary occlusion in a difficult aneurysm.

Anterior Clinoid Process. Problems caused by this bony obstacle during dissection and clipping may not be obvious on the angiogram. The anterior clinoid process itself allows the neck of the aneurysm to appear narrow and clippable, but in its proximal side the neck may be firmly adherent to the clinoid process. The clinoid process can be drilled away with a high-speed drill, but the risk of premature rupture should be borne in mind.

Optic Nerve. In view of the close association of the aneurysm with the optic nerve, the functional integrity of this nerve must be protected during dissection. The nerve can be mobilised to some extent by unroofing the optic canal with the drill.

Cavernous Sinus. Aneurysms projecting downwards invariably have an extension into the cavernous sinus. In this situation, total obliteration is not possible without opening the sinus. If part of the neck appears intracavernous, it is safer to occlude only the intracranial part, if possible, since a tear in the sinus leads to catastrophic problems.

A considerable proportion of these aneurysms, however, may not present any of these specific problems, and direct obliteration of the aneurysm should be the first line of consideration. Aneurysms which pose a significant hazard from direct surgery are better treated with carotid ligation and extracranial–intracranial vascular shunt. The choice should depend on the size, shape and projection of the aneurysm and the skill and experience of the surgeon.

Results of Treatment

Because of unusual morphological features, the method of treatment for these aneurysms has been variable (Table 10.32). Of the 49 patients, 37 had symptomatic aneurysm and were treated surgically (Table 10.34). During the early seventies, we carried out elective cervical carotid ligation in four patients in whom direct surgery was considered hazardous. In seven patients complete occlusion was not feasible at surgery and so the aneurysm was either partially clipped or wrapped with muslin, and carotid ligation carried out at a later date. In four other patients rupture of aneurysm at surgery required trapping, by both extra- and intracranial internal carotid ligation. In only 14 patients was satisfactory clipping possible. In recent years, where direct surgery was deemed difficult we combined carotid ligation with simul-

Table 10.32. Carotid ophthalmic aneurysms: surgical procedures (*n* = 37)

	No.
Primary cervical carotid ligation	4
Craniotomy partial clip or wrap followed by carotid ligation	7
Forced trapping	4
Clip	14
Carotid ligation + EC/IC shunt	8

taneous extracranial–intracranial anastomosis. Eight patients were treated with this combined approach. The age incidence is shown in Table 10.33.

The outcome in relation to the method of treatment is shown in Table 10.34. There was one death, three patients had a poor outcome, but 30 patients did well.

Table 10.33. Carotid-ophthalmic aneurysms: age incidence

Age (years)	10–19	20–29	30–39	40–49	50–59	60–69	Total
	1	3	7	16	19	3	49

Table 10.34. Carotid ophthalmic aneurysms: outcome versus method of procedure

	Good	Fair	Poor	Dead
Primary carotid ligation	4	–	–	–
Secondary carotid ligation	6	1	–	–
Forced trapping	–	1	2	1
Clip	12	1	1	–
Carotid ligation EC/IC	8	–	–	–

Aneurysms of the Posterior Circulation

The incidence of aneurysms in the posterior circulation is fortunately less, since direct surgical treatment is indeed difficult. The natural history of a ruptured posterior circulation aneurysm is no less gloomy than that of a ruptured aneurysm in the anterior circulation.

Special Problems

1. Lying deep in front of the brain stem or posterior fossa, these aneurysms pose considerable problems of access.
2. Posterior circulation contributes blood supply to the brain stem, hypothalamus and other vital structures of the brain. Manipulation of these vessels during surgery may lead to profound disturbances of these structures.
3. During dissection or clipping of the aneurysms, temporary proximal control is not always possible.
4. Significantly, the low incidence of these aneurysms does not give adequate experience to any individual surgeon in dealing with them.

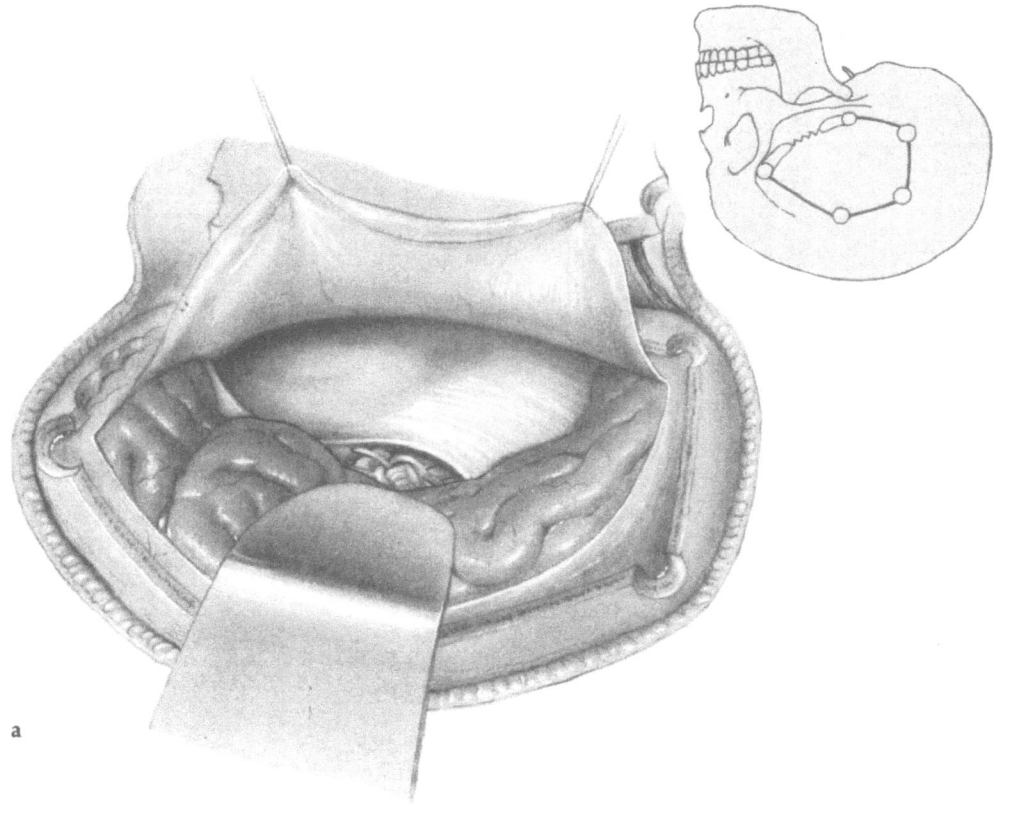

a

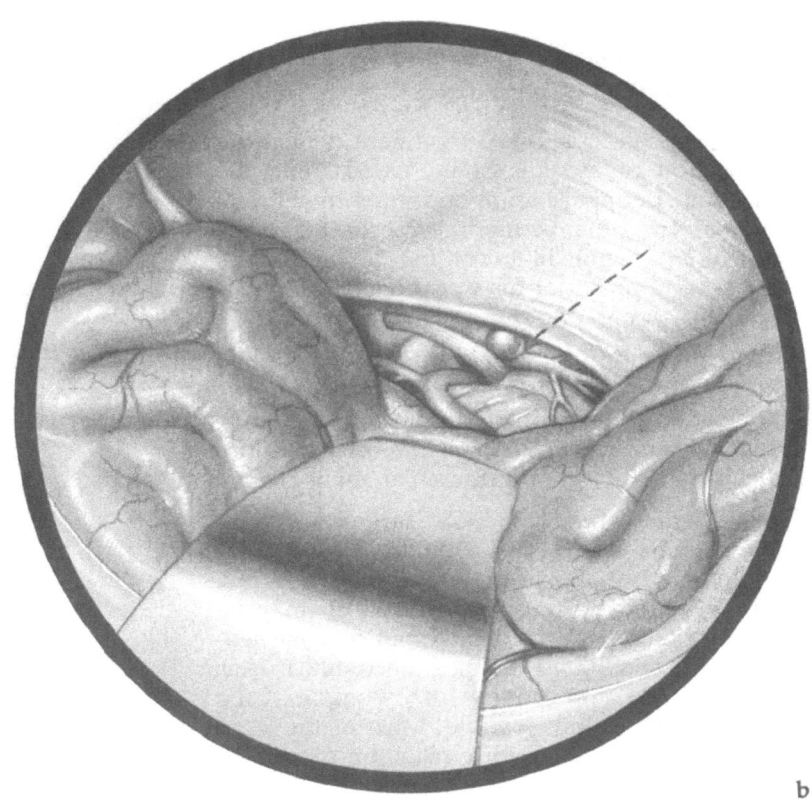

Fig. 10.33. a Subtemporal approach
to basilar-superior cerebellar
aneurysm, showing the tentorial edge
and cisterna ambiens. *Inset*: position
of craniotomy. **b** Further dissection in
the cisterna ambiens exposes the third
nerve and the posterior cerebral and
superior cerebellar arteries. Note the
location of the aneurysm at the origin
of the superior cerebellar artery. The
basilar artery is not visualised. *Broken
line* indicates the division of the
tentorium to expose the aneurysm of
the basilar trunk. **c** After division of
the tentorium, structures in the
posterior fossa, including the fourth
and fifth nerves and cerebellum, can
be seen. Note that only part of the
basilar trunk will be seen from this
viewpoint.

Fig. 10.33c *overleaf*

b

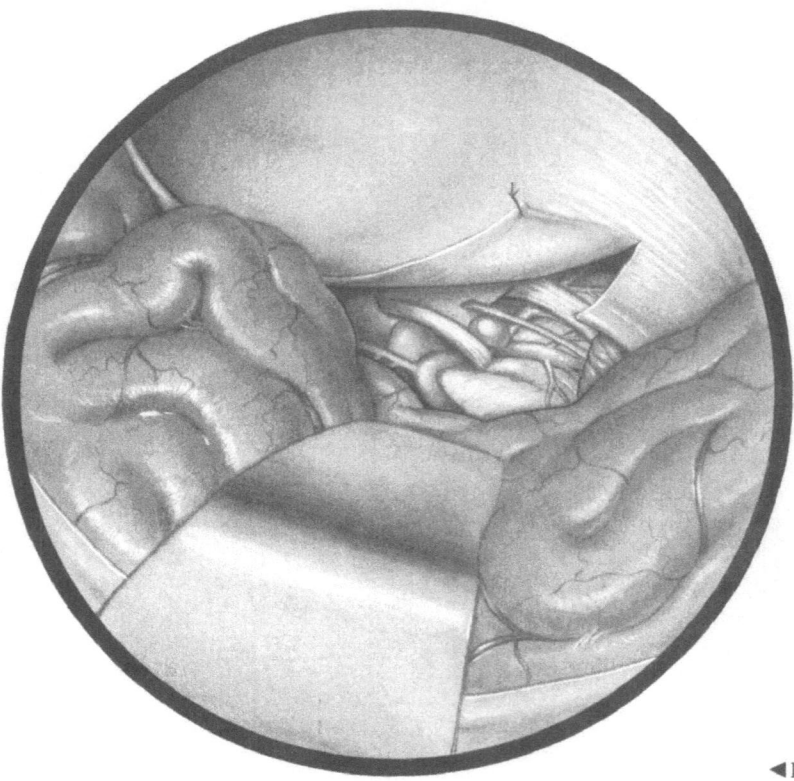

◀ Fig. 10.33c

Factors Influencing Direct Surgical Treatment

Problems in direct surgical treatment depend on the location of the aneurysm, its size and the projection. In upper basilar and superior cerebellar aneurysms, a subtemporal approach is used (Fig. 10.33), while in lower basilar and PICA aneurysms, a posterior fossa approach is applied.

Location of the Aneurysm. Aneurysms at the basilar bifurcation and the vertebrobasilar junction are the most difficult to obliterate. On the other hand, aneurysms of the posterior inferior cerebellar artery (PICA) region are no more difficult than any other intracranial aneurysm.

Size of the Aneurysm. A large or giant aneurysm in the posterior circulation is very difficult to obliterate by direct surgery. Apart from a large vertebral artery aneurysm, which may be satisfactorily treated with proximal arterial ligation, these aneurysms are not amenable to this method. The procedure of wrapping the aneurysms is also not feasible. Most of the large aneurysms in the posterior circulation present as mass lesions, rather than with SAH.

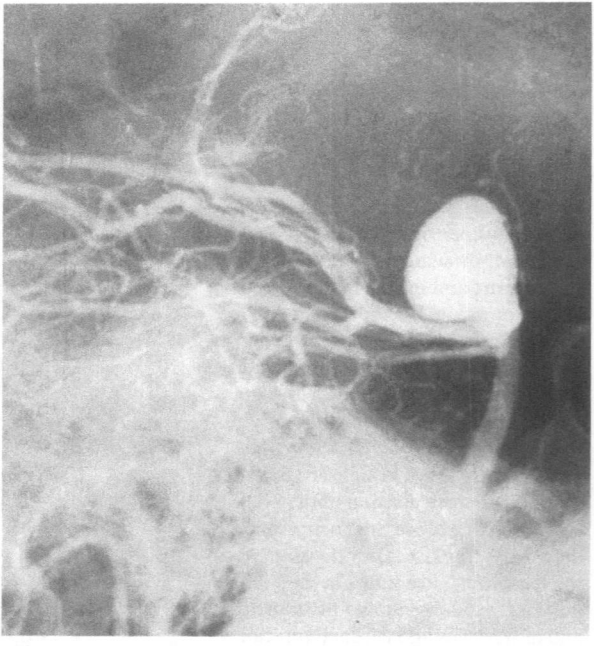

Fig. 10.34. Lateral vertebral angiogram showing basilar bifurcation aneurysm projecting posteriorly. Note the close relationship between the perforating vessels and the aneurysm.

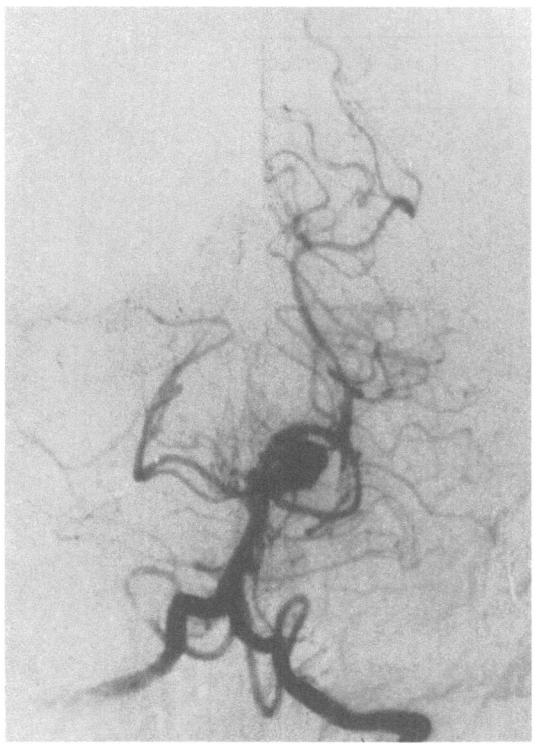

Fig. 10.35. Vertebral angiogram (AP projection) showing a basilar bifurcation aneurysm, which projects laterally so that its sac comes into close anatomical relationship with the left posterior cerebral artery. Note that the aneurysm sac is displacing the posterior cerebral artery upwards.

Projection. Aneurysms projecting backwards from the basilar bifurcation provide difficult surgical access, as they lie buried within the cerebral peduncle and the neck is often invested with blood vessels of the brain stem (Fig. 10.34). Some of the basilar bifurcation aneurysms projecting laterally may form an intimate relationship with the ipsilateral posterior cerebral artery, requiring difficult dissection before clipping (Fig. 10.35).

Level of Basilar Bifurcation. Surgical approach to basilar bifurcation aneurysms is more difficult if the basilar bifurcation is low (Fig. 10.36). This necessitates a greater retraction of the temporal lobe and division of the tentorium.

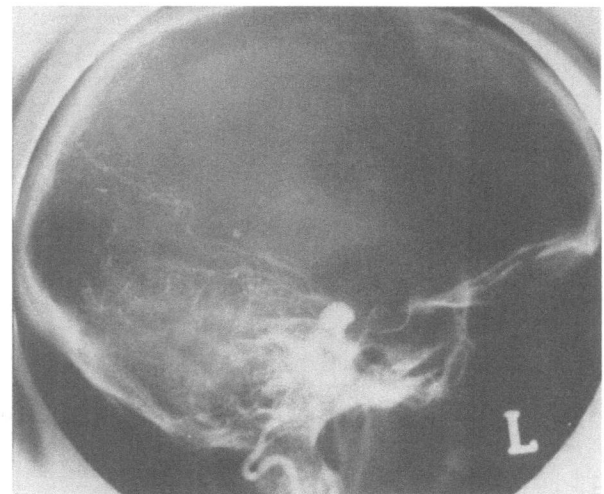

Fig. 10.36. Lateral vertebral angiogram showing a low basilar bifurcation aneurysm.

Results of Treatment

There were 30 patients with aneurysms in the posterior circulation which were operated on in this series. In 14 patients the aneurysm was at the basilar bifurcation, in two it was on the posterior cerebral artery, and in two it was at the origin of the superior cerebellar artery. In nine patients the aneurysm was located at the origin of the PICA, in one at the peripheral PICA and in two others at the vertebrobasilar junction (Table 10.35). There were 13 males and 17 females (Table 10.36), and the age incidence is shown in Table 10.37. Thir-

Table 10.35. Vertebrobasilar aneurysms: location

Aneurysm site	No.
Basilar bifurcation	14
PICA	10
Basilar origin	2
Basilar/superior cerebellar	2
Posterior cerebral (peripheral)	2
	30

Table 10.36. Vertebrobasilar aneurysms: sex incidence

	Superior cerebellar	VB junction	PICA	Post. cerebral	Basilar Bifurc.	Total
Male	1	1	3	1	7	13
Female	1	1	7	1	7	17
	2	2	10	2	14	30

Table 10.37. Vertebrobasilar aneurysms: age incidence

Age (years)	Sup. cerebellar	VB junction	PICA	Post. cerebral	Basilar bifurc.	Total
10–19	–	–	1	–	–	1
20–29	–	–	1	–	1	2
30–39	1	–	–	1	4	6
40–49	–	2	4	–	7	13
50–59	–	–	4	1	1	6
60–69	1	–	–	–	1	2
	2	2	10	2	14	30

Table 10.38. Vertebrobasilar aneurysms: neurological grade at operation (Hunt and Hess)

Grade	Sup. cerebellar	VB junction	PICA	Post. cerebral	Basilar bifurc.	Total
I	1	2	2	–	8	13
II	–	–	6	1	5	12
III	–	–	2	1	1	4
IV	1	–	–	–	–	1
	2	2	10	2	14	30

Table 10.39. Vertebrobasilar aneurysms: timing of surgery

Days since last SAH	Sup. cerebellar	VB junction	PICA	Post. cerebral	Basilar bifurc.	Total
0– 4	–	–	–	–	–	–
5– 7	–	–	2	1	2	5
8–11	–	–	4	1	3	8
12–14	1	–	2	–	–	3
15–18	1	–	–	–	2	3
19–21	–	–	–	–	–	–
> 21	–	2	2	–	7	11
	2	2	10	2	14	30

Table 10.40 Vertebrobasilar aneurysms: outcome at discharge

Outcome	Sup. cerebellar	VB junction	PICA	Post. cerebral	Basilar bifurc.	Total
Good	–	–	9	1	7	17
Fair	2	–	–	–	5	7
Poor	–	–	–	–	–	–
Dead	–	2	1	1	2	6
	2	2	10	2	14	30

teen patients were in grade 1, 12 in grade 2, four in grade 3 and 1 in grade 4 at the time of operation (Table 10.38). Six PICA aneurysms, five basilar bifurcation aneurysms and both the posterior cerebral aneurysms were operated upon before the 12th day of the last haemorrhage. Seven basilar bifurcation aneurysms and two each of the PICA and vertebrobasilar junction aneurysms were operated upon more than 3 weeks after the last haemorrhage (Table 10.39).

Of the 30 patients operated upon by direct surgery on the posterior circulation aneurysms, there were six deaths: two patients in the basilar bifurcation group, one each in the posterior cerebral and PICA groups, and both the patients with aneurysm at the vertebrobasilar junction. Of the surviving 24 patients, 17 had a good outcome at the time of discharge. Five of the seven patients who had only a fair outcome were operated on for basilar bifurcation aneurysms (Table 10.40).

References

Bailey WL, Loeser JD (1971) Intracranial aneurysms. JAMA 216:1993–1996

Debrun G, Lacour B, Caron JP et al. (1978) Detachable balloon and calibrated-leak balloon techniques in the treatment of cerebral vascular lesions. J Neurosurg 49:635–649

Dott NM (1933) Intracranial aneurysms: cerebral arterio-radiography surgical treatment. Edin Med J 40:219–240

Drake CG (1975) Ligation of the vertebral (unilateral or bilateral) or basilar artery in the treatment of large intracranial aneurysms. J Neurosurg 43:255–274

Drake CG (1979) Giant intracranial aneurysms: Experience with surgical treatment in 174 patients. Clin Neurosurg 26:12–95

Falconer MA (1951) The surgical treatment of bleeding intracranial aneurysms. J Neurol Neurosurg Psychiatry 14:143–186

Fox JL (1978) Intracranial aneurysms: intracranial and intraspinal arterio-venous malformations. Neurosurgery 3:305–320

Gillingham FJ (1967) The management of ruptured intracranial aneurysms. Scott Med J 12:377–383

Gillingham FJ (1975) Twenty-five years experience with middle cerebral aneurysms. J Neurol Neurosurg Psychiatry 38:404–413

Hamby WB (1952) Intracranial aneurysms. Charles C. Thomas, Springfield, Ill., pp 321–339

Hori S, Suzuki J (1979) Early intracranial operations for ruptured aneurysms. Acta Neurochir 46:93–104

Hunt WE, Miller CA (1977) The results of early operation for aneurysm. Clin Neurosurg 24:208–215

Kempe L (1968) Operative neurosurgery, vol 1. Cranial, cerebral and intracranial vascular diseases. Springer, Berlin Heidelberg, New York, pp 22–75

Kirgis HD, Llewellyn RC, Peebles EMcC (1960) Functional trifurcation of the internal carotid artery and its potential clinical significance. J Neurosurg 17:1062–1072

Locksley HB (1966) Natural history of subarachnoid haemorrhage, intracranial aneurysms and arteriovenous malformations. J Neurosurg 25:321–368

Logue V (1956) Surgery in spontaneous subarachnoid haemorrhage. Br Med J I:473–479

Martindale BV, Garfield J (1978) Subarachnoid haemorrhage above the age of 59. Br Med J I:465–467

Mount LA, Brisman R (1974) Treatment of multiple intracranial aneurysms—symptomatic and asymptomatic. Clin Neurosurg 21:166–170

Mullan S (1974) Experiences with surgical thrombosis of intracranial berry aneurysms and carotid-cavernous fistula. J Neurosurg 41:657–670

Mullan S, Raimondi AJ, Dobson G, Vailati G, Hekmatpanah J (1965) Electrically induced thrombosis in intracranial aneurysms. J Neurosurg 22:539–547

Norlen G, Barnum AS (1953) Surgical treatment of aneurysms of the anterior communicating artery. J Neurosurg 10:634–650

Paterson A, Bond MR (1973) Treatment of multiple intracranial arterial aneurysms. Lancet I:1302–1304

Pool JL (1961) Aneurysms of the anterior communicating artery. Bifrontal craniotomy and routine use of temporary clips. J Neurosurg 18:98–111

Romodanov AP, Shcheglov VI (1979) Endovascular method of excluding from the circulation saccular cerebral arterial aneurysms, leaving intact vessels patent. Acta Neurochir 28:312–315

Sano K, Saito I (1978) Timing and indication of surgery for ruptured intracranial aneurysms with regard to cerebral vasospasm. Acta Neurochir 41:49–60

Schmidek HH, Sweet WH (1982) Operative neurosurgical technique—indication, method and result. Grune and Stratton, New York, pp 819–932

Sengupta RP (1975) Anatomical variations in the origin of the posterior cerebral artery demonstrated by carotid angiography and their significance in the direct surgical treatment of posterior communicating aneurysms. Neurochirurgia 18:33–42

Sengupta RP (1977) Anterior communicating aneurysms and their management after subarachnoid haemorrhage. M.Sc. Thesis, University of Newcastle upon Tyne

Sengupta RP (1982a) Special indications for external/internal by-pass operations. Neurosurg Rev 5:107–112

Sengupta RP (1982b) Management of large and giant aneurysms. Neurosurg Rev 5:173–178

Sengupta RP, Lassman LP (1974) Identification of the source of bleeding in multiple intracranial aneurysms. Vasc Surg 8:177–183

Sengupta RP, Lassman LP, Hankinson J (1978) Scope of surgery for intracranial aneurysm in the elderly. A preliminary report. Br Med J II:246–247

Serbinenko PB (1974) Balloon catheterisation and occlusion of major cerebral vessels. J Neurosurg 41:125–144

Spetzler RF, Schuster H, Roski RA (1980) Elective extracranial-intracranial arterial by-pass in the treatment of inoperable giant aneurysms of the internal carotid artery. J Neurosurg 53:22–27

Suzuki J, Yoshimoto T (1979) The effect of mannitol in prolongation permissible occlusion time of cerebral artery. Clinical data of aneurysm surgery. In: Suzuki J (ed) Cerebral aneurysms. Neuron, Tokyo, pp 330–337

Symon L (1980) (ed) Neurosurgery. Rob C, Smith R (gen eds) Operative surgery, edn III. Butterworth, London, Boston, pp 225–306

Tonnis W (1936) Erfolgreiche Behandlung eines Aneurysma der Arteria communicans anterior cerebri. Zentralbl Neurochir 1:39–42

Winn HR, Almaani W, Berga S, Jane J, Richardson AE (1983) The longterm outcome in patients with multiple aneurysms. Incidence of late haemorrhage and implication for treatment in incidental aneurysms. J Neurosurg 59:642–651

Yasargil MG (1969) Microsurgery—applied to neurosurgery. Thieme, Stuttgart

11 Results of Surgical Treatment of Intracranial Aneurysms

Written in conjunction with V.R. Sastry Kolluri

Natural History of Intracranial Aneurysms

The natural history of ruptured and unruptured aneurysms must be clearly understood to evaluate rationally the surgical management of ruptured intracranial aneurysms. The clinical course of the untreated cases and the factors which influence the prognosis in patients with SAH must be clearly defined, so that the risks of mortality and morbidity implied in the treatment can be fully assessed against the risk of subsequent haemorrhage.

Ruptured intracranial aneurysms accounted for a quarter of all cerebrovascular deaths in a defined area of Surrey, England, over a 12-month period (Crawford and Sarner 1965). Each year about 28 000 patients suffer from SAH due to ruptured aneurysms in the United States (Kassel and Drake 1982). Thirty to forty per cent of patients with SAH succumb to the initial haemorrhage (Ask-Upmark and Ingvar 1950; Pakarinen 1967). There have been a number of studies on SAH, but the information in them depends upon the admission policy of that particular hospital, and is not representative of the disease in general. For example, Crawford and Sarner (1965) noticed that only 36 out of 57 patients with SAH had survived to reach a neurosurgical centre. Seven died at home, 47 were admitted to the district or local hospital, and three directly to the neurosurgical centre. Fourteen out of the 47 patients died before they could be transferred to a neurosurgical centre. Of the 36 patients reaching the centre, only 22 survived for more than a month. Overall, 27 of the initial 57 patients died within a week, and 35 within a month. The clinical picture presented at the neurosurgical centre is quite different to that obtained in the community study. Fifteen males and 21 females were admitted to the centre, but 10 men and 11 women died before admission, i.e. more men died early. As far as the age of the patient population is concerned, only 25 out of the 45 patients in the older age group and 11 out of the 12 patients in the younger age group survived to reach the centre. The site of the ruptured aneurysm also presented a different picture. In 48 patients the origin of the SAH was known. Only 9 (25%) of the 36 cases admitted to the neurosurgical centre had a middle cerebral artery aneurysm, whereas 7 (55%) of the 12 patients who died before reaching the centre had such aneurysms. Thus, a completely different picture may emerge from analysis of the patients presenting at a neurosurgical centre.

Brewis et al. (1966) in a survey at Carlisle, England, over a 5-year period (1955–1961) found the incidence of SAH to be 10.9 per 100 000 population. Phillips et al. (1980) in the United

States found a similar incidence of 10.8 per 100 000 population over a 30-year period in a well defined population of Rochester, Minnesota. However, Pakarinen (1967) noticed the incidence to be as high as 15.7 per 100 000 population in Helsinki over an 8-year period. Subarachnoid haemorrhage was responsible for 1.2% of all deaths, and 9.2% of deaths due to cerebrovascular disease in his study.

Subarachnoid haemorrhage due to rupture of an intracranial aneurysm is both an acute illness and a chronic disease, as the risk of rebleeding is both short- and long-term. Excellent long-term studies carried out during the last two decades allow us to predict with reasonable accuracy the incidence of both early and late rebleed, and their outcome in a given patient population (Locksley 1966; Jane et al. 1977; Winn et al. 1977).

The incidence of rebleeding is 10% in the first week and 12% in the second. It is reduced to about 7% in the third week and 8% in the fourth. The rate falls sharply to 1.8% per week up to 3 months after the initial bleed (Locksley 1969). Overall, in the first 6 months, at least 50% of the patients will rebleed. Thereafter, the rebleeding rate is about 3% per year in the first decade (Jane et al. 1977).

The rate of rebleeding was reported to increase to a peak at 7 days after SAH by Locksley (1969) and Graf (1971). On the other hand, studies in recent years (Jane et al. 1977; Kassell and Torner 1983; International Cooperative Study on Timing of Aneurysm Surgery, Kassell and Torner 1985, personal communication) have suggested that rebleeding is maximum on the day of the initial haemorrhage. However, it is difficult to diagnose a recurrent bleed within 24 h after a major haemorrhage.

In a follow-up of 364 non-surgically treated patients with single cerebral aneurysm over a 21-year period, Winn et al. (1973) found the incidence of rebleed in posterior communicating artery aneurysms to be greater than in anterior communicating artery aneurysms. The risk of rebleed in the acute stage increases, especially if the size of the aneurysm is more than 9 mm. Posterior communicating aneurysms rebleed more in women (Richardson et al. 1966b). Anterior communicating aneurysms have a very low rebleed rate after 3 years (Richardson et al. 1964). Middle cerebral artery aneurysms are less frequent after 60 years of age. The incidence of rebleed is least frequent following middle cerebral aneurysm rupture (Hudson and Raaf 1968).

There is little relationship between the age of the patient or the size of the aneurysm and the occurrence of late haemorrhage. However, Winn et al. (1977) did find a difference in the time interval to average rebleeding in relation to age. For patients 40 years and older it was 4.4 years, while it was twice as long for younger patients.

Forty percent of deaths due to first bleed occur within a week, and 67% by 3 weeks (Locksley 1969). Mortality after the second bleed is about 42% (Locksley 1969). As a rule, late mortality averages 2% annually during the first decade (Winn et al. 1977).

On the basis of the U.S. population and available data on incidental aneurysms, Dell (1982) calculated the risk of haemorrhage depending upon the age of the patient at the time of diagnosis. The risk of rupture during lifetime is around 16% when diagnosed at 20–30 years of age, 10% at 50 years, and less than 5% at 60 years.

The natural history of symptomatic but unruptured aneurysms is again different from asymptomatic or incidental aneurysms. In a follow-up study (Graf 1971) of 35 patients with symptomatic unruptured aneurysms over 2–12 years, nine subsequently died of SAH, while only two patients bled in a follow-up of 52 patients with asymptomatic or incidental aneurysms. Asymptomatic aneurysms in the vertebral circulation are twice as common as in the carotid circulation (Housepian and Pool 1958). The incidence and distribution of symptomatic unruptured aneurysms are different to those which rupture: There is a high incidence of supracavernous internal carotid aneurysms when compared with anterior communicating and middle cerebral artery aneurysms, and symptomatic unruptured aneurysms are more frequent in females (Locksley 1966).

Multiple aneurysms are associated with a higher mortality than a single aneurysm (Shepherd 1983), but recurrent haemorrhage usually occurs from the original lesion (McKissock et al. 1964). Recurrent haemorrhage in these patients is more frequent and earlier than in patients with a single aneurysm. Though typically only one aneurysm ruptures in patients with multiple aneurysms, very rarely two aneurysms may bleed at the same time (Leo et al. 1982). In a follow-up of 84 patients with multiple aneurysms, over periods ranging from 4 months to 11 years, Heiskanen and Marttila (1970) noted recurrent haemorrhage in eight patients, due to rupture of a previously unruptured aneurysm. Winn et al. (1983) found that the risk of haemorrhage from an incidental aneurysm is 1% per year.

After a thorough investigation the source of haemorrhage may not be found if a small aneurysm is either completely destroyed at the time of haemorrhage or has undergone thrombosis. Prognosis in these patients is better (Hayward 1977).

McKissock et al. (1962) in a controlled study of both conservatively and surgically treated patients found no significant difference in mortality in patients who were unconscious at the time of inclusion in the trial. In their study, males treated surgically faired better than those treated conservatively. In another controlled trial of conservative and surgical treatment in patients admitted on an average of 7 weeks after the haemorrhage, Troupp and Bjorkesten (1971) found no statistical difference between the two groups. However, careful analysis of their data indicated some benefit with surgical treatment. Nine of the 92 conservatively treated patients died of recurrent haemorrhage during a 3.5-year period. Although 5 of the 86 patients treated surgically also died during the same period, none of these patients had ligature at the neck of the aneurysm. There was only one postoperative death, this in a patient who had carotid ligation after the aneurysm ruptured during direct surgery. The rest died 1 month to 4 years after the operation. In a further follow-up study of these patients (Kaste and Troupp 1978) there were significantly more late rebleeds in the conservatively treated patients.

In the Co-operative Study (Sahs et al. 1981) the mortality in patients treated with bed-rest was highest in patients admitted within 7 days of the last bleed. The overall mortality was 55%. It was highest in patients with anterior communicating aneurysms, and lowest in those with internal carotid aneurysms. The middle cerebral artery aneurysm group occupied an intermediate position, but this difference was not statistically significant.

Alvord et al. (1972) constructed predictability tables for survival after SAH, utilising the duration of survival from the first haemorrhage or the last haemorrhage and the neurological state at the time of examination. These tables are very useful in the management of patients with SAH (Fig. 11.1).

Having reviewed the natural history of both ruptured and unruptured aneurysms, we will now discuss the outcome of surgical treatment in patients with aneurysmal SAH. First, a clinical profile of the patients operated on for ruptured intracranial aneurysm by one of the authors between 1969 and 1980 will be presented, and then the results will be analysed and discussed in the light of other reported series.

Finally, the factors which have an influence on the outcome after surgery will be reviewed. The surgical outcome was analysed at the time of

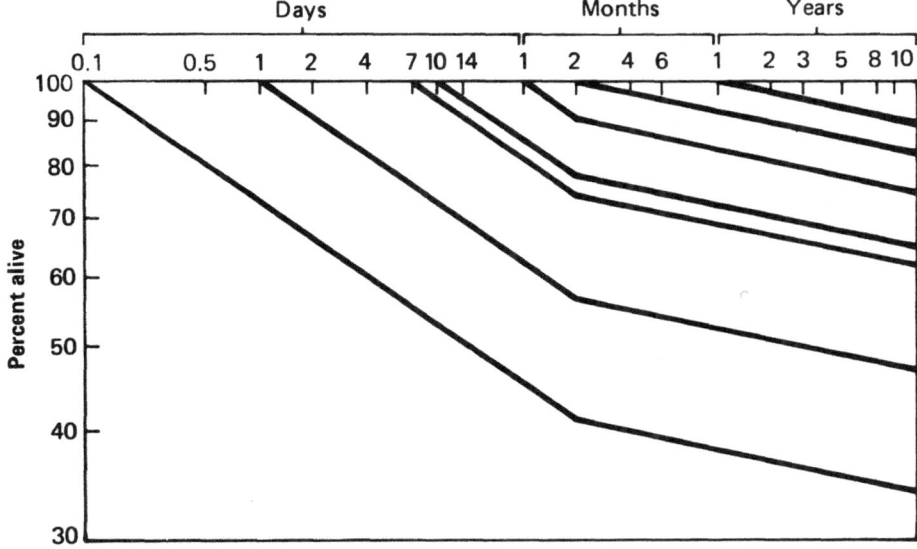

Fig. 11.1. Survival rates of patients admitted to study at particular times after their initial major subarachnoid haemorrhage (Adapted from Alvord et al. 1972)

discharge from the neurosurgical centre and at follow-up. At discharge, the residual neurological deficit and the functional independence were taken into account, to group the patients as good, fair or poor:

Good—no residual neurological deficit, or mild residual deficit but with normal mentation.

Fair—moderate neurological deficit. Able to take care of oneself.

Poor—severe neurological deficit. Not able to be self-supportive or needing institutional care.

The outcome at follow-up was measured on the basis of capacity for employment:

1. Employed
2. Capable but unemployed
3. Unfit for work

Clinical Profile of Surgical Patients

Five hundred patients were operated on for intracranial aneurysms; all but 13 presented with SAH. Patients who were treated conservatively or who died before surgery are not included in this study.

There were 203 males and 297 females—a ratio of 2:3. The age of the patients ranged from the second to the eighth decade (Table 11.1). Seventy-seven per cent (384) of the patients were in the fourth, fifth and sixth decades of life. There were 57 patients in the second and third decades, 53 in the seventh decade, and only six patients in the eighth decade. There was also a difference in the distribution of age in relation to sex. Thirty-five per cent of the males were in the second, third and fourth decades, while only 20% of the females were in these age groups ($P < 0.001$).

Table 11.1. Incidence of aneurysmal SAH: age vs sex

	Male	Female	Total
< 19	8	5	13
20–29	23	21	44
30–39	45	31	76
40–49	48	85	133
50–59	62	113	175
60–69	15	38	53
70–79	2	4	6
Total	203	297	500

An internal carotid aneurysm was responsible for SAH in 197 patients, and an anterior cerebral aneurysm in 174 patients. A middle cerebral artery aneurysm was the underlying cause of haemorrhage in 99 patients. Only 30 patients had an aneurysm in the posterior circulation. The location of the aneurysm varied in relation to both sex and age. Anterior cerebral aneurysms were more frequent in males (42%) ($P < 0.005$), while internal carotid aneurysms were more common in females (45.1%) ($P < 0.001$) (Table 11.2). Internal carotid aneurysms were more common in younger patients, while middle cerebral aneurysms were infrequent in extremes of age ($P < 0.001$) (Table 11.3).

Table 11.2. Type of aneurysm vs sex

	Internal carotid	ACA	MCA	Post. circ.	Total
Male	54	87	49	13	203
Female	143	87	50	17	297
Total	197	174	99	30	500

Abbreviations: ACA, anterior communicating artery; MCA, middle cerebral artery; Post. circ., posterior circulation

Table 11.3. Age vs distribution of aneurysm

	Internal carotid	ACA	MCA	Post. circ.	Total
10–19	6	4	2	1	13
20–29	18	19	5	2	44
30–39	22	26	22	6	76
40–49	52	37	31	13	133
50–59	70	62	37	6	175
60–69	25	25	2	1	53
70–79	4	1	–	1	6
Total	197	174	99	30	500

The symptomatology at the onset of SAH in patients with different types of aneurysm is shown in Table 11.4. The majority of the patients (80%) had sudden severe headache, the like of which they had never experienced before. In 73% of the patients the haemorrhage was not related to any specific activity. They were either reading, walking in the house, gardening, shopping, or working in the office (Table 11.5). 19.6% (98) of patients had a previous history of headache, and 14.4%

Table 11.4. Symptoms at the time of initial SAH

	Internal carotid	ACA	MCA	Post. circ.	Total
Headache	151	145	82	21	399
Loss of consciousness	77	80	51	12	220
Disturbance of vision	48	18	8	1	75
Convulsions	11	9	9	2	31
Dizziness	14	19	9	2	44
Confusion	12	14	15	2	43
Limb weakness	19	26	15	2	62
Sensory disturbance	4	14	4	–	22

Table 11.5. Activity related to the onset of SAH

	Internal carotid	ACA	MCA	Post. circ.	Total
At work	32	32	16	4	84
Sleep	15	13	12	1	41
Intercourse	3	2	2	1	8
Strenuous work	16	22	6	2	46
Other times	131	105	63	22	321

(72) were being treated for hypertension. s with chronic bronchitis and heart disease accounted for 3.8% (19 patients) each. 5.6% (28 patients) gave a past history of other major illness. Ninety-one patients had a previous history of confirmed SAH before admission to the regional centre.

The neurological condition of each patient was graded according to the Hunt and Hess classification (1968). However, no consideration was given to systemic illness. There were 106 patients in grade 1, 240 in grade 2 and 109 in grade 3. Grades 4 and 5 accounted for 43 and 2 patients respectively at the time of admission (Table 11.6). All of the 13 patients who did not have SAH were included in grade 1 for analysis.

Table 11.6. Neurological grade on admission

Neurological grade	Internal carotid	ACA	MCA	Post. circ.	Total
1	31	55	15	5	106
2	114	68	43	15	240
3	36	37	28	8	109
4	15	13	13	2	43
5	1	1	–	–	2
Total	197	174	99	30	500

The majority of the patients (75%) had angiography within 10 days of the last haemorrhage. Multiple aneurysms were noted in 24.8% of the cases. One patient had as many as seven aneurysms. Two hundred and four patients had some degree of spasm in pre-operative angiograms. The spasm was classified as generalised, localised or segmental, depending on its extent (see Chap. 12). Seventy-seven patients had generalised, 102 localised and 25 segmental angiographic spasm.

Thirty-five patients had further haemorrhage while awaiting surgery. Overall, 98 patients had two bleeds, 23 patients three bleeds, and four patients four bleeds before surgery. One patient had a total of seven haemorrhages. Fifty-one patients developed pre-operative ischaemic complications (Table 11.7), and 31 of these showed

Table 11.7. Incidence of ischaemic complications and hydrocephalus related to the site of aneurysm

	Internal carotid	ACA	MCA	Post. circ.	Total
Ischaemic complications					
Pre-op.	16	19	14	2	51
Postop.	44	23	17	1	85
Hydrocephalus					
Pre-op.	14	26	7	2	49
Postop.	8	28	6	5	47

evidence of some degree of spasm. Forty-nine patients developed hydrocephalus in the pre-operative period and 68% of these patients had cerebral vasospasm of variable degree. In seven patients, external ventricular drain had to be inserted before definitive surgery on the aneurysm.

By the time of operation, there was an overall improvement in the condition of the patients (Table 11.8). There were 145 patients in grade 1

Table 11.8. Neurological grade at operation vs type of aneurysm

Neurological grade	Internal carotid	ACA	MCA	Post. circ.	Total
1	64	44	24	13	145
2	93	88	40	12	233
3	38	36	27	4	105
4	2	6	8	1	17
Total	197	174	99	30	500

and 233 patients in grade 2. Neurological grades 3 and 4 accounted for 105 and 17 patients respectively. Fifty-seven per cent of the patients were operated on within 12 days of the last haemorrhage (Table 11.9).

Table 11.9. Timing of surgery vs type of aneurysm

	Interval between last SAH and operation							
	0 < 4	5–7	8–11	12–14	15–18	19–21	> 21	Total
C. ophth.	4	6	7	2	1	2	2	24
Post. comm. a.	16	29	24	19	7	5	16	116
Ant. choroidal	–	4	1	–	2	–	3	10
Bifurcation ICA	7	7	7	1	3	1	6	32
Cavernous ICA	1	1	–	–	–	–	1	3
Non-specific ICA	3	1	6	1	1	–	–	12
Ant. comm. a.	14	33	45	24	12	12	20	160
Proximal ACA	–	1	2	–	–	–	1	4
Perical.	2	3	2	1	–	1	1	10
MC trifurcation	6	23	19	15	10	7	16	96
Proximal MCA	–	1	–	–	1	–	1	3
VB junction	–	–	–	–	–	–	2	2
PICA	–	2	4	2	–	–	2	10
Bas. bifurc.	–	2	3	–	2	–	7	14
Sup. cerebral	–	–	–	1	1	–	–	2
Post. cerebral	–	1	1	–	–	–	–	2
Total	53	114	121	66	40	28	78	500

Abbreviations: C. ophth., carotid óphthalmic; Post. comm. a., posterior communicating artery; Ant. choroidal, anterior choroidal; Ant. comm. a., anterior communicating artery; Perical., pericallosal; MC trifurcation, middle cerebral artery trifurcation; VB junction, vertebrobasilar junction; PICA, posterior inferior cerebellar artery; Bas. bifurc., basilar bifurcation; Sup. cerebral, superior cerebral; Post. cerebral, posterior cerebral

The ideal method of treatment for ruptured intracranial aneurysm is to exclude it from the cerebral circulation, either by clip or ligature, effectively eliminating the risk of recurrent haemorrhage from the aneurysm. It was not, however, always feasible to occlude the neck of an aneurysm, because of factors such as shape and size, and occasionally location. In such cases, alternative procedures were undertaken. The aneurysm was covered with muslin or histoacrylic glue in some, to strengthen the aneurysmal wall. In a few, the aneurysm was trapped, and in others only proximal ligation of the carotid artery in the neck was undertaken, with EC/IC anastomosis in recent years (Table 11.10).

Table 11.10. Methods of treatment

Clipping	441
Wrapping	41
Trapping	6
Proximal ligation	4
Proximal ligation with EC/IC anastomosis	8
Total	500

Outcome

At Discharge from Hospital. At the time of discharge from hospital, 375 patients (75%) had a good outcome, 80 (16%) a fair, and 13 (2.6%) a poor outcome. Thirty-two patients (6.4%) had died (Table 11.11).

Table 11.11. Type of aneurysm vs condition at discharge

	Good	Fair	Poor	Dead	Total
C. ophth.	18	5	1	–	24
Post. comm. a.	86	17	5	8	116
Ant. choroidal	8	–	–	2	10
Bifurcation ICA	25	5	1	1	32
Cavernous ICA	3	–	–	–	3
Non-specific ICA	9	2	–	1	12
Ant. comm. a.	127	23	5	5	160
Proximal ACA	4	–	–	–	4
Perical.	7	–	–	3	10
MC trifurcation	68	21	1	6	96
Proximal MCA	3	–	–	–	3
VB Junction	–	–	–	2	2
PICA	9	–	–	1	10
Bas. bifurc.	7	5	–	2	14
Sup. cerebral	–	2	–	–	2
Post. cerebral	1	–	–	1	2
Total	375	80	13	32	500

At Follow-up. Of the 468 survivors, 22 patients were lost to follow-up. Of the remaining 446, 326 (73%) returned to their previous occupation, 57 (12.5%) were capable but unemployed, while 63 (14.5%) were unfit for work (Table 11.12).

Analysis of Patients with Fatal Outcome

The clinical profile of the 32 patients who died in this series is given in Table 11.13. There were 7 males and 25 females. There was no mortality in patients in the second and third decades and only one of the 76 patients in the fourth decade died. Mortality was almost equal between patients who were in the fifth, sixth and seventh decades of life. Two of the six patients who were in the eighth decade did not survive the operation. Mortality was also similar in the three different aneurysm groups in the anterior circulation. Thirteen patients had a massive infarction confirmed either on CT scan or at post-mortem, due to ischaemia. Six patients had rebled in the postoperative period; in five the clip was not occluding the aneurysm properly, and in one patient only wrapping was done. In two patients with multiple aneurysms, the initial operation was done on an incidental aneurysm as there was difficulty in identifying the source of haemorrhage. At operation, technical difficulty was encountered in four patients, and the aneurysm ruptured during dissection. One patient developed postoperative haematoma. Wound infection or ventriculitis developed in four patients. Eight patients developed epilepsy, and three had pulmonary embolism in the postoperative period. Overall, in ten patients there was more than one factor which contributed to the death.

Table 11.12. Type of aneurysm vs occupational status at follow-up

	Employed	Capable but unemployed	Unfit	Not stated	Total
C. ophth.	16	2	6	–	24
Post. comm. a.	74	13	16	5	108
Ant. choroidal	6	1	–	1	8
Bifurcation ICA	23	3	4	1	31
Cavernous ICA	3	–	–	–	3
Non-specific ICA	7	–	3	1	11
Ant. comm. a.	112	20	14	9	155
Proximal ACA	4	–	–	–	4
Perical.	6	1	–	–	7
MC trifurcation	60	9	18	3	90
Proximal MCA	2	1	–	–	3
VB Junction	–	–	–	–	–
PICA	6	2	–	1	9
Bas. bifurc.	5	5	1	1	12
Sup. cerebral	1	–	1	–	2
Post. cerebral	1	–	–	–	1
Total	326	57	63	22	468

Table 11.13. Analysis of 32 patients who died following surgery

Serial no.	Age	Sex	Grade on admission	Grade at operation	Further SAH	Pre-operative ischaemia	Site of aneurysm	Angiographic spasm	Condition of brain at operation	Rupture of aneurysm at operation	Day of operation	Associated illness	Intra- and postoperative problems—cause of death
035	40	F	3	4	No	No	Ant. comm. a.	Generalised	Infarcted	No	13	None	Difficult dissection. Postop. ischaemia and oedema. Excision of bone flap. Fits. Tracheostomy. Infarct
043	62	F	2	3	No	No	Ant. comm. a.	Localised	Ischaemic	No	11	None	Postop. ischaemia with oedema. Excision of bone flap. Tracheostomy. Infarct
104	53	F	2	2	Yes	No	Post. comm. a. (Rt.)	None	—	No	14	Hypertension	Postop. ischaemia. Stormy course. Cardiac arrest. Death. P.M.—Moderate subdural haematoma with brain shift. Aneurysm clip in good position
105	48	F	3	3	No	No	Post. comm. a.	—	Normal	No	15	Hypertension	Postop. ischaemia. Oedema. Infarct
135	44	F	3	3	No	No	Perical. (R) MCA (L)	Localised	Normal	No	12 and 29	None	Patient had clipping of pericallosal aneurysm on 12th day followed by clipping of incidental MCA on 29th day. 12 days after second surgery she suddenly became unconscious and died. Autopsy—Fresh bleed from pericall. Clip not occluding the aneurysm completely.
136	59	F	2	2	No	No	Post. cereb.	None	Ischaemia	No	8	None	Patient had rebled. Postop. intracerebral haematoma. Evacuated. Clip O.K. Fits.
142	61	M	2	2	No	No	MC tri. (R) Post. comm. a.	None	Infarcted	Yes	8	None	Difficult dissection. Rupture at operation. Unsatisfactory recovery. Ischaemia. Infarct
239	40	F	1	1	Yes	Yes	Post. comm. a.	None	Congested	No	2	None	Foetal PCA. Postop. ischaemia. Angiogram showed generalised spasm. Clip O.K. Did not respond to treatment. Infarct
286	42	F	2	2	No	Yes	MC tri.	None	Congested	No	12	None	As craniotomy was being closed after clipping, sudden bleeding. Re-opened. Bleeding from aneurysm. Reapplication of clip. Wrapped in muslin and glue. Fits day 2—post-op patient deteriorated. Death
305	57	M	4	3	No	No	Post. comm. a.	Localised	Congested	No	14	None	Patient had pre-operative CSF drainage. Post-op. ventriculitis and chest infection. Meningitis. Tracheostomy. Cardiorespiratory arrest
334	53	F	2	2	No	No	Ant. comm. a.	None	Ischaemic	No	5	Hypertension	Postop. ischaemia. Oedema. Excision of bone flap. Tracheostomy. Infarct

Table 11.13. (continued)

Serial no.	Age	Sex	Grade on admission	Grade at operation	Further SAH	Pre-operative ischaemia	Site of aneurysm	Angiographic spasm	Condition of brain at operation	Rupture of aneurysm at operation	Day of operation	Associated illness	Intra- and postoperative problems—cause of death
367	70	M	3	4	No	Yes	Post. comm. a.	None	Infarcted	No	2 and 11	None	Patient deteriorated day after admission. Intracerebral haematoma. Evacuated. Deteriorated tenth day. Craniotomy. Evacuation of haematoma, clipping of aneurysm. Persistent neurological deficit. Chest infection. Postoperative fits. Deteriorated.
379	65	F	2	2	No	Nil	Post. comm. a.	None	Congested	No	13	Hypertension	Immediate postoperative bleed. Recraniotomy. Clip. Patient did not recover
385	45	F	3	2	No	No	MC tri.	None	Normal	No	9	Hypertension	Postoperative convulsions, ischaemia and œdema. Infarct
386	37	M	4	4	Yes	No	MC tri.	Localised	Congestion	No	6	None	Also had haematoma. Evacuated and clipped. Postoperative ischaemia. Responded to isoprenaline/lignocaine. Improved. Hydrocephalus. External drainage. Later ventriculoperitoneal shunt. Sudden death 15 days after original operation for aneurysm. ?Pulmonary embolism
412	70	F	2	2	No	No	Car. bif.	Segmental	–	No	28	None	Following craniotomy did not recover
432	50	F	2	1	No	Yes	IC ant. chor.	None	Ischaemic	No	25	Obstructive airway disease	Pre-operative bronchospasm. Ischaemic symptoms. Isoprenaline/lignocaine. Improved. Craniotomy. Immediate postop. fits. Elective ventilation. Bronchospasm. Tracheal stenosis. Repair done. Sudden respiratory arrest 3 weeks after craniotomy
444	56	F	2	4	No	No	Ant. comm. a.	Generalised	Normal	No	20	None	Deteriorated 7th day postop. Bulging flap. Excision of bone flap with subdural haematoma and subfrontal external ventricular drainage. Tracheostomy. Infarct. Death on 13th day
445	58	F	2	2	No	No	Perical.	None	Ischaemic	No	4	Hypertension	Postoperative ischaemia, hemiparesis. Isoprenaline/lignocaine. No response. External ventricular drainage. No change. Infarct
463	63	F	Non-SAH presentation	–	–	–	IC an.	None	Normal	No	Non-SAH	None	Aneurysm trapped. Internal carotid ligation in neck and multiple clip occlusion of aneurysm. Ventricular drain left. Bleeding same day. Blood in temporal lobe. Died following day

Table 11.13. (continued)

Serial no.	Age	Sex	Grade on admission	Grade at operation	Further SAH	Pre-operative ischaemia	Site of aneurysm	Angiographic spasm	Condition of brain at operation	Rupture of aneurysm at operation	Day of operation	Associated illness	Intra- and postoperative problems—cause of death
160	56	F	3	2	No	No	PICA Ant. comm. a. C. ophthal.	None	Normal	Yes	8 27	Chronic bronchitis	Multiple lesions. CT. No blood. Spasm of ACA Ant. comm. a. thought to be offending lesion. On 8th day, clipping of Ant. comm. a. Site of bleed not confirmed at surgery. Postoperative vert. angio. PICA aneurysm. Reoperated. Clipped (27th day). Difficult dissection, large lesion. Intraoperative rupture. Postop. lower cranial nerve palsies, hemiparesis. Postop. hydrocephalus. Shunt done. Gastro-duodenal haemorrhage. Laparotomy and "over-sewing" of bleeding duodenal ulcer.
165	46	F	3	2	Yes	No	Bas. bif. Car. bif.	–	–	No	11	None	External ventricular drain. Poor general condition. Tracheostomy. Ventriculoperitoneal shunt. DVT hypostatic pneumonia.
166	40	M	2	2	No	No	Bas. bif.	None	Oedematous	No	8	None	Postoperative septicaemia. Scan. hydrocephalus. External ventricular drain. Subdural haematoma. Evacuated. Ventriculitis. Fits
170	41	F	3	1	Yes	No	VB junct.	Localised	–	No	48	Hypertension	DVT in pre-operative period. At surgery, wrapping and glueing. Could not be clipped. Postoperative chest infection. Sudden unconsciousness. "Rebled" (confirmed). Death
177	44	M	4	4	No	No	VB junct.	Non-SAH	Normal	Yes	–	None	Admitted in 1974 for SAH. VB junction aneurysm found. Opted for conservative treatment. Presented in 1977 causing space-occupying effects. Operated. Intraoperative rupture. Patient did not recover. Died same day
212	57	F	3	3	Yes	No	Ant. comm. a.	None	–	No	3	Hypertension, chronic bronchitis	Postoperative day 2: Deteriorated. Had intracerebral haematoma. Evacuated. Aneurysm reclipped. Ventilated. Wound sepsis. Infarction of frontal lobe seen on scan. Bronchospasm and tracheostomy. Death

Table 11.13. (continued)

Serial no.	Age	Sex	Grade on admission	Grade at operation	Further SAH	Pre-operative ischaemia	Site of aneurysm	Angiographic spasm	Condition of brain at operation	Rupture of aneurysm at operation	Day of operation	Associated illness	Intra- and postoperative problems—cause of death
224	46	F	2	4	Yes	Yes	Perical. and car. bif.	None	Oedematous	No	15	None	While preparing for surgery, sudden unconsciousness, twice. Surgery postponed. Operation a day after second attack of unconsciousness. One week later patient deteriorated. Postoperative ischaemia. Infarct
225	53	F	3	2	No	No	IC ant. chor.	None	Normal	Yes	16	None	Postoperative ischaemia. Infarct
227	55	F	2	2	No	No	MC tri.	Generalised	Ischaemic	No	7	Hyper-tension	Bilateral carotid angiogram showed multiple aneurysms with probable bleed from right MCA, which was clipped. In postop. period patient had fatal rebleed. At postmortem a previously unrecognised basilar bifurcation aneurysm was found to be responsible for the haemorrhage
464	67	F	2	2	No	No	Post. comm. a.	Generalised	Normal	No	9	Hyper-tension	Had postoperative external ventricular drainage. Rebled from aneurysm. Died. Incomplete occlusion of aneurysm at post-mortem
482	46	F	3	4	No	No	MC tri.	None	Congested	No	4		Had subdural and intracerebral haematoma evacuation. No improvement. Clipping done. Pulmonary embolism on 5th day. Confirmed at post-mortem
491	58	M	2	2	No	No	Post. comm. a.	None	Ischaemic	No	39	Labile hyper-tension	Grand-mal fits postoperatively. Scan. Large infarct.

Abbreviations: Ant. comm. a., anterior communicating artery; Post. comm. a., posterior communicating artery; Perical., pericallosal; Post. cereb., posterior cerebellar; MC tri., middle cerebral trifurcation; Car. bif., carotid bifurcation; IC ant. chor., internal carotid anterior choroidal; IC an., internal carotid aneurysm; PICA, posterior inferior cerebellar artery; C. ophthal., carotid ophthalmic; Bas. bif., basilar bifurcation; VB junct., vertebrobasilar junction

Outcome in Relation to the Site of the Aneurysm

Internal Carotid Artery Aneurysms

There were 197 patients with internal carotid artery aneurysms. The age incidence varied from the second to the eighth decade. They were more common in females, and varied with the location of the aneurysm on the internal carotid artery (Table 11.14). As the origin of the aneurysms proceeded distally, the incidence gradually became less in women. In females, carotid ophthalmic aneurysms were five times as frequent as in men, while posterior communicating artery aneurysms were three times more so, and the aneurysms of the carotid bifurcation were in the ratio of 2:1. In the pre-operative period, seven patients had a further haemorrhage; five of them had posterior communicating artery aneurysms. Seventy-two patients had some degree of angiographic spasm. Sixteen patients developed ischaemic complications. Of the 14 patients who developed symptomatic hydrocephalus, six had posterior communicating artery aneurysms, and in another six the aneurysm was at the carotid bifurcation.

Table 11.14. Location of internal carotid aneurysms in relation to sex

	Male	Female	Total
Carotid ophthalmic	4	20	24
Posterior communicating artery	29	87	116
Anterior choroidal	6	4	10
Bifurcation	11	21	32
Cavernous	1	2	3
Non-specific	3	9	12
Total	54	143	197

One hundred and forty-five patients were in neurological grades 1 and 2, and 52 patients in grades 3 and 4 on admission. However, by the time of operation, the number of patients in grades 1 and 2 had increased to 157. One hundred and twenty-three of the 197 patients were operated within 12 days of the last haemorrhage. Ten patients developed epilepsy in the postoperative period; eight of them had a posterior communicating aneurysm. Forty-four patients had postoperative ischaemic complications. Twenty-nine of these were operated upon for posterior communicating aneurysm. Eight patients had symp-

tomatic hydrocephalus in the postoperative period. The overall mortality for internal carotid aneurysms was 6%.

Specific aneurysms of the internal carotid artery will now be discussed.

Carotid Ophthalmic Aneurysms

According to Drake et al. (1968a) carotid ophthalmic aneurysms arise from the internal carotid artery at the origin of the ophthalmic artery, while Kothandaram et al. (1971) included in this group all aneurysms arising between the origin of the ophthalmic artery and the carotid bifurcation. In our series, we have included only those aneurysms arising in the region of the ophthalmic artery. Sengupta et al. (1976) studied 32 cases of carotid ophthalmic aneurysms. Multiplicity was found to be a common factor in these aneurysms. In ten cases of multiple aneurysms, eight carotid ophthalmic aneurysms were incidental. However, the tendency to rebleed from a ruptured carotid ophthalmic aneurysm is similar to that from other aneurysms, and hence they pose a risk to both life and vision.

Yasargil and Smith (1982) reported 26 patients with carotid ophthalmic aneurysms. Twenty-four had a good and two a fair outcome. There was no operative mortality. Crowell and Ojemann (1983b) operated 15 cases without mortality, and only two patients had a poor outcome.

In our present series, 24 carotid ophthalmic aneurysms were operated. Eighteen patients had a good and five patients a fair outcome. One patient was graded as poor at the time of discharge from hospital. There was no mortality. There were five patients whose presenting symptom was only visual deterioration without SAH. In four patients there was a varying degree of improvement in vision postoperatively. In one of these patients the improvement was dramatic immediately after surgery. In another patient, who presented with bilateral visual loss due to a giant aneurysm, the vision in the contralateral eye improved enormously. On the ipsilateral side, the optic nerve had to be sacrificed while dealing with the aneurysm.

Ferguson and Drake (1980) analysed the surgical results in 19 patients with visually symptomatic, but intact, aneurysms. Of these, 12 patients had no persisting neurological signs, other than visual symptoms. Of the six patients who had persistent deficit, four had mild and two major deficits. There was one death, as a result of anoxic encephalopathy. The visual function improved in nine patients, remained unchanged in five, and became worse in four patients. Postoperative visual deterioration can be immediate or delayed. When delayed, the expansion of the aneurysm by the thrombus may be responsible. Though the outcome of surgery in terms of visual recovery is unpredictable, certain factors, such as a short history of illness, avoidance of injury to the ophthalmic artery at operation, good decompression of the nerve and evacuation of the sac at operation, result in a good outcome. Neither optic pallor nor initial deterioration of vision post-operatively precludes complete recovery of vision, which may take as long as 2 years (Ferguson and Drake 1980).

Posterior Communicating Aneurysms

There were 116 patients with posterior communicating artery aneurysms in this series of 197 internal carotid aneurysms. In five patients there were further episodes of SAH, and seven had ischaemic complications before surgery. In 15 patients there was generalised and in 25 localised vasospasm in the pre-operative angiograms. In four patients the spasm was segmental, while there was no evidence of spasm in 72 patients. At the time of operation, 39 patients were in grade 1 and 58 patients in grade 2; there were only 17 patients in grade 3, and two in grade 4. Fifty-eight per cent (68 patients) were operated upon within 12 days of the last haemorrhage. Twenty-eight per cent (29 patients) had postoperative ischaemic complications. Eighty-six patients had a good outcome while in 17 patients it was fair. There were eight (7%) operative deaths.

In a controlled study, McKissock et al. (1960) treated 42 patients with posterior communicating artery aneurysm conservatively, and 41 patients surgically, 37 of whom had common carotid ligation. Fifteen patients (35%) in the conservative group died, but only four in the surgical group. One hundred and thirty-six posterior communicating artery aneurysms were operated on in the series reported by Yasargil and Smith (1982). Ninety-nine patients were in grades 1 and 2 at surgery. Eighty-nine per cent of these patients had a good outcome with only one death. Six patients had a fair and four patients a poor outcome. Mortality was 16% in 37 patients who were in a poor grade, and only 65% of these patients had a good outcome.

Anterior Choroidal Aneurysms

There were ten anterior choroidal aneurysms in this series of 197 internal carotid aneurysms with two operative mortalities. All eight who survived had a good outcome.

In operating on anterior choroidal aneurysms, the artery should be preserved. Inadvertent injury may result in severe neurological deficit (Drake et al. 1968b). Though at surgery it may look as if the artery is preserved, in some cases postoperative angiogram fails to show the patency of the artery (Yasargil et al. 1978; Viale and Pau 1979). In the series reported by Yasargil and Smith (1982) there were 14 patients with anterior choroidal aneurysm. Ten were in grades 1 and 2 and four in grade 3 at the time of surgery. Eleven patients had a good outcome, and there were two operative deaths.

Carotid Bifurcation Aneurysms

In the present series, 32 carotid bifurcation aneurysms were operated on. There were 11 males and 21 females. One patient had ischaemic neurological deficit, and only three patients had vasospasm in the pre-operative period. Twenty-three patients were in grades 1 and 2, and nine patients in poor grades on admission. However at operation, 9 were in grade 1, 17 in grade 2, and 6 in grade 3. Of the 32 patients 21 were operated on before 12 days. Six patients developed ischaemic complications in the postoperative period. In 75% (25 patients) the outcome was good, and in five patients it was fair. One patient died.

There were 44 patients with carotid bifurcation aneurysm in a series of 638 patients reported by Yasargil and Smith (1982). Twenty-eight patients were in grades 1 and 2, and 16 in poorer grades. Eighty-six per cent had a good outcome. There was only one operative death. In four patients the outcome was fair.

Anterior Cerebral Artery Aneurysms

Anterior Communicating Artery Aneurysms

One-hundred and seventy-four patients with aneurysms on the anterior cerebral artery were operated on. The majority, 160 patients, had an anterior communicating artery aneurysm, and only four had a proximal A_1 segmental aneurysm.

In ten patients the aneurysm was located on the pericallosal artery. The pericallosal aneurysms, also known as distal anterior cerebral aneurysms, are analysed separately. The four patients with an aneurysm on the proximal anterior cerebral artery are included with those with an anterior communicating artery aneurysm, giving a total of 164 patients in this analysis. The age distribution ranged from the second to the eighth decade. Anterior communicating artery aneurysms were slightly more frequent in males. Thirty-two patients had a past history of SAH. On admission, 115 patients were in grades 1 and 2, and 49 patients in the lower grades. Thirteen patients had a recurrent haemorrhage during their stay in hospital before surgery. In the preoperative period, 17 patients had ischaemic complications. Seventy patients had some degree of spasm on pre-operative angiograms. Twenty-six patients had generalised, 32 localised, and 12 segmental vasospasm. Twenty-four patients showed symptomatic hydrocephalus in the pre-operative period. Ninety-three patients were operated on within 12 days of the last haemorrhage.

The majority, 125 patients, were in grades 1 and 2 at the time of surgery. In the postoperative period 23 patients developed ischaemic complications and 17 patients epilepsy. The operative mortality was 5%. Seventy-eight per cent had a good outcome, and in 14% it was fair.

In a controlled study by McKissock et al. (1965) there was no overall long-term difference between surgically and conservatively treated patients, whereas Logue (1956) found long-term mortality to be significantly higher in conservatively treated patients. In his series, the majority of the patients were operated upon 2 weeks after SAH. Seventy per cent of the patients were in a favourable grade at the time of surgery. Durity and Logue (1971) analysed the effect of proximal ligation in the management of anterior communicating aneurysms in 43 patients. In 90% of the patients, the postoperative angiograms were done within 1 month, and in the rest, subsequently. In 14 patients there was a decrease in the size of the aneurysm, and in ten it was not visualised at all. In 37% (16 patients) there was no change in the size of the aneurysm. However, in 7% (three patients) an increase in the size of the aneurysm was noticed.

Hori and Suzuki (1979) studied 346 cases operated on for anterior communicating artery aneurysm. The mortality was 5%, and 75% had a good to excellent outcome.

Nornes and Wikerby (1979) operated on 175 patients with anterior cerebral aneurysms.

Although this figure is similar to ours, they had slightly more aneurysms on the proximal and distal segments of the artery. In 146 patients the aneurysm was located on the anterior communicating artery, and in ten patients, on the proximal anterior cerebral artery. There were 19 patients in whom the aneurysm was on the distal anterior cerebral artery (pericallosal). The outcome after surgery was graded as good in 76% of the patients.

Yasargil and Smith (1982) reported 291 patients with anterior communicating artery aneurysms in a series of 638 patients with SAH. At the time of surgery 131 patients were in grades 1 and 2, and 105 in grade 3. Mortality was 3% in grades 1 and 2, and 7% in grade 3. Four of the 55 patients (7%) in grade 4 also died. Overall, 12 patients (8%) had a poor outcome. All were in grades 3 and 4 at the time of surgery.

Crowell and Ojemann (1983a) operated on 52 cases of anterior communicating artery aneurysms. There were 41 patients in grades 1 and 2, and 11 patients in poorer grades. There was one death in each group. Forty-five per cent (five patients) in lower grades had a poor outcome, compared with 5% of patients in good grades. Overall, the mortality was 4% and the morbidity rate 13% in their series.

In a study of 26 patients with ruptured anterior communicating artery aneurysm selected for surgery, Sengupta et al. (1975) found no change in the quality of survival after direct surgical treatment of the aneurysm. Artiola et al. (1981a), in an analysis of 265 patients with SAH, found patients with anterior communicating artery aneurysms to have least residual neurological deficit.

Pericallosal Aneurysms

Ten patients with pericallosal artery aneurysms were operated on in this series. Nine patients were in the fifth and sixth decades, and only one patient in the second decade of life. The majority were female. On admission, eight patients were in grade 2, and one patient each in grades 3 and 4. Two patients had a past history of SAH. Two patients had further episodes of SAH during their stay in hospital before surgery. Four patients showed angiographic spasm: one generalised, one segmental, and two localised. One patient developed hydrocephalus in the pre-operative period. At the time of operation, seven patients were in grades 1 and 2, and two patients in grade

3. One patient in grade 4 was operated on as he was not showing any further improvement. Eight patients were operated on within 12 days of the last haemorrhage. Two patients developed postoperative epilepsy, and three patients postoperative ischaemic complications. Two patients were treated for symptomatic hydrocephalus. There were three operative deaths. All the seven surviving patients had a good outcome.

Pericallosal aneurysms constitute 2%–5% of cerebral aneurysms (Fisher and Ciminello 1966). Yasargil and Carter (1974) preferred to call them distal anterior cerebral aneurysms. They give credit to Sugar and Tinsley for the first successful treatment of this aneurysm in 1948. In their series of 13 cases, there was no mortality, but four cases were classified as failures. Nine patients went back to work.

Yoshimoto et al. (1979b) operated on 34 cases of distal anterior cerebral aneurysms between 1961 and 1975. Twenty-seven patients (79%) were in a good grade at surgery. The majority were operated on 14 days after SAH. Only three patients were operated on within the first week and nine within the second week. There was only one operative mortality. Seventy-six per cent of the patients had a good to excellent outcome.

Middle Cerebral Artery Aneurysms

In our series of 500 cases, a middle cerebral artery aneurysm was seen in 96 patients at the bifurcation or trifurcation, and in three on the proximal M_1 segment. These are considered as one group. The age of the patient varied from the second to the seventh decade. However, the aneurysms were less frequent below 30 years. Similarly, they were least observed in patients over 60 years of age. There was an almost equal incidence amongst the sexes. Of the 99 patients, six had further SAH before definitive surgery could be carried out. Fifteen patients developed preoperative ischaemic complications. Forty-nine patients showed angiographic evidence of cerebral vasospasm pre-operatively. There were 58 patients in grades 1 and 2, 28 in grade 3, and 13 in grade 4 on admission. By the time of operation, only eight patients were in grade 4, and 27 patients were in grade 3. Sixty-four patients were in grades 1 and 2. Seven patients had preoperative and six patients postoperative hydrocephalus. Thirty patients were operated upon within 7 days, and 34 patients between 8 and 14 days. Only 17 patients were operated on after 21 days. Postoperative ischaemic complications were

noted in 17%, and the incidence of postoperative epilepsy was 12%. The mortality for this group was 6%, with 71% of the patients having a good outcome.

Krayenbuhl et al. (1972) operated on 48 patients with middle cerebral aneurysm. The operative mortality was 10%, and in 70% of patients the outcome was good. Nornes and Wikerby (1979b) operated on 151 middle cerebral artery aneurysms. One hundred and seven (71%) had a good and 13% a poor outcome. The operative mortality was a 6%. In Suzuki's series reported by Yoshimoto et al. (1979a) 174 patients with a ruptured middle cerebral aneurysm were operated on. The mortality was 5%. In 72% of the patients the outcome was good. Eighteen patients (10%) had a poor outcome in their series. Of 62 patients with middle cerebral aneurysm reported by Symon (1982), 29 were in grades 1 and 2, 20 in grade 3, 12 in grade 4, and 1 in grade 5. Those in grades 4 and 5 were not operated on until their neurological condition had improved. Forty-five of the 62 patients were operated on within 15 days. Mortality was 4.8% (three patients). Yasargil and Smith (1982) reported 132 patients with similar aneurysms with recent haemorrhage. Seventy-three patients were in grades 1 and 2, and 40 patients in grade 3. In grades 4 and 5, there were 11 and 8 patients respectively. Seven of the eight patients in grade 5 died. Overall, the mortality was 8%. Seventy-four per cent had a good outcome and in 14% it was fair.

The result of surgical outcome in our series is comparable to the other series reviewed above. In 70% of patients a good outcome can be expected after direct surgical treatment of middle cerebral artery aneurysms.

Posterior Circulation Aneurysms

In this series, only 30 patients with posterior circulation aneurysms were operated on. The age distribution varied from the second to the eighth decade, as in the anterior circulation. The majority were in the fourth, fifth and sixth decades of life. There was a higher incidence in females (Table 11.15). Five patients had a past history of SAH before admission. Twenty patients were in grades 1 and 2, and ten patients in grades 3 and 4 on admission. Two patients developed pre-operative ischaemic complications: one with a superior cerebellar aneurysm and the other with a basilar bifurcation aneurysm. Of the nine patients who showed angiographic evidence of spasm, four had

Table 11.15. Location of posterior circulation aneurysms in relation to sex

	Male	Female	Total
PICA	3	7	10
Vertebrobasilar junction	1	1	2
Superior cerebellar	1	1	2
Basilar bifurcation	7	7	14
Posterior cerebral	1	1	2
Total	13	17	30

a PICA aneurysm. Only two patients had pre-operative hydrocephalus. Twenty-five patients were in grades 1 and 2, four in grade 3 and one in grade 4 at the time of surgery. Only 13 patients were operated on within 12 days of the last haemorrhage. Four patients developed post-operative epilepsy and only one patient had ischaemic complications. The mortality was 20%.

Both patients with vertebrobasilar aneurysms died. Two of the 14 patients with basilar bifurcation aneurysm and one of the two patients with posterior cerebral aneurysm also died. There was only one death amongst ten patients with PICA aneurysm. Twenty-three per cent (seven patients—five with basilar bifurcation and two with superior cerebellar artery aneurysms) had a fair outcome. Overall, 57% (17 patients) had a good outcome at the time of discharge from hospital.

The surgical mortality is considerably higher in this group of aneurysms compared with the whole series (6.4%). The problems encountered in surgical treatment of these aneurysms has been discussed in the previous chapter. Yoshimoto et al. (1979a) reported only 23 patients with aneurysms on the vertebrobasilar system in their series of 1000 cases. Fifty-seven per cent of these patients had a good to excellent outcome. Six patients (26%) had a poor outcome. Mortality was 8.7%. In Nornes and Wikerby's (1979) study of 468 patients, there were only 12 with vertebro-basilar aneurysms. Six of them had a good and four a fair outcome. There was only one death. One patient was classified as having a poor outcome. Drake (1979), with his enormous experience in treating posterior circulation aneurysms, stressed the importance of size and vascular anatomy in influencing the operative result. Mortality in his patients was only 4% with smaller aneurysms and 15% with giant aneurysms.

Quality of Survival

In recent reports (Artiola et al. 1981a; Ropper and Zervas 1984), evaluation of the quality and functional status of patients following surgery for ruptured intracranial aneurysms has been stressed.

In the present series, the outcome at follow-up was assessed according to the patient's capacity for employment. Twenty-two patients (4.7%) were lost to follow-up. The remaining 446 were assessed in the out-patient clinic for a minimum of 6 months after the operation. Overall, 73% had returned to work, 12.5% were capable but unemployed and 14.5% were unfit for any employment. Significantly, functional recovery was found to be related to the location of the aneurysm. Twenty-five per cent of patients operated on for carotid ophthalmic aneurysm and 19% for middle cerebral aneurysm were unfit for employment. The patients operated on for anterior communicating artery aneurysm were the least disabled (9%) (Table 11.12).

Factors Which Influence Outcome

Age

There is considerable controversy about the rationale of investigating and treating elderly patients with SAH (Martindale and Garfield 1978). In a preliminary report, Sengupta et al. (1978) found 75% of the 32 patients treated surgically to have a satisfactory outcome. However, they advised that the risks of surgery should be balanced against advancing age on an individual basis, and stressed the importance of physiological rather than chronological age in evaluating a patient for surgery.

In the present series of 500 patients, the neurological grade of the patients on admission according to age is shown in Table 11.16. There were 57 patients below 30 years, and 59 patients over 60. In these combined age groups, 29 patients were in grade 3 or worse on admission, and 87 in grades 1 and 2. A significantly high number of patients in grades 3 and 4 were over 60 years of age ($P < 0.025$). Fifty-one patients had angiographic spasm, with no significant difference between the two groups (Table 11.17). By the time of operation, there had been a further improvement in the

Table 11.16. Age vs clinical grade on admission

Age	1	2	3	4	5	Total
10–19	5	8	–	–	–	13
20–29	10	25	8	–	1	44
30–39	16	33	16	11	–	76
40–49	27	58	35	13	–	133
50–59	35	90	38	12	–	175
60–69	12	24	9	7	1	53
70–79	1	2	3	–	–	6
Total	106	240	109	43	2	500

Table 11.19. Age vs ischaemic neurological complications

Age	None	Pre-op.	Postop.	Both	Total
10–19	10	2	1	–	13
20–29	39	2	2	1	44
30–39	58	10	7	1	76
40–49	96	7	28	2	133
50–59	131	14	25	5	175
60–69	36	6	10	1	53
70–79	4	–	2	–	6
Total	374	41	75	10	500

Table 11.17. Age vs spasm

	Generalised	Localised	Segmental	Total
10–19	–	4	–	4
20–29	5	15	3	23
30–39	16	11	4	31
40–49	17	27	7	51
50–59	30	35	6	71
60–69	10	8	4	22
70–79	–	1	1	2
Total	78	101	25	204

Table 11.20. Outcome vs age

	Good	Fair	Poor	Died	Total
10–19	12	1	–	–	13
20–29	42	2	–	–	44
30–39	63	12	–	1	76
40–49	98	19	4	12	133
50–59	123	34	6	12	175
60–69	35	11	2	5	53
70–79	2	1	1	2	6
Total	375	80	13	32	500

Table 11.18. Age vs neurological grade at operation

Age	1	2	3	4	Total
10–19	7	5	1	–	13
20–29	14	26	4	–	44
30–39	22	24	24	6	76
40–49	34	68	27	4	133
50–59	52	76	41	6	175
60–69	15	30	8	–	53
70–79	1	4	–	1	6
Total	145	233	105	17	500

neurological condition of the patients; thus there were only 14 patients in grades 3 and 4 (five patients below 30 years of age and nine patients over 60 years) (Table 11.18).

The brain looked abnormal in 46 patients at surgery, and the abnormality was more marked in patients over 60 years. Twelve patients had pre-operative ischaemic complications; seven were over 60 years and five below 30 years. This difference was not significant. Fifteen patients developed postoperative ischaemic complications. Of these, 13 were over 60 years. Thus, there is a significant correlation ($P < 0.001$) between surgical manipulation and the occurrence of postoperative ischaemic complications in patients over 60 years (Table 11.19). The overall mortality in this series is 6.4%. However, if the under 30 and over 60 age groups are considered separately, there is a significant variation. Of the 116 patients in these two age groups, seven patients died, and all were over 60 years of age (12%) ($P < 0.001$). Ninety-one patients had a good outcome and the majority of these were under 30 years of age ($P < 0.005$) (Table 11.20).

Amacher et al. (1977) assessed the role of surgery in 93 good risk patients over 60 years of age. In their series, old patients (60 years or more) tolerated surgery as well as young patients. However, unexpected deaths, unrelated to aneurysm, were common in the older age group. The overall mortality was 17.2% (16 patients) in the older age group, compared with 8.9% in the younger age group. There was also a difference in outcome when the location of the aneurysm was considered. Younger patients with posterior circulation aneurysms had a significantly favourable outcome.

Shepherd (1978) analysed 75 patients over 60 years old among a group of 694 patients who presented with SAH due to an aneurysm or angioma. Forty-two patients were operated on, and nine (22%) died within 3 months. Thirty-three patients were treated conservatively, and ten (30%) died. The survivors in both groups were followed for 6.3 years on average. The quality of life was distinctly better in the operated group of patients. Nornes and Wikerby (1979) studied 468 patients who underwent surgery for aneurysmal SAH. There were 72

Table 11.21. Age vs occupational status at follow-up

	< 19	< 29	< 39	< 49	< 59	< 69	< 79	Total
Employed	11	36	58	87	104	29	1	326
Capable but unemployed	0	5	7	13	24	7	1	57
Unfit	1	1	8	15	29	7	2	63
Lost to follow-up	1	2	2	6	6	5	–	22
Total	13	44	75	121	163	48	4	468

patients in the first three decades, and 75 in the seventh decade of life. In 88% of patients in the younger age group, and 67% in the older age group, the outcome was good after surgery. There were only four deaths, three of which were in the older age group. The overall mortality in his series was 5%.

In an analysis of 1000 cases by Yoshimoto et al. (1979a), 39 patients were below 30 years, and 164 patients in the seventh and eighth decades of life. Eighty-seven per cent of the younger age group of patients had a good to excellent outcome, compared to 61% of the older age group. The mortality was 3% in the younger age group of patients, and three times as high in the older age group.

Artiola et al. (1980), in an analysis of 265 patients with SAH, found an overall mortality of 20%. Mortality was proportional to the age of the patients. In patients below 30 there were no deaths. Mortality increased to 34.4% in patients over 60 years of age.

In summary, with increasing age the postoperative morbidity and mortality increase. However, the outcome of surgical treatment is better than the natural history, even in the older age group, if selection for surgery is made on the basis of the physiological rather than the chronological age (Table 11.21).

Sex

The prognosis in males treated surgically for ruptured intracranial aneurysms is better than in females (Richardson et al. 1966a; Artiola et al. 1981a, b).

Of the 85 patients with postoperative ischaemic complications in our series, 25 were male and 60 female (Table 11.22). Of the 32 patients who died postoperatively, 7 were male and 25 female. Although our results are in agreement with the other reported series, the reason for this sex difference is not clear.

Table 11.22. Sex vs ischaemic neurological complications

	None	Pre-op.	Postop.	Both	Total
Male	156	22	21	4	203
Female	218	19	54	6	297
Total	374	41	75	10	500

Site of Aneurysm

There is no significant difference in the mortality after surgery for different groups of aneurysms in the anterior circulation. However, when certain subgroups are examined, some difference can be noted. There was no mortality in the 24 patients with a carotid ophthalmic aneurysm, and only one death in the 32 with a carotid bifurcation aneurysm. Two of the ten patients with an anterior choroidal aneurysm died. Mortality in patients with posterior circulation aneurysms is three times (20%) greater than among those with anterior circulation aneurysms. This may partly reflect the difficult access and rarity of the posterior circulation aneurysms.

Yoshimoto et al. (1979a) also found a slight increase in mortality in patients undergoing surgery for vertebrobasilar aneurysms.

In relation to the quality of survival, the outcome was good in 76% of internal carotid and 78% of anterior cerebral artery aneurysm patients in our series. It was reduced to 71% in middle cerebral artery aneurysm and 57% in posterior circulation aneurysm patients (Table 11.23).

In Yasargil and Smith's series (1982), the middle cerebral aneurysm group had the highest (8%) mortality. There were no deaths among 26 carotid ophthalmic and 20 pericallosal aneurysm patients.

Drake (1981) reported 35 patients with aneurysms in all locations over 60 years of age. All were in Botterell grades 1, 2 and 3. There were no operative deaths in 21 patients with anterior circulation aneurysms, while only one of

Table 11.23. Outcome vs type of aneurysm operated on

Outcome	Internal carotid	ACA	MCA	Post. circ.	Total
Good	149	138	71	17	375
Fair	29	23	21	7	80
Poor	7	5	1	–	13
Died	12	8	6	6	32
	197	174	99	30	500

Table 11.25. Neurological grade at operation vs outcome

Grade	Good	Fair	Poor	Died	Total
1	122	16	3	4	145
2	184	25	8	16	233
3	65	33	1	6	105
4	4	6	1	6	17
5	–	–	–	–	–
Total	375	80	13	32	500

the 14 patients operated on for posterior circulation aneurysm died. There was one poor result in each group.

Neurological Condition of the Patient

The neurological condition of the patient at admission and the time of operation has an important bearing on the prognosis (Botterell et al. 1956; Hunt and Hess 1968; Nishioka 1966; Nibbelink et al. 1977).

In the present series, there were 106 patients in grade 1, 240 patients in grade 2, and 109 and 43 in grades 3 and 4 respectively on admission (Table 11.24). Eighty-seven per cent of grade 1 and 77% of grade 2 patients had a good outcome, while the mortality in these two grades was 1% and 7% respectively. Of the 109 patients in grade 3, only 67% had a good outcome, and the mortality was as high as 11%.

When the neurological grade at operation was taken into consideration, 84% of grade 1 and 79% of grade 2 patients had a good outcome, compared to only 62% and 24% in grades 3 and 4 respectively ($P < 0.001$) (Table 11.25). Six out of 17 patients who were in grade 4 at the time of operation died (35%). Patients in good grades had a significantly better outcome ($P < 0.001$).

In the series of Yoshimoto et al. (1979a) about 73% of patients operated on were in grade 2 or better. Twenty per cent were in grade 3 and 3.5% in grade 4. Mortality was 12% in poorer grades,

Table 11.24. Neurological grade on admission vs outcome at discharge

Grade	Good	Fair	Poor	Dead	Total
1	92	9	4	1	106
2	184	35	5	16	240
3	73	20	4	12	109
4	24	16	–	3	43
5	2	–	–	–	2
Total	375	80	13	32	500

compared to the overall mortality of 6.1%. Of the patients considered as having a good to excellent outcome at discharge, 85% were in favourable grades and 15% in poorer grades at surgery.

In Krayenbuhl et al.'s (1972) series of 231 anterior circulation aneurysm patients, there were 42 in grade 1 and 70 in grade 2 at surgery. In grades 3 and 4 there were 74 and 39 patients respectively, while six patients were in grade 5. There was no operative mortality in grade 1 and 2 patients. Five of the six patients in grade 5 died and one had a poor outcome. Of the patients who were in grade 3 at operation, 12.5% died, compared with the overall mortality of 5%.

In Yasargil and Smith's 1982 series of 638 patients with SAH, from the same centre as above, 160 were in grade 1, 202 in grade 2, and 189 in grade 3 at the time of surgery. Grades 4 and 5 included 75 and 12 patients respectively. Ninety-six per cent of patients in grades 1 and 2 had a good outcome, compared to 68% in poorer grades. The mortality was only 1% for patients in grades 1 and 2, while it rose to 9% for patients in poorer grades.

Of the 466 patients with recent SAH analysed by Sundt et al. (1982), 232 were in grade 1, 110 in grade 2, and 104 in grade 3. There were only 20 patients in grade 4 at operation. Mortality was highest (13%) in grade 4 patients and lowest in grade 1 patients. It was 3.6% and 4.8% in grades 2 and 3 respectively. As the main difference between grades 1 and 2 is the presence or absence of meningeal reaction, these authors concluded that an inflammatory reaction about the vessels predisposes to vasospasm and infarction. Our observations are similar, particularly in relation to postoperative ischaemic neurological deficit.

The surgical outcome in patients with various neurological grades is also considerably influenced by the timing of surgery. However, the overall management mortality can be reduced by submitting the patients in a favourable neurological condition to early surgery (Hunt and Hess 1968). Mortality in patients who are drowsy and operated on 1 week after the last haemorrhage is half that of those operated on within a week (Drake 1968). Poor outcome after surgery in grade 3 patients may be due to cerebral ischaemia and vasospasm. Surgical manipulation in these patients with brain oedema makes things worse (Hunt and Kosnik 1974).

Time of Admission to Neurological Centre

There are few reports in the literature concerning the influence of the interval between SAH and admission to the neurological centre on the final outcome after surgery. Recently, in a co-operative study Kassell et al. (1981) analysed 511 patients with verified SAH. They divided the patients into two groups. Two hundred and forty-nine patients were admitted on days 0–3 post-haemorrhage, and 262 patients on days 4–7. The patients were further subdivided into good condition (grades 1, 2 and 3) and poorer condition (grades 4 and 5). These two groups were comparable with regard to the time interval between SAH and surgery, and the type of operation. There was a slightly smaller number of good condition patients in the days 0–3 group (76% vs 84%) ($P < 0.05$). There was a higher rebleed rate in patients admitted on days 0–3, irrespective of the neurological condition on admission. Overall, the outcome was also less favourable in patients admitted on days 0–3. Thirty-four per cent of patients admitted on days 0–3 and 24% of patients admitted on days 4–7 died by 90 days post-haemorrhage. Thus, a natural selection takes place in those patients who are admitted later to a neurological centre.

Adams et al. (1981) analysed 249 patients admitted within 3 days of SAH. All the patients were operated on after 2 weeks. During the first 2 weeks, 9.2% of patients in a good condition and 25% of those in a poor condition rebled. Proven rebleeds also occurred in nine good and four poor condition patients up to 90 days after the initial haemorrhage. The mortality during this period was 6.5% among patients in a good grade and 32.8% among those who were in a poor condition at the time of admission. The two major causes of death were rebleed and progressive neurological deterioration.

Timing of Surgery

There is controversy regarding the optimum time for surgical treatment of ruptured intracranial aneurysms. An operation performed during the early days after SAH would be ideal to prevent recurrence of bleeding. However, because of altered cerebrovascular physiology there are risks of complications after early surgery. Hence, when electing the time of surgery, the risks of re-bleeding should be balanced against the probable complications following surgery. An operation performed many weeks later, though helpful in preventing a late recurrence of bleed and reducing the operative mortality and morbidity, does not help in the immediate postictal period.

Mullan et al. (1978) managed 97 patients with similar neurological conditions on admission by means of antifibrinolytics, hypotension, intracranial pressure control and respiratory support where needed, in the pre-operative period. On average they operated 10 days after SAH, when lumbar CSF pressure came down to around 200 mm H_2O. There was no operative mortality, but nine patients deteriorated and six patients rebled before operation, and all of these 15 patients died. The overall management mortality was thus 15%.

In 56 patients with SAH analysed by Giannotta et al. (1979), 39 were in grades 1 and 2 at operation, and 7 in grade 3. Grades 4 and 5 included ten patients. Five patients died before surgery. Twenty-nine patients were operated on within 7 days. There was no operative death in patients who were in grades 1 and 2. Two patients operated on in grades 4 and 5 died. One patient in grade 3 also died. The overall operative mortality was 5.8%, and the total management mortality was 14.2%.

Weir and Aronyk (1981) studied 224 patients admitted to hospital on day 0 or day 1 after SAH. One hundred and forty-nine patients had surgery for aneurysm. Fifty-seven were operated upon within 3 days, 59 between 4 and 9 days, and the remaining 33 patients after 9 days. Seventy-five patients died without definitive operation. They found that when operation was delayed, postoperative mortality decreased but the management mortality increased, as more patients awaiting surgery died. This difference was evident especially in grades 3 and 4 patients ($P < 0.005$). Grade 1 and 2 patients had a better operative and management mortality than grade 3 and 4 patients.

Drake (1981) also noticed an increased incidence of rebleed and cerebral ischaemia with vasospasm in a significant number of patients, resulting in a higher overall mortality if surgery was delayed.

Some of the reports in the literature do not include overall management mortality. However, the following reviews give a good indication of the influence of timing or surgery on outcome.

Krayenbuhl et al. (1972) analysed 231 patients with anterior circulation aneurysms to indicate the timing of surgery. Twenty-four percent were operated on within 1 week and 52% within the second week. Of the 56 patients operated on in the first week, 23 were in grades 1 and 2, 11 in grade 3, and 16 in grade 4. In the second week, 34 of the 65 patients operated upon were in grades 3 and 4. Only 68% of the patients operated on in the first week had a good outcome, while the percentage of patients having such an outcome increased to 80% in the second week and 90% after 2 weeks. Mortality was 12% in the first week and 8% in the second week.

Hunt and Miller (1977) studied 104 patients with SAH. Patients in good grades only were operated on early. Thirty patients were admitted in grades 1 and 2; 15 were operated on within a week. Three out of the 30 patients in good grades died without operation because of rebleed or infarction. There was only one operative death in a patient who was in grade 3. They found no difference in the mortality with early or later operation.

Adams et al. (1976) operated on 100 cases over a 2-year period. Sixty-five patients were in Botterell grade 1, 17 in grade 2, and 18 in grade 3. Fifty-eight patients were operated on in the first week, and 22 in the second week. Mortality was highest in patients operated on in the first week. Thirty-five patients operated on in the first week were in grade 1, and five patients died, while there were no deaths among the 14 grade 1 patients who were operated on in the second week. Adams et al. stressed the importance of operating after 1 week.

Samson et al. (1979) evaluated morbidity in 106 grade 1 and 2 patients undergoing early (less than 8 days) or late (more than 8 days) surgery following SAH. There was no significant difference in the incidence of either intra-operative complications or morbidity. However, there was a slight increase in postoperative ischaemic complications in the group operated on earlier. Interestingly, the incidence of recurrent haemorrhage was high in patients operated on after 8 days, though they were on antifibrinolytic drugs, highlighting the limitations of this therapy. Twenty-three per cent of the patients with early surgery had a poor or fair outcome on discharge, but at 6 months there were only 8% in a similar condition.

In Suzuki's series (Yoshimoto et al. 1979a) the mortality was highest (20.2%) in patients operated upon on days 3–7, and least (3.8%) in those

operated on 15 days after SAH. In only 50% of the patients operated on in the first week was the outcome good to excellent, compared with 65% or more after the second week. Though the results of surgery in the first week were poor, they differed strikingly according to the day of operation (Suzuki et al. 1979).

Similarly, Sano (1979) analysed 403 patients; 60 patients (15%) were operated on within the first week after SAH, and 343 patients (85%) later. The mortality was 15% in the patients operated on in the first week, while only 3.7% of patients operated on later, died. The operative mortality was highest (14.3%) between days 4 and 8 post-SAH. There were no deaths among 18 patients operated on within 3 days.

In Yasargil and Smith's 1982 series, 38% were operated on within 14 days, and 31% 4 weeks or more after SAH. Seventy-four per cent (180 patients) of the early operated group had a good outcome after surgery, with a mortality of 8%, while 90% of the patients operated on 2 weeks after SAH had a good outcome, with only 2% mortality.

Nornes and Wikerby (1979) operated on grade 1 and 2 patients as soon as possible, but delayed the operation in grade 3 patients until they improved or became stable. Mortality in patients operated on within 3 days was high (26%). There was no significant difference between days 4 and 14. After 2 weeks, the mortality was considerably less.

Peerless (1979) advocated surgery 1 week after haemorrhage, as the condition of the brain, i.e. brain swelling and fragility of the aneurysm, make operating conditions difficult if the patient is submitted to surgery earlier.

Early operation in patients with multiple haemorrhages was associated with a high mortality in the series reported by Shepherd (1983). In the single haemorrhage group, mortality was highest (19%) in those operated on between days 5 and 7 post-haemorrhage. The overall mortality was 13%. In the multiple haemorrhage group, mortality was highest in patients operated on between days 1–4 (39%) with an overall mortality of 25%.

In an attempt to reduce the overall management mortality, early surgery is gaining favour with some surgeons. Taneda (1982) found significantly less mortality and morbidity in patients operated on within 48 h. However, Ljunggren et al. (1981) operated on 81 grade 1, 2 and 3 patients within 48 h, with a mortality of 16%. Seventeen of the 81 patients developed delayed ischaemic complications. Seventy-four per cent had a good, and 10% a fair outcome at discharge. Four of the 13 patients over 60 years of the age died, and three had a fair outcome.

Mizukami et al. (1982) operated on 64 patients within 4 days of SAH. There were seven patients in grade 1 and 24 in grade 2 at the time of surgery. In grades 3 and 4 there were 20 and 13 patients respectively. They aggressively removed the clot from the basal cistern, as far as possible. At 3 months follow-up, all the grade 1 patients had an excellent result. Eighty-four per cent (20 patients) in grade 2 and 85% (17 patients) in grade 3 also had similar results. In only one (7.8%) patient in grade 4 was the outcome excellent. Overall, 18 patients (28%) had a poor to fair outcome.

Hugenholtz and Eldie (1982) reviewed 100 grade 1, 2 and 3 patients at operation in different periods. Mortality was lower in patients operated on within 48 h after SAH than in those operated on after 7 days. It was maximum in patients operated on between days 3 and 7.

The International Cooperative Study on Timing of Aneurysm Surgery involved a study of 3521 patients (Kassel and Torner 1985, personal communication). Of these patients, 45.3% were operated on during the first 3 days, 10.6% between 4 and 6 days, 17.7% between 7 and 10 days, 12.3% between 11 and 14 days and 7% between 15 and 32 days. In 7.1% no surgery was carried out. In the surgical group there was good recovery in 67.9% of patients; 10.4% were moderately disabled, 5.7% were severely disabled, 1.7% had a vegetative survival and 14.3% died.

In our study of 500 patients, 57% were operated on within 12 days of the last haemorrhage: 10% within 4 days, 23% between 5 and 7 days, and 24% between 8 and 11 days. Less than 16% were operated upon beyond 21 days after the last haemorrhage. The neurological condition of the patients at the time of operation is shown in Table 11.26. Patients operated on within 14 days were significantly more often in grades 1 and 2 than in the lower grades ($P < 0.05$). The majority of grade 3 patients (55%) were operated on after 11 days, while only 34% of grade 2 patients had late

Table 11.26. Clinical grade vs timing of surgery

Days	0–4	5–7	8–11	12–14	15–18	19–21	> 21	Total
1	21	30	27	17	14	6	30	145
2	20	66	69	29	15	10	24	233
3	7	16	24	16	8	10	24	105
4	5	2	1	4	3	2	–	17
5	–	–	–	–	–	–	–	–
	53	114	121	66	40	28	78	500

Table 11.27. Timing of operation vs ischaemic complications

	0–4	5–7	8–11	12–14	15–18	19–21	> 21	Total
Yes	10	21	28	10	8	4	4	85
No	43	93	93	56	32	24	74	415
	53	114	121	66	40	28	78	500

Table 11.28. Timing of surgery vs outcome

	0–4	5–7	8–11	12–14	15–18	19–21	> 21	Total
Good	39	94	89	48	31	18	56	375
Fair	6	13	22	9	7	7	16	80
Poor	1	3	2	4	0	2	1	13
Died	7	4	8	5	2	1	5	32
	53	114	121	66	40	28	78	500

operation ($P < 0.005$). Fifty-seven per cent of patients operated on between days 5 and 11 were in neurological grade 2. Two hundred and thirty-five patients were operated on between days 5 and 11. Ischaemic complications were found more frequently in patients operated on during this period than at any other time (Table 11.27). Fourteen per cent of patients operated upon within 4 days died, compared with only 5% operated upon between 5 and 11 days (Table 11.28). However, a detailed analysis of Table 11.13 will indicate that surgery alone did not influence the mortality within 4 days of SAH.

Possible Measures for Selection of Ideal Time for Surgery

Apart from the neurological condition of the patient, there are no definite parameters for electing the optimum time for surgical intervention in patients with aneurysmal SAH. However, there are several factors which have been studied for this purpose.

Klafta and Hamby (1969) were the first to measure intracranial pressure and correlate it with the neurological grade at operation and the final outcome. They measured lumbar CSF pressure in 123 patients undergoing surgery for recent haemorrhage. Patients were graded according to the Hunt and Hess system and were subdivided into two groups on the basis of CSF pressure— CSF pressure less than 200 mm H_2O and more than 200 mm H_2O. The mortality was significantly higher in grade 3 patients with a CSF pressure more than 200 mm H_2O. The pre-operative CSF pressure did not influence outcome in the other grades.

In patients unfit for immediate surgery, continuous intracranial pressure monitoring has been used to determine the optimum time (Nornes 1973) By waiting until the extradural pressure fell to about 200–400 mm H_2O, the operative conditions became satisfactory (Nornes and Magnaes 1972).

Kelly et al. (1977) carried out dynamic perfusion studies using Tc^{99m}. They found that the extent of cerebral perfusion had a bearing on both the pre-operative and the postoperative course. Although the incidence of rebleeding in patients with normal perfusion is high, in general the outcome is satisfactory. Patients with low perfusion have a high incidence of ischaemic complications, especially after aneurysm surgery.

The presence of angiographic spasm is regarded as a contraindication to surgery by some. Parks and James (1971) measured cerebral blood flow and EEG in patients with SAH. They noticed an increase in the theta activity in severely ill patients and correlated this observation with the presence of spasm. They advised serial EEG to judge the reversal of spasm and to decide on the timing of surgical intervention.

Voldby and Enevoldsen (1982c) found high CSF lactate levels with the increase in intracranial pressure and the presence of vasospasm. As the outcome in these patients is poor, they suggested pre-operative estimation of CSF lactate levels, which may help in the timing of operation.

The cerebral autoregulatory capacity is impaired to a variable degree following subarachnoid haemorrhage. Bohm and Hugosson (1979) used I 131-labelled para-aminohippuric acid intravenously, as an indicator to measure cerebral circulation. Operation was performed only after the blood flow reached normal values.

Symon et al. (1972) found a good correlation between cerebral blood flow and the neurological condition of the patients. Cerebral blood flow studies within a day of operation were also found to be helpful by Hunt and Miller (1977). Cerebral conduction time has also been used to select the appropriate time for surgery by Symon et al. (1979).

Cerebral blood flow measurements were found to be prognostic indicators in some studies. An increase in cerebral blood flow on the day following surgery, relative to the pre-operative values, gave a better prognosis (Merory et al. 1979). Intra-operative measurement of cerebral blood flow response to drug-induced hypotension helps to identify patients at risk of developing complications. Pickard et al. (1980) studied 20 patients; in 15 there was increased cerebral blood flow,

and only one patient in this group developed late ischaemia. Of the five patients in whom cerebral blood flow fell, four developed ischaemic problems.

Condition of the Brain at Operation

Postoperative neurological deterioration is more frequent in patients in whom a hyperaemic and swollen brain is seen at surgery (Peerless 1979). However, the neurological condition of the patient before surgery will not always reflect the condition of the brain to be found at surgery (Voldby and Enevoldsen 1982b).

The pre-operative lactate levels were high in patients in whom the brain looked red and swollen at surgery (Voldby and Enevoldsen 1982).

In our series of 500 patients, the brain looked abnormal (tense, oedematous or infarcted) in 197 patients at operation (39%). In patients over 50 years the brain was normal in 56%, compared to 65% of patients below 50 years ($P < 0.05$) (Table 11.29). In 35% of grade 1 and 2 patients and 64% of those in grade 3 or worse on admission, the brain looked abnormal at surgery ($P < 0.001$). There was a significantly greater number of patients in grade 3 or less at surgery in whom the brain was abnormal ($P < 0.001$) (Table 11.30).

It is also interesting to note that there was a significant difference in the condition of the brain between patients in grades 1 and 2 at the time of surgery ($P < 0.001$) (Table 11.31). In only 23%

Table 11.29. Age vs brain appearance at surgery

	Normal	Abnormal	Not stated	Total
10–19	9	4	–	13
20–29	28	16	–	44
30–39	45	26	5	76
40–49	74	47	12	133
50–59	90	78	7	175
60–69	23	23	7	53
70–79	2	3	1	6
	271	197	32	500

Table 11.30. Grade on admission vs brain appearance

	Normal	Abnormal	Not stated	Total
1	82	21	3	106
2	133	93	14	240
3	49	49	11	109
4	7	32	4	43
5	–	2	–	2
	271	197	32	500

Table 11.31. Neurological grade at operation vs brain appearance

Neurological grade	Normal	Abnormal	Not stated	Total
1	106	32	7	145
2	126	92	15	233
3	37	59	9	105
4	2	14	1	17
5	–	–	–	–
	271	197	32	500

Table 11.32. Pre-operative spasm vs brain appearance

Type of spasm	Normal	Abnormal	Not stated	Total
Generalised	34	36	8	78
Localised	52	45	4	101
Segmental	10	14	1	25
None	175	102	19	296
	271	197	32	500

Table 11.33. Brain appearance vs outcome

	Normal	Abnormal	Not stated	Total
Good	228	124	23	375
Fair	32	44	4	80
Poor	3	10	–	13
Died	8	19	5	32
	271	197	32	500

to 69% of patients in whom the brain looked abnormal ($P < 0.001$) (Table 11.33).

Cerebral Vasospasm

Diffuse intracranial spasm is associated with increased intracranial tension. The incidence of spasm is high in patients who rebleed, and the prognosis in these patients is poor (Strornelli and French 1964). However, the effects of intracranial arterial spasm on surgical outcome have not been clearly defined. The outcome is also complicated by the pathophysiological variables, such as pre-ictal health, severity of the haemorrhage and possible autonomic and endocrine dysfunction due to SAH (Wilkins 1977). Krayenbuhl et al. (1972) stressed the importance of clinical condition and not the presence of spasm in patients undergoing surgery for aneurysmal SAH. In their opinion, in an alert and intact patient the presence of spasm is no contraindication to surgery, and we agree with their view.

Adams et al. (1978) studied postoperative angiographically confirmed spasm and intracranial pressure, and correlated their effect on the neurological condition. There were ten patients with vasospasm. In eight patients there was evi-

of grade 1 patients did the brain look abnormal, compared to 42% of patients in grade 2. The brain was abnormal in only 34% of patients without angiographic spasm, compared to 47% with spasm ($P < 0.001$) (Table 11.32). Post-operative ischaemic complications were significantly more frequent when the condition of the brain was not favourable ($P < 0.001$). In about 50% of patients operated on between days 5 and 8, the brain looked abnormal, compared to 33% before and 35% after this period (Fig. 11.2). In 59% of the patients who died, the brain was abnormal at surgery ($P < 0.01$). Eighty-nine per cent of the patients whose brain appearance was normal at surgery had a good outcome, compared

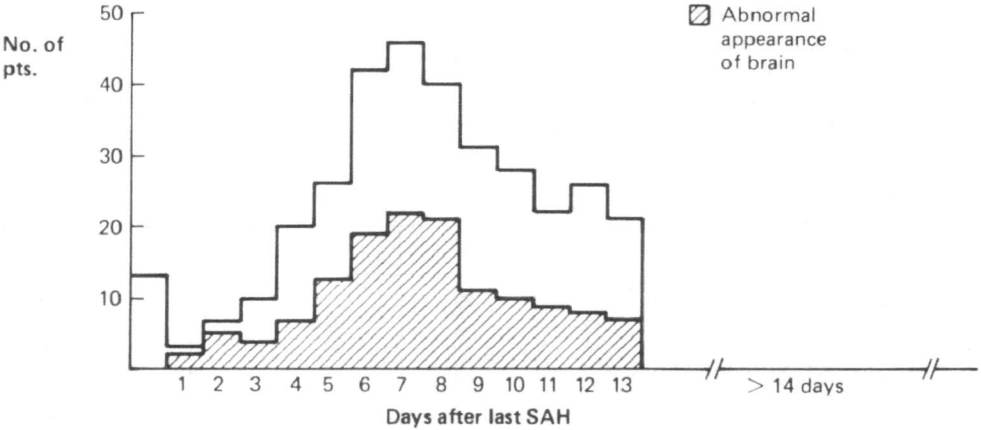

Fig. 11.2. Condition of the brain in relation to the timing of surgery.

dence of neurological deterioration and in three of these the intracranial pressure was high in addition. Of the 18 patients without spasm, six deteriorated, and all of these had increased intracranial pressure.

Mizukami et al. (1980) could predict the development of cerebral vasospasm to a very high level (85%) when high density collections of blood could be seen on CT scan performed within 4 days of SAH. The predictability was not so high when the scan was done more than 4 days after SAH. Similar observations were also made by Fisher et al. (1980). Artiola et al. (1981a–c) found that generalised vasospasm rather than the localised type had an important bearing on the long-term results. A significantly smaller number of patients with generalised postoperative spasm are likely to be fully independent compared to those with localised spasm or no spasm at all.

In our series, there was no correlation between pre-operative angiographic spasm and mortality (Table 11.34). However, the incidence of ischaemic complications was higher in patients with vasospasm (68%) (Table 11.35). Sixty per cent of the patients who had a good outcome did not have pre-operative spasm. Further analysis of the effects of vasospasm on surgical outcome in out series is included in Chap. 12.

Table 11.34. Pre-operative spasm vs condition at discharge

	Good	Fair	Poor	Died	Total
No spasm	227	40	7	22	296
Generalised	59	12	3	4	78
Local	73	20	3	5	101
Segmental	16	8	–	1	25
	375	80	13	32	500

Table 11.35. Spasm vs ischaemic complications

	None	Pre-op.	Postop.	Both	Total
Generalised	48	15	9	6	78
Localised	73	9	17	2	101
Segmental	18	2	5	–	25
None	235	15	44	2	296
	374	41	75	10	500

Ischaemic Complications

The most important feature of the ischaemic syndrome is the temporal profile of the neurological deficit with cerebral blood flow alterations. It starts with a relatively minor deficit, which is often slow in evolution, and may culminate over a period of hours or days in major focal deficit, coma or death (Sundt 1975). Focal cerebral ischaemia can occur both before and after operation. Pre-operatively it is seen frequently in patients with a severe degree of meningeal reaction (Sundt 1975). Postoperative deficits may be immediate or delayed (Sundt and Whisnant 1978). In the immediate group, the patients wake up from anaesthesia with a deficit, which was not present previously, and is usually due to vascular trauma at surgery. In the delayed group, they are not present on recovery from anaesthesia, but develop subsequently, presumably due to vasospasm.

We have classified ischaemic complications into pre- and postoperative groups depending upon the time of onset. One hundred and twenty-six patients developed ischaemic complications during their stay in hospital. In 51 patients it was in the pre-operative period and in 75 patients in the postoperative period, whereas ten patients had ischaemic complications in both the pre- and the postoperative period. Only 26 patients were below 40 years of age. When the extremes of age groups were taken into consideration, eight patients below 30 years (14%) and 19 patients (32%) above 60 years had these complications ($P < 0.025$).

Thirty per cent of patients who had pre-operative ischaemic complications were operated on within 10 days of the last haemorrhage, while 51% who had postoperative complications were operated on in the same period ($P < 0.001$). Some degree of angiographic cerebral vasospasm was noted in 34 (68%) of the 51 patients with ischaemic complications in the pre-operative period ($P < 0.001$). Angiography was not performed after the onset of the ischaemic complications, and hence no comment can be made regarding the onset of angiographically confirmed cerebral vasospasm. Fifty-one per cent of the patients who had ischaemic complications in the pre-operative period were in neurological grade 2, and only 10% in grade 1 on admission. Thirty per cent were in grade 3 (Table 11.36). Ten patients who had pre-operative ischaemic changes developed further neurological deterioration postoperatively. Nine of these patients were in grades 3 and 4 at the time of operation, and only one patient was in grade 2. Forty-six per cent of the patients who had postoperative ischaemia were in grade 2 at the time of surgery, while only 24% each were in grades 1 and 3 (Table 11.37). It should be pointed out that in general, grade

Table 11.36. Grade on admission vs ischaemic complications

	None	Pre-op.	Postop.	Both	Total
1	91	5	10	–	106
2	171	21	41	7	240
3	75	12	19	3	109
4	35	3	5	–	43
5	2	–	–	–	2
	374	41	75	10	500

Table 11.37. Grade at operation vs postoperative ischaemic complications

	Ischaemic complications		
Neurological grade	No	Yes	Total
1	125	20	145
2	194	39	233
3	85	20	105
4	11	6	17
5	–	–	–
Total	415	85	500

Table 11.38. Postoperative ischaemic complications vs condition at discharge

	Ischaemic complications		
	Yes	No	Total
Good	33	342	375
Fair	30	50	80
Poor	9	4	13
Dead	13	19	32
Total	85	415	500

3 patients were operated on later. Only 39% of the patients who developed postoperative ischaemia had a good outcome, while 82% of patients without such complications had a similar result. The mortality in patients with postoperative ischaemic complications was 15% compared to only 5% in patients without such complications (Table 11.38).

In Sundt et al.'s series (1982) the incidence of delayed ischaemia was not influenced by the timing of surgery in grade 1 patients. However, in grade 2 patients the incidence increased with early surgical intervention. Symon et al. (1980) classified CT scan findings of basal cisterns into hyperdense or isodense. The ischaemic complications were high in the hyperdense group, and all the patients who died had a hyperdense lesion.

Mizukami et al. (1982) removed the subarachnoid clot at operation as far as possible, and measured the residual clot by follow-up CT scan. Delayed neurological deficit occurred only in patients in whom subarachnoid blood clot remained in the cisterns, thus suggesting that removal of clot from the subarachnoid space will prevent intracranial arterial spasm and associated neurological deterioration.

Recently, Gurusinghe and Richardson (1984) used the amount of blood in the basal cisterns, seen on the CT scan, as an indicator of ischaemic neurological complications. They devised a score for the amount of blood. It ranged from 0 (no clot at all) to 9+. In patients with a CT scan score of 8, 9 or 9+, only 10% had a good outcome, compared to 90% with a score of zero. It was difficult to evaluate patients with scores between 4 and 7. In this group 50% had ischaemic neurological deficit, and half of them recovered.

Epilepsy

Forty-five patients had postoperative epilepsy in our series. Epilepsy was less in younger age groups (Table 11.39). It developed in a smaller number of women (8%) than men (10.3%), though women outnumber men in the total population (Table 11.40). Thirty-one patients had convulsions at the time of SAH, but additional seizures in the postoperative period were seen in only four of these patients. The timing of surgery in patients who did not develop seizures was not significantly different. However, epilepsy was significantly higher in patients who were in grades 3

Table 11.39. Epilepsy vs age

Age	Postop. epilepsy	No epilepsy	Total
10–19	1	12	13
20–29	1	43	44
30–39	6	70	76
40–49	11	122	133
50–59	20	155	175
60–69	6	47	53
70–79	0	6	6
	45	455	500

Table 11.40. Epilepsy vs sex

	Postop. epilepsy	No epilepsy	Total
Male	21	182	203
Female	24	273	297
	45	455	500

Table 11.41. Grade at operation vs postoperative epilepsy

Neurological grade	Epilepsy	No epilepsy	Total
1	15	130	145
2	12	221	233
3	12	93	105
4	6	11	17
	45	455	500

Table 11.42. Type of aneurysm vs epilepsy

	Epilepsy	No epilepsy	Total
ACA	19	155	174
MCA	12	87	99
Internal carotid	10	187	197
Post. circ.	4	26	30
	45	455	500

Table 11.43. Outcome vs postoperative epilepsy

	Epilepsy	No epilepsy	Total
Good	22	353	375
Fair	11	69	80
Poor	4	9	13
Dead	8	24	32
	45	455	500

and 4 at the time of surgery ($P < 0.001$) (Table 11.41). In only 17 patients with seizures did the brain look normal at operation; this was less than in other patients ($P < 0.025$). In 11.5% of patients with intracerebral haematoma, postoperative epilepsy was noted. It also developed in about 16% with pre-operative ischaemic complications, and 13% with postoperative ischaemic complications. Twelve per cent of the patients operated on for middle cerebral artery aneurysm and 11% of patients with anterior communicating artery aneurysm developed epilepsy. It was least common after internal carotid aneurysm. Four patients with posterior circulation aneurysm also developed epilepsy (Table 11.42). In three, the aneurysm was located at the basilar bifurcation, and in one, on the posterior cerebral artery. Excessive brain retraction and temporal lobe resection at surgery may be contributory factors for epilepsy in these cases. Angiographic spasm did not influence the incidence of epilepsy. Epilepsy in the postoperative period was associated with high morbidity and mortality. Only 49% of the patients who had seizures were graded as having a good outcome, compared to 75.5% of patients who were free of seizures ($P < 0.001$) at the time of discharge (Table 11.43). Of the 45 patients who experienced early postoperative seizures, eight died, as opposed to 24 of the 455 patients who were seizure free ($P < 0.005$).

Hypertension

The prognosis of aneurysmal SAH in untreated hypertensive patients is poor (Adams et al. 1976), and hypertensive disease has a significant influence on the surgical outcome. Good results were obtained in 93% of normotensive patients and only 67% of patients with hypertension in Krayenbuhl et al.'s series of 1972. In an analysis of 256 patients, Artiola et al. (1980) found the mortality (23.4%) in normotensive patients to be less than that in those with hypertension (31.5%). When the patients were divided into subgroups according to age, the mortality was found to be higher in those above 50 years old. A high mortality was also found in the study of Robinson (1971). Interestingly, Artiola et al. grouped their patients into hypertensive and non-hypertensive on the basis of systemic blood pressure at the time of admission alone. Thus, patients with chronic hypertension controlled with medication were grouped as normotensive, whereas some patients with reactionary hypertension following SAH were defined as hypertensive.

There were 18 patients with hypertension in a group of 81 patients reported by Ljunggren et al. (1981). Nine patients (50%) developed delayed ischaemic deficit in contrast to six patients (13%) who were normotensive. Eight hypertensive patients were under treatment, and six of these developed delayed ischaemic deficit.

In a controlled study, Rosenwasser et al. (1983) found that preliminary volume expansion and control of blood pressure in patients with known hypertension reduced the incidence of clinical vasospasm significantly ($P < 0.01$). The volume depletion associated with standard diuretic therapy in hypertensive patients with recent SAH may have a deleterious effect, and may precipitate a clinical vasospastic crisis.

In the present series, there were 72 patients with known hypertension who had SAH. Mortality in this group was 14% (eleven) compared to 5.8% in normotensive patients ($P < 0.05$).

Hydrocephalus

In the acute phase of SAH resistance to CSF outflow contributes to increased intracranial pressure (Kostel Janetz 1984), and in the majority the severity of the neurological condition is related to the disturbance of CSF circulation (Doczi et al. 1983). Early surgery and removal of blood clots lessen the risks of fibrosis and impaired CSF flow (Ljunggren et al. 1981). Mortality in patients who develop hydrocephalus is higher.

In the present series, 82 patients developed hydrocephalus either pre- or postoperatively. In seven patients, an external ventricular drain was inserted prior to surgery on the aneurysm. One of these patients developed ventriculitis in the postoperative period and died. In three patients, an external ventricular drain was left at the time of craniotomy for aneurysm, because of either cerebral oedema or hydrocephalus. In one of these patients it was later converted into a ventriculoperitoneal shunt. In four other patients an external ventricular drain was inserted postoperatively, as the neurological condition deteriorated. All four of these died. The causes of death were ventriculitis in one, pulmonary embolism in one, and massive cerebral infarction in two. Overall, 29 patients needed permanent drainage operation (Table 11.44). Only 50% of the patients who developed postoperative hydrocephalus had a good outcome at discharge.

Table 11.44. Incidence of symptomatic hydrocephalus after SAH

Type of aneurysm	Total	Patients needing permanent drainage procedure
Ant. comm. a. complex	44	15
Int. car. a. complex	21	7
MCA	12	4
Posterior circulation	5	3
Total	82	29

Intracerebral Haematoma

Prognosis in patients with intracerebral haematoma following rupture of an aneurysm is directly related to the size of the haematoma. The site also has an influence. It is interesting to note that Wheelock et al. (1983) found a poor prognosis when haematoma involved the parietal lobe. The role of surgery on the offending aneurysm in the acute stage in patients with haematoma is debatable. We prefer to decompress the haematoma only if the space-occupying effect is life threatening. The aneurysm is treated later on, when the brain has recovered from the initial insult.

Surgical Procedures for Aneurysm

It has already been stressed that obliteration of the aneurysm from the circulation is the ideal method of treatment. When the aneurysm was difficult to clip, one of the alternative methods, such as proximal ligation or wrapping, was considered. Therefore, the influence of these procedures on the surgical outcome, other than recurrent haemorrhage, should be measured against the difficulty of direct obliteration. However, Artiola et al. (1981a–c) found the mortality in patients with clipping to be half that among those with wrapping. This was thought to be due partly to damage to the small perforators.

In the present series of 500 cases, 88% (441) of the aneurysms were clipped. Forty-one patients (8%) had wrapping, and in six the aneurysm was trapped. Twelve patients had carotid ligation, of whom eight had simultaneous EC/IC anastomosis in recent times.

In a review of 186 consecutive patients by Paul and Arnold (1970), a major vessel clipping was the major cause of morbidity in good risk patients. In 23 of the 31 patients who died, a major vessel was clipped. There was evidence of infarction at autopsy in 10 of the 16 patients with vessel occlusion.

The aneurysm may remain incompletely occluded following clipping. The incidence of this varies from 4% to 17% in the literature (Zlotnik et al. 1977). If the clip is not in position on check angiography, the patient should be reoperated on as quickly as possible. Delay in surgery makes dissection difficult, and may result in postoperative neurological deficit (Drake and Allcock 1973). Moreover, there is a risk of rebleeding or growth of the aneurysm if it is not treated.

Conclusions

Weir et al. (1975) found that independent variables, such as neurological grade at angiography and at operation, exhibited the highest correlation with the dependent variable of surgical outcome. There was a modest correlation with preoperative spasm, and only a limited relationship with the timing of surgery. Artiola et al. (1981a–

c) devised a discriminant score for predicting outcome, depending upon certain pre-operative and postoperative factors, such as neurological grade, age, blood pressure, timing of operation and site of aneurysm.

In conclusion, the most important factor which contributes to the success of surgical outcome is early surgery in neurologically stable patients. A sound clinical judgement for electing the timing of surgery is required for the others. The overall management mortality can be improved by taking a flexible attitude to each individual patient by taking account of the various factors previously discussed. Early surgery not only prevents recurrent haemorrhage but may prove to be an important step in the prevention of vasospasm by removing the perivascular blood clots. Adequate management of intracranial pressure, both pre- and postoperatively, is another important factor in the prevention and treatment of cerebral ischaemia from vasospasm.

References

Adams CBT, Loach PB, O'Laoire SA (1976) Intracranial aneurysms: Analysis of results of microsurgery. Br Med J II:607–609

Adams CBT, Fearnside MR, O'Laoire SA (1978) An investigation with serial angiography into the evolution of cerebral arterial spasm following aneurysm surgery. J Neurosurg 49:805–815

Adams PH, Kassell NF, Torner JC, Nibbelink DW, Sahs AL (1981) Early management of aneurysmal subarachnoid haemorrhage. A report of the Co-operative Aneurysm Study. J Neurosurg 54:141–145

Alvord EC, Loeser JD, Bailey WL, Copass MK (1972) Subarachnoid haemorrhage due to ruptured aneurysm—a simple method of estimating prognosis. Arch Neurol 27:273–284

Amacher AL, Ferguson GG, Drake CG, Girvin JP, Barr HWK (1977) How old people tolerate intracranial surgery for aneurysm. Neurosurgery 3:242–244

Artiola IL, Fortuny I, Adams CBT, Briggs M (1980) Surgical mortality in an aneurysm population: effects of age, blood pressure and pre-operative neurological state. J Neurol Neurosurg Psychiatry 43:879–882

Artiola IL, Fortuny I, Adams CBT (1981a) Predicting outcome in patients with intracranial aneurysm with the help of microsurgery. J Neurol Neurosurg Psychiatry 44:615–620

Artiola IL Fortuny I, Prieto-Valiente L (1981b) Long-term prognosis in surgically treated intracranial aneurysms. Part 1, Mortality. J Neurosurg 54:26–34

Artiola IL, Fortuny I, Priesto-Valiente L (1981c) Long-term prognosis in surgically treated intracranial aneurysms. Part 2, Morbidity. J Neurosurg 54:35–43

Ask-Upmark E, Ingvar D (1950) A follow-up examination of 138 cases of subarachnoid haemorrhage. Acta Med Scand 138:15–31

Bohm E, Hugosson R (1979) Results of surgical treatment of 200 consecutive cerebral artery aneurysms. Acta Neurol Scand 46:43–52

Botterell EH, Loughead WM, Scott JW, Vanenwafer SL (1956) Hypothermia and interruption of carotid or carotid and vertebral circulation in the surgical management of intracranial aneurysms. J Neurosurg 13:1–42

Brewis M, Poskanzer DC, Rolland C, Miller H (1966) Neurological disease in an English city. Acta Neurol Scand [Suppl] 24:42

Crawford MD, Sarner M (1965) Ruptured intracranial aneurysm—community study. Lancet II:1254–1257

Crowell RM, Ojemann RG (1983a) Surgical treatment of anterior communicating artery aneurysms. In: Schmidek HH, Sweet WH (eds) Operative neurosurgical techniques. Grune and Stratton, New York, pp 829–854

Crowell RM, Ojemann RG (1983b) Surgical treatment of carotid ophthalmic aneurysms. In: Schmidek HH, Sweet WH (eds) Operative neurosurgical techniques. Grune and Stratton, New York

Dell S (1982) Asymptomatic cerebral aneurysm. Assessment of its risk of rupture. Neurosurgery 10:162–166

Doczi T, Nemessanyi Z, Szeguary Z, Huszkar E (1983) Disturbances of cerebrospinal fluid circulation during the acute stage of subarachnoid haemorrhage. Neurosurgery 12:435–438

Drake CG (1968) Comments. J Neurosurg 28:19

Drake CG (1979) The treatment of aneurysms of the posterior circulation. Clin Neurosurg 26:96–144

Drake CG (1981) Management of cerebral aneurysms. Stroke 12:273–283

Drake CG, Allcock JM (1973) Postoperative angiography and the "slipped" clip. J Neurosurg 39:683–689

Drake CG, Vanderlinden RG, Amacher AL (1968a) Carotid-ophthalmic aneurysms. J Neurosurg 29:24–31

Drake CG, Vanderlinden RG, Amacher AL (1968b) Carotid-choroidal aneurysms. J Neurosurg 29:32–36

Durity F, Logue V (1971) The effect of proximal anterior cerebral occlusion on anterior communicating artery aneurysms. J Neurosurg 35:16–19

Ferguson GG, Drake CG (1980) Carotid-ophthalmic aneurysm; the surgical management of those cases presenting with compression of the optic nerve and chiasma alone. Clin Neurosurg 27:263–308

Fisher RG, Ciminello V (1966) Pericallosal aneurysm. J Neurosurg 25:512–515

Fisher CM, Kistler JP, Davis JM (1980) Relation of cerebral vasospasm to subarachnoid haemorrhage. Visualised by computerised tomographic scan. Neurosurgery 6:1–9

Giannotta SL et al. (1979) Total morbidity and mortality rates of patients with surgically treated intracranial aneurysms. Neurosurgery 4:125–128

Graf C (1971) Prognosis for patients with non-surgically treated aneurysms. Analysis of the co-operative study of intracranial aneurysms and subarachnoid haemorrhage. J Neurosurg 35:438–443

Gurusinghe NT, Richardson AE (1984) The value of computerised tomography in aneurysmal subarachnoid haemorrhage. J Neurosurg 60:763–770

Hayward RD (1977) Subarachnoid haemorrhage of unknown aetiology. A clinical and radiological study of 51 cases. J Neurol Neurosurg Psychiatry 40:926–931

Heiskanen O, Marttila I (1970) Risk of rupture of second aneurysm in patients with multiple aneurysms. J Neurosurg 32:295–299

Hori S, Suzuki J (1979) Early and late results of intracranial direct surgery of anterior communicating artery aneurysm. J Neurosurg 50:433–440

Housepian EM, Pool JL (1958) Systemic analysis of intracranial aneurysm from the autopsy file of Presbyterian Hospital—1914–1956. J Neuropathol Exp Neurol 17:409–423

Hudson CH, Raaf J (1968) Timing of angiography and operation in patients with ruptured intracranial aneurysm. J Neurosurg 29:37–41

Hugenholtz H, Eldie RG (1982) Consideration in early surgery on good risk patients with ruptured intracranial aneurysm. J Neurosurg 56:180–185

Hunt WE, Hess RM (1968) Surgical risk as related to time of intervention in the repair of intracranial aneurysm. J Neurosurg 28:14–19

Hunt WE, Kosnik EJ (1974) Timing and peri-operative care in intracranial aneurysm surgery. Clin Neurosurg 21:79–89

Hunt WE, Miller CA (1977) The results of early operation for aneurysm. Clin Neurosurg 24:208–215

Jane JA, Winn HR, Richardson AE (1977) The natural history of intracranial aneurysm. Rebleeding rate during the acute and long-term period and implication for surgical management. Clin Neurosurg 24:176–184

Kassel NF, Drake CG (1982) Timing of aneurysm surgery. Neurosurgery 10:514

Kassel NF, Torner JC (1983) Aneurysmal re-bleeding—a preliminary report from the Co-operative Aneurysm Study. Neurosurgery 13:479–481

Kassel NF, Adams HP, Torner JC, Sahs AL (1981) Influences of timing of admission after aneurysmal subarachnoid haemorrhage on overall outcome. A report of the Co-operative Study. Stroke 12:620–623

Kaste M, Troupp H (1978) Subarachnoid haemorrhage. Long-term follow-up results of late surgical versus conservative treatment. Br Med J I:1310–1311

Kelly PJ, Gorten RJ, Grossman RG et al. (1977) Cerebral perfusion—vascular spasm and outcome in patients with ruptured intracranial aneurysm. J Neurosurg 47:44–49

Klafta LA Jr, Hamby WB (1969) Significance of CSF pressure in determining time for repair of intracranial aneurysm. J Neurosurg 31:217–219

Kostel Janetz M (1984) CSF dynamics in patients with subarachnoid and/or intraventricular haemorrhage. J Neurosurg 60:940–946

Kothandaram P, Dawson BH, Krupt RC (1971) Carotid-ophthalmic aneurysm; a study of 19 patients. J Neurosurg 34:544–548

Krayenbuhl HA, Yasargil MG, Flamm ES et al. (1972) Microsurgical treatment of intracranial saccular aneurysm. J Neurosurg 37:678–686

Leo RD, Mielke B, Allen P (1982) Letters to the Editor, Neurosurgery 11:330

Ljunggren B, Brandt L, Kagstrom E et al. (1981) Results of early operation for ruptured aneurysm. J Neurosurg 54:473–479

Locksley HB (1966) Natural history of subarachnoid haemorrhage, intracranial aneurysm and AVM based on 6,368 cases in the Co-operative Study. J Neurosurg 25:219–239

Locksley HB (1969) Natural history of subarachnoid haemorrhage, intracranial aneurysm and AVM In: Sahs AL, Perret GE, Locksley HB, Nishioka H (eds) Intracranial aneurysm and subarachnoid haemorrhage. A Co-operative Study. JB Lippincott, Philadelphia Toronto, pp 37–57

Logue V (1956) Surgery in spontaneous subarachnoid haemorrhage. Operative treatment of aneurysm on the anterior cerebral and anterior communicating arteries. Br Med J I:473–479

Martindale BV, Garfield J (1978) Subarachnoid haemorrhage above the age of 59. Are intracranial investigations justified? Br Med J I:465–466

McCallum JC, Gendell H, Jannetta P, Wilkins RH (1976) Pre-infarction diuresis following subarachnoid haemorrhage. Presented at the 28th Annual Meeting of the South Neurological Society, New Orleans, Louisiana, 20th Feb. (Quoted by Wilkins RH, Clin Neurosurg, vol 24).

McKissock W, Richardson A, Walsh L (1960) Posterior communicating aneurysm. A controlled trial of the conservative and surgical treatment of ruptured aneurysm of the internal carotid artery at or near the point of origin of the posterior communicating artery. Lancet I:1203–1206

McKissock W, Richardson A, Walsh L (1962) Middle cerebral aneurysm. Further results in control trial of conservative and surgical treatment of ruptured intracranial aneurysm. Lancet II:417–421

McKissock W, Richardson A, Walsh L et al. (1964) Multiple intracranial aneurysms. Lancet I:623–626

McKissock W, Richardson A, Walsh L (1965) Anterior communicating aneurysm—a trial of conservative and surgical treatment. Lancet I:873–876

Merory J, du Boulay GH, Marshall J et al. (1979) Cerebral blood flow following aneurysmal surgery after subarachnoid haemorrhage. Acta Neurochir (Abstr) 46:180

Mizukami M, Takemae T, Tazawa T, Kawase T, Matenzaki T (1980) Value of computerised tomography in the prediction of cerebral vasospasm after aneurysm rupture. Neurosurgery 7:583–586

Mizukami M, Kawasi T, Usani T, Tazawa T (1982). Prevention of vasospasm by early operation with removal of subarachnoid blood. Neurosurgery 10:301–307

Mullan S, Hanlon K, Brown F (1978) Management of 136 consecutive supratentorial berry aneurysms. J Neurosurg 49:794–804

Nibbelink DW, Torner JC, Henderson WG (1977) Intracranial aneurysms and subarachnoid haemorrhage—A report on a randomized treatment study. Stroke 8:202–218

Nishioka H (1966) Evaluation of the conservative management of ruptured intracranial aneurysm. J Neurosurg 25:574–592

Nornes H (1973) The role of intracranial pressure in the arrest of haemorrhage in patients with ruptured intracranial aneurysm. J Neurosurg 39:226–234

Nornes H, Magnaes B (1972) Intracranial pressure in patients with ruptured saccular aneurysm. J Neurosurg 36:537–547

Nornes H, Wikerby P (1979) Results of microsurgical management of intracranial aneurysm. J Neurosurg 51:608–614

Pakarinen S (1967) Incidence, aetiology and prognosis of primary subarachnoid haemorrhage. Acta Neurol Scand [Suppl] 29:1–128

Parks JD, James IM (1971) Electro-encephalographic and cerebral blood flow changes following spontaneous subarachnoid haemorrhage. Brain 94:69–76

Paul RL, Arnold JG Jr (1970) Operative factors influencing mortality in intracranial aneurysm surgery. Analysis of 186 consecutive cases. J Neurosurg 32:289–294

Peerless SJ (1979) Pre- and post-operative management of cerebral aneurysms. Clin Neurosurg 26:209–231

Phillips LH, Whisnant JP, O'Fallon WM Sundt TM Jr (1980) The unchanging pattern of subarachnoid haemorrhage in a community. Neurology (New York) 30:1034–1040

Pickard JD, Matheson M, Patterson J, Wyper D (1980) Prediction of late ischaemic complications after cerebral aneurysm surgery by the intra-operative measurement of central blood flow. J Neurosurg 53:305–308

Richardson AE, Jane JA, Payne PM (1964) Assessment of the natural history of anterior communicating artery aneurysms. J Neurosurg 21:266–274

Richardson AE, Jane JA, Payne PM (1966a) The prediction of morbidity and mortality in anterior communicating aneurysms treated by proximal anterior carotid ligation. J Neurosurg 25:280–283

Richardson AE, Jane JA, Yashow D (1966b) Prognostic factors in the untreated course of posterior communicating aneurysms. Arch Neurol 14:172–176

Robinson RG (1971) Ruptured aneurysm of the middle cerebral artery. J Neurosurg 35:25–33

Ropper AH, Zervas NT (1984) Outcome one year after subarachnoid haemorrhage from cerebral aneurysm. Management, morbidity, mortality and functional status in 112 consecutive good risk patients. J Neurosurg 60:909–915

Rosenwasser RH, Delgado TE, Buchheit WA, Freed MH (1983) Control of hypertension and prophylaxis against vasospasm in cases with subarachnoid haemorrhage. A preliminary report. Neurosurgery 12:658–661

Sahs AL, Nibbelink DW, Torner JC (1981) Aneurysmal subarachnoid haemorrhage: report of the Co-operative Study. Urban & Schwarzenberg, Baltimore Munich

Samson DS, Hodosh RM, Reid WR et al. (1979) Risk of intracranial aneurysm surgery with good grade patients—early versus late operation. Neurosurgery 5:422–426

Sano K (1979) Personal experiences. In: Pia HW, Langmaid C, Zierski J (eds) Cerebral aneurysms. Advances in diagnosis and therapy. Springer, Berlin Heidelberg New York, pp 428–432

Sengupta RP, Chiu JSP, Brierley H (1975) Quality of survival following direct surgery for anterior communicating artery aneurysm. J Neurosurg 43:58–64

Sengupta RP, Gryspeerdt GL, Hankinson J (1976) Carotid-ophthalmic aneurysm. J Neurol Neurosurg Psychiatry 39:837–853

Sengupta RP Lassman LP, Hankinson J (1978) Scope of surgery for intracranial aneurysm in the elderly. A preliminary report. Br Med J II:246–267

Shephard RH (1978) Subarachnoid haemorrhage in patients over 59 (letter). Br Med J I:921

Shephard RH (1983) Ruptured cerebral aneurysm: early and late prognosis with surgical treatment—a personal series 1958–1980. J Neurosurg 59:6–15

Strornelli SA, French JD (1964) Subarachnoid haemorrhage—factors in prognosis and management. J Neurosurg 21:769–779

Sundt TM (1975) Management of ischaemic complications after subarachnoid haemorrhage. J Neurosurg 43:418–425

Sundt TM Jr, Whisnant JP (1978) Subarachnoid haemorrhage from intracranial aneurysm. Surgical management and natural history of disease. N Engl J Med 299:116–122

Sundt TM, Kobayashi S, Fodi NL, Whisnant JP (1982) Results and complications of surgical management of 809 intracranial aneurysms in 722 cases. J Neurosurg 56:753–765

Suzuki J, Ozuma T, Yoshimoto T (1979) Results of early operation on cerebral aneurysm. Surg Neurol 11:407–412

Symon L (1982) Surgical management of middle cerebral artery aneurysm. In: Schmidek HH, Sweet WH (eds) Operative neurosurgical techniques. Grune and Stratton, New York, pp 891–908

Symon L, Acherman R, Bull JWD et al. (1972) The uses of the xenon clearance method in subarachnoid haemorrhage. Post-operative studies with clinical and angiographic correlation. Eur Neurol 8:8–14

Symon L, Haragadine J, Zawirski M, Branston N (1979) Central conduction time as an index of ischaemia in subarachnoid haemorrhage. J Neurol Sci 44:95–103

Symon L, Bell BA, Kendall B (1980) Relationship between effused blood, clinical course and prognosis in aneurysmal subarachnoid haemorrhage. A preliminary computerized tomographic scan study. In: Wilkins RH (ed) Cerebral arterial spasm. Proceedings of the second international workshop. Williams and Wilkins, Baltimore, pp 409–411

Taneda M (1982) Effect of early operation for ruptured aneurysm in prevention of delayed ischaemic symptoms. J Neurosurg 57:622–628

Troupp H, Bjorkesten G (1971) Results of a controlled trial of late surgical versus conservative treatment of intracranial arterial aneurysm. J Neurosurg 35:20–24

Viale GL, Pau A (1979) Carotid-choroidal aneurysm: remarks on surgical treatment and outcome. Surg Neurol 11:141–145

Voldby B, Enevoldsen EM (1982a) Intracranial pressure changes following aneurysm rupture. Part 3, Recurrent haemorrhage. J Neurosurg 56:784–789

Voldby B, Enevoldsen EM (1982b) Changes following aneurysm rupture. Part 1, Clinical and angiographic correlation. J. Neurosurg 56:186–196

Voldby B, Enevoldsen EM (1982c) Intracranial pressure changes following aneurysm rupture. Part 2, Associated CSF lactacidosis. J Neurosurg 56:197–204

Weir B, Rothberg C, Graem M et al. (1975) Relative prognostic significance of vasospasm following subarachnoid haemorrhage. Can J Neurol Sci 2:109–114

Weir B, Aronyk K (1981) Management mortality and the timing of surgery for supratentorial aneurysm. J Neurosurg 54:146–150

Wheelock B, Weir R, Mohr G et al. (1983) Timing of surgery for intracranial haematoma due to aneurysm rupture. J Neurosurg 58:476–481

Wilkins RH (1977) The role of intracranial arterial spasm in the timing of operation for aneurysm. Clin Neurosurg 24:185–207

Winn HR, Richardson AE, Jane JA (1977) The long-term prognosis in untreated cerebral aneurysms. 1. The incidence of later hemorrhage in cerebral aneurysms: A 10 year evaluation of 364 patients. Ann Neurol 1:358–370

Winn HR, Almaani W, Berga S, Jane J, Richardson AE (1983) The long-term outcome in patients with multiple aneurysms. Incidence of later haemorrhage and implication for treatment of incidental aneurysm. J Neurosurg 59:642–651

Yasargil MG, Carter LP (1974) Saccular aneurysm of the distal anterior cerebral artery. J Neurosurg 39:218–223

Yasargil MG, Smith RD (1982) Management of aneurysm of anterior circulation by intracranial procedure. In: Youmans JR (ed) Neurological surgery, vol 3. WB Saunders, Philadelphia London Toronto Mexico City Sydney Tokyo, pp 1663–1696

Yasargil MG, Yonas H, Gasser JC (1978) Anterior choroidal artery aneurysms; their anatomy and surgical significance. Surg Neurol 9:129–138

Yoshimoto T, Uchida K, Kaniko U, Kayama T, Suzuki J (1979a) An analysis of follow-up results of 1000 intracranial aneurysms with definitive surgical treatment. J Neurosurg 50:152–157

Yoshimoto T, Uchida K, Suzuki J (1979b) Surgical treatment of distal anterior cerebral aneurysm. J Neurosurg 50:40–44

Zlotnik EI, Olishkevich FV, Stolkarts JZ (1977) Microsurgical technique in the treatment of intracranial aneurysm. J Neurosurg 46:591–595

12 Vasospasm

Introduction

Vasospasm is a major problem in the management of patients with aneurysmal SAH. The surgical obliteration of the aneurysm is the goal; however, the timing of surgery is influenced by the neurological condition of the patient, as well as by the presence of vasospasm. Too long a delay in treatment may result in further bleeds. It is common knowledge that not all patients who exhibit vasospasm develop neurological deficit, and the reverse is also true. One has to weigh up the pros and cons of waiting for the spasm to disappear or of obliterating the aneurysm as early as possible. Our policy is to operate on patients with a stable neurological condition as soon as possible.

Cerebral infarcts following SAH were found to be related to ischaemia produced by cerebral vasospasm (Robertson 1949). Ecker and Riemenschneider (1951) were the first to demonstrate angiographic evidence of arterial spasm following SAH. They were of the opinion that spasm played an important role in preventing fatal recurrent bleed. This angiographic term "vasospasm" is, however, undesirable for three reasons:

1. Many cases of confirmed angiographic vasoconstriction are unaccompanied by ischaemic infarction or any other evidence of brain dysfunction.

2. The term has often been used by the physicians to explain vascular phenomena associated with a variety of clinical syndromes, such as migraine and cephalgia, with an altogether different pathological process.

3. Vasospasm can occasionally be seen in a variety of other conditions, such as trauma, infection and surgery in the region of the hypothalamus and pituitary (Wilkins et al. 1968; Peerless 1979).

For these reasons, it was agreed at the Second International Workshop on cerebral vasospasm in Amsterdam (Wilkins 1979) to define cerebral vasospasm as angiographic narrowing of the cerebral vessels, which may be symptomatic or asymptomatic.

For proper management of patients with cerebral vasospasm in aneurysmal SAH, a background understanding of cerebral blood flow, its autoregulation, and its alteration in SAH is necessary.

Cerebral Blood Flow

Roy and Sherrington (1890) suggested the existence of an intrinsic control of cerebral circulation, depending upon the local metabolic and functional needs. Bayliss et al. (1895) were of the opinion that the circulation of the whole of the body was regulated to meet the circulatory demands of the brain, as they could not find any evidence of vasomotor control of cerebral vessels. Meyer and Denny-Brown (1957) found that the smooth muscles of the cerebral vessels were like the smooth muscles elsewhere, and responded to stretch by contraction. They termed this phenomenon "the Bayliss effect". Carbon dioxide and oxygen were thought to play minor roles. Functionally important anastomoses between the cerebral arteries of all sizes were found from the internal arterial network to the circle of Willis, suggesting that the intraluminal pressure played an important role in controlling the compensatory adjustment in the collateral vessels, especially cortical arterioles 50–250 mμ in size within 30 s. Thereafter, slower circulatory adjustments appeared to be mediated by a combination of local metabolic factors. The reactive hyperaemia after prolonged ischaemia is partly due to localised accumulation of acid metabolities (Meyer and Denny-Brown 1957). Shalit et al. (1967) suggested an intrinsic neural reflex mechanism which responds to increases in carbon dioxide and thus alters the cerebral blood flow. Pool (1958) thought that the cerebral vasoconstriction might be regulated by a brain stem mechanism. Harper et al. (1972) suggest that there is dual control of cerebral circulation, the extraparenchymal vessels being influenced by the sympathetic nervous system while the intraparenchymal vessels are under local intrinsic metabolic regulation, with the pial vessels possibly being influenced by both.

The normal cerebral blood flow is 50 ml/100 g/min. The cortical electrical activity and the release of intracellular potassium in the brain depend on the degree of cerebral blood flow. When the cerebral blood flow is 30 ml/100 g/min or above, there is no change in the electroencephalogram, and between 18 and 30 ml there are only minor changes. However, with a flow below 17 ml/100 g/min, there is a marked reduction in cortical activity (Sharbrough et al. 1973), and when the flow falls below 16 ml/100 g/min, the cortical evoked potentials are significantly depressed (Branston et al. 1976). At about 8–11 ml/100 g/min of cerebral blood flow, there is a massive release of intracellular potassium (Astrup et al. 1977). If the local cerebral blood flow falls below 12 ml/100 g/min for over 2 h, infarction sets in (Morawetz et al. 1978). By increasing the mean arterial pressure, complete recovery of evoked potential and partial recovery of potassium can be obtained (Astrup et al. 1977; Hope et al. 1977b), supporting the concept that the neurones remain structurally intact, although functionally inactive, in the ischaemic penumbra.

Cerebral Autoregulation

Cerebral autoregulation is the capacity of the cerebral circulation to maintain a constant flow despite changes in the blood pressure. The calibre of the cerebral vessels can alter to compensate for changes in blood pressure within a wide range (from 60 to 170 mmHg systolic in normotensive persons) (Lassen 1959). Below this normal range, the brain compensates the low flow by increasing the extraction of oxygen, but when the pressure falls below 40 mmHg systolic, this mechanism fails, and symptoms of brain hypoxaemia develop. In hypertensive patients, both the limits are shifted to the right, possibly as a consequence of hypertrophy of the arterial wall, and this may explain the intolerance of these patients to a rapid lowering of blood pressure (Strandgaard et al. 1973). This observation has a practical implication for the management of hypertensive patients.

Harper (1966) studied the influence of blood pressure on cerebral blood flow in dogs, and came to the conclusion that the mean arterial blood pressure can fall by at least one-third without affecting the cerebral blood flow. A passive pressure flow relationship in hypercapnic animals was noticed. This observation may have a bearing on dealing with patients with relative ischaemia of the brain, because the cerebral vessels are already dilated to compensate for the ischaemia and any reduction in the pressure of the blood perfusing the ischaemic area will result in a decrease in blood flow, leading to uncompensated ischaemia. The degree of autoregulatory loss to reduced perfusion pressure depends upon the severity of the ischaemia (Symon et al. 1976). The autoregulation is partially preserved when the flow is greater than 40% of basal flow, but absent when the flow is less than 20%. Pickard et al. (1980) in a preliminary report suggested that measurement of cerebral blood flow in response to drug-induced hypotension may identify those patients who are at risk of developing late cerebral ischaemia after SAH.

Cerebral Blood Flow in Subarachnoid Haemorrhage

Both pre- and postoperative studies of regional cerebral blood flow in patients with aneurysmal SAH showed evidence of local impairment of autoregulation (Heilbrun et al. 1972; Hashi et al. 1972b). The cerebral blood flow is decreased following SAH (James 1968; Pitts et al. 1977), and this reduction is marked in patients with a poor neurological condition. There is a good correlation between the cerebral blood flow and the degree of vasospasm (James 1968). Zingesser et al. (1968) confirmed that there is a global cerebral blood flow reduction in patients with SAH, but a poor correlation between regional blood flow and the presence or absence of vasospasm. In experimental SAH, Petruk et al. (1972) found a decrease in cerebral perfusion pressure and a good correlation between the degree of decreased blood flow and neurological deficit.

For a significant reduction in cerebral blood flow, angiographic constriction of cerebral arteries needs to be more than 50% of the control value. Cerebral blood flow studies should be carried out to complement the angiographic studies while assessing the efficacy of treatment for vasospasm (Simeone et al. 1972). Kelly et al. (1977) showed that adequate cerebral perfusion is the critical factor in the prevention of cerebral infarction, and cerebral vasospasm plays an important part in determining the outcome, as it may affect the cerebral perfusion. Cerebral blood volume is increased in grade 3 and 4 patients with severe diffuse spasm. Angiographically demonstrable vasospasm is due to constriction of large extraparenchymal vessels, while there is a massive dilatation of intraparenchymal vessels, which accounts for the increase in blood volume (Grubb et al. 1977). Martins et al. (1975) studied the cerebral blood flow in the rhesus monkey, using hydrogen clearance methods, before and after experimental SAH. They found the blood flow to be stable, unless the SAH was associated with a fall in cerebral perfusion pressure, and the cerebrovascular resistance was not increased. Hashi et al. (1972a) found an increased cerebral blood flow and a decreased cerebrovascular resistance in SAH, despite angiographic spasm, and came to the conclusion that other factors related to cerebral metabolism might exert a greater influence on cerebral blood flow than arterial spasm in the main vessels during the early stages of SAH.

Fein (1975) noted a primary depression of oxidative metabolism unrelated to ischaemia and glucose supply after SAH. A decrease in cerebral metabolic rate, as well as in cerebral blood flow, was seen after SAH (Grubb et al. 1977). This reduction, however, was also seen in patients with good clinical condition without vasospasm.

Aetiology and Pathophysiology

Florey (1925) gives credit to Schultz for observing under the microscope in 1886 the contraction of cerebral vessels in reponse to electrical stimulation. Florey (1925) noted that the main arteries and capillaries reacted by constriction to both mechanical and electrical stimuli, and that a refractory period, lasting up to 15 min, existed after the first contraction. Local application of adrenalin failed to produce constriction of arteries, and in some cases dilatation was noted. There are species variations in the response to both mechanical and electrical stimulation of the pial vessels (Echlin 1942). The pial vessels of cats are most sensitive, and those of monkeys least. Harvey and Rasmussen (1951) observed general contraction of the middle cerebral arteries in monkeys following manipulation. The constriction was usually localised to the vessels manipulated, but occasionally it spread to the internal carotid artery as well. Within a few minutes, however, the vessels regained their normal calibre.

Brawley et al. (1968) and Nagai et al. (1974) demonstrated a biphasic response of cerebral vasospasm in experimental SAH. The acute phase starts within minutes, and lasts up to 1 hour. The chronic phase begins 4–24 hours after the SAH. According to Brawley, the acute phase has three possible causes:

1. Local reduction of intra-arterial pressure, due to escape of blood
2. Local mechanical distortion of cerebral arteries
3. Release of strong vasoconstrictors from platelets

Phases of spasm have been induced by repeated injections of blood into the subarachnoid space in monkeys (Weir et al. 1970), but in man a second phase of spasm has not been documented after a second haemorrhage if the spasm has already appeared and subsided after the first bleed.

Three phases in the evolution of chronic cerebral vasospasm have recently been proposed (Kapp et al. 1982): initial muscular contraction, secondary injury to the arterial wall due to denuded internal elastic laminae, and their repair process.

The aetiology of vasospasm remains unknown, though many factors have been incriminated from time to time. So far, vasospasm appears to be related to the amount of blood in the subarachnoid space enclosing the circle of Willis. For a long time it has been noted that vasospasm does not occur without a significant amount of blood around the major vessels in the base of the brain (Pool 1958; Echlin 1965; Kapp et al. 1968; Boullin et al. 1976; Symon 1978; Weir et al. 1980; Bell et al. 1980; Fisher et al. 1980; Mizukami et al. 1980; Espinosa et al. 1982). Kistler (1982) reported that he could predict the development of vasospasm in 92% of cases on the basis of the amount of blood in the subarachnoid space as assessed on the CT scan. Nonaka et al. (1979) thought that oxyhaemoglobin (or its allied polypeptide) produced in the process of clot lysis or as the breakdown product of blood corpuscles was the main cause of vasospasm.

, According to Suzuki (1979), early spasm is induced by mechanical stimulation and serotonin. The second phase of the vasospasm is induced by oxyhaemogloblin following haemolysis of blood in the subarachnoid space. The production of oxyhaemogloblin reaches its peak by the seventh day; it is slowly converted to methaemogloblin and then breaks down further to haem and globlin. These are absorbed by the fifteenth day.

The onset of cerebral vasospasm and its resolution correspond to the time taken for the lysis of erythrocytes in the subarachnoid space and the clearance of the breakdown product from the CSF. Handa et al. (1980) and Asano et al. (1980) showed indirect evidence that clot lysis plays a role in the genesis of chronic vasospasm. Watts (1977) could not produce vasospasm by pretreating dogs with reserpine, a phosphodiesterase inhibitor, and then injecting 5-day-old clotted blood into the subarachnoid space. In the controls, however, there was evidence of spasm. Pennink et al. (1972) found prostaglandin $F_{2\alpha}$ to be spasmogenic, but not its E_1 fraction. However, Yamamoto et al. (1972) found that both prostaglandin E_1 and prostaglandin $F_{2\alpha}$ were spasmogenic, and the spasmogenic property of prostaglandin E_1 could be blocked by ethanol. Kapp et al. (1968) found that the spasmogenic substance was a fraction of platelets, other than serotonin or angiotensin. Delayed chronic vasospasm might be caused by the release of vasoactive substances

from the platelets during the disintegration of platelet lysosome, producing an injurious effect on the vessel wall (Rice-Edwards et al. 1975). Simeone et al. (1968) suggested that mechanical injury to the vessel wall is sufficient to induce long-standing constriction, and they did not think that blood products could produce vasoconstriction lasting for several days. According to other workers (Peerless and Griffiths 1972; and Neil-Dwyer et al. 1974) SAH results in variable sympatho-adrenal discharge, and the increase in circulating catecholamines is correlated with the degree of vasospasm. In experiments on animals, intradural blood vessels are found to be devoid of vasa vasorum, but contain a rete vasorum in the adventitia that is permeable to large protein and is in continuity with the subarachnoid space (Zervas et al. 1982). These vessels derive their nutrition through the retevasorum, which are analogous to systemic vasavasorum. It is possible that blood clot around the vessels mechanically blocks the nutrient pathways and causes morphological changes in the segment of the arterial tree, and that this initiates a series of biochemical changes which act upon the vessel wall, giving rise to the morphological changes seen in the various experimental models. Considering the vast experimental evidence of the different spasmogenic substances in the blood, White (1980) commented that more than one factor is responsible for the cerebral vasospasm. The experimental models so far do not provide a satisfactory parallel to human cerebral vasospasm (Fraser 1980).

Pathological Changes in Vasospasm

The morphological structure of arteries in spasm may be indistinguishable from that of normal arteries under light microscopy. Histological examination under an electron microscope, however, shows evidence of focal medial necrosis in large arteries which correlates with the site of angiographic narrowing in chronic spasm (Fien et al. 1974; Alksne and Greenhoot 1974; Tani et al. 1978; Peerless et al. 1978). There is also evidence of focal narrowing in parenchymal arteries and capillaries, without changes in the walls, in patients who suffer fatal SAH and show angiographic evidence of vasospasm (Peerless et al. 1978).

Mayberg et al. (1978) studied the feline basilar arterial endothelium under scanning electron microscope after SAH, and found longitudinal furrows that correlated with angiographically demonstrated vasospasm. There was, however, no evidence of changes in the endothelial cell morphology or thrombogenesis, even 1 week after SAH.

Crompton (1963) described ischaemic and haemorrhagic lesions in the hypothalamus in 61% of patients dying after SAH. The highest incidence of cerebral infarction was found in posterior communicating artery aneurysms, followed by those in the distal middle cerebral artery. Anterior communicating artery aneurysms were much less associated with infarction. The infarction was most extensive in the distribution of the artery to which the aneurysm was closely related (Crompton 1964a; Schneck 1964). It has been suggested that the cerebral vasospasm by itself is not the only cause of cerebral infarction, but a combination of other factors, such as hypotension, atheroma, haematoma and surgical manipulation, is also responsible for converting initial ischaemia to infarction (Crompton 1964a; Schneck 1964; Graham et al. 1983).

Incidence

The incidence of vasospasm following aneurysmal SAH varies in different series from 20% to 40% (Wilkins et al. 1968; Millikan 1975; Saito et al. 1977; Peerless 1977; Fleischer and Tindall 1980). In the author's series of 500 patients, 204 (40.8%) showed a variable degree of vasospasm in preoperative angiograms (Table 12.1). The incidence of vasospasm was equally distributed in all age groups (Table 12.2). There was no sex predilec-

Table 12.1 Incidence of vasospasm in pre-operative angiograms

No spasm	296
Spasm	204 (40.8%)
Generalised	78 (38.2%)
Localised	101 (49.5%)
Segmental	25 (12.2%)

Table 12.2. Spasm as related to age

	No spasm group	Spasm group
10–19	9	4
20–29	21	23
30–39	45	31
40–49	82	51
50–59	104	71
60–69	31	22
70–79	4	2
	296	204

tion: out of 203 males, 79 (39%) showed vasospasm, compared to 125 (42%) females in a total of 297. Vasospasm seems to appear at about the third day after SAH, and reaches a maximum at about 6–8 days (Weir et al. 1978). However, Sano and Saito (1978) found that in 66% of cases vasospasm was observed between 6 and 9 days after SAH. In the authors' series, angiography was carried out in 75% of patients within 10 days of the last SAH (Fig. 12.1). The incidence of vasospasm was maximum on the seventh day of the haemorrhage. It is interesting to note that the incidence had increased by approximately 9% per day until the seventh day, as demonstrated in Fig. 12.2. However, it was not related to the number of haemorrhages. Vasospasm usually subsides within 3 weeks after SAH (du Boulay 1963).

Cerebral vasospasm can be localised or diffuse, and varies in severity. Zingesser et al. (1968)

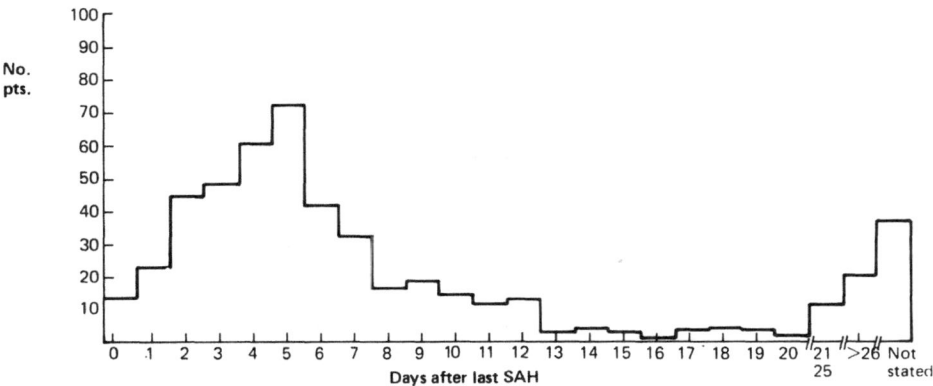

Fig. 12.1. Time interval from last subarachnoid haemorrhage to angiographic investigation.

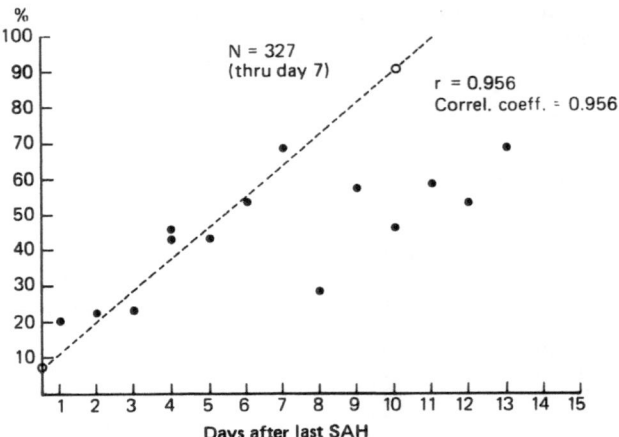

Fig. 12.2. Incidence of vasospasm related to the time interval (days) since the last subarachnoid haemorrhage.

divided spasm into three grades on the basis of its severity. In grade one, the vessels are narrowed but still retain 50% of their calibre. In grade two, the narrowing is more than 50%, and in grade three the vessels are barely visible. Sano and Saito (1978) classified vasospasm into three types—extensive, multisegmental and focal. In the Newcastle series, vasospasm was divided into generalised, local and segmental types, according to the extent of vascular territory involved. In the generalised type, there was spasm in at least two major vessels. In the local type, spasm was limited to one artery, and in the segmental type only a part of the artery was involved (Figs. 7.36–7.38). Of the 204 patients who demonstrated spasm, in 38.2% the spasm was generalised, in 49.5% local and in 12.2% segmental. Cerebral vasospasm was most commonly seen when an aneurysmal sac arose from the carotid siphon and least frequently when it was on the middle cerebral artery (Allcock and Drake 1965). Wilkins et al. (1968) could not find any correlation between the site of the aneurysm and vasospasm. In our series vasospasm was more commonly seen in middle cerebral artery aneurysms

and was least common in aneurysms of the posterior circulation (Table 12.3). It is generally believed that vasospasm is a protective phenomenon against further bleed; however, du Boulay and Gado (1974) and Nibbelink et al. (1975) did not feel that vasospasm conferred any degree of protection against rebleed.

Vasospasm and Neurological Condition of the Patient

The correlation between vasospasm and the clinical neurological grade on admission and at the time of operation was analysed in the present series. There were significantly more patients in grades 1 and 2 who did not have vasospasm. Of 296 patients without vasospasm, 221 (75%) were in grades 1 and 2 on admission, compared to 125 (61%) patients with vasospasm in these grades. A similar difference was also noted when the clinical grade at operation was compared to the vasospasm. There were 243 patients (82%) without vasospasm in grades 1 and 2, whereas only 135 patients (66%) with vasospasm were in these grades (Table 12.4). Allock and Drake (1965), Saito et al. (1977) and Weir et al. (1978) noted that patients with vasospasm have a significantly higher mortality and morbidity than those without this condition. Wilkins et al. (1968) and Millikan (1975) could not find any consistent correlation with known cerebral vasospasm, and came to the conclusion that cerebral vasospasm had no effect on the mortality from SAH due to ruptured aneurysms. In the authors' series, vasospasm demonstrated in pre-operative angiograms

Table 12.3. Vasospasm in relation to the type of aneurysm

Type of aneurysm	No spasm group	Spasm group	Total
Internal carotid artery	125	72	197
Anterior cerebral artery	100	74	174
Middle cerebral artery	50*	49*	99
Posterior circulation	21	9	30
	296	204	500

* $P < 0.05$

Table 12.4. Vasospasm as related to the neurological status

	On admission		At operation	
Grade[a]	Non-spasm group	Spasm group	Non-spasm group	Spasm group
1	71 }*	35 }*	103 }**	42 }**
2	150	90	140	93
3	54	55	47	58
4	20	23	6	11
5	1	1	–	–
	296	204	296	204

[a] Hunt and Hess classification
*$P < 0.005$
**$P < 0.001$

Table 12.5. Outcome as related to vasospasm

	No spasm group	Spasm group
Good	227 (76.6%)	148 (72.5%)
Fair	40	40
Poor	7	6
Dead	22	10
	296	204

Table 12.6. Outcome as related to the extent of vasospasm

	Good	Fair	Poor	Dead	Total
No spasm	227	40	7	22	296
Generalised spasm	59	12	3	4	78
Localised spasm	73	20	3	5	101
Segmental spasm	16	8	–	1	25

did not influence the mortality or morbidity in patients at the time of discharge from hospital. A good outcome was obtained in 72.5% of patients with pre-operative vasospasm, compared to 76.6% without vasospasm (Table 12.5). It should be pointed out that the vasospasm was grouped according to the extent of vascular territory involved, rather than its severity. There was, however, no correlation between the extent of vasospasm and the outcome (Table 12.6).

Fisher et al. (1977) analysed 50 patients with cerebral vasospasm and divided them into five grades according to the severity of the spasm seen on the angiogram. Eighty per cent of their patients with grade 3 and 4 spasm showed ischaemic deficit, and, more significantly, all patients with progressive neurological deterioration had a grade 3 or 4 type of vasospasm. In the authors' series, ischaemic neurological deterioration was noted in 51 patients (10%) in the pre-operative period and 85 patients (21%) in the postoperative period. Thirty-four patients (66.5%) in the pre-

operative group and 39 patients (46%) in the postoperative group showed some degree of pre-operative vasospasm. In 64% of the patients who developed pre-operative hydrocephalus, vasospasm was also noted. In 160 patients (54%) without vasospasm and 93 patients (45%) with spasm, operation was carried out within 10 days of the last SAH. Richardson (1976) and Adams et al. (1978) stressed the importance of post-operative vasospasm in the development of neurological deterioration. The influence of post-operative vasospasm in our series has not been analysed, since angiography was felt undesirable in the ischaemic phase. Peerless (1977) studied the angiograms of 250 patients with SAH prospectively for detection of progressive neurological deterioration. He noted significant spasm in 39% of the patients, but only in 22% was the arterial narrowing associated with neurological deterioration. He suggested that progressive neurological deterioration was multifactorial, involving increased intracranial pressure, brain oedema, low perfusion pressure, disturbance of rheology of microcirculation, and low cerebral blood flow. Voldby and Enevoldsen (1982) correlated cerebral vasospasm, intracranial pressure and the neurological condition of the patient. They found that patients with elevated intraventricular pressure in the postictal period had developed vasospasm more often than those with normal pressure. Congenital anomaly of the circle of Willis also adversely affects the surgical result in patients with vasospasm (Sengupta 1975). The role of congenital variations of the circle of Willis in SAH and vasospasm has been discussed in Chaps. 3 and 10.

Management of Cerebral Vasospasm

The pathogenesis of this malevolent condition remains an enigma and the solution to the problem of vasospasm remains equally unresolved. Wilkins (1973, 1980) exhaustively reviewed the literature on the various approaches to the prevention and treatment of intracranial arterial spasm. During the past 30 years, approaches to this problem have been made on two fronts and with two aims: first, to prevent or reverse the narrowing of the cerebral vessels, and second, to prevent or reverse the effect of diminished blood flow to the involved territory.

As the cause of vasospasm is still unknown, application of various measures to prevent or reverse the narrowing of the vessels is largely empirical. Treatment of cerebral ischaemia has consisted in various manoeuvres directed towards increasing the perfusion pressure in the affected area. The reason for these manoeuvres is the understanding that cerebral blood flow is closely related to cerebral perfusion pressure and cerebrovascular resistance. The cerebral perfusion pressure is equal to the difference between the mean arterial pressure and the intracranial pressure. Therefore, the perfusion pressure could be increased by increasing the mean arterial pressure, by decreasing the intracranial pressure, or by decreasing the cerebrovascular resistance.

More than 25 years ago Denny-Brown and Meyer (1957) carried out considerable experimental work and came to the following conclusions, which still remain very significant. They thought that cortical ischaemia can proceed to the point of failure of electrical activity, with the production of injury potentials which can still recover rapidly and almost completely, with little damage to vessels. Beyond this point, however, any further prolongation of anoxia leads to stasis in the small vessels emerging from the cerebral cortex. This microstasis is reversible, provided that blood pressure is increased within 15–30 min. Depending upon the severity of anoxic insult, the extent and number of ischaemic foci leading to infarction vary. The infarction from anoxia is primarily due to damage to the vascular endothelium, with resulting oedema, haemo-concentration, sludging and stasis. The final effect of anoxic anoxia is the same as that due to ischaemic anoxia.

Cerebral blood flow is dependent upon systemic blood pressure and vascular resistance in the cerebral vessels (Farhat and Schneider 1967). The vascular resistance in turn is dependent upon intracranial pressure, viscosity of the blood, and other chemical factors and the calibre of the vessels. With an increase in blood pressure there is an associated increase in vascular resistance to control cerebral blood flow, but clinical elevation of blood pressure outweighs the factor of resistance. Due to local lactacidosis, the vessels are dilated in an ischaemic area, and an increase in blood pressure allows a reasonable flow. Wise et al. (1972) found that the response to hypertension therapy was usually noticed within an hour after starting the therapy, and they recommended discontinuing the therapy if no response could be observed after several hours. In 5 out of 13 patients showing clinical features of cerebral

vasospasm, they found an improvement in brain function by giving levarterenol 1–6 μg/cc and noted that a deterioration of the neurological state occurred whenever the blood pressure was allowed to fall by decreasing the infusion rate. Levarterenol has a brief duration of action, and has both an alpha constrictor and a beta inotrophic effect. Kosnik and Hunt (1976) gave credit to Denny-Brown (1951) for recognising the benefit of elevation of arterial blood pressure in the management of brain ischaemia. They recommended elevation of blood pressure by 40–60 mmHg systolic with the use of noradrenalin, and cautioned on "too little or too late" use of induced hypertension. Once cerebrovascular damage has occurred, a further increase in perfusion caused by overzealous treatment might lead to brain swelling, and even cardiac failure. Blood volume expansion with plasma and whole blood transfusion is recommended, since vasoconstriction alone produces volume depletion (Wise et al. 1972; Kosnik and Hunt 1976).

The two main problems in the use of drug-induced hypertension and volume expanders were appreciated by Kosnik and Hunt (1976) and Pritz et al. (1978). These are, the risk of recurrent bleeding from the aneurysm before surgical obliteration, and cardiopulmonary compromise. Pritz et al. (1978) advocated monitoring of intravascular volume and cardiac function by the indicator dilution technique in order to assess the state of hydration and other cardiovascular parameters. These authors also recommended the use of digoxin to protect cardiac function during prolonged hypervolaemic therapy. Kassell et al. (1982) used a combination of hypervolaemia, induced hypertension, antidiuretic hormone and steroids in 58 patients with ischaemic symptoms. There was a satisfactory response in 74% of these patients. Hypovolaemia might play a critical role in the pathophysiology of ischaemic syndrome in patients with aneurysmal SAH (Giannotta et al. 1977; Maroon and Nelson 1979). Maroon and Nelson (1979) studied the red cell mass and total blood volume in 15 patients with SAH and found them to be significantly low, whereas the plasma volume had not changed. Bed-rest, negative nitrogen balance, decreased erythropoiesis and iatrogenic blood loss were thought to be responsible for these changes. Maroon and Nelson also reported an excellent result from volume expansion in three patients out of a total of five who had developed pre-operative ischaemic syndrome following SAH. None of their patients suffered recurrent haemorrhage as a result of volume expansion.

Lowe and Gilboe (1971) showed the presence of α- and β-adrenergic receptors in the cerebrovascular bed, and that the cerebrovascular resistance could be increased with adrenalin and noradrenalin. The action of these agents could be reversed after pretreating the animals with phenoxybenzamine hydrochloride, an α-adrenergic blocking drug. The cerebrovascular resistance is also reduced with isoproterenol, a β-adrenergic drug, and this reduction could be reversed with propranolol, a β-adrenergic blocking agent. On the suggestion of H.E. Garrett (1968), quoted by Sundt et al.), Sundt et al. (1973) started using isoproterenol in the treatment of cerebral vasospasm. They favoured the drug as it caused less peripheral hypotension and is easily controllable when compared with an α-adrenergic blocking agent. Isoproterenol acts by increasing the heart rate and cardiac output. It dilates peripheral arterioles and decreases the arterial pressure. However, it also decreases the venous reservoir, with a marked increase in venous return to the heart. The potential risk of cardiac arrhythmia can be offset by the simultaneous use of lignocaine hydrochloride (Xylocaine). Sundt et al. advocated the use of isoproterenol in a dose of 0.4–0.8 mg in 150 cc of 5% glucose at the rate of 10–20 microdrops per minute, with the simultaneous administration of lignocaine 2 g in 450 cc of 5% glucose, in 0.20% saline with 20 mEq potassium chloride at the rate of 20 microdrops per minute. Since this report, we have used the regime in Newcastle for ischaemic complications following SAH, in both pre- and postoperative periods, with satisfactory results.

Meyer et al. (1965) and Brawley et al. (1967), in an experimental study, showed that the systemic vasopressors increased blood pressure and flow to an ischaemic area, but carbon dioxide inhalation decreased the flow, as the capillaries and arterioles in the ischaemic area are already dilated and a further increase in carbon dioxide tension dilates the vessels only in the non-ischaemic brain, resulting in a drop in the collateral circulation to the ischaemic area—a local steal phenomenon. A developing cerebral infarct in an ischaemic zone may increase if systemic hypotension is allowed to develop.

Little (1978) studied the effect of mannitol on focal cerebral ischaemia in cats. Pretreating the cats with 1.2 g/kg mannitol had a protective effect on cerebral tissue during the primary phase of acute focal ischaemia. Considerable preservation of neurones was noted in the treated cats, compared to those without treatment. The beneficial effect of mannitol is due to a combination of prevention of capillary narrowing and suppression of ischaemic cerebral oedema. Suzuki and Yoshimoto (1979) advocated the use of routine mannitol during aneurysm surgery. They believe that this therapy reduces the risk of postoperative ischaemic vasospasm, in spite of temporary occlusion of a major artery during surgery. Mannitol improves the intracranial compliance within minutes of administration, resulting in better cerebral blood flow (Allen and Gross 1976; Brown et al. 1978). Brown et al. (1978) used dopamine with mannitol in four patients with hemiplegia caused by SAH. They used dopamine to increase the mean arterial pressure, and mannitol for the reasons stated by Little (1978). In low doses (less than 5 μg/kg per minute), dopamine produces peripheral vasodilatation secondary to β-adrenergic stimulation. However, in high doses (greater than 10 μg/kg per minute) it produces peripheral vasoconstriction secondary to α-adrenergic stimulation, and an increase in mean arterial pressure results (Brown et al. 1978). Brown et al. found a remarkable degree of clinical improvement in all four of their patients with the combined use of dopamine in high doses and mannitol in a dose ranging from 3.5 g to 6 g/kg per 24 h. They stressed the importance of high fluid replacement with central venous pressure monitoring.

Aminophylline is a potent vasoconstrictor of normal blood vessels. However, in focal ischaemic areas this response is abolished with the increase of local flow, inverting the intracranial steal phenomenon (Skinhoj and Paulson 1970). Flamm and Ransohoff (1976) used aminophylline in combination with isoproterenol. They found these drugs to be more effective when given together than when either of them was given alone. After using aminophylline 125 mg per hour and isoproterenol 125 μg per hour in 12 patients, a clinical improvement was seen in nine patients, and in eight of these the response was noticeable within 24 h of starting the treatment.

Patten et al. (1972) found the beneficial effect of corticosteroids in acute stroke with severe neurological deficit. They used dexamethasone 16 mg per day during the double-blind study.

Gilroy et al. (1969) found dextran to be useful in patients with stroke. The decrease of blood viscosity, with an increase in plasma volume and consequent decrease of packed cell volume, as well as a reduction in the aggregation of blood elements, was supposed to be the cause of the beneficial effect of dextran. We do not use dextran at present, as we have encountered bleeding problems in the postoperative period.

Serotonin is one of the primary vaso-constrictors stored in the platelets and plays an active role in the acute phase of vasospasm. Zervas et al. (1973) observed that reserpine prevents the storage of vasoactive amines, including serotonin, by platelets. Consistent and complete prevention of the development of experimental vasospasm by pretreatment of the animals with reserpine was noticed by these authors. A similar observation was also made by Watts (1977). Zervas found that specific depletion of serotonin with kanamycin also prevented the development of vasospasm in experimental SAH. They combined reserpine 0.1 mg subcutaneously three times daily and kanamycin 1 g orally three times daily in patients with SAH, and noted a significant reduction in cerebral ischaemia (Zervas 1979).

Trapedil, an antagonist and selective inhibitor of thromboxane A_2 synthesis, was also used in patients with SAH, with a considerable reduction in morbidity from symptomatic vasospasm (Suzuki et al. 1981). The latest efforts to treat cerebral vasospasm involve the use of calcium antagonists. It has been shown that extracellular calcium is required in the process of smooth muscle contraction with noradrenalin, angiotensin, histamine (Van Breeman et al. 1972), phenylephrine, serotonin and prostaglandin $F_{2\alpha}$ (Allen et al. 1976). Nifedipine, a calcium channel blocker, inhibited the action of serotonin and phenyl-ephrine, as well as potassium-induced spasm on canine arteries in in vitro and in vivo experiments (Allen and Baughart 1979; Allen and Bahr 1979). Nimodipine, another calcium antagonist, has selective affinity for the calcium receptors of the brain vessels and prevents serotonin-induced vasospasm (Kazda and Towart 1982). It causes redistribution of blood flow in an ischaemic hemisphere by decreasing the flow in the hyper-aemic penumbra and increasing the flow in the ischaemic umbra, without affecting the total hemisphere blood flow (Symon et al. 1982). The loss of cerebral autoregulatory mechanism and the accumulation of water in the ischaemic zone were also noted by Symon et al. in experimental animals. Allen et al. (1982) reported the use of nimodipine on patients with cerebral vasospasm in a double-blind study, with a significant reduction of ischaemic neurological deficits, although there was no difference in the angiographic appearance of cerebral vasospasm with the use of this agent.

In summary, in the management of patients with symptomatic vasospasm, hypertensive therapy with volume expansion remains the mainstay of treatment, and calcium antagonists promise beneficial effects. Overzealousness or delay in the institution of hypertensive therapy may not result in the desired beneficial effects.

References

Adams CBT, Fearnside MR, O'Laoire SA (1978) An investigation with serial angiography into the evolution of cerebral arterial spasm following aneurysm surgery. J Neurosurg 49:805–815

Alksne JF, Greenhoot JH (1974) Experimental catecholamine induced chronic cerebral vasospasm. Myonecrosis in vessel wall. J Neurosurg 41:440–445

Allcock JM, Drake CG (1965) Ruptured intracranial aneurysms. The role of arterial spasm. J Neurosurg 22:21–29

Allen GS, Bahr AL (1979) Cerebral arterial spasm, Part 10. Reversal of acute and chronic spasm in dogs with orally administered nifedipine. Neurosurgery 4:43–47

Allen GS, Baughart SB (1979) Cerebral arterial spasm, Part 9. In vitro effects of nifedipine on serotonin, phenylephrine and potassium induced contraction of canine basilar and femoral arteries. Neurosurgery 4:37–42

Allen GS, Gross CJ (1976) Cerebral arterial spasm. Part 7. In vitro effects of alpha adrenergic agents on canine arteries from six anatomical sites and six blocking agents on serotonin induced contractions of the canine basilar artery. Surg Neurol 6:63–70

Allen GS, Gross CJ, Henderson LA, Chou SN (1976) Cerebral arterial spasm. Part 4. In vitro effects of temporary serotonin, serotonin analogues, large non-physiological concentrations of serotonin and extra-cellular calcium and magnesium on serotonin induced contractions of the canine basilar artery. J Neurosurg 44:585–593

Allen GS, Batty ER, Boone S, Chou S, Kelly D, Weir B (1982) Preliminary results of multi-central double blind prospective study of nimodipine in the prevention of delayed neurological lypsis for cerebral arterial spasm. Proceedings of the Congress of Neurological Surgeons, Toronto, p 98

Asano T, Tanishima T, Sasaki T, Sano K (1980) Possible participation of the free radical reaction initiated by clot lysis in the pathogenesis of vasospasm following subarachnoid haemorrhage. In: Wilkins RH (ed) Cerebral arterial spasm. Williams and Wilkins, Baltimore pp 190–201

Astrup J, Symon L, Branston NM, Lassen NA (1977) Cortical evoked potential and extracellular potassium and hydrogen at critical levels of brain ischaemia. Stroke 8:51–57

Bayliss WM, Hill L, Gulland GL (1895) On the intracranial pressure and the cerebral circulation. J Physiol (Lond) 18:334–364

Bell BA, Kendal BE, Symon L (1980) Computed tomography in aneurysmal subarachnoid haemorrhage. J Neurol Neurosurg Psychiatry 43:522–524

Boullin DJ, Mohan J, Grahame-Smith DG (1976) Evidence for the presence of a vaso-active substance (possibly involved in the aetiology of cerebral vasospasm) in cerebro-spinal fluid from patients with subarachnoid haemorrhage. J Neurol Neurosurg Psychiatry 39:756–766

Branston NM, Symon L, Crockard HA (1976) Recovery of the cortical evoked response following temporary middle cerebral arterial occlusion in baboons in relation to local blood flow and PO_2. Stroke 7:151–157

Brawley BS, Strandness BE, Kelly WA (1967) The physiological response to therapy in experimental cerebral ischaemia. Arch Neurol 17:180–187

Brawley BW, Strandness BE, Kelly WA (1968) The biphasic response of cerebral vasospasm in experimental subarachnoid haemorrhage. J Neurol 28:1–7

Brown FD, Hanlon K, Mullan S (1978) Treatment of aneurysmal hemiplegia with dopamine and mannitol. J Neurosurg 49:525–529

Crompton MR (1963) Hypothalamic lesions following the rupture of cerebral berry aneurysms. Brain 86:301–314

Crompton MR (1964a) Cerebral infarction following the rupture of cerebral berry aneurysms. Brain 87:263–279

Crompton MR (1964b) The pathogenesis of cerebral infarction following the rupture of cerebral berry aneurysms. Brain 87:491–510

Denny-Brown D (1951) The treatment of recurrent cerebrovascular symptoms and the question of "vasospasm". Med Clin North Am 35:1457–1474

Denny-Brown D, Meyer JS (1957) The cerebral collateral circulation 2. Production of cerebral infarction by ischaemic anoxia and its reversibility in early stages. Neourology 7:567–579

du Boulay G (1963) Distribution of spasm in the intracranial arteries after subarachnoid haemorrhage. Acta Radiol [Diagn] 1:256–266

du Boulay G, Gado M (1974) The protective value of spasm after subarachnoid haemorrhage. Brain 97:153–156

Echlin FA (1942) Vasospasm and focal cerebral ischaemia: an experimental study. Arch Neurol Psychiatry 47:77–96

Echlin FA (1965) Spasm of basilar and vertebral arteries caused by experimental subarachnoid haemorrhage. J Neurosurg 23:1–11

Ecker A, Riemenschneider PA (1951) Arteriographic demonstration of spasm of the intracranial arteries with special reference to saccular arterial aneurysm. J Neurosurg 8:660–667

Espinosa F, Weir B, Boisvert D, Overton T, Castor W (1982) Chronic cerebral vasospasm after large subarachnoid haemorrhage in monkeys. J Neurosurg 57:224–232

Farhat SM, Schneider RC (1967) Observations on the effect of systemic blood pressure on intracranial circulation in patients with cerebrovascular insufficiency. J Neurosurg 27:441–445

Fein JM (1975) Cerebral energy metabolism after subarachnoid haemorrhage. Stroke 6:1–8

Fein JM, Flor WJ, Cohan SL, Parkhurst J (1974) Sequential changes of vascular ultrastructure in experimental cerebral vasospasm, myonecrosis of subarachnoid arteries. J Neurosurg 41:49–58

Fisher CM, Robson EH, Ojemann RG (1977) Cerebral vasospasm with ruptured saccular aneurysm. The clinical manifestations. Neurosurgery 1:245–248

Fisher CM, Kistler JP, Davies JM (1980) Relation of cerebral vasospasm to subarachnoid haemorrhage, visualised by computerized tomographic scanning. Neurosurgery 6:1–9

Flamm ES, Ransohoff J (1976) Treatment of cerebral vasospasm by control of cyclic adenosine monophosphate. Surg Neurol 6:223–226

Fleischer AS, Tindall GT (1980) Cerebral vasospasm following aneurysm rupture: a protocol for therapy and prophylaxis. J Neurosurg 52:149–152

Florey H (1925) Microscopical observations on the circulation of blood in the cerebral cortex. Brain 48:43–64

Fraser RAR (1980) Cerebral vasospasm—after 15 years in laboratory assessment of animal models. In: Wilkins RH (ed) Cerebral arterial spasm. Williams and Wilkins, Baltimore, pp 287–290

Giannotta SL, McGillicuddy JE, Kindt GW (1977) Diagnosis and treatment of postoperative cerebral vasospasm. Surg Neurol 8:286–290

Gilroy J, Arnhart MI, Meyer JS (1969) Treatment of acute stroke with dextran 40. JAMA 210:293–298

Graham DI, MacPherson P, Pitts LH (1983) Correlation between angiographic vasospasm, haematoma and ischaemic brain damage following subarachnoid haemorrhage. J Neurosurg 59:223–230

Grubb RL, Raichle ME, Eichling JO, Gado MH (1977) Effects of subarachnoid haemorrhage on cerebral blood volume, blood flow and oxygen utilization in humans. J Neurosurg 46:446–453

Handa H, Osaka K, Okamoto S (1980) Breakdown products of erythrocytes as a cause of cerebral vasospasm. In: Wilkins RH (ed) Cerebral arterial spasm. Williams and Wilkins, Baltimore.

Harper AM (1966) Autoregulation of cerebral blood flow—influence of the arterial blood pressure on the blood flow through the cerebral cortex. J Neurol Neurosurg Psychiatry 29:398–403

Harper AM, Deshmukh VD, Rowan JO, Jennett WB (1972) The influence of sympathetic nervous activity on cerebral blood flow. Arch Neurol 27:1–6

Harvey J, Rasmussen T (1951) Occlusion of the middle cerebral artery—an experimental study. Arch Neurol Psychiatry 66:20–29

Hashi K, Meyer JS, Shinmaru S, Welch KMA, Teraura T (1972a) Cerebral haemodynamic and metabolic changes after experimental subarachnoid haemorrhage. J Neurol Sci 17:1–14

Hashi K, Meyer JS, Shinmaru S, Welch KMA, Teraura T (1972b) Changes in cerebral vasomotor reactivity in CO_2 and autoregulation following experimental subarachnoid haemorrhage. J Neurol Sci 17:15–22

Heilbrun MP, Olesen J, Lassen NA (1972) Regional cerebral blood flow studies in subarachnoid haemorrhage. J Neurosurg 37:36–44

Hope TD, Branston NM, Symon L (1977a) Restoration of neurological function with hypertension in acute experimental cerebral ischaemia. Acta Neurol Scand 56 (Suppl 64):506–507

Hope TD, Branston NM, Symon L (1977b) Restoration of neurological function with induced hypertension in acute experimental cerebral ischaemia. In: Ingvar DH, Lassen NA (eds) Cerebral function, metabolism and circulation. Munksgaard, Copenhagen, pp 506–507

James IM (1968) Changes in cerebral blood flow and systemic arterial pressure following spontaneous subarachnoid haemorrhage. Clin Sci 35:11–22

Kapp J, Mahaley MS Jr, Odom GL (1968) Cerebral arterial spasm. Part II: Experimental evaluation of mechanical and humoral factors in pathogenesis. J Neurosurg 29:339–349

Kapp JP, Neill WR, Neill CL, Hodges LR, Smith RR (1982) The three phases of vasospasm. J Surg Neurol 18:40–45

Kassel NF, Peerless J, Durward TJ, Beck DW, Drake CG, Adams HP (1982) Treatment of ischaemic deficits from vasospasm with intravascular volume expansion and induced arterial hypertension. Neurosurgery 11:337–343

Kazda S, Towart R (1982) Nimodipine, a new calcium antagonist drug with preferential cerebrovascular action. Acta Neurochir 63:259–265

Kelly PJ, Gorton RJ, Grossman RG, Eisenberg HM (1977) Cerebral perfusion, vascular spasm and outcome in patients with ruptured intracranial aneurysm. J Neurosurg 47:44–49

Kistler JP (1982) Predicting symptomatic vasospasm in patients with SAH from a ruptured saccular aneurysm. Advances in Neurosurgery No 1–5. Harvard Medical School,

Department of Continuous Medical Education, 25 Shattuck Street, Boston, M.A.

Kosnik EJ, Hunt WE (1976) Postoperative hypertension in the management of patients with intracranial arterial aneurysms. J Neurosurg 45:148–154

Lassen NA (1959) Cerebral blood flow and oxygen consumption in man. Physiol Rev 39:183–238

Little JR (1978) Modification of acute focal ischaemia by treatment with mannitol. Stroke 9:4–9

Lowe RF, Gilboe DD (1971) Demonstration of alpha and beta adrenergic receptors in canine cerebral vasculature. Stroke 2:193–200

Maroon JC, Nelson PB (1979) Hypovolaemia in patients with subarachnoid haemorrhage. Therapeutic implications. Neurosurgery 4:223–225

Martins AN, Doyle TF, Newby N, Kobrine AI, Ramirex A (1975) The effect of a simulated subarachnoid haemorrhage on cerebral blood flow in the monkey. Stroke 6:664–672

Mayberg MR, Houser OW, Sundt TM Jr (1978) Ultrastructural changes in feline arterial endothelium following subarachnoid haemorrhage. J Neurosurg 48:49–57

Meyer JS, Denny-Brown D (1957) The cerebral collateral circulation (1) Factors in influencing collateral blood flow. Neurology 7:447–458

Meyer JS, Gotoh F, Gilroy J et al. (1965) Improvement in brain oxygenation and clinical improvement in patients with stroke treatment with papaverine hydrochloride. JAMA 194:957–961

Millikan GH (1975) Cerebral vasospasm and ruptured intracranial aneurysm. Arch Neurol 32:433–449

Mizukami M, Takemae T, Tazawa T, Kawase T, Matsuzaki T (1980) Value of computerized tomography in the prediction of cerebral vasospasm after aneurysm rupture. Neurosurgery 7:583–586

Morawetz RB, deGirolami U, Ojemann RG, Marcoux W, Crowell RM (1978) Cerebral blood flow determined by hydrogen clearance during middle cerebral artery occlusion in unanaesthetised monkeys. Stroke 9:143–149

Nagai H, Suzuki Y, Sugiura M, Noda S, Mabe H (1974) Experimental cerebral vasospasm. Part 1—Factors contributing to early spasm. J Neurosurg 41:285–292

Neil-Dwyer G, Cruickshank J, Stott A, Brice J (1974) The urinary catecholamine and plasma cortisol levels in patients with subarachnoid haemorrhage. J Neurol Sci 22:375–382

Nibbelink DW, Torner JC, Henderson WG (1975) Intracranial aneurysms and subarachnoid haemorrhage—a co-operative study. Antifibrinolytic therapy in recent onset subarachnoid haemorrhage. Stroke 6:622–629

Nonaka T, Watanabe S, Chigasaki H, Miyacka M, Ishu S (1979) Aetiology and treatment of vasospasm following subarachnoid haemorrhage. Neurol Med Chir (Tokyo) 19:55–60

Patten BM, Mandell J, Braun B et al. (1972) Double blind study of the effects of dexamethasone on acute stroke. Neurology 22:337–383

Peerless SJ (1977) Comments on cerebral vasospasm. Neurosurgery 1:248

Peerless SJ (1979) Pre- and post-operative management of cerebral aneurysms. Clin Neurosurg 26:209–231

Peerless SJ, Griffiths JC (1972) Plasma catecholamines following subarachnoid haemorrhage. Ann R Coll Phys Surg Can 5:48–49

Peerless SJ, Hunter I, Drake CG (1978) Structural changes in the human cerebral artery following subarachnoid haemorrhage and spasm. Stroke 9:103

Pennink M, White RP, Crockarell JR, Robertson JT (1972) Role of prostaglandin F2 alpha in the genesis of experimental cerebral vasospasm—angiographic study in dogs. J Neurosurg 37:398–406

Petruk KC, West GR, Marriott MR, McIntyre JW, Overton TR, Weir BKA (1972) Cerebral blood flow following induced subarachnoid haemorrhage in the monkey. J Neurosurg 37:316–324

Pickard JD, Matheson M, Patterson J, Wyper D (1980) Prediction of late ischaemic complications after cerebral aneurysm surgery by the intraoperative measurement of cerebral blood flow. J Neurosurg 53:305–308

Pitts LH, MacPherson P, Wyper DJ, Jennett WB (1977) Cerebral blood flow, cerebral vasospasm and subarachnoid haemorrhage. Acta Neurol Scand 56 (Suppl 64):334–335

Pool J (1958) Cerebral vasospasm. N Engl J Med 259:1259–1264

Pritz MB, Giannotta SL, Kindt WG et al. (1978) Treatment of patients with neurological deficit associated with cerebral vasospasm by intravascular volume expansion. Neurosurgery 3:364–368

Rice-Edwards JM, Bull B, Thompson J, Austin G (1975) Role of platelets in causation of cerebral vasospasm. J Neurol Neurosurg Psychiatry 38:828

Richardson JTE (1976) Arterial spasm and recovery from subarachnoid haemorrhage. J Neurol Neurosurg Psychiatry 39:1134–1136

Robertson EG (1949) Cerebral lesions due to intracranial aneurysms. Brain 72:150–185

Roy CS, Sherrington CS (1890) On the regulation of blood supply of the brain. J Physiol (Lond) 11:85–108

Saito I, Ueda Y, Sano K (1977) Significance of vasospasm in the treatment of ruptured intracranial aneurysm. J Neurosurg 47:412–429

Sano K, Saito I (1978) Timing and indications of surgery for ruptured intracranial aneurysm with regard to vasospasm. Acta Neurochir 41:49–60

Schneck SA (1964) On the relationship between ruptured intracranial aneurysm and cerebral infarction. Neurology 14:691–702

Sengupta RP (1975) Anatomical variations in the origin of the posterior cerebral artery demonstrated by carotid angiography and their significance in the direct surgical treatment of posterior communicating aneurysms. Neurochirurgia 18:33–42

Shalit MN, Shimojyo S, Reinmuth OM (1967) Carbon dioxide and cerebral circulatoryy control. 1. The extra-vascular effect. Arch Neurol 17:298–303

Sharbrough FW, Messick JM, Sundt TM Jr (1973) Correlation of continuous electro-encephalograms with cerebral blood flow measurements during carotid endarterectomy. Stroke 4:674–683

Simeone FA, Ryan KG, Cotter JR et al. (1968) Prolonged experimental cerebral vasospasm. J Neurosurg 29:357–366

Simeone FA, Trepper PPJ, Brown DJ (1972) Cerebral blood flow evaluation of prolonged experimental vasospasm. J Neurosurg 37:302–311

Skinhoj E, Paulson O (1970) Mechanism of action of aminophylline upon cerebrovascular disorder. Acta Neurol Scand 46:129–140

Strandgaard S, Olesen J, Skinhoj E, Lassen NA (1973) Autoregulation of brain circulation in severe arterial hypertension. Br Med J I:507–510

Sundt TM, Onofrio BM, Merideth J (1973) Treatment of cerebral vasospasm from subarachnoid haemorrhage with isoproterenol and lidocaine hydrochloride. J Neurosurg 38:557–560

Suzuki J (1979) Cerebral vasospasm—prediction, prevention and protection. In: Pia HW, Langmaid C, Zierski J (eds) Cerebral aneurysms. Advances in diagnosis and therapy. Springer Berlin Heidelberg New York, pp 155–161

Suzuki J, Yoshimoto T (1979) The effect of mannitol in prolongation of permissible occlusion time of cerebral arteries: Clinical data of aneurysm surgery. In: Suzuki J (ed) Cerebral aneurysms. Neuron, Tokyo, pp 330–337

Suzuki S, Sobata E, Iwabuchi T (1981) Prevention of cerebral ischaemic symptoms in cerebral vasospasm with trapidil, an antagonist and selective synthesis inhibitor of thromboxane A_2. Neurosurgery 9:679–685

Symon L (1978) Disordered cerebrovascular physiology in aneurysmal subarachnoid haemorrhage. Acta Neurochir 41:7–22

Symon L, Branston NM, Strong AJ (1976) Autoregulation in acute focal ischaemia—an experimental study. Stroke 7:547–554

Symon L, Harris RJ, Branston NM (1982) Calcium ion and calcium ion antogagonist in ischaemia. Acta Neurochir 63:272–275

Tani E, Yamagata S, Ito Y (1978) Intracellular granules and vesicles in prolonged cerebral vasospasm. J Neurosurg 48:179–189

Van Breeman C, Farinas BR, Girba P et al. (1972) Excitation, contraction coupling in rabbit aorta—studied by Lantharum method for measuring cellular calcium inflow. Circ Res 30:44–45

Voldby B, Enevoldsen EM (1982) Intracranial pressure changes following aneurysm rupture. Part I. Clinical and angiographic correlation. J Neurosurg 56:186–196

Watts C (1977) Reserpine and cerebral vasospasm. Stroke 8:112–114

Weir B, Erasmo R, Miller J et al. (1970) Vasospasm in response to repeated subarachnoid haemorrhage in the monkey. J Neurosurg 33:395–405

Weir B, Grace M, Hansen J, Rothberg C (1978) Time course of vasospasm in man. J Neurosurg 48:173–178

Weir BKA, Okwuasava SK, Cook DA, Krueger CA (1980) Pharmacology of vasospasm—effects of various agents including blood on isolated cerebral artery. In: Wilkins RH (ed) Cerebral arterial spasm. Williams and Wilkins, Baltimore, pp 237–243

White RP (1980) Overt view of the pharmacology of vasospasm. In: Wilkins RH (ed) Cerebral arterial spasm. Williams and Wilkins, Baltimore, pp 229–236

Wilkins RH (1973) Attempts at treatment of intracranial arterial spasm in animals and human beings. Surg Neurol 1:148–159

Wilkins RH (1979) Proceedings of the second international workshop on cerebral vasospasm. Amsterdam, July 11–14

Wilkins RH (1980) Attempted prevention or treatment of intracranial arterial spasm—a survey. Neurosurgery 6:198–210

Wilkins RH, Alexander JA, Odom GL (1968) Intracranial arterial spasm—a clinical analysis. J Neurosurg 29:121–134

Wise G, Sutter R, Burkholder J (1972) The treatment of brain ischaemia with vasopressor drugs. Stroke 3:135–142

Yamamoto YL, Feindel W, Wolfe LS, Katoh H, Hodge CP (1972) Experimental vasoconstriction of cerebral arteries by prostaglandins. J Neurosurg 37:385–397

Zervas NT (1979) Vasospasm—up-date. Clin Neurosurg 26:643–656

Zervas NT, Kuwayama A, Rosoff CB, Salzman ES (1973) Cerebral arterial spasm. Modification by inhibition of platelet function. Arch Neurol 28:400–404

Zervas NT, Liszezak TM, Mayberg MR, Black P McL (1982) Cerebro-spinal fluid may nourish cerebral vessels through pathways in the adventitia that may be analogous to systemic vasa vasorum. J Neurosurg 56:475–481

Zingesser LH, Schechter MM, Dexter J et al. (1968) On the significance of spasm associated with rupture of a cerebral aneurysm. The relationship between spasm as noted angiographically and regional blood flow determinations. Arch Neurol 18:520–528

13 Arteriovenous Malformations

Introduction

Arteriovenous malformations (AVMs) or angiomas are defined as a "congenital non-neoplastic vascular abnormality, consisting essentially of a coiled mass of arteries and veins, partially separated by sclerotic tissue, lying in a bed formed by displacement of, rather than invasion of, normal brain tissue" (Anderson and Korbin 1958). The veins are enlarged and tortuous and may be difficult to distinguish from arteries because of the shunting of blood. Pool (1972) noticed evidence in the literature about Egyptians having recognised AVMs as early as 1500 B.C. He gives credit to Steinheil in 1895 for making the first clinical diagnosis of a cerebral AVM. Few were diagnosed, however, until the introduction of cerebral angiography by Egaz Moniz in 1927. Angiographic diagnosis of AVMs was first reported by Bergstrand et al. in 1936. An AVM was first successfully excised in 1932 in Stockholm (Olivecrona and Riives 1948). Recent advances in angiography and surgical techniques have broadened the indications for surgical treatment of these lesions.

Incidence

The true incidence of AVMs is difficult to assess and figures vary with the source of the material examined. Olivecrona and Riives (1948) found 46 AVMs while examining 3206 brain tumours, giving an incidence of 1.4%. In the Co-operative Study, the incidence varied from 1.5% to 4% of verified intracranial tumours (Perret and Nishioka 1966). The prevalance of AVMs in the Co-operative Study was estimated to be one-seventh of that of intracranial aneurysms. As the incidence of aneurysms in the general population is 1%, the estimated incidence of AVMs is about 0.14% (Michelsen 1979). Arteriovenous malformations rarely produce clinical symptoms before 10 years of age and commonly present in the second and third decades of life (Olivecrone and Riives 1948; McKenzie 1953; Paterson and McKissock 1956). The majority present before the fourth decade (Moody and Poppen 1970; Pia 1975). Though a higher incidence of AVMS has been found in males (Olivecrona and Riives 1948; Forster et al. 1972; Pia 1975), the sex incidence was almost equal in the Co-operative Study (Perret and Nishioka 1966) and in the series reported by Amacher et al. in 1972.

Natural History

The natural history of AVMs is still under investigation but there are good long-term studies reported in the literature. Unsuspected and silent AVMs may be detected on computerised tomography (carried out for unrelated reasons) and at autopsy.

Some AVMs increase in size and inflict progressive damage on the brain tissue (Hook and Johanson 1958; Forster et al. 1972). In this connection, low resistance–high flow fistulae predispose to enlargement of AVMs (Parkinson and Bachers 1980) although larger AVMs may rarely diminish in size (Waltimo 1973b). The presenting symptom is commonly a bleed with small AVMS, and epilepsy with larger AVMs (McKenzie 1953; Paterson and McKissock 1956; Waltimo 1973a; Drake 1979; Parkinson and Bachers 1980). Forster et al. (1972) could not find any relation between patient age, sex and size of AVMs and haemorrhage, although the size of the AVMs can be related to the duration of symptoms (Moody and Poppen 1970). In patients over 30 years old, 70% present with large AVMs, compared to only 59% below 30 years old (Paterson and McKissock 1956). The prognosis of these lesions depends upon the age of the patient when the diangosis is first established. Beyond 40 years of age the likelihood of an AVM bleeding rapidly diminishes, irrespective of previous haemorrhage (Luessenhop and Ross 1984). At 55 years there is a 50% chance of having a normal expectancy of life (Luessenhop 1975). AVMs occasionally disappear completely, either due to thrombosis, arteriosclerosis or haemodynamic disturbances (Hook and Johanson 1958; Amojola et al. 1982); at present ten such cases have been reported in the literature (Nukiu et al. 1982).

In the Co-operative Study reported by Perret and Nishioka (1966), 32% of the AVMs had not bled at the time of admission. This contrasts with 9.7% of cerebral aneurysms. In fact, over 50% of AVMs bled before 30 years of age; the risk of death from the first bleed was 10%, and the risk of rebleeding, 23%. However, fatalities increased to only 12% after the second haemorrhage and to 20% after the third haemorrhage. A similar risk of rebleeding was also found by Svien and McRae (1965). Troupp (1976) followed 137 patients with an AVM over a 25-year period, with a median time of 8 years. They found that fatal haemorrhage could occur at any time, without any set pattern and in any subgroup of patients. The prognosis with frontal, temporal and occipital AVMs was better than with parietal, central and infratentorial ones. By analysing over a 15-year follow-up period the occurrence of bleeding in 106 patients with AVMs who had bled once, 30 patients who had bled twice, and 46 patients with AVMs suffering from epilepsy alone, Forster et al. (1972) came to the following conclusions: Without surgical intervention a patient who has epilepsy but no history of bleeding has a 25%

chance of bleeding in 15 years. Patients who have a single episode of bleeding have a 25% chance of bleeding again in 4 years, while patients who have bled twice have a 25% chance of bleeding again within 1 year. Graf et al. (1983), in a recent review, studied the tendency to bleed in 191 patients with AVMs. They observed that the initial bleeding occurred mostly in the second, third and fourth decades, and often with a small lesion. The time interval of recurrent bleeding was irregular and not related to age, sex or site of the lesion. The risk of first recurrent haemorrhage was 2% per year after the first year.

Pathology

The term "arteriovenous malformation" is generally used to describe all vascular malformations, as well as the specific type containing both arterial and venous structures. They have been classified into the following groups by McCormick (1966):

1. Capillary angiomas (telangiectasia)
2. Cavernous angiomas
3. Arteriovenous malformations (angiomas)
4. Venous angiomas
5. Varices

It should be noted, however, that many lesions contain histological features of one or more groups.

In addition, Crawford and Russell (1956) have coined the term cryptic AVM for a sixth group, i.e. those small AVMs which can produce haemorrhage and yet on angiography or autopsy are difficult to find.

Capillary Angiomas (Telangiectasia)

Capillary angiomas are typically small solitary groups of abnormally dilated capillaries, separated by normal neural tissue. They present macroscopically as small areas of red softening, with ill-defined borders. Sometimes they resemble a cluster of petechiae. Microscopically the thin-walled capillaries are devoid of smooth muscle or elastic fibres. The brain parenchyma between the capillaries may be gliotic and mineralised. Capillary angiomas are usually found at autopsy; they are especially frequent in the brain stem, particularly the pons (Fig. 13.1). They rarely give rise to spontaneous haemorrhage.

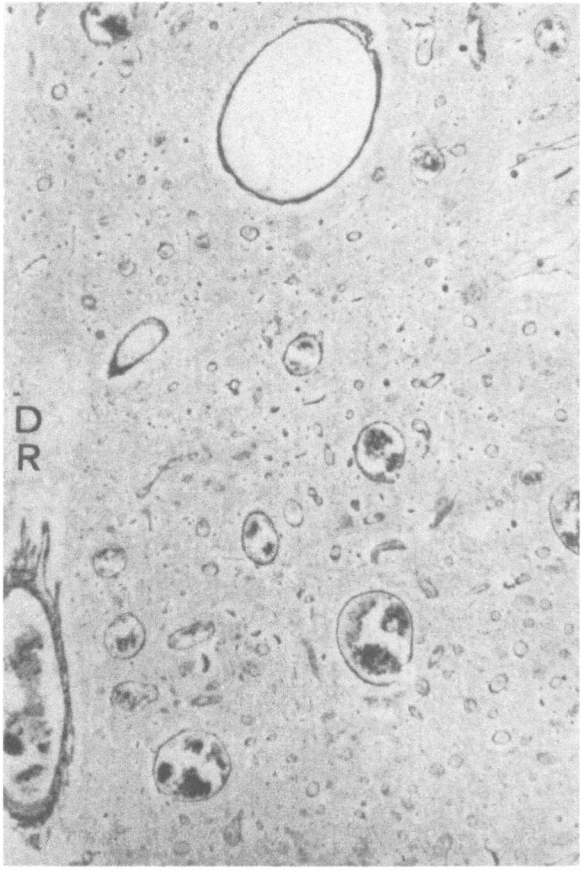

Fig. 13.1. Thin-walled capillaries characterise this pontine angioma which was visible macroscropically as a haemorrhagic lesion adjacent to the dorsal raphe (*DR*) of the mid pons. Neurons in the adjacent parenchyma showed iron incrustation but otherwise the intervening neural tissue was surprisingly normal. No clinical symptoms had been associated with this capillary angioma, which was an incidental postmortem finding.

Cavernous Angiomas

Cavernous angiomas are composed of closely clustered sinusoidal, thin-walled vessels, with no intervening parenchyma. They vary greatly in size. Small ones may appear to be of a petechial nature, while the larger ones appear as a purple-red, well circumscribed or even encapsulated mass. The microscopic appearance consists of large sinusoidal vascular spaces (Fig. 13.2). Like capillary angiomas, these thin-walled vessels are devoid of smooth muscle or elastic tissue. Hyalinization of the vessel wall and calcification may be seen. Thrombosis of the vessels may lead to complete or, more usually, partial obliteration of the lesion. Cavernous angiomas may be found

in all parts of the central nervous system, and may be multiple. From the surgical point of view, because of their partial encapsulation they are relatively easy to excise. They produce severe haemorrhage on rupture.

Arteriovenous Malformations

Arteriovenous malformations constitute the most frequent type of angioma in the central nervous system, with greatly dilated and thickened vessels. Macroscopically they form a wedge-shaped mass extending from the leptomeninges deep into the parenchyma (Fig. 13.3a), often reaching the ventricles. The overlying leptomeninges are thickened and opacified. Calcification in the gliotic parenchyma may be seen. At surgical exploration, the large draining veins look bright red (due to arterialised blood), and both feeding arteries and veins are widely dilated. Microscopically a variable appearance in the vessels is characteristic (Fig. 13.3b). Some are well differentiated as dilated normal arteries and veins while others have thin-walled, hyalinised vessels with segmental dilatations. Degeneration of the parenchyma with calcification and haemosiderin pigment from minor haemorrhages is commonly found.

Arteriovenous malformations vary in size, ranging from a few centimetres to extensive areas covering a large part of the brain. They may occur in all parts of the central nervous system, but the larger ones commonly involve areas supplied by the middle cerebral artery. Occasionally, large AVMs occur in the choroid plexus of the lateral ventricles.

Venous Angiomas

Venous angiomas are composed entirely of veins. They are smaller than AVMs but resemble them except for the absence of arterial structures. The vessels are devoid of normal quantities of smooth muscle and elastic tissue. They occur throughout the central nervous system but are more common in the spinal cord.

Varices

This vascular abnormality usually consists of a single dilated vein, though occasionally several veins may be involved. They are found in the parenchyma of the brain, but may not be identified on gross post-mortem examination. They

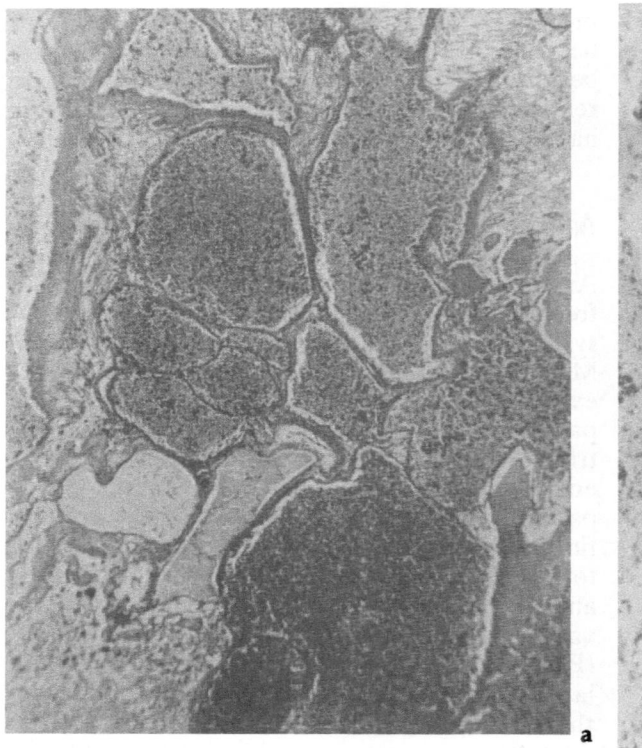

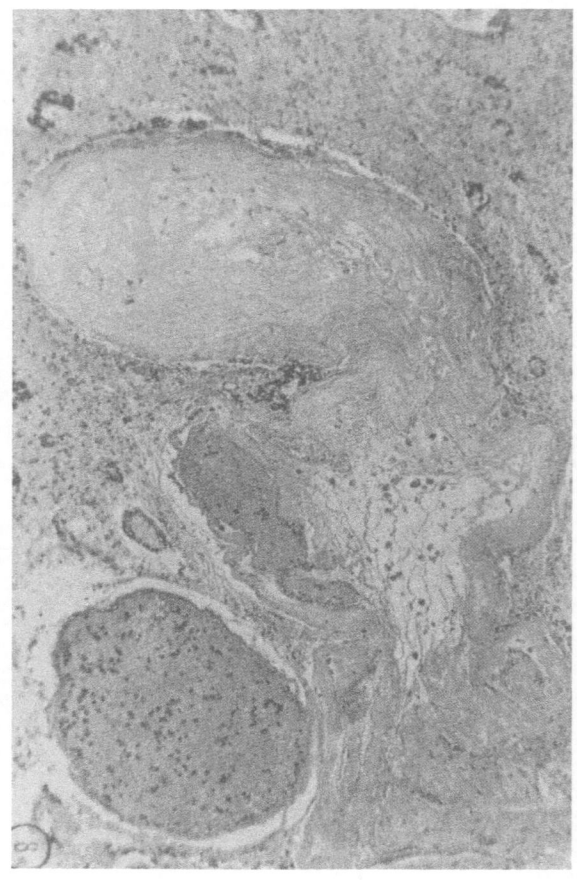

Fig. 13.2.a Histology of a cavernous angioma showing sinusoidal thin-walled vessels. There is no neural parenchyma between the component vessels. **b.** Histological section taken at the edge of a cavernous angioma. There is hyalinization and thickening of vessels, gliosis of adjacent neural parenchyma and haemosiderin deposition from previous minor haemorrhages. (By courtesy of Dr. W.F. McCormick 1969).

can give rise to massive haemorrhage, although gliosis and calcification are uncommon. Certain malformations in the vein of Galen may be included in this group.

Cryptic Angiomas (Micro-Angiomata)

The term cryptic has been used for those malformations which, due to haemodynamic or pathological changes, such as thrombosis, fail to be demonstrated at cerebral angiography. They consist of a small microscopic collection of vessels which may show a variety of histological structures. They may occur in any part of the central nervous system and require a meticulous search for detection in pathological examination.

Surgical Pathology

From the management point of view, the location and size of the lesion and the vascular supply are the important factors to consider in surgical excision. Waltimo (1973a) divided AVMs into small (less than 7 cm³) and large (more than 7 cm³). Drake (1979) classified AVMs into three grades—small (smaller than 2.5 cm in diameter), medium (between 2.5 and 5 cm) and large (above 5 cm). Luessenhop and Rosa (1984) classified them into four grades, depending upon the size in the lateral projection on the angiograms—grade 1, less than 2 cm; grade 2, 2–4 cm; grade 3, 4–6 cm; grade 4, more than 6 cm. The import-

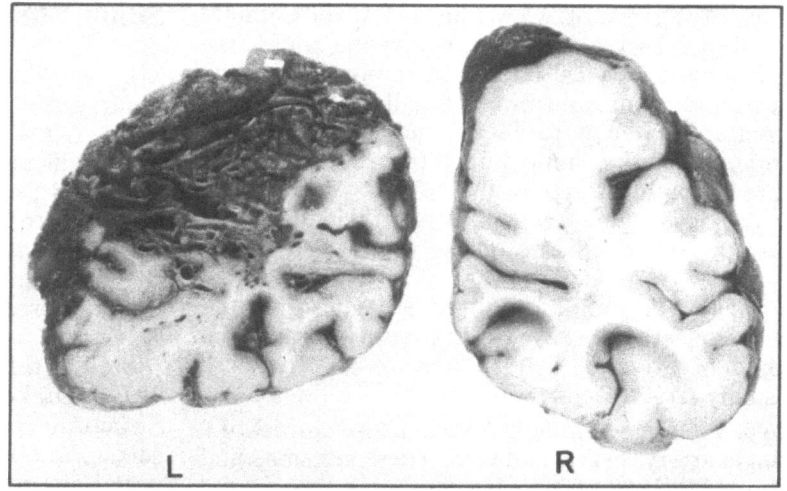

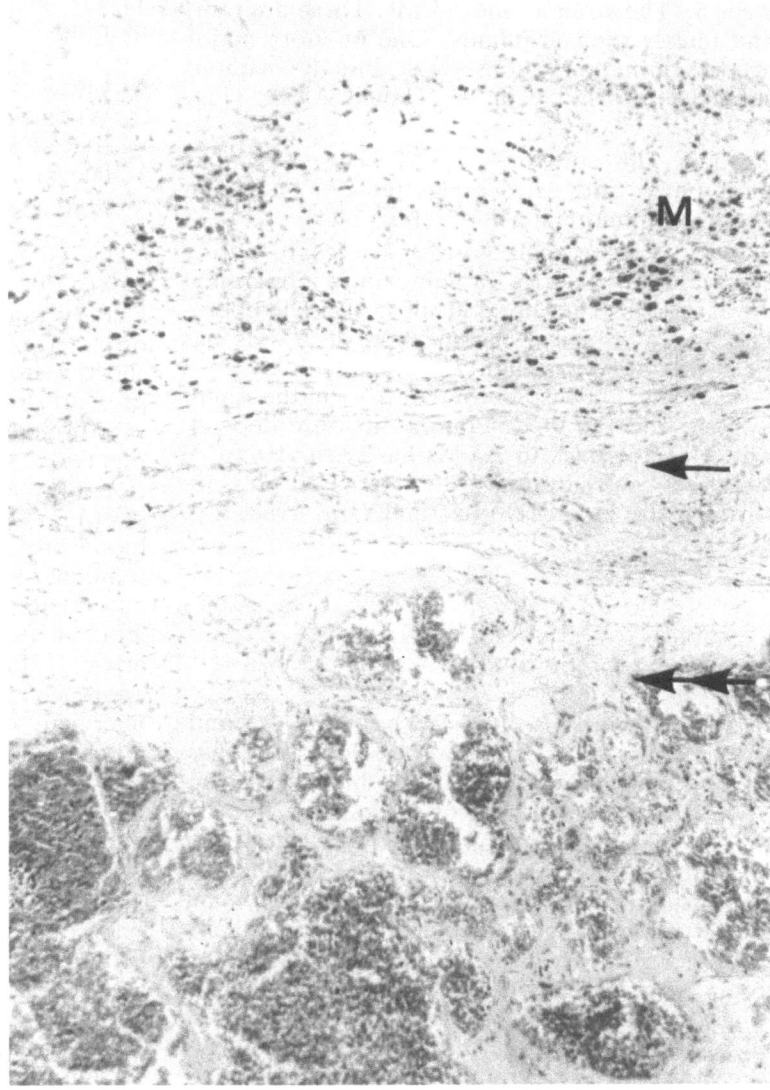

Fig. 13.3. a An AVM occupies the superior-lateral surface of the parietal/occipital lobe. Adjacent cortex is gliosed and the vascular lesion extends into deep white matter. Subarachnoid haemorrhage occurred terminally in this patient, extending across the midline to involve part of the right hemisphere. **b** Recurrent minor bleeding from this AVM has resulted in considerably thickened and haemosiderin-pigmented meninges (*M*). A major feeding artery is shown in tangential section (*arrow*) whilst beneath this multiple vessels of varying calibre are present (*double arrow*).

ance of the size of AVMs has been well summarised by Drake (1979). The bigger the AVM, the greater the surgical hazard in removal from the surrounding normal brain. Small AVMs have a greater tendency to bleed and the danger of removal of the sump effect (see below) varies directly with the size of the AVM.

Parkinson and Bachers (1980) divided AVMs into five groups, based on the vascular supply:

Type 1. The multiple unit AVM. These are the commonest type (82%). They consist of multiple units of arteries, fistulae and veins. They are usually large (Fig. 7.47).

Type 2. The single unit AVM. These consist of a single artery, fistula and vein. These are small and constitute 10% of AVMs (Fig. 7.45).

Type 3. The straight line AVMs. These are rare, and mostly seen in infants. One or more major arteries join the venous sinus directly, without subdivision, e.g. vein of Galen AVM (Fig. 13.17).

Type 4. The combined AVM. The AVM has both intra- and extracranial feeders but drain through intracranial sinuses (Fig. 7.44).

Type 5. Venous wall AVMs. These are purely extracerebral arteries draining into intracranial dural sinuses. They are difficult to excise at operation. A radiological classification of AVMs has been described in Chap. 7.

There is no vasomotor control in the shunt system, and the flow is purely pressure dependent. Haemorrhage in AVMs has been attributed to a venous origin due to the increased pressure through the shunt (Nornes and Grip 1980).

Hazards of Removal of Large AVMs

A large angioma is often fed by many "secondary" feeders which remain undisclosed at angiography due to variations in the blood flow pattern. Inadvertent tearing of any of these feeding vessels may lead to profuse haemorrhage within the brain as a consequence of the feeder itself retracting into the brain tissue. Identification and cautery or clipping of the bleeding source is liable to add further surgical insult to the functioning brain. Occasionally it may be difficult to distinguish between arteries and veins in an AVM. Cardiac green injected through the catheter into the carotid artery intraoperatively will help in the differentiation (Wilson et al. 1979).

Sump Effect of Large AVMs

Massive brain oedema often occurs after excision of large AVMs. Occasionally, following resection of an AVM, the chronically ischaemic adjacent brain will not be able to tolerate the increased perfusion pressure due to the loss of the "sump effect" of the AVM. This leads to loss of capillary integrity with resulting oedema and haemorrhage. Such an event has been termed "normal pressure break-through" by Spetzler et al. (1978). Since this report, similar cases have been reported by others (Wilson et al. 1979; Mullen et al. 1979; Drake 1979; Nornes and Grip 1980). Structural changes in the media of resistance vessels upon elimination of pressure load have been noted in experimental animals (Folkow et al. 1971). This break-through phenomenon is common in:

1. Large AVMs
2. When there is rapid shunt with non-visualisation of normal cerebral circulation in the ipsilateral hemisphere
3. Patients with ischaemic neurological deficit (Wilson et al. 1979).

Arteriovenous malformations fed by vessels 8 cm or longer from the circle of Willis are more prone to postoperative oedema than those with short vessels (Nornes and Grip 1980). Normal pressure break-through can be counteracted by careful management of these cases. This consists in a two-stage approach of embolisation or occlusion of the major feeders and excision of the AVM 2 weeks later. Further lowering of the blood pressure in the postoperative period after removal of the AVMs (to the lower limits of the autoregulatory curve) has been suggested (Spetzler et al. 1978). Ipsilateral occlusion of the carotid artery (Mullen et al. 1979) and a combined approach of reducing the size of the AVM with bucrylate and then excising it (Cromwell and Harris 1980) have also been advocated.

Site of the Lesion

From the surgical point of view, the location of the AVM is important for the following reasons:

1. The relationship of the AVM to functionally significant areas of the brain will influence whether surgery is indicated.

Table 13.1. Anatomical locations of AVMs in various reported series

	*Perret and Nishioka (1966)[a]	Anderson and Korbin (1958)	Troupp et al. (1970)	Waltimo (1973a)	Pia (1975)	Wilson et al. (1979)	Authors (unpublished)
Site/total no.	453	37	137	45	124	83[b]	44[c]
Parietal	107	12	39	16	40[a]	20	12
Frontal	102	7	23	–	5	11	6
Temporal	82	7	19	14	17	9	8
Parieto-occipital	18	6	–	–	–	–	–
Occipital	23	3	–	7	6	10	4
Midline	–	2	36	1	–	15	5[d]
Posterior fossa	32	–	10	3	21	14	6
Sylvian fissure	–	–	–	–	9	–	–
Interhemispheric	–	–	–	–	15	–	–
Deep (includes ventricular and basal ganglia)	81	–	–	–	11	–	–

[a] Numbers are modified according to the main location of the AVM
[b] Four cases are extracerebral
[c] Three cases are extracerebral
[d] Cases include basal ganglia and thalamus

2. The site of the AVM will determine the specific arterial supply and venous drainage, and may make resection more difficult than usual.
3. The morphological type of the AVM may vary with the location; for example, vascular malformations are usually capillary in type in the pons, whereas malformations of the spinal cord are venous angiomas, and angiomas of the cerebral hemisphere are usually arteriovenous in type.

The anatomical location of AVMs in different reported series is shown in Table 13.1.

Cerebral Hemisphere

Sixty-five to eight-five per cent of AVMs involve the cerebral hemisphere (Anderson and Korbin 1958; Svien and McRae 1965; Kelly et al. 1969; Waltimo 1973a; Pia 1975). Most convexity AVMs, as mentioned previously, are visible on the surface of the brain, from where they extend as a wedge of abnormal vessels to the subcortical white matter (Fig. 13.4). A number of AVMs, although commonly seen at or near the surface of the cortex, may lie deeply (hidden in the interhemispheric fissure), medially in the hippocampal region or above the tentorium (Fig. 13.5). Arteriovenous malformations in the watershed areas of the cerebral vasculature are always fed by more than one major artery (Fig. 13.6). Thus temporal lobe AVMs, with their major supply from the middle cerebral artery, may have secondary feeders from the posterior cerebral artery (Fig. 13.7). Frontal lobe AVMs have a dominant supply from the anterior cerebral artery, but may have an associated supply from the middle cerebral artery and opposite anterior cerebral artery (Fig. 13.8). Arteriovenous malformations over the parieto-occipital region are notorious for having a multiple arterial supply. In large AVMs all three major arteries may be involved. The superficial AVMs are drained by passively enlarged cortical veins, and the deeply located ones, by the vein of Galen via the internal cerebral vein (Fig. 13.4).

Basal Ganglia, Ventricles and Corpus Callosum

About 8%–12% of all AVMs are located deep in the cerebral hemisphere (Anderson and Korbin 1958; Svien and McRae 1965; Kelly et al. 1969; Waltimo 1973a). Basal ganglia AVMs are usually fed by the lenticulostriate arteries (Fig. 13.9) and ventricular AVMs by branches of the posterior choroidal and posterior cerebral arteries. Basal ganglia AVMs may be confined to the lenticular nucleus, thalamus or periventricular region, but may involve large central areas of both hemispheres with extension into the basal ganglia and the brain stem. Haemorrhage into the basal ganglia or ventricular system is a common presentation of cryptic AVMs.

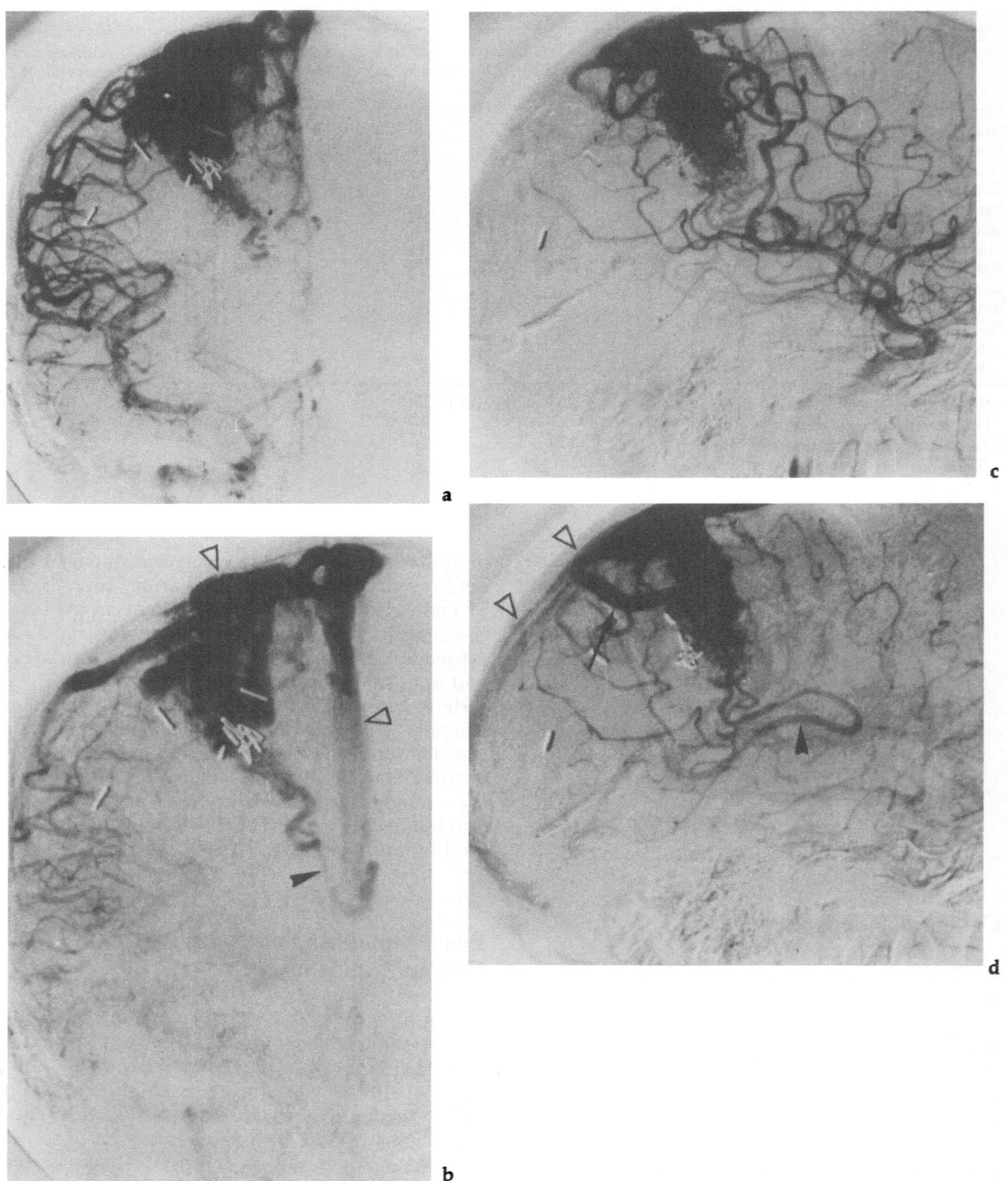

Fig. 13.4. a Townes arterial phase, showing the wedge-shaped appearance of the AVM fed by superficial feeding vessels from the middle cerebral artery. **b** Townes venous phase, showing superficial drainage into the sagittal sinus (*open arrowheads*) and deep venous drainage into the internal cerebral vein (*black arrowhead*). **c** Lateral arterial phase showing a wedge-shaped AVM in the parietal region. **d** Lateral venous phase showing superficial venous drainage into the sagittal sinus (*open arrowheads*) and a cortical vein (*black arrow*). There is a deep venous drainage into the internal cerebral vein (*black arrowhead*).

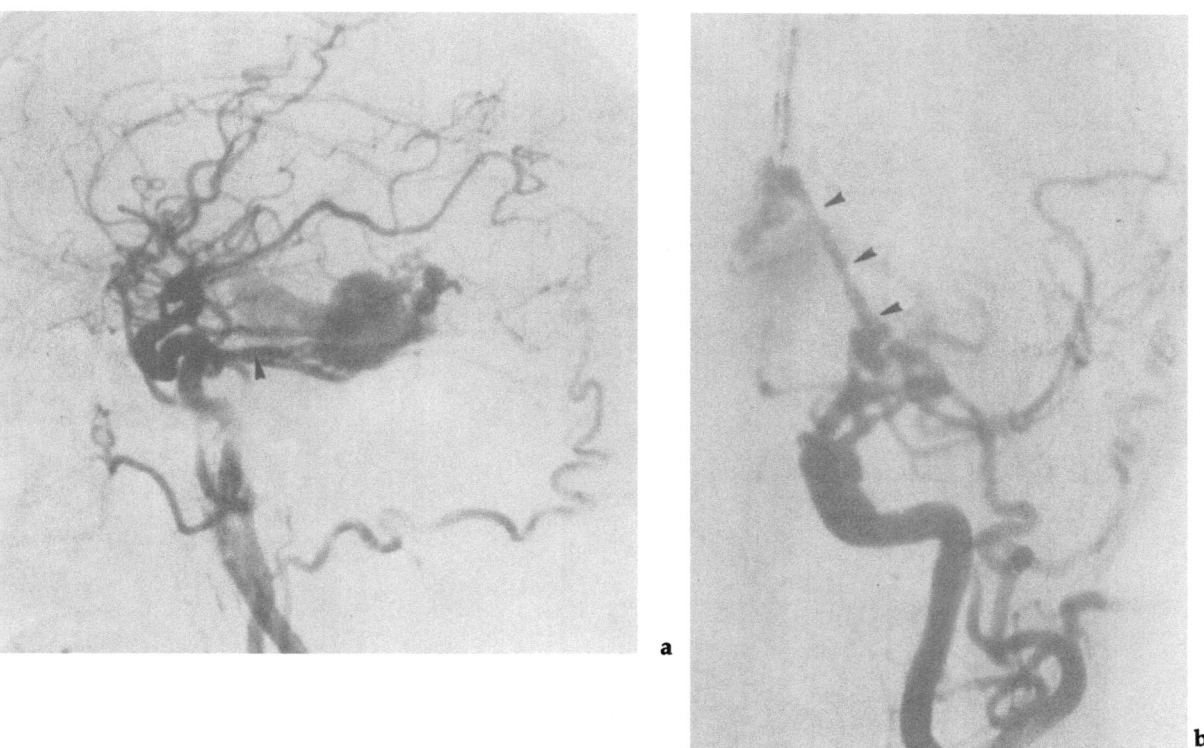

Fig. 13.5. Right carotid angiogram (**a** lateral and **b** Townes projection) showing a midline tentorial AVM. The major feeding vessel is an enlarged tentorial artery (*arrowheads*). There is aneurysmal dilatation of the internal cerebral vein.

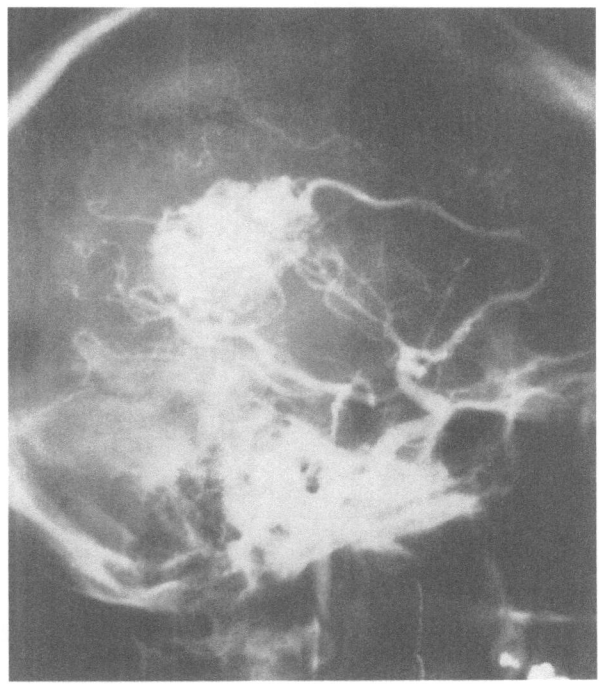

Fig. 13.6. Parietal AVM fed by both the anterior cerebral artery and the posterior cerebral artery.

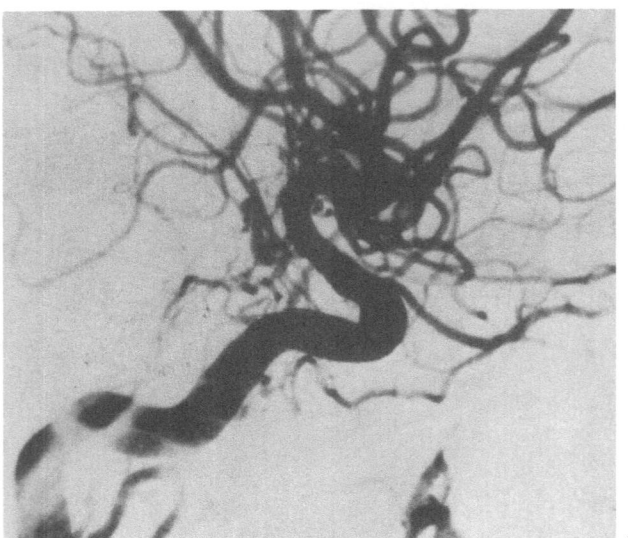

a

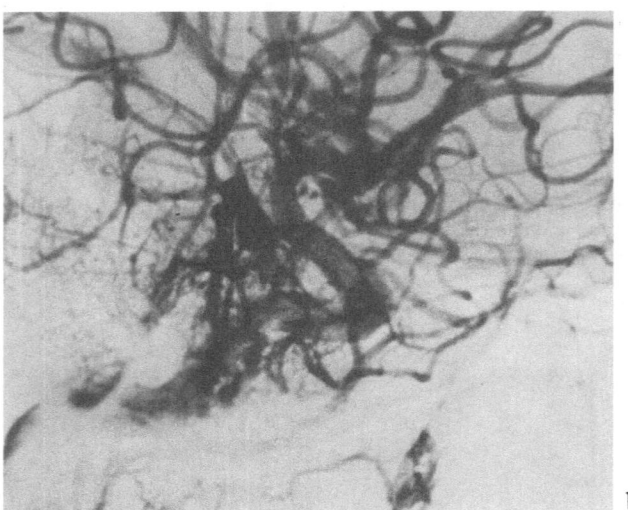

b

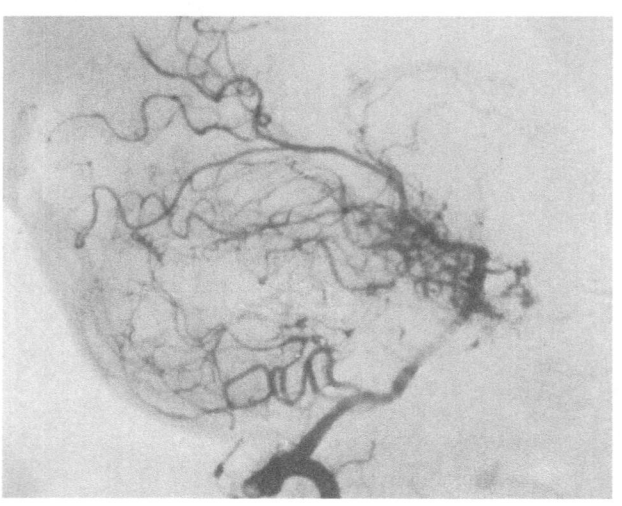

c

Fig. 13.7. a, b Temporal lobe AVM. Lateral carotid angiogram (a arterial and b venous phase) showing feeding vessels
from the middle cerebral artery and early draining veins.
c Lateral vertebral angiogram showing feeding vessels from
the posterior cerebral and posterior communicating arteries.

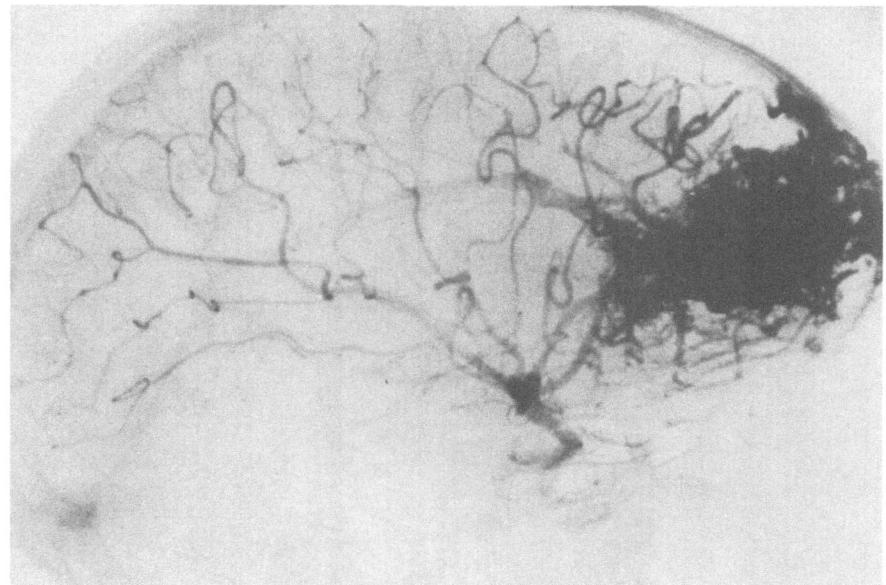

a

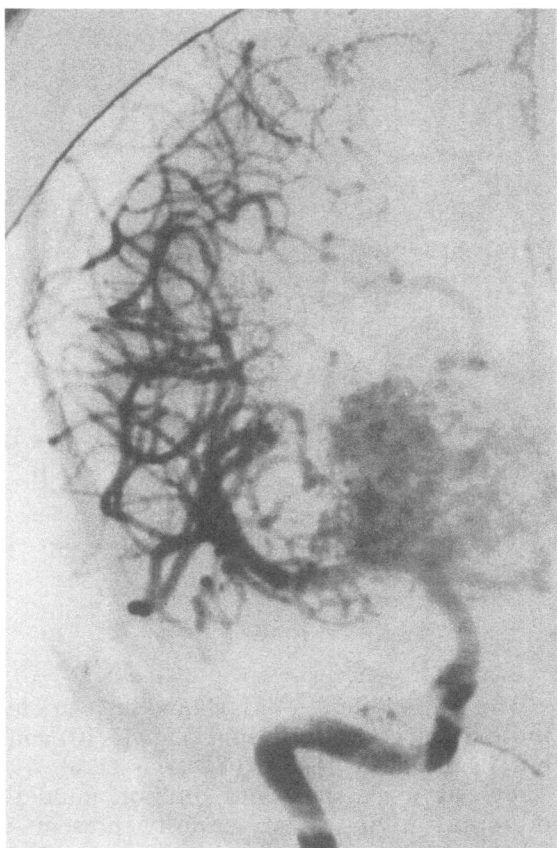

b

Fig. 13.8a, b. Frontal lobe AVM. Carotid angiography (**a** lateral and **b** Townes projection) shows a large midline frontal arch with early venous drainage into the superior sagittal and inferior sagittal sinuses.

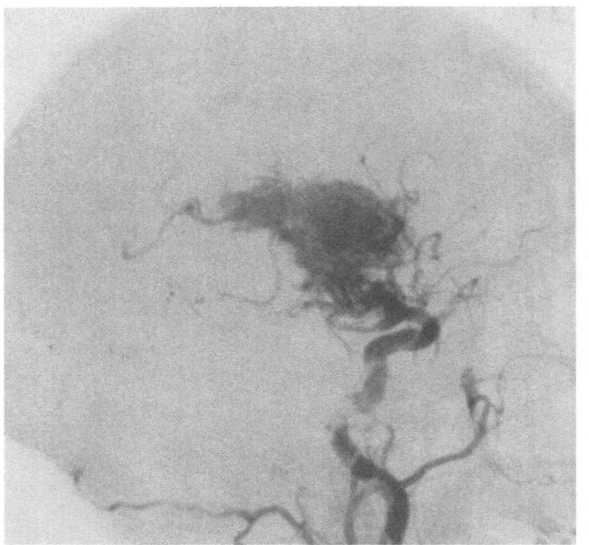

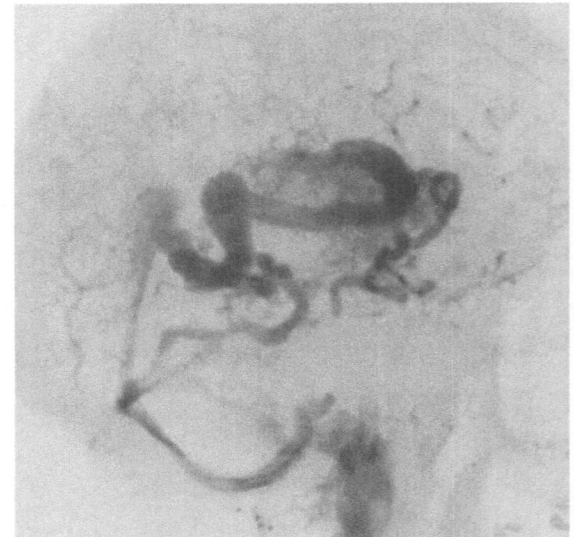

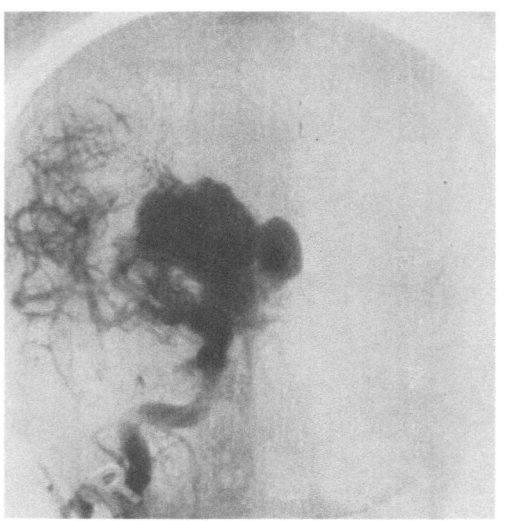

Fig. 13.9a–c. Deep thalamic AVM. Right carotid angiogram (**a** lateral and **b** Townes projection) showing large deeply situated thalamic AVM supplied by enlarged lenticulostriate arteries. **c** Lateral venous phase showing prominent venous drainage into an enlarged internal cerebral vein and vein of Galen.

The term midline AVMs should be restricted to those in the corpus callosum (Fig. 13.10) and the interhemispheric fissure (Yasargil et al. 1976). They can be classified into anterior, middle and posterior groups. The majority present with SAH. They occur in the young and are more common in males. The neurological deficits are more severe with the posterior group (Yasargil et al. 1976a). Occasionally the middle group may occlude the aqueduct and present with obstructive hydrocephalus (De Feo et al. 1976).

Brain Stem

Vascular malformations in the midbrain are often limited to the mesencephalic tectum and may extend into the thalamus (Fig. 13.11). Mechanical obstruction of the aqueduct may occur with resulting intermittent or progressive hydrocephalus. A cavernous angioma in this region may remain undisclosed by angiography, having no special vessel of supply. Aneurysms of the vein of Galen will be discussed later.

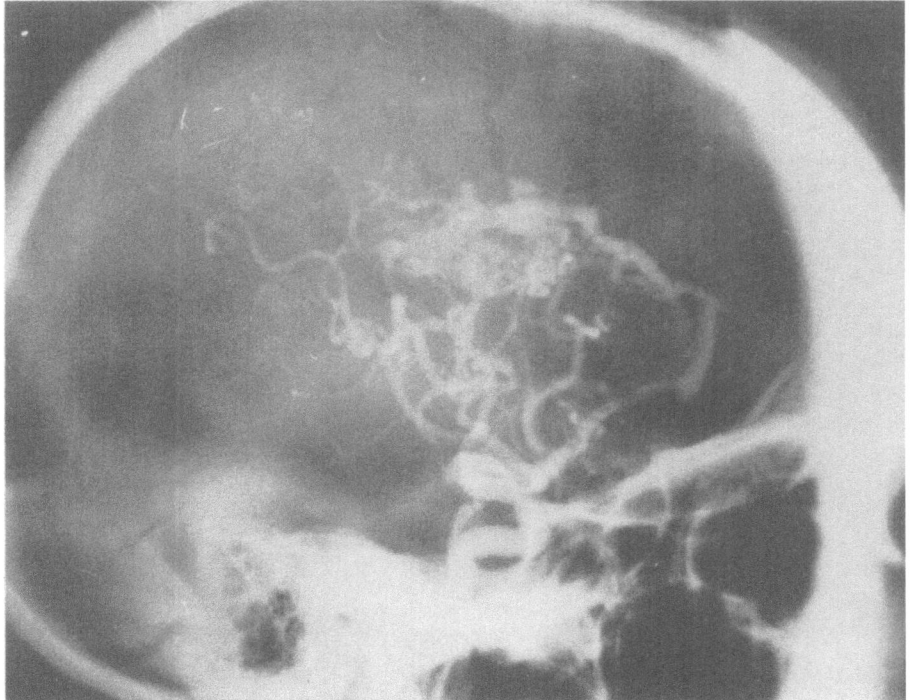

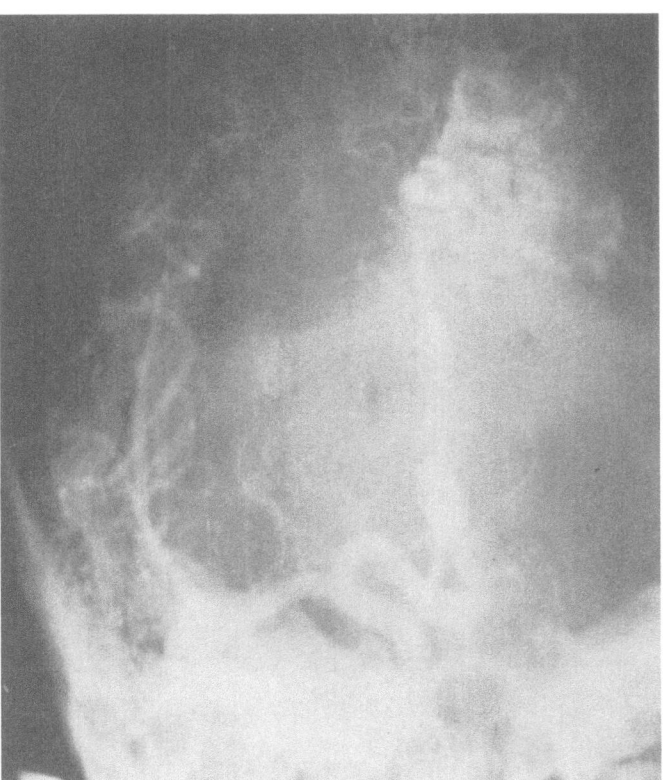

Fig. 13.10a, b. Corpus callosum AVMs. Right carotid angiogram (**a** lateral and **b** Townes projection) showing midline AVM in the corpus callosum supplied by both enlarged pericallosal arteries.

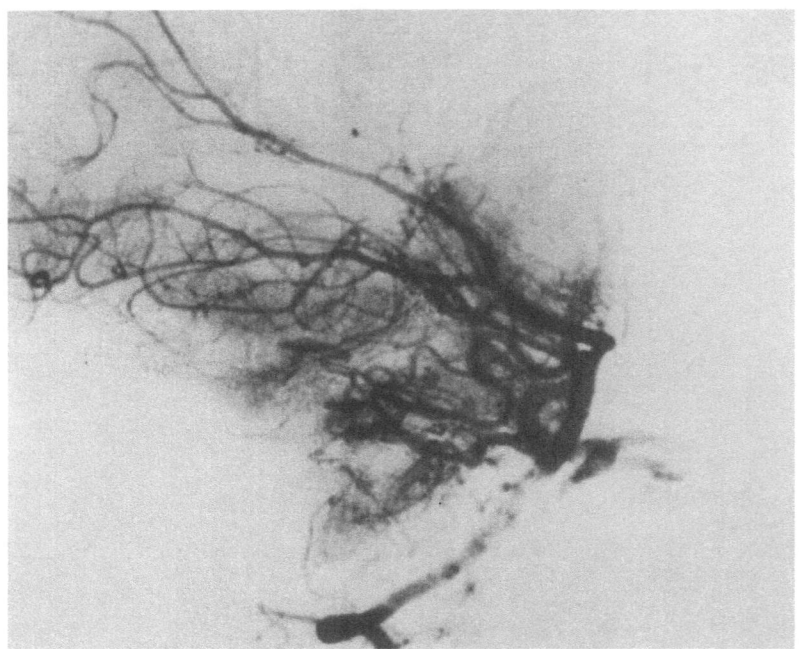

a

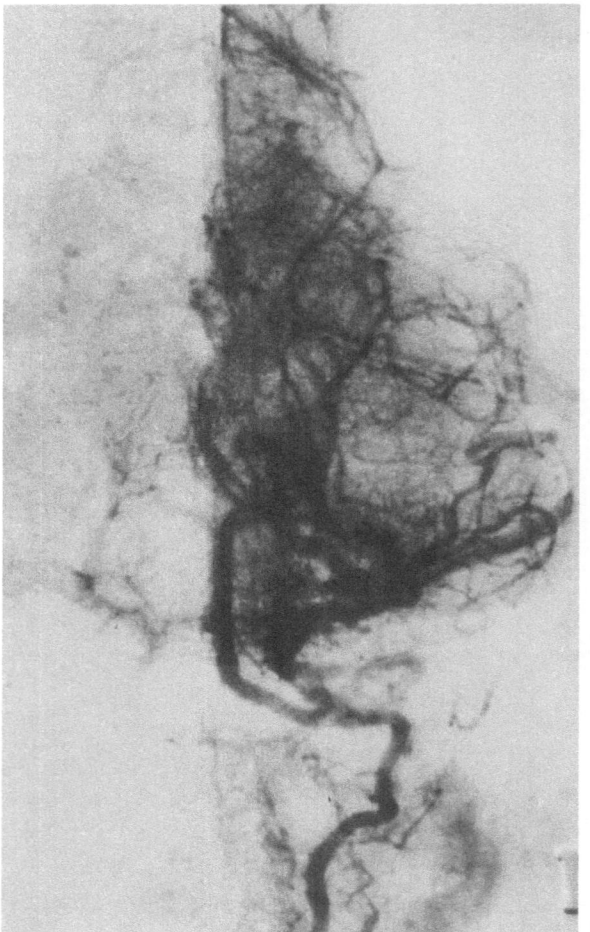

Fig. 13.11a, b. Vertebral angiogram showing extensive brain
b stem AVM which extends into the thalamic region.

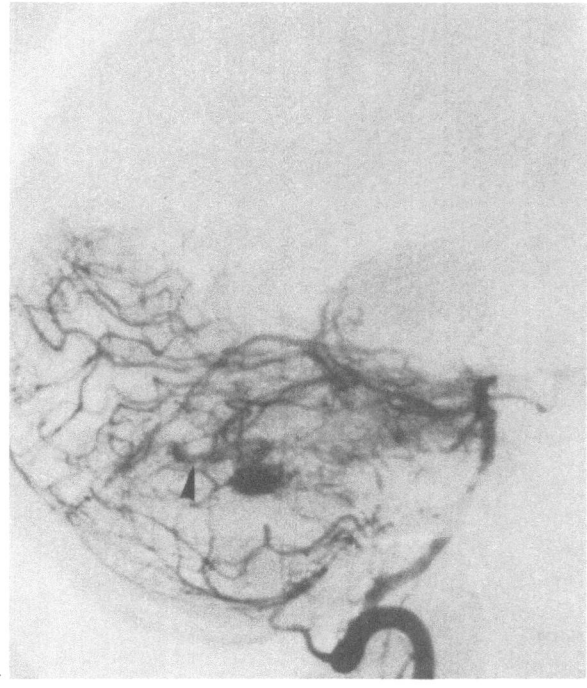

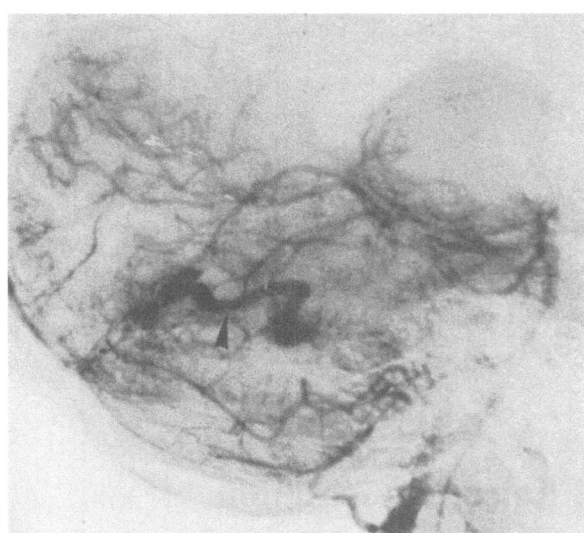

Fig. 13.12a, b. Vertebral angiogram (lateral projection) showing a small cerebellar AVM supplied by the superior cerebellar artery with a prominent draining vein (*arrowheads*).

Cerebellum

Arteriovenous malformations are more frequent in the cerebellar hemisphere than in the brain stem (Svien and McRae 1965; Kelly et al. 1969; Waltimo 1973a; Pia 1975). Deep AVMs within the cerebellar white matter tend to be small (Fig. 13.12), but those over the midline within the vermis, extending to the tentorium, are largest and clinically significant. They may extend to the brachium conjunctivum and the tegmental region of the pons, the arterial contribution coming from the terminal branches of the superior cerebellar arteries and the venous drainage being into the transverse or straight sinuses. The cerebello-pontine angle AVMs usually lie extrapially or are loosely subpial in the brain stem. They therefore may be in close contact with cranial nerves. Apart from haemorrhage, they also produce pressure effects and may present with trigeminal neuralgia or hemifacial spasm. Such a 28-year-old female with a 2-year history of trigeminal neuralgia has been seen in our centre. Six months prior to seeking a medical opinion, she developed headache and mild unsteadiness of gait. Vertebral angiography revealed a large cerebellar hemisphere AVM extending into the cerebellopontine angle (Fig. 13.13).

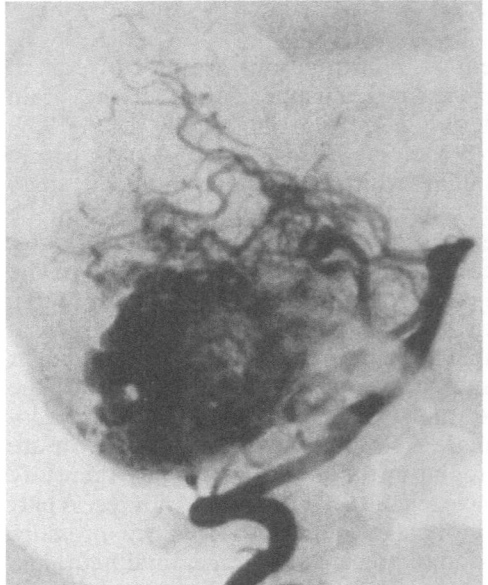

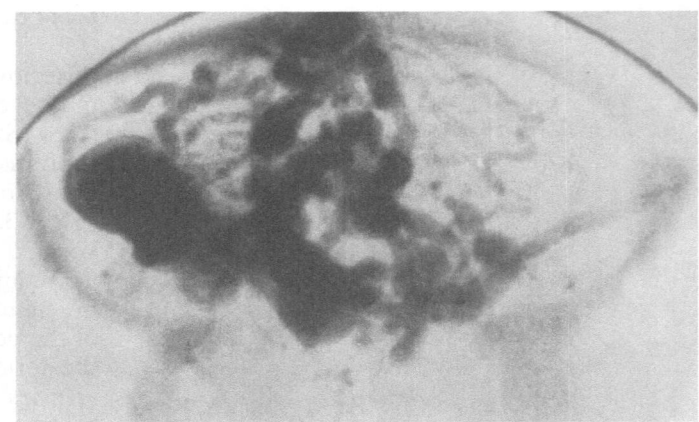

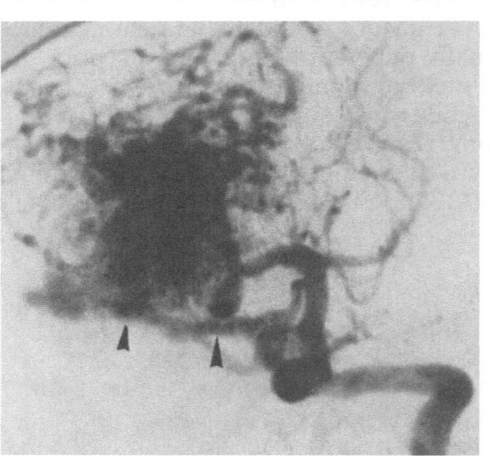

Fig. 13.13a–c. Vertebral angiogram (**a** lateral and **b, c** Townes projection) showing a large right cerebellar hemisphere AVM which extends into the cerebellopontine angle. The AVM has numerous feeding vessels, including an enlarged right AICA (*arrowheads*) as well as superior cerebellar artery branches.

Dural AVM

Dural AVMs are supplied exclusively by branches of the carotid or vertebral arteries before they penetrate the dura (Fig. 13.14).

The majority of dural AVMs arise within or adjacent to a major venous sinus and have predominantly dural venous drainage. They infrequently cause intracranial haemorrhage. Dural AVMs lying outside a major sinus and which have a primary leptomeningeal venous drainage are uncommon but they have a propensity for serious intracranial haemorrhage (Malik et al. 1984).

Clinical Presentation

Arteriovenous malformations present in one or more of the following ways:

1. Intracranial haemorrhage
2. Epilepsy
3. Headache
4. Focal neurological deficit
5. Impairment of higher cerebral functions

The incidence of such presentations is outlined in Table 13.2.

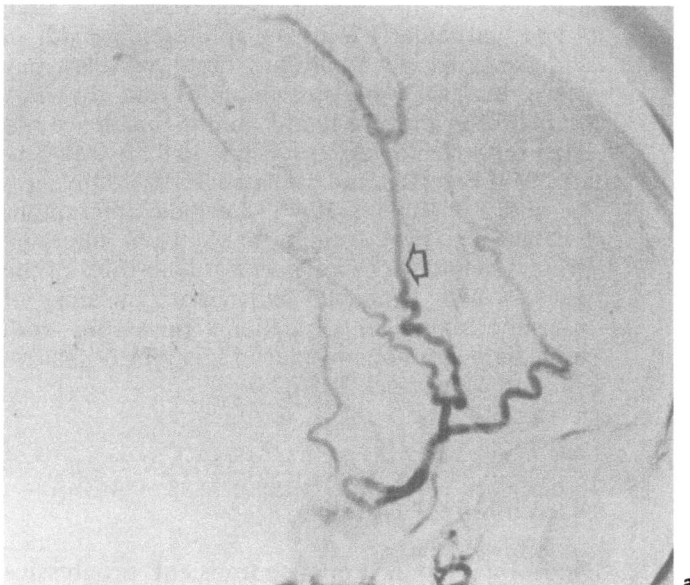

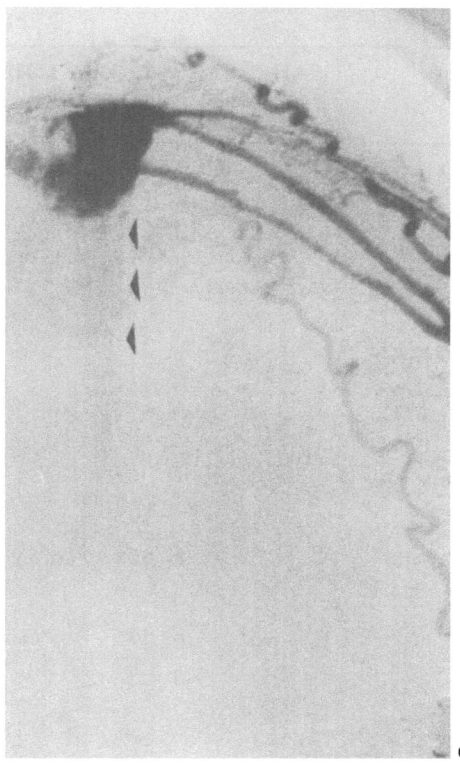

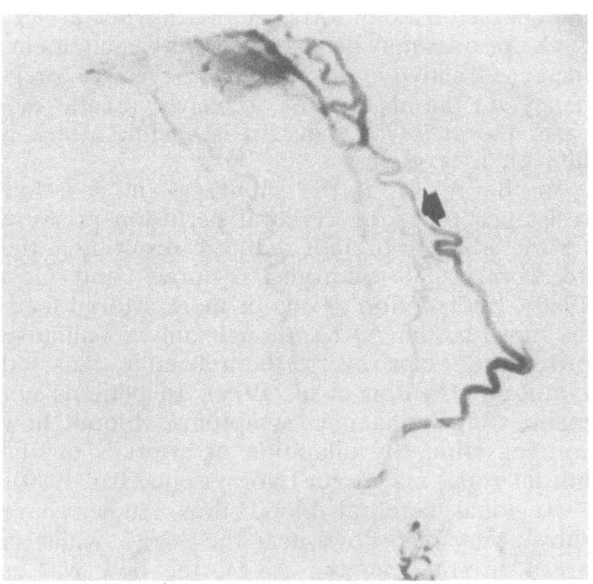

Fig. 13.14. a, b Lateral and **c** Townes carotid angiography showing a dural AVM supplied by the middle meningeal (*open arrow*) and superficial temporal arteries (*closed arrow*) with early drainage into the sagittal sinus (*arrowheads*). A right carotid angiogram also showed feeding vessels from the middle meningeal artery.

Intracranial Haemorrhage

Depending upon the site, AVMs may produce intracerebral, intraventricular or subarachnoid haemorrhage. Minor repeated haemorrhages occur more often than is clinically appreciated, since clinically silent AVMs at autopsy clearly show evidence of minor bleeds. As previously described, following the first major bleed fatalities occur in about 10% of patients. It is unusual for such lesions to bleed in the first decade, and the most common age of presentation is the second to fourth decade.

Epilepsy

Epilepsy is more common in superficial AVMs (McKenzie 1953), and patients with convulsions have a low risk of bleeding (McKenzie 1953; Graf et al. 1983). From the Co-operative Study (Perret and Nishioka 1966) it was deduced that generalised seizures are as common as focal seizures. Generalised seizures are more frequent if the lesion is in the frontal lobe, while focal seizures

Table 13.2. Presenting symptoms of AVMs (figures in percentages)

Author	SAH	SAH and ICH	Epilepsy	HA	PND
McKenzie (1953) 50 cases	–	30	32	24	14
Paterson and McKissock (1956) 110 cases	42	4	29	13	7
Anderson and Korbin (1958) 37 cases	–	54	24	13	8
Svein and McCrae (1965) 95 cases	–	53	46	34	21
Kelly et al. (1969) 70 cases	51	–	37	9	3
Moody and Poppen (1970) 105 cases	40	–	50	38	37
Troupp et al. (1970) 137 cases	58	–	25	8	9
Amacher et al. (1972) 50 cases	11	32	4	3	–
Waltimo (1973a) 45 cases	–	49	51	–	–
Luessenhop (1975) 55 cases	–	38.1	34.5	27	22
Authors' series 44 cases	73	9	7	4	7

Abbreviations: SAH, subarachnoid haemorrhage; ICH, clinically diagnosed intracerebral haematoma; HA, headache; PND, progressive neurological deterioration

predominate when the lesion involves the parietal lobe. The incidence of seizures increases when both the frontal and the temporal lobe are involved.

Headache

Continuous headache, or a migrainous type headache, is a distressing symptom seen in a minority of patients with AVMs. When associated with minor bleeds or hydrocephalus, as evidenced by CT scan, the cause of the headache is to a certain extent understandable, but in the absence of such features the cause has not been defined. A large AVM, particularly in the occipital region with an additional supply from the dural vessels, may cause headache by stretching of the dura. A cranial bruit may be heard, and its incidence has been reported to vary from 10% to 82% (McKenzie 1953; Paterson and McKissock 1966; Olivecrona and Ladenheim 1957). Periodic migrainous headache is not distinguishable from migraine (Paterson and McKissock 1956). One-third of the patients with headache had a family history of migraine, and 67% of patients presenting with periodic migrainous headache had a bruit (Paterson and McKissock 1956).

Neurological Deficit

Neurological deficit may be transient, progressive or permanent. The transient deficit commonly has the characteristic of a transient ischaemic attack. Such episodes may be associated with excitement, increased activity, the menstrual cycle or pregnancy. In the absence of occlusive vascular disease, the cause of transient ischaemic attack is difficult to explain.

In the AVM, if the shunt system is a low resistance type, the cerebral perfusion pressure for the adjacent brain is reduced, resulting in the "cerebral steel syndrome" (Nornes and Grip 1980). Interruption of one or more arterial feeders close to the AVM, though only a palliative procedure, helps reverse the ischaemic signs and symptoms (Wilson et al. 1979). In patients not manifesting ischaemic symptoms, blood flow compensation (by dilatation of arterials on the border zone) may occur (Nornes and Grip 1980).

Regional cerebral blood flow studies have shown very high flows near the AVM, whilst in areas distant from the AVM, the flow was as low as 20 ml/100 g per minute, despite angiographically normal vasculature (Heiss et al. 1970).

Impairment of Higher Cerebral Functions

Impaired cognitive function in association with AVM is well recognised. Improvement in behavioural and intellectual performance in young children after excision of AVMs would indicate that haemodynamic deprivation of the brain might be responsible. Normal pressure hydrocephalus, resulting from minor bleeds, may also be responsible for dementia.

Management

When central nervous system vascular malformations present with complications, such as life-threatening haematoma or hydrocephalus, the management is clearly surgical and poses no dilemma in its application. Apart from these situations, the following factors should be considered in relation to surgical treatment.

1. Clinical syndrome presented by the AVM
2. Natural history of the AVM
3. Feasibility of surgical obliteration
4. Expertise of the surgeon
5. Facilities available

Clinical Syndrome

The management of the patient will depend upon the type of clinical presentation.

Haemorrhage. The risk of further haemorrhage from an AVM has already been discussed. In about 50% of AVMs in neurosurgical practice, the patient presents with an intracerebral haematoma. If the haematoma is life threatening or neurological function is compromised, it should be evacuated. This was necessary in 11% of our cases. It is relatively straightforward to excise an AVM in the presence of a haematoma, but the optimal timing of the operation is more debatable. In this centre, operative procedures are performed 2–3 weeks after the haemorrhage if there is no life-threatening haematoma. This is at a time when the brain is recovering from the initial insult and any haematoma that is present is resolving.

Epilepsy. It should be noted that excision of an AVM does not necessarily remove the threat of further epilepsy (Anderson and Korbin 1958; Svien and McRae 1965), but a 14%–44% decrease in seizure activity with drug therapy has been observed after excision of the malformation (Paterson and McKissock 1956; Forster et al. 1972; Guidetti and Delitala 1980). In some cases epilepsy may be due to a minor haemorrhage,

which may be confirmed by CT scanning. Transient ischaemic attacks can occur with AVM, and must be differentiated from focal epilepsy.

Headache. When there is no evidence of haemorrhage or hydrocephalus, headache is rarely an indication for surgery. However, if the headache is due to distended dural supply, excision may help. Luessenhop and Presper (1975) noted relief of headache following embolisation of feeding arteries.

Neurological Deficit. Well established neurological deficit is usually due to past haemorrhage from an AVM, and neurological function cannot be improved by excision of the AVM. The role of surgery in progressive neurological deterioration is debatable and embolisation has been found to be useful in its management (Luessenhop and Presper 1975).

Natural History

The need for surgical treatment of AVMs largely depends on their natural history, which has been discussed previously. It has been noted that incidentally discovered AVMs may continue to remain static in size and asymptomatic, and, unlike unruptured aneurysms, pose very little threat to life or neurological function.

Feasibility of Surgical Obliteration

Incomplete excision of AVMs or their feeding arteries in an attempt to decrease the blood flow through the AVM is of no benefit. These procedures may aggravate the patient's condition by depriving the normal brain of an adequate blood supply. Ligation of superficially visible feeding arteries at operation is also futile, as deeply situated vessels will enlarge to fill the lesion. Total excision of an AVM, where feasible, is the only way to guarantee that it will not be a future risk to the patient. Excision is difficult in the following cases:

1. Midline lesions in the medulla, midbrain or diencephalon and vein of Galen aneurysms
2. AVMs in the basal ganglia
3. Huge AVMs in functionally important areas of the cerebral hemispheres (especially the dominant side) or in the posterior fossa

It should be borne in mind that excision of a very large AVM carries the risk of postoperative oedema or haemorrhage. The results of complete excision or obliteration must therefore be weighed against the natural history of the disorder.

Surgical Expertise

It is well known that the skill of a surgeon improves with experience, but these formidable lesions usually present to the surgeon only occasionally. Some surgeons, such as Yasargil and Drake, have accrued enormous expertise with cases referred worldwide. What is surgically feasible and possible in their hands may prove not to be so for other neurosurgeons, even those with an interest in vascular surgery. Such lack of expertise may improve if angiomas from a particular region are referred to a team of neurosurgeons with a special interest in vascular malformations.

Facilities Available

Recent advances in neurosurgical techniques have improved the outcome of surgery on AVMs. A team dealing with these lesions should have considerable skill in microvascular surgery, and well trained theatre personnel. Such a unit should work in collaboration with radiologists able to perform superselective angiography and embolisation techniques in selected cases. A unit lacking such facilities is limited to the management of simple cases, especially those with acute life-threatening haematomas.

Principles of Direct Surgical Treatment

The ideal treatment of AVMs is complete separation from the cerebral circulation. This is often possible with microvascular technique, bipolar coagulation, steroid therapy and hypotensive anaesthesia. In practice, however, total excision of AVMs is not always feasible. It is useful to consider the following factors during surgery:

1. The contribution of cerebral arteries to the malformation
2. The contribution of dural and scalp vessels from the external carotid artery to the malformation

3. Draining veins from the malformation
4. The presence of haematoma within the malformation
5. The presence of hydrocephalus
6. Associated vascular anomalies of the cerebral vessels
7. Clinical syndrome requiring surgical treatment

Feeding Cerebral Arteries

An AVM is usually fed by one or more of the three major cerebral arteries. If the AVM is located well within the territory of a major cerebral artery, then the supply to the AVM usually comes from that vessel but in the borderline area the supply often comes from more than one source. An AVM within the ventricle may receive blood from both the anterior and the posterior choroidal arteries. Prior identification of all possible sources of supply is vital to successful surgery. Complete four vessel angiography, with the subtraction technique, is essential to define all the feeding arteries requiring obliteration (Fig. 13.15). Intraoperative angiography is also occasionally useful.

External Carotid Supply

Occasionally the large AVMs lying over the brain surface may receive a vascular supply from dural and scalp vessels (Fig. 13.16). Large AVMs causing epilepsy, the cerebral steal phenomenon or intense headache are particularly liable to have an additional external carotid blood supply. The supply from the external carotid artery can be removed by careful planning of the scalp flap to include these vessels. A further reduction of the external carotid artery supply can be obtained by excising the dura over the AVM.

Draining Veins

The presence of large and extensive venous drainage in the angiogram may look ominous, but it does not necessarily preclude successful excision of the AVM. Such drainage only indicates rapid shunting of blood from the malformation. The significance of extensive venous drainage lies in the fact that the loss of the sump effect following excision is related to the size of the AVM and the extent of venous drainage (Fig. 13.17).

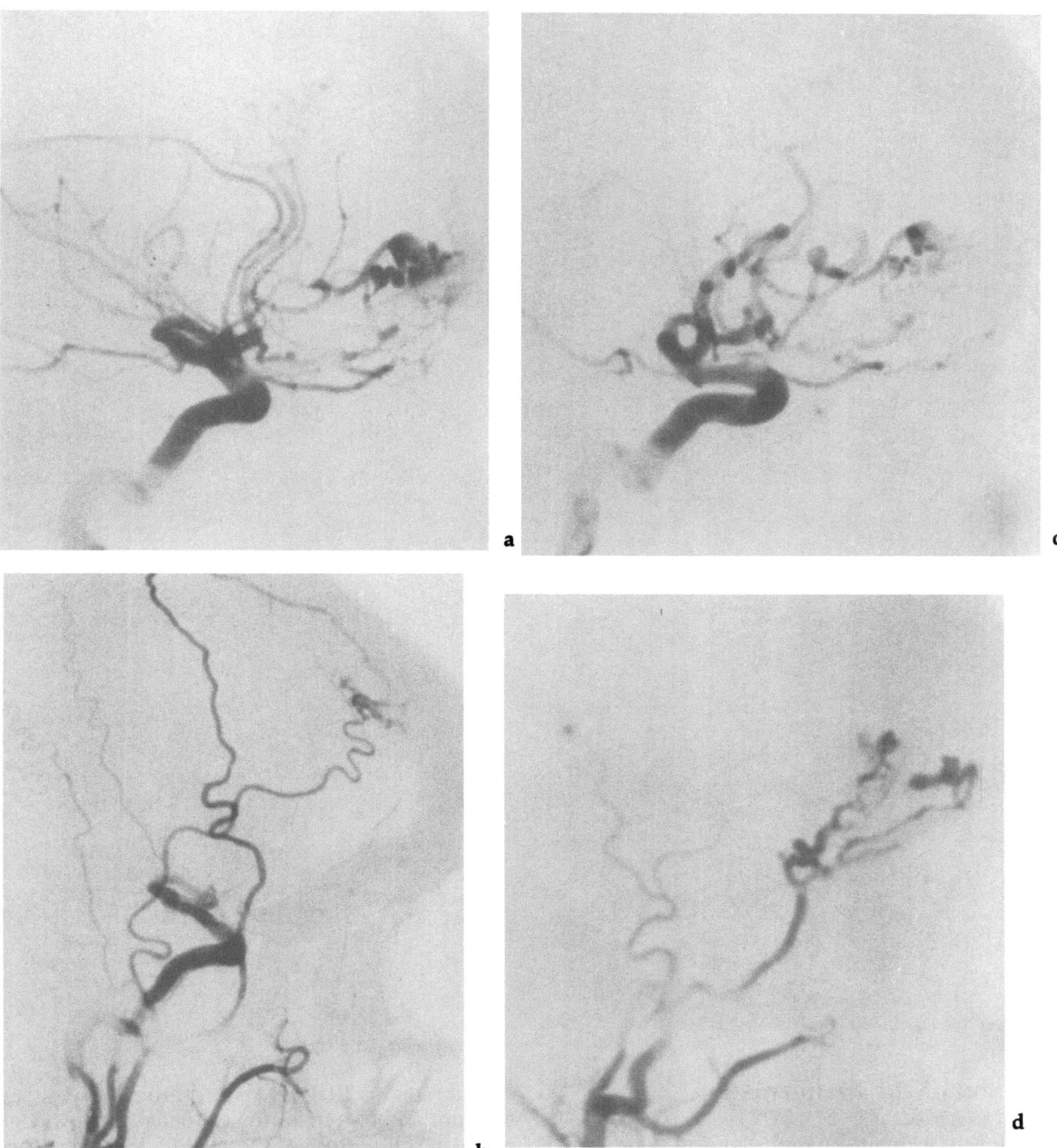

Fig. 13.15a–f. Large midline frontal AVM. **a** Selective right internal carotid angiogram; **b** selective right external carotid angiogram; **c** selective left internal carotid angiogram; **d** selective left external carotid angiogram. These clearly define the feeding vessels (see legend to Fig. 7.44). **e** Postoperative RT common carotid angiograph and **f** postoperative LT common carotid angiography shows complete removal of the AVM.

Fig. 13.15e,f *overleaf*

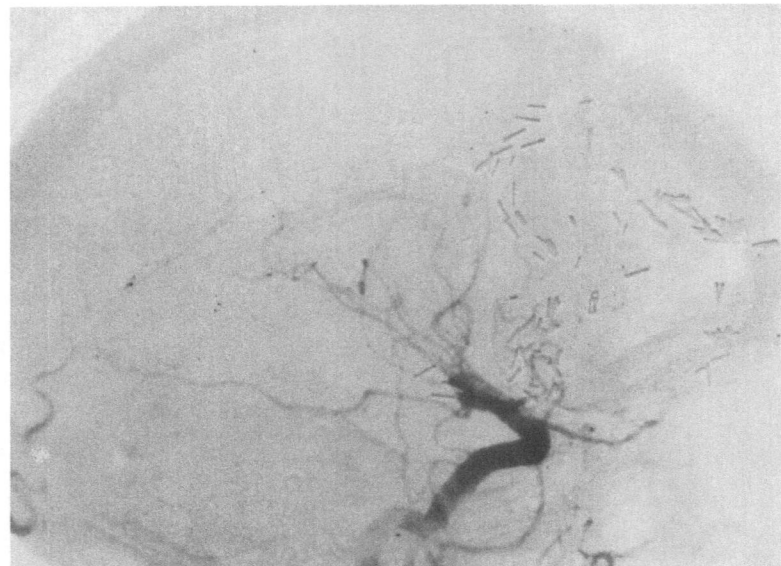

Fig.13.15e

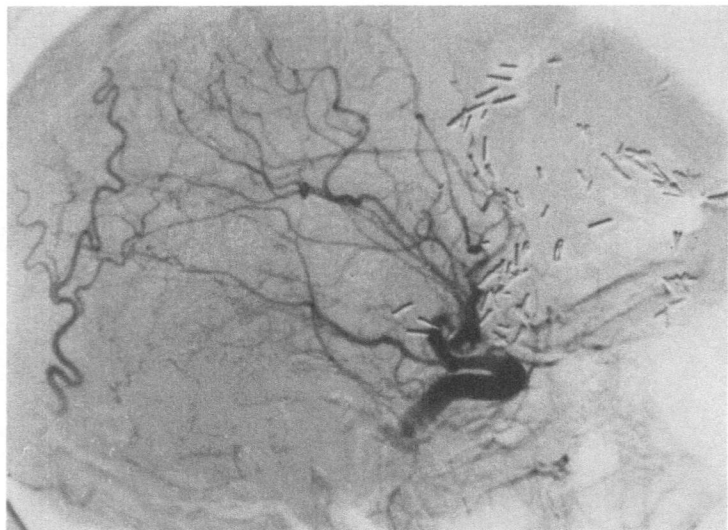

Fig. 13.15f

Location of the Malformation

Arteriovenous malformations lying at the poles of frontal or temporal lobes can be totally excised by performing simple lobectomy. Resection of non-vital areas in the right frontal or temporal lobes that harbour an AVM can also be performed without any resulting neurological deficit. An AVM in the dominant hemisphere or in the sensory or motor cortex requires careful excision to minimise damage to the surrounding brain. It is fortunate that brain tissue in the immediate neighbourhood of the AVM is usually non-functioning, so that dissection through this tissue may not add to a neurological deficit. Knowledge of the exact location of the AVM is also necessary for the planning of surgical access, e.g. an AVM of the tentorium or superior portion of the cerebellum is best approached by the subtemporal route, while intraventricular AVMs are best approached through the midtemporal gyrus or by a combined subtemporal and midtemporal route. Brain stem malformations may look inoperable on angiograms, but they often lie on the surface of the brain stem and a plan of dissection may be available to excise them completely.

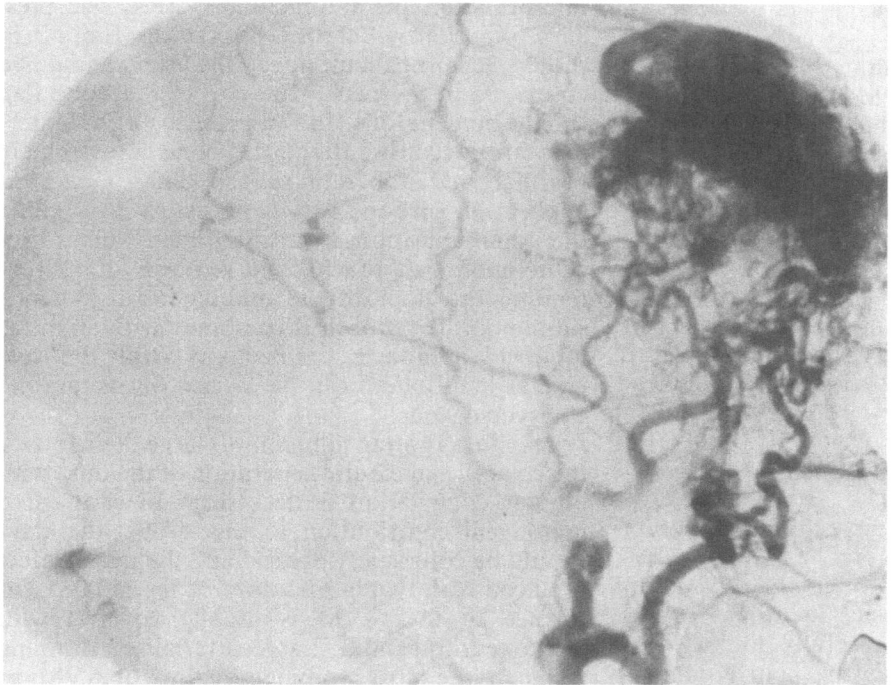

Fig. 13.16. Selective right external carotid angiogram in a patient with a frontal AVM showing very extensive external carotid supply through the superficial temporal and middle meningeal vessels.

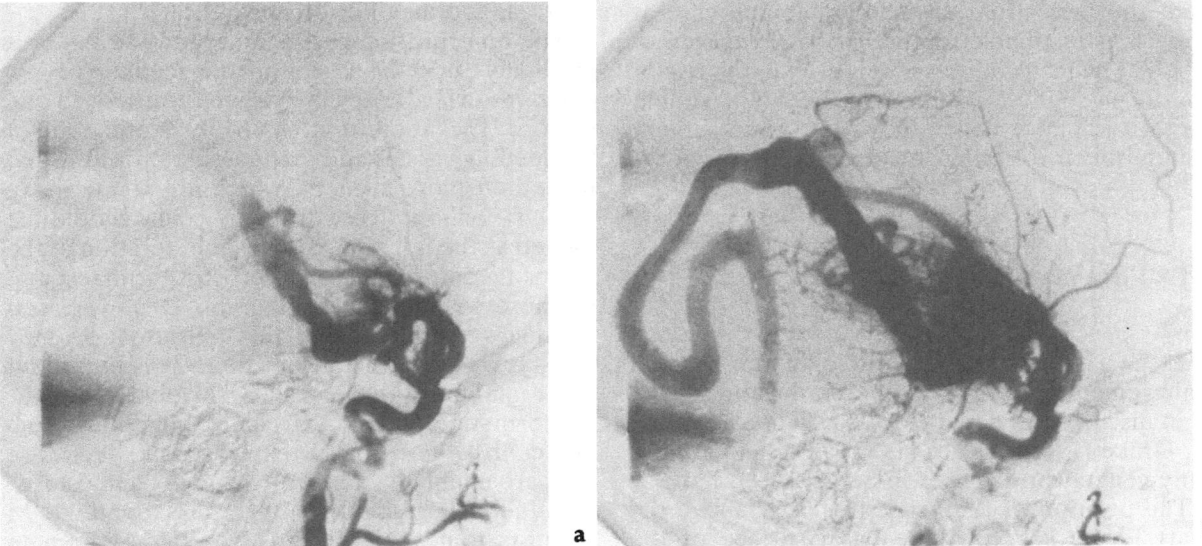

Fig. 13.17a, b. Lateral carotid angiogram showing an AVM with very extensive venous drainage. There is very poor filling of the intracranial vessels (sump effect of AVM).

Presence of Haematoma

Excision of an AVM is facilitated by the presence of a haematoma. The AVM usually lies in the wall of the haematoma, which should be evacuated as a preliminary step (Fig. 13.18).

Hydrocephalus

If the pre-operative scan shows the presence of hydrocephalus, a preliminary shunting procedure to alleviate this should be performed.

Associated Vascular Anomalies

The presence of cerebral aneurysms in association with AVMs is well known (Figs. 7.51, 7.52). Because of the rapid flow through the AVM, an aneurysm may not be easily identified angiographically and must be carefully looked for. Normal cerebral vessels may be poorly demonstrated due to rapid shunting of blood through the AVM. Any anomalies of the circle of Willis (preventing redistribution of cerebral blood flow following excision of the AVM) should be noted since they pose an additional hazard.

Clinical Syndrome Requiring Surgical Treatment

During the operation it is essential to bear in mind the indications for surgery in the case at hand. It is justifiable to attempt total excision of an AVM which produces SAH, even at the risk of certain morbidity. Excision of an AVM should not lead to major deficit, however, when surgery is undertaken for either headache or epilepsy.

Operative Procedures

The special techniques required in the surgical management of AVMs in different locations have been discussed in depth by Yasargil et al. (1976a, b), Drake (1979), Heros (1982) and Stein (1984). Only general principles will be discussed here.

The position of the head should be above the heart level. To reach the basal surface of the brain, the neck should be kept slightly extended. The craniotomy should allow total access to the

malformation and the feeding vessels. The presence of external carotid supply to the AVM should be borne in mind, and the artery should be accessible in the neck. The size of the bone flap should be generous. In the presence of an external carotid contribution, the bone is extremely vascular and adherent to the dura. Generous application of bone wax is necessary to occlude the communications with the diploic veins. In a subtemporal approach bone removal should extend to the floor of the middle fossa. When a subtemporal approach is combined with an infratentorial approach, craniectomy over the cerebellar hemisphere can be carried out across the transverse sinus.

The dura is often adherent to large AVMs over the cortex, and careful separation of the dura with bipolar coagulation is necessary. In cases of a meningeal contribution to the AVM, the dura should be completely excised and the dural defect replaced with lyophilised dura or fascia lata. The surface of the AVM is usually covered with thickened arachnoid. Large arterialised draining veins are the most prominent feature of AVMs at operation, and avoidance of any trauma to these veins is essential. If the angiogram shows a single feeder to the AVM, the initial step is to locate this feeder as close as possible to the AVM. The feeding artery is usually greyish pink. A trial application of a clip to the feeding vessel changes the colour of the draining veins from bright red to dark. In such an ideal situation, the major feeding artery is ligated and the malformation can be excised without any difficulty. In most instances, however, the feeding arteries come from multiple sources, and may not be apparent.

The non-functioning brain around the AVM is gradually sucked away until the feeding vessels come into view. They are clipped, cauterised and divided. Elevation of an AVM by ligating one of the feeding vessels and gradual suction will reveal more and more feeders, which are treated in a similar fashion. The draining veins should be ligated as the last step. Surgical obliteration of the major feeding vessels should broadly correspond to those seen in the angiogram. Deeply placed feeding vessels reaching the malformation may tear, and disappear out of vision. It is important to remember that vessels involved in the malformation may be extremely thin and without any contractile tissue in their wall, in which case they are unable to contract to obtain haemostasis. Continuous oozing from the bed of an AVM suggests that some feeding vessels still remain unoccluded. These should be identified and ligated.

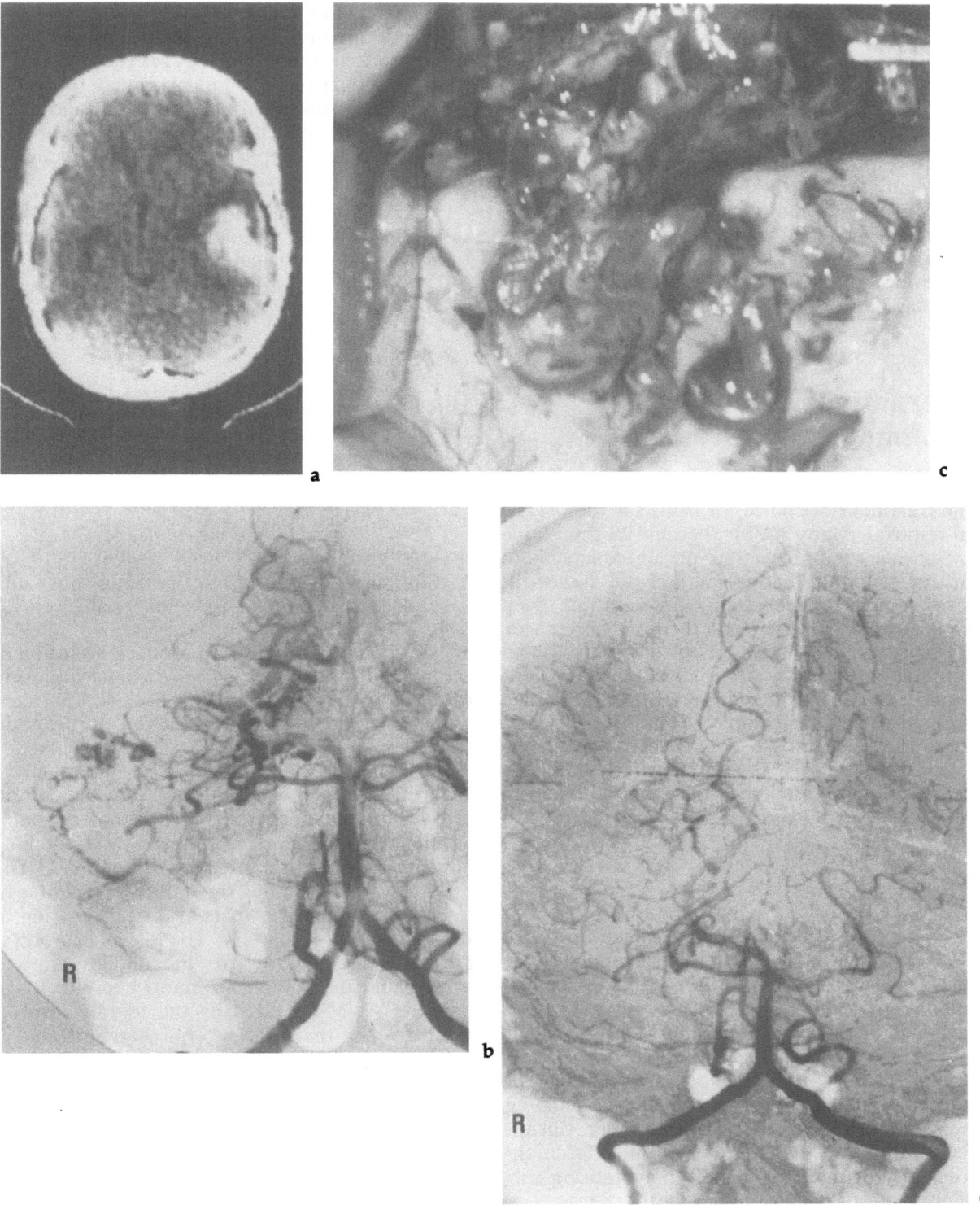

Fig. 13.18a–d. A 25-year-old female, 12 weeks pregnant, with SAH. **a** CT scan shows a large temporal lobe haematoma. **b** Bilateral carotid angiography was negative but vertebral angiography showed a small AVM in the posterior temporal region supplied by the posterior cerebral artery. **c** Operative photograph showing cystic cavity within the temporal lobe created by previously removed haematoma. The AVM is lying in the wall of this cavity. Excision of this malformation was carried out easily through this cavity. **d** Postoperative vertebral angiogram showing satisfactory removal of the AVM.

Postoperative Care

In spite of meticulous haemostasis, minor feeding vessels may escape detection at operation and may produce bleeding as the blood pressure rises in the postoperative period. Some advocate elective ventilation for 48 h to avert this problem. Anticonvulsants and steroid therapy should be continued. Check angiography in the postoperative period will indicate the completeness of the surgical excision of an AVM. Further operation may be necessary to complete the excision.

Alternative Methods of Treatment

The treatment of choice for AVMs is total surgical removal. Many AVMs, because of their large size or inaccessible location, are not amenable to surgery, and alternative methods of treatment have been introduced (e.g., embolisation, deep X-ray therapy, proton beam therapy, stereotactic radiosurgery, cryosurgery, electrothrombosis and stereotactic obliteration). Each of these methods requires extreme skill and special facilities. None of them has so far completely fulfilled expectations. However, they have a special place in the management of AVMs and clinicians should be aware of these methods, their limitations and their value.

Embolisation

Luessenhop and Spence (1960) first introduced the technique of embolisation of silicone beads to an AVM in 1960. Further progress in the embolisation method was made in 1974, when Serbinenko showed the feasibility of introducing catheters with a detachable balloon percutaneously into the feeding arteries of the malformation. Although the detachable balloons themselves offered no advantage over silicone beads, this selective catheterisation offered the possibility of injecting rapidly polymerising substances into the malformation itself.

Indications

Indications for embolisation include:

1. Surgically inoperable AVMs. There are, however, some limitations to the use of embolisation to treat inoperable AVMs (Seeger 1975), i.e. (a) recurrence or enlargement of an incompletely occluded malformation, and (b) a paradoxical effect of improvement in the angiographic appearance without clinical benefit.
2. Cases anatomically unsuitable for surgery.
3. Clinical manifestations, predominantly headache, or neurological deficit.
4. As an adjunct to radical surgical excision.

Technique

Three main methods have been used for embolisation:

1. Embolisation with particles (Silastic spheres, Gelfoam, Lyodura or polyvinyl alcohol film (Ivalon)
2. Embolisation with detachable balloons
3. Embolisation with fast polymerising substances, e.g. isobutyl-2-cyanoacrylate

The aim of treatment is to produce occlusion of the nidus of the AVM, since proximal occlusion of the AVM arterial feeders is useless. The technique can be used alone or as an adjuvant to surgery.

Radiopaque Silastic spheres of different size are available, and when injected into the carotid arteries in the neck they are flow dependent, tending to pass into high-flow AVMs, taking advantage of the sump effect of the AVM. The main factor determining the intracranial course of injected emboli is the angle at the termination of the internal carotid artery. The internal carotid is normally directed towards the middle cerebral artery, and the emboli are more likely to lodge into the AVM supplied by the middle cerebral artery rather than the anterior cerebral artery. Similarly, the bifurcation of the basilar artery and the origin of the posterior cerebral artery is variable, and the basilar artery is directed towards one of the posterior cerebral arteries (Wolpert and Stein 1979). Another important factor is the length, tortuosity and size of the feeding artery itself. If the ratio is below 4:1, there is a 90% chance that the emboli will stray and at 4:1 the chances of emboli straying away are reduced to 50% (Wolpert and Stein 1979). The spheres are injected one at a time and their position located by X-ray. One selects the size of sphere which can reach the nidus of the AVM without passing into the venous outlet. The injection of spheres is discontinued when flow in the feeding artery is dramatically decreased, when a sphere is seen in a normal artery, or when neurological deficit occurs. Some authors advocate carrying out the technique under local anaesthesia so that a deterioration in neurological status is quickly appreciated. In the short-term this technique will reduce the flow and size of an AVM prior to surgery. In the long-term, collaterals develop and recanalisation of the nidus may occur. Serbinenko (1974, 1979) has reported on the use of balloon occlusion of the major vessels supplying AVMs.

Latex and silicone detachable balloons are now available. Serbinenko (1983) reports 110 cases of AVM in which balloon occlusion of the feeding arteries has been carried out. He claims very favourable results as regards treatment of epileptic fits, stabilisation of neurological deficit, and frequency of rebleed.

Recently isobutyl-2-cyanoacrylate, a fast polymerising liquid, has been used for embolisation (Kerber 1980). The technique requires super-selective catheterisation of the individual feeding arteries by means of a special calibrated leak balloon catheter system which can be flow guided into third and fourth order branches of the intracranial arteries, through which controlled amounts of the polymerising liquid can be injected. The balloon is placed closed to the nidus of the AVM and about 0.2–0.9 cc of the polymerising liquid rendered opaque by the addition of tantalum powder injected under screen control. The polymerising time can be varied by the addition of iophendylate, depending on the arteriovenous transit time of the AVM shown at angiography. Intra-operative embolisation of a cerebral AVM, making use of a 50% mixture of isobutyl-2-cyanoacrylate and Duroliopaque, has been reported by Deruty et al. (1983).

Complications

Potential complications of transvascular embolisation with isobutyl-2-cyanoacrylate include:

1. Glueing of the balloon in place
2. Subarachnoid haemorrhage produced by bursting of the balloon in small arterial feeders to the AVM
3. Damage to the internal carotid artery resulting from the use of large axial catheters

4. Postembolic severe brain hyperaemia and swelling
5. Permanent neurological deficit by occlusion of normal cortical arteries

Results

Vinuela et al. (1983) report on the use of transvascular embolisation with isobutyl-2-cyanoacrylate in 69 patients with large brain AVMs. The transfemoral and/or intraoperative approaches were used, depending on the size and location of the AVM. In 28 cases 70%–99% of the AVM was obliterated by embolisation alone; in 17 cases complete obliteration of the AVM was obtained, and 10 of these cases had final surgical resection. They report a long-term morbidity for the technique of 14.5% and a mortality of 4.5%.

Deep X-Ray Therapy (Megavoltage)

The role of radiotherapy in the treatment of AVMs is still debatable. Paterson and McKissock (1956) followed 11 patients for 14 years, who had deep X-ray therapy only. Four patients died due to subsequent haemorrhage, and three developed progressive neurological deficit. Johnson (1975) reported on the follow-up of 100 cases treated with 4000–5000 rads over a 3-week period at the Radium Institute, Manchester. This follow-up is continuing; by 1975 20 of these cases had been studied with serial angiography at intervals of 2–20 years. Nine had been totally cured, five improved, and five had shown no change in the size of the angioma. In only one patient did the angioma increase in size. He found medially placed medium size angiomas had been cured, but large cortically placed angiomas did not show any change.

Stereotactic Radiosurgery

Leksell in 1971 developed the stereotactic radiosurgical technique and this has been further developed by Steiner (1977). The technique allows fields of up to 25 mm in diameter to be covered by a sufficient dose. The location and the target volume are taken into consideration in making the dose planning by computer. This also helps to shape the radiation field to be found spatially congruate to the malformation, and to obliterate the AVM without opening the skull. This can be done as an out-patient procedure. Steiner et al.

(1977) reviewed 24 patients treated with the ^{60}Co gamma unit. The dose ranged from 5 to 12 krads over a period of 30 min, and the cases were divided into four groups:

1. The irradiation field covered, completely or almost completely, the nidus of the AVM.
2. The irradiation included only part of the nidus of the AVM.
3. The beam was directed to the feeding arteries.
4. The field included only some of the multiple feeders.

In groups 1 and 2, they found a decrease in the size of the feeding arteries and the rate of blood flow through the malformation in four cases, and total obliteration or a successive decrease in the size of the AVM in 13 cases. In group 3, obliteration of the AVM occurred in one case, a slight decrease in size in one case, and no change in the third. There were no changes observed in the four patients who belonged to group 4, and there were no untoward effects of the treatment.

Bragg Peak Proton Beam Therapy

Kjellberg et al. (1977), who are using Bragg Peak Proton Beam treatment for pituitary tumours, applied it to AVMs in patients in whom conventional surgical excision was either unwanted or had been unsuccessful. The technique involves delivery of carefully defined and graded doses of proton radiation to precisely defined intracranial target lesions by stereotactic techniques, under local anaesthesia, in one session lasting less than 2 h. In this procedure, the radiation to the scalp and brain is less than 1/20th of that to the target lesion. This procedure can be done on an outpatient basis. The proton beam induces subendothelial deposition of hyaline, resulting in narrowing of the lumen of the vessels. The resultant thickness of the vessel walls protects against haemorrhage.

Protons enter the nucleus of the endothelial cells of small vessels and produce ionization in the DNA, with resultant inactivation of the DNA chain. With further ionization, the cells become physiologically impaired. This phenomenon is called endotheleitis. The impaired endothelial cells produce collagen and hyaline in the subendothelial space, leading to narrowing of the lumen of small vessels. It takes 1–2 years for the pathological changes to take place and for the treatment to be effective. This period is termed the "incubation period", during which the AVM may bleed (Kjellberg 1983). A recent survey by Kjellberg et al. (1984) in 206 patients who presented with haemorrhage showed that three patients died and six patients experienced 13 episodes of recurrent haemorrhage during this incubation period.

In the 134 patients with a follow-up longer than the 2-year incubation period there were no deaths (the predicted death rate from exponential probability function employing published mortality rates would be approximately three to five). There were seven recurrent haemorrhages (2.4% per year), which is significantly lower than the haemorrhage rate of the same patients in the years preceding therapy (7.25% per year) ($P = 0.005$).

In 260 patients presenting with haemorrhage, headache, seizures or progressive neurological deficit as a first symptom and with a follow-up of more than 2 years, check angiography was carried out in 57%; it showed total obliteration of the AVM in 22% and nearly total obliteration in 29% of cases.

Cryosurgery

Walder (1975a, b) reported his experience in cryosurgery in the treatment of AVMs. Indications were large sized AVMs situated in functionally important areas and inoperable by orthodox surgical procedures. Certain precautions should be taken during the procedure—the cryoprobe should be immobile during freezing, and it must be entirely above freezing point when it is withdrawn to avoid rupture of the vascular wall. This process results in proliferation of the intima and thrombosis at a subsequent stage.

Electrothrombosis

Handa et al. (1977) used electrothrombosis to overcome troublesome bleeding and facilitate radical excision of AVMs. The technique involves inserting copper electrodes 0.25 mm in diameter into the feeding arteries after formal craniotomy and with the aid of stereotactic methods, into the nidus. Depending upon the size of the AVM, as many as 30–60 electrodes are used. Between 0.5 and 10 mA direct current is applied for a period of 5–60 min, and peroperative angiography is performed to confirm the disappearance of the nidus. Thereafter, the AVM can be excised easily.

Stereotactic Obliteration

Riechert (1975) used a combined open and stereotactic method for deep angiomas to avoid functional deficit caused by resection of brain tissue and uncertainty in localisation of the angioma and its feeding vessels. In 18 patients with AVMs in the region of the basal ganglia and third ventricle, there was no immediate post-operative death. Late results were evaluated in 14 patients; eight returned to their occupation, one patient died 23 days after operation from fatal haemorrhage while waiting check angiogram, and another, $2\frac{1}{2}$ years later from bronchopneumonia.

Aneurysms of the Vein of Galen

In 1964 Gold et al. reviewed aneurysms of the vein of Galen in the world literature. Recently Hoffman et al. (1982) added 29 cases of their own to the literature. These aneurysms (Fig. 13.19) are common in boys. Depending upon the age of onset, and the symptoms and signs, they have been divided into three clinical syndromes (Gold et al. 1964).

1. *Neonatal*: The new-born presents with cyanosis and/or respiratory distress. There is

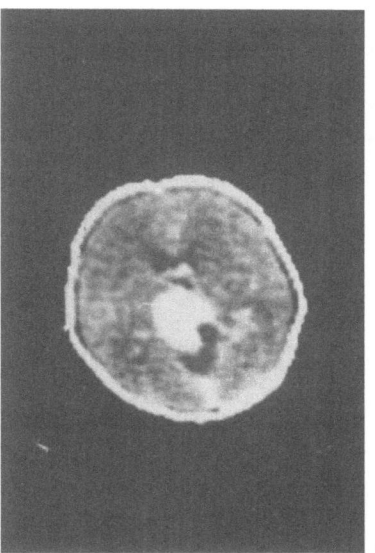 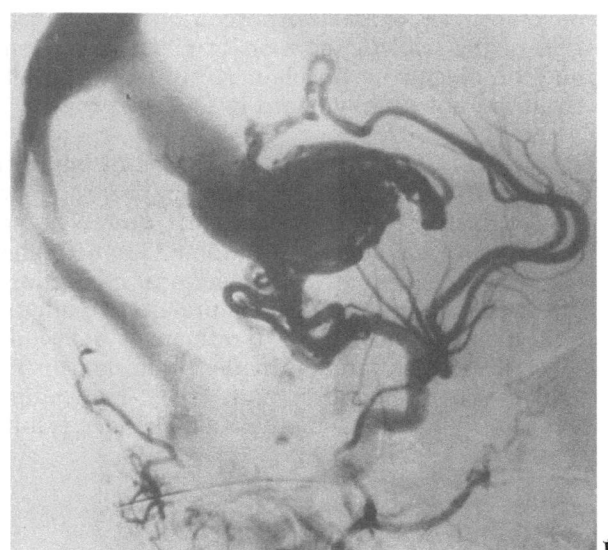

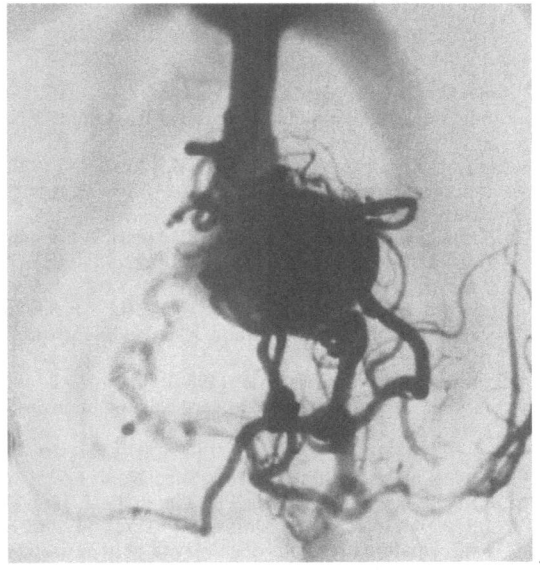

Fig. 13.19. a CT scan showing an enhancing mass at the posterior end of the third ventricle. Carotid angiogram (**b** lateral and **c** Townes projection) showing a typical aneurysm of the vein of Galen which is supplied by the anterior and posterior cerebral arteries.

evidence of congestive heart failure, often refractory to digitalis therapy. The syndrome is more common in males. Most cases die, due to cardiovascular decompensation. Other complications, such as marked hypoglycaemia and convulsions, also influence the prognosis.

2. *Infancy*: Hydrocephalus and/or convulsions are the usual presentations in this group. One should also look for other signs, such as psychomotor retardation, pyramidal involvement, cardiomegaly or proptosis, which may develop subsequently. The important diagnostic sign in this age group is an intracranial bruit.

3. *Older children and adults*: Headache or signs and symptoms of SAH may be the presenting features. Subsequently cerebellar signs may develop. The characteristic concentric calcification in the wall of the vein of Galen aneurysm may be diagnostic on plain X-rays of the skull. Bruit are not usually heard in this age group.

Prognosis. This depends on the age of onset of symptoms and the therapeutic approach. The prognosis is best in the older age group owing to the relatively small size of the shunt. In neonates the prognosis is poor. After surgical correction, hypervolaemia and cardiac failure are two important complications. Early treatment is advisable to prevent (a) infarction of the brain due to the "steal phenomenon" and (b) myocardial ischaemia due to haemodynamic changes (Hoffman et al. 1982).

References

Amacher AL, Allcock JM, Drake CG (1972) Cerebral angiomas: the sequelae of surgical treatment. J Neurosurg 37:571–575

Amojola MF, Fox AJ, Vinuela FV, Drake CG (1982) Spontaneous regression of intracranial AVMs. A report of three cases. J Neurosurg 57:818–822

Anderson FM, Korbin MA (1958) Arteriovenous malformations of the brain—a review and presentation of 37 cases. Neurology 8:89–101

Crawford JB, Russell DS (1956) Cryptic arteriovenous and venous hamartomas of brain. J Neurol Neurosurg Psychiatry 19:1–11

Cromwell LD, Harris AB (1980) Treatment of cerebral AVMs. A combined neurosurgical and neuroradiological approach. J Neurosurg 52:705–708

De Feo DR, Kusslu JA, Rush JL, Pribram H (1976) Aqueduct occlusion by midline AVMs. Surg Neurol 5:59–62

Deruty R, Lapras CL, Bret PH, Capdville J, Hor FR (1983) Intraoperative embolisation of cerebral arteriovenous malformation by means of a delayed polymerisation mixture (16 cases). Abstract from Proceedings of the 7th European Congress of Neurosurgery, Brussels, p 6

Drake CG (1979) Cerebral AVMs. Considerations for and experience with surgical treatment in 166 cases. Clin Neurosurg 26:145–208

Folkow B, Gurevich M, Hallbac Y, Lundren Y, Weiss L (1971) The haemodynamic consequences of regional hypotension in spontaneously hypotensive and normotensive rats. Acta Physiol Scand 83:532–541

Folkow B (1971) Haemodynamic consequences of adaptive structural changes of the resistance vessels in hypertension. Clin Sci 41:1–12

Forster DMC, Steiner L, Hakanson S (1972) Arteriovenous malformation of the brain. A long term clinical study. J Neurosurg 37:562–570

Gold AP, Ransahoff J, Carter S (1964) Vein of Galen malformation. Acta Neurol Scand 40 [Suppl 11]:1–31

Graf CJ, Perret GE, Torner JC (1983) Bleeding from cerebral AVM: As a part of their natural history. J Neurosurg 58:331–337

Guidetti B, Delitala A (1980) Intracranial AVMs. Conservative and surgical treatment. J Neurosurg 53:149–152

Handa H, Yoneda S, Matsuda M et al. (1977) The surgical treatment of deep seated or large AVMs of the brain with the aid of electrically induced thrombosis. In: Carrea R (ed) Abstracts of papers in Sixth International Congress of Neurological Surgery, Sao Paulo, June, 1977. Excerpta Medica No. 418, Amsterdam, p 2

Heiss WD, Kvicala V, Prosenz P et al. (1970) The importance of arterial shunting in areas of brain stem from an AVM (Abstr). Neurology 20:376

Heros RC (1982) Arteriovenous malformations of the medial temporal lobe. Surgical approach and neuroradiological characterisation. J Neurosurg 56:44–52

Hoffman HJ, Chuang S, Hendrick D, Humphreys RB (1982) Aneurysms of the vein of Galen. Experience at the Hospital for Sick Children, Toronto. J Neurosurg 57:316–322

Hook O, Johanson G (1958) Intracranial arteriovenous aneurysms. Follow-up study with particular attention to the growth. Arch Neurol Psychiatry 80:39–54

Johnson RT (1975) Radiotherapy of cerebral angiomas. With a note on some problems in diagnosis. In: Pia HW, Gleave JRW, Grote E, Zierski J (eds) Cerebral angiomas. Advances in diagnosis and therapy. Springer, Berlin Heidelberg New York, pp 256–259

Kelly DL Jr, Alexander EJ Jr, Davis CH Jr et al. (1969) Intracranial arteriovenous malformations. Clinical review and evaluation of brain scans. J Neurosurg 31:422–428

Kerber C (1980) Use of balloon catheters in the treatment of cranial arterial abnormalities. Stroke 11:210–216

Kjellberg RN (1983) Advances in neurosurgery. Harvard Medical School, Dept of Continuous Education

Kjellberg RN, Poletti CE, Adams RD (1977) Bragg Peak proton beam treatment of AVMs and certain brain tumours. Sixth international congress of neurological surgeons, Sao Paulo

Kjellberg RN, Davis KR, Lyons S, Butler W, Adams RD (1984) Bragg Peak proton beam therapy for arteriovenous malformations of the brain. In: (ed) Clinical neurosurgery. Williams and Wilkins, Baltimore London, pp 248–290

Luessenhop AJ (1975) Operative treatment of AVMs of the brain. In: Morley (DP (ed) Current controversies in neurosurgery. WB Saunders, Philadelphia London Toronto, pp 203–209

Luessenhop AJ, Presper JH (1975) Surgical embolisation of cerebral arteriovenous malformations through internal carotid and vertebral arteries. J Neurosurg 42:443–451

Luessenhop AJ, Spence WT (1960) Artificial embolisation of cerebral arteries. Report of use in a case of arteriovenous malformation. JAMA 172:1153–1155

Luessenhop AJ, Rosa L (1984) Cerebral arteriovenous malformations. Indications for and results of surgery and the role of intravascular techniques. J Neurosurg 60:14–22

Malik GM, Pearce JE, Ausman JI, Mehta B (1984) Dural arteriovenous malformations and intracranial haemorrhage. Neurosurgery 15:332–339

McCormick WF (1966) The pathology of vascular (arteriovenous) malformation. J Neurosurg 24:807–812

McCormick WF (1969) The pathology of vascular (arteriovenous) malfirmations, In: Sahs AL, Perret GE, Locksley HB, Nishioka H (eds) Intracranial aneurysm and subarachnoid haemorrhage. A Co-operative Study. JB Lippincott, Philadelphia Toronto, pp 194–199

McKenzie I (1953) The clinical presentation of cerebral angiomas. A review of 50 cases. Brain 76:184–214

Michelsen WJ (1979) Natural history and pathophysiology of AVMs. Clin Neurosurg 26:307–313

Moody RA, Poppen JL (1970) Arteriovenous malformations. J Neurosurg 32:503–508

Mullen S, Brown FD, Patronas NJ (1979) Hyperaemic and ischaemic problems of surgical treatment of AVMs. J Neurosurg 51:757–764

Nornes H, Grip A (1980) Haemodynamic aspects of cerebral AVMs. J Neurosurg 53:456–464

Nukiu H, Miyaji O, Tamada J et al. (1982) Longterm follow-up study of cerebral angiography in cases with AVM of the brain with special reference to spontaneous disappearance of AVMs in cerebral angiography. Neurol Med Chir 22:125–132

Olivecrona H, Riives J (1948) Arteriovenous aneurysms of the brain, their diagnosis and treatment. Arch Neurol Psychiatry 59:567–603

Olivecrona H, Ladenheim J (1957) Congenital arteriovenous aneurysms of the carotid and vertebral artery systems. Springer, Berlin Heidelberg New York

Parkinson D, Bachers G (1980) AVMs. Summary of 100 consecutive supratentorial cases. J Neurosurg 53:285–299

Paterson JH, McKissock W (1956) A clinical survey of intracranial angiomas with special reference to their modes of progression and surgical treatment. Report of 110 cases. Brain 79:233–266

Perret G, Nishioka H (1966) AVMs. An analysis of 545 cases of cranio-cerebral AVMs and fistulae. Report of the Co-operative Study. J Neurosurg 25:467–490

Pia HW (1975) The acute treatment of cerebral AVMs associated with haematomas. In: Pia HW, Gleave JRW, Grote E, Zierski J (eds) Cerebral angiomas—Advances in diagnosis and treatment. Springer, Berlin Heidelberg New York, pp 155–177

Pool JL (1972) AVMs of the brain. In: Vinken PG, Bruyn GW (eds) Handbook of clinical neurology. North Holland, Amsterdam, pp 227–266

Riechert T (1975) Stereotactic treatment of cerebral angiomas. In: Pia HW, Gleave JRW, Grote E, Zierski J (eds) Cerebral angiomas—Advances in diagnosis and treatment. Springer, Berlin Heidelberg New York, pp 129–135

Seeger W (1975) The artificial embolisation of inoperable angiomas. In: Pia HW, Gleave JRW, Grote E, Zierski J (eds) Cerebral angiomas—advances in diagnosis and treatment. Springer, Berlin Heidelberg New York, pp 213–221

Serbinenko FA (1974) Balloon catheterisation and occlusion of major cerebral vessels. J Neurosurg 41:125–145

Serbinenko FA (1979) Six hundred endovascular neurosurgical procedures in vascular pathology. A ten year experience, Acta Neurochir [Suppl] 28:310–311

Serbinenko FA (1983) The endovascular treatment of arteriovenous malformations in the brain. Abstract from Proceedings of the 7th European Congress of Neurosurgery, Brussels, p 6

Spetzler RF, Wilson CB, Weinsten B et al. (1978) Normal perfusion pressure break-through theory. Clin Neurosurg 25:671–672

Stein BM (1984) Arteriovenous malformations of medial hemisphere and the limbic system. J Neurosurg 60:23–31

Steiner L (1977) Radiosurgery in intracranial AVMs—technique. Sixth International Congress of Neurological Surgery, Sao Paulo. Excerpta Medica no. 148

Steiner L, Greitz T, Leksell L, Noren C, Rahn T et al. (1977) Radiosurgery in intracranial AVMs—a follow-up study. Sixth International Congress of Neurological Surgery, Sao Paulo. Excerpta Medica no. 148

Svien HJ, McRae JA (1965) Arteriovenous anomalies of the brain: fate of patients not having definitive surgery. J Neurosurg 23:23–28

Troupp H (1976) AVMs of the brain. What are the indications for operation? In: Morley TP (ed) Current controversies in neurosurgery. WB Saunders, Philadelphia London Toronto

Troupp H, Morttila I, Halonen V (1970) Arteriovenous malformations of the brain: Prognosis without operation. Acta Neurochir 22:125–128

Vinuela FV, Debrun GM, Fox AJ, Girvin JP, Peerless SJ (1983) Dominant hemisphere AVMs. Therapeutic embolisation with isobutyl-2-cyanoacrylate. Am J Neuroradiol 4:959–966

Walder HAD (1975a) Cryocoagulation of deep AVMs. In: Pia HW, Gleave JRW, Grote E, Zierski J (eds) Cerebral angiomas—advances in diagnosis and treatment. Springer, Berlin Heidelberg New York

Walder HAD (1975b) Freezing arteriovenous anomalies in the brain. In: Pia HW, Gleave JRW, Grote E, Zierski J (eds) Cerebral angiomas—advances in diagnosis and treatment. Springer, Berlin Heidelberg New York, pp 183–193

Waltimo O (1973a) The relationship of size, density and localisation of intracranial AVMs to the type of initial symptom. J Neurol Sci 19:13–19

Waltimo O (1973b) The change in size of intracranial arteriovenous malformations. J Neurol Sci 19:21–27

Wilson CB, Sang Ho, Domingo J (1979) Microsurgical treatment of intracranial vascular malformations. J Neurosurg 51:446–454

Wolpert SM, Stein BM (1979) Factors governing the cause of embolisation in the therapeutic embolisation of cerebral AVMs. Radiology 131:125–131

Yasargil MG, Jain KK, Antic J, Laciga R (1976a) AVMs of the splenium of the corpus callosum: Microsurgical treatment. Surg Neurol 5:5–14

Yasargil MG, Jain KK, Antic J, Laciga R, Kletter G (1976b) AVMs of the anterior and the middle portions of the corpus callosum: Microsurgical treatment. Surg Neurol 5:67–80

14 Subarachnoid Haemorrhage in Pregnancy

Introduction

Subarachnoid haemorrhage is an unusual event during pregnancy, labour or the puerperium. This association, however, is significant for several reasons.

1. Maternal mortality from non-obstetric causes, such as SAH, has attracted increasing attention in recent years, as mortality from obstetric causes has decreased considerably due to improved obstetric care (Hunt et al. 1974; Barno and Freeman 1976).

2. Subarachnoid haemorrhage is the most serious cerebrovascular complication of pregnancy and is often confused with eclampsia, since both conditions have certain clinical features in common (Cannell and Botterell 1956; Pedowitz and Perell 1957; Dimsdale 1962).

3. Since there is a considerable physiological change in the body, particularly of the cardiovascular system, during pregnancy, the occurrence of SAH at this period has aroused interest as to a possible causal relationship between the two events.

4. Management of pregnancy or SAH requires highly skilled knowledge on the part of a specialist working in an unrelated field of medicine, and an understanding of each field's problems. The routine management of either condition requires to be altered, not only for the safety of the mother but also for the well-being of the foetus.

5. Finally, since the association of these two events is rare, any team of neurosurgeons or obstetricians is unlikely to come across more than a few cases in their working life. Therefore, clear guidance on the subject is helpful.

Incidence

The Department of Health and Social Security (1982) reported that 5.6% of maternal deaths between 1976 and 1978 in England and Wales were attributable to spontaneous intracranial haemorrhage, excluding those from cerebral haemorrhage associated with hypertensive diseases of pregnancy. The incidence is estimated to be one in 2000 deliveries (Cannell 1959; Copelan and Mabon 1962). However, the accuracy of any estimate is influenced by a number of factors, including the interest of the neurosurgical staff in such cases, the vascular problems involved and the obstetrician's awareness of this condition, as it can easily be mistaken for eclampsia. According to many workers, pregnancy per se has no effect on the incidence of SAH (Walton 1953; Cannell 1959; Barno and Freeman 1976), but labour may increase the risk (Barno and Freeman 1976).

Robinson et al. (1974) found arteriovenous malformations (AVMs) as a source of SAH in the younger age group. In a study of SAH during pregnancy, Amias (1970) found a preponderance

Table 14.1. Profile of the cases of SAH

Patient	Age	Stage of pregnancy	Cause of SAH	Treatment and outcome[a]
S.D.	25	16 weeks	AVM	Was treated conservatively. Delivered by Caesarean section. Rebled 4 years later and underwent operation. Was given prophylactic phenobarbital.
B.S.	34	31 weeks	AVM	Delivered immediately by Caesarean section. Underwent excision of AVM. Improved gradually, but had ataxia and nystagmus. Underwent second operation to remove residual AVM. Improved markedly.
A.S.	15	26 weeks	AVM	Underwent excision of AVM. Continued pregnancy to term. Delivered by Caesarean section. Was given prophylactic anticonvulsant. Had no focal neurological signs when last seen.
J.M. *1st SAH*	25	2nd trimester	AVM	Had pre-eclampsia and underwent Caesarean section and tubal ligation at 36 weeks. Resumed normal activities, but had intermittent occipital headaches.
2nd SAH	31	Not pregnant	AVM	Underwent excision of AVM. Was given prophylactic anticonvulsant. Was asymptomatic when last seen.
S.R.[b]	18	16 weeks	AVM	Underwent excision of AVM. Had physiotherapy and speech therapy. Continued with pregnancy. Was given prophylactic anticonvulsant. Had residual impairment of position sense in right arm.
S.C.	30	38 weeks	2 aneurysms	Was given aminocaproic acid. Delivered by Caesarean section. One week later both aneurysms were clipped. Was treated with isoprenaline and lignocaine for postoperative left hemiparesis. Was asymptomatic when last seen.
L.F.	26	36 weeks	Aneurysm	Went into labour and delivered by Caesarean section. *First operation:* Aneurysm ruptured prematurely; procedure abandoned. VP shunt installed to treat hydrocephalus. *Second operation:* Aneurysm clipped successfully. Had postoperative infection of abdominal wound; otherwise recovery was uneventful. Was given prophylactic anticonvulsant. Was fully alert and without focal neurological signs at discharge.
L.E. *1st SAH*	34	27 weeks	AVM	SAH with large intracerebral haematoma. Angiogram showed a large basal ganglia AVM fed by middle cerebral and lenticulostriate arteries. AVM felt to be inoperable and patient made a good recovery.
2nd SAH	36	Not pregnant	AVM	Patient readmitted with massive SAH. CT showed a large left intracerebral haematoma with rupture into the ventricular system. Patient's condition was critical and the haematoma was evacuated and AVM excised. Patient died soon after surgery.
A.S.	31	SAH 6 h after delivery	?Thrombosed cryptic AVM	Normal delivery of twins followed by dense left hemiplegia and left homonymous hemianopia. There was no loss of consciousness. CT showed a large right posterior parietal haematoma. Angiography was normal. The haematoma was evacuated and the patient's neurological condition improved markedly. On discharge her only complaint was difficulty in focussing, probably related to resolving papilloedema.
L.B. *1st SAH*	24	12 weeks	—	Unconscious 3 h, dense left homonymous hemianopia. CT showed temporo-parietal haematoma. Bilateral carotid angiogram normal. Haematoma evacuated and patient made a good postoperative recovery.
2nd SAH	25	6 months	AVM	Recurrent SAH. CT showed a right temporal haematoma. Repeat bilateral carotid angiogram was again normal but vertebral angiogram showed a small AVM in the right postero-temporal region. Delivered normal baby at 38 weeks by caesarian section. AVM successfully excised (12/3/84). Postoperative course uneventful. No neurological deficit apart from residual left homonymous hemianopia.

Continued on opposite page

Table 14.1. (*continued*)

Patient	Age	Stage of Pregnancy	Cause of SAH	Treatment and outcome
L.O.	25	12 weeks	Aneurysm	ICA bifurcation aneurysm successfully clipped. Good post-operative recovery. Plan is to continue pregnancy to term and carry out a normal delivery.

ᵃ All infants were healthy at birth.
ᵇ This patient had had an abortion several months previously.

of primigravida in the group with aneurysms, whereas Robinson et al. (1972) and Minielly et al. (1979) found no relation between cause of SAH and parity.

We have personal experience of 11 cases of SAH during pregnancy. The source of the haemorrhage was an AVM in eight cases and an aneurysm in three. Eight were primigravida at the time of the first haemorrhage. The mean age was 25.7 years for patients with AVM and 27 years for patients with aneurysmal SAH (Table 14.1).

Cause

Secondary subarachnoid bleeding associated with pre-eclampsia and eclampsia is well known. Subarachnoid haemorrhage in pregnancy is equally likely to be due to an aneurysm or AVM. Other rarer causes of SAH in pregnancy are outlined in Table 14.2.

Time of Occurrence

It appears that the time of occurrence of SAH varies with the basic underlying cause. Arteriove-

Table 14.2. Rarer causes of spontaneous SAH in pregnancy (modified from Donaldson 1978)

Haematological disorders (e.g. anticoagulants, leukaemia, thrombocytopenia, disseminated intravascular coagulation)
Subacute bacterial endocarditis (mycotic aneurysm)
Metastatic choriocarcinoma
Vasculitis
Eclampsia
  Early—hypertensive intracerebral haematomas
  Late—cerebral infarction and multiple petechial haemorrhages
Cerebral venous thrombosis
Spinal SAH—AVMs, aneurysms, ectopic endometriosis

nous malformations may bleed at any time during pregnancy, though there are two peak periods of increased incidence, one at 16–20 weeks and the other at 30–40 weeks. With aneurysms, the incidence of haemorrhage rises steadily during pregnancy. Cannell (1959) found that aneurysmal rupture was equally distributed in the first and second halves of pregnancy. Copelan and Mabon (1962), Robinson et al. (1972) and Hunt et al. (1974) found the majority of SAHs occurred in the third trimester.

Course of Haemorrhage

Cannell (1959) and Copelan and Mabon (1962) reported that with untreated ruptured aneurysms the maternal death rate is at least 50%. Robinson et al. (1972) found a similar risk (46%) in cases of recurrent haemorrhage from conservatively treated aneurysms. Robinson et al. (1972) found that a patient with AVM who never becomes pregnant has a 10% risk of sustaining SAH. However, if such a woman does become pregnant, the chances of haemorrhage at some time increase to 87%. If SAH due to an AVM occurs during pregnancy, the risk of recurrent haemorrhage during the same pregnancy is estimated to be 27%. Recurrent haemorrhage from sources other than an aneurysm or AVM is extremely unusual.

Physiological Changes During Pregnancy Relevant to Subarachnoid Haemorrhage

The cardiovascular stresses of pregnancy have been incriminated as factors that could cause a vascular lesion, such as an AVM or aneurysm, to bleed.

Cardiac output increases by about 30%–60% in the first trimester, reaching a peak at the twelfth week which is maintained until term (Kerr 1968).

In the first stage of labour, in association with uterine contractions there is a rise in cardiac output accompanied by some rise in arterial pressure (Hansen and Ueland 1966).

The cooperative study found that at least one-third of SAHs due to an AVM occurred during activities involving bearing down. It seems likely that the vigorous valsalva manoeuvre during delivery could produce rupture of an aneurysm or AVM. The exact relationship of an SAH to such a Valsalva manoeuvre has not been documented, but it seems likely that it would occur after release of straining, when a sudden thrust of blood at high pressure could rupture an enlarged or weakened vessel (Donaldson 1978). "Bearing down" can be prevented by keeping the glottis open, e.g. by panting exercises, which are often taught in antepartum classes. Lumbar epidural anaesthesia will also have the same effect.

Immediately after delivery, a rise in cardiac output, related to the administration of oxytocic drugs, may occur. Robinson et al. (1974) have shown that the peak incidence for SAH due to a ruptured AVM corresponds with times of greatest change in cardiac output, e.g. the first 12 weeks of pregnancy, during labour and delivery. However, the peak time of SAH due to aneurysm rupture is at 30–40 weeks, and in the post-partum period from 2 days to 6 weeks; thus it does not correspond with the times of greatest change in cardiac output.

It is not clear why AVMs should rupture during the second trimester. There could be a hormonal factor, with increased circulating oestrogens and progesterones causing dilatation of the abnormal vessels and feeding arteries, with constriction of the draining vessels (Newman 1958). Thus, flow through the AVMs may increase at a time when resistance in draining vessels also increases, contributing to the rupture of the AVM. Donaldson believes, on indirect grounds, that one can reasonably assume that either AVMs enlarge or shunting increases during pregnancy. He cites two facts to support this. Firstly, vascular tumours, such as meningiomas or skin and gum tumours, enlarge during pregnancy. Secondly, an inference can be drawn from the vascular spider naevi which appear in the majority of caucasian women during early pregnancy, and which increase in number and size throughout pregnancy and fade away within days after delivery.

Diagnosis

The outcome of SAH depends on the appropriate management of the source of the haemorrhage. Hence, it is essential to confirm the diagnosis and the underlying cause. Symptoms of SAH due to aneurysmal rupture are similar to those in non-pregnant patients, e.g. severe headache, vomiting, loss of consciousness or seizures. The presence and severity of meningeal and other neurological signs depend on the site and extent of the haemorrhage. Robinson et al. (1972) identified certain features that distinguish between the rupture of an AVM and an aneurysm in a pregnant woman. If the patient is multiparous, over 30 years old and in the third trimester, the source of haemorrhage is usually an aneurysm. Rupture of an AVM is more common in younger primigravida. Bleeding tends to occur in early pregnancy or during labour and puerperium.

The diagnosis of pre-eclampsia is made by the coincidence of certain physical signs detected after the 20th week of pregnancy. A blood pressure in excess of 140/90 mmHg or a rise of 20 units in the diastolic value is commonly the earliest manifestation. Overt oedema or excessive weight gain may develop due to fluid retention. The subsequent development of more infective proteinuria indicates a severe disease, even when the blood pressure is only moderately elevated. Symptoms such as headache, photophobia and epigastric pain signal imminent eclampsia. The whole progression may develop slowly or very rapidly within 24 h, and post-partum eclampsia is common. Kirby and Jaindyl (1984) report two cases of eclampsia in which CT showed diffuse cerebral oedema and basal ganglia involvement. Rare causes of spontaneous SAH, such as are outlined in Table 14.2, should be excluded before a definitive investigation, e.g. angiography, is carried out. Haematological disorders as a cause of SAH can be excluded by routinely estimating the haemogloblin, platelet count and partial thromboplastin time. Fatal SAH has been reported in association with disseminated intravascular coagulation (Heron et al. 1974), and is a well recognised complication of anticoagulant therapy (Weigle 1955; Hirsh et al. 1972).

In patients with subacute bacterial endocarditis with haemorrhage from a mycotic aneurysm, there is usually evidence of cardiac disease and other stigmata, such as splinter haemorrhages, splenic enlargement and microscopic haematuria.

Choriocarcinoma may present as an intracranial haemorrhage either during or after normal pregnancy (including spontaneous abortion) or molar pregnancy.

Cerebral venous thrombosis may present like an SAH. It commonly occurs during the puerperium, when it may present as an unexplained puerperal pyrexia. It may also occur in early pregnancy. Whilst the diagnosis can be suspected clinically, angiography or digital subtraction angiography is usually the definitive diagnostic test.

In spinal SAH there is usually sudden onset of back pain followed by headache and neck stiffness. Lombardo et al. (1968) reported a case of SAH due to ectopic endometrioma of the cauda equina, while Garcia et al. (1979) described a case of spinal SAH during pregnancy due to rupture of an aneurysm of the artery of Adamkiewicz.

In patients with suspected SAH lumbar puncture is essential to confirm the diagnosis unless there is evidence of a life-threatening space-occupying haematoma. CT scanning is often helpful in elucidating the size of the haemorrhage and its probable aetiology. If CT is non-contributory, angiography alone may help in the final diagnosis. The value of lumbar puncture and CT scanning in a pregnant woman with unexplained seizures and severe headache cannot be overemphasised.

Angiography is performed early, usually during normal working hours and within 24 hours of admission. It may be carried out under local anaesthesia, using the new non-ionic water-soluble contrast media (iopamidol or iohexol). Additional lead screening to protect the foetus is used. On the basis of the CT scan findings, limited angiography should be carried out to identify the source of haemorrhage. If CT scan is non-contributory, bilateral carotid angiography is done initially, and if this is negative vertebral angiography is also carried out. Pregnant patients with SAH are more likely than the average non-pregnant patient to have a demonstrable lesion, with AVMs and aneurysms occurring about equally. Robinson et al. (1972) reported that angiography was positive in 93% of cases. In the present series angiography showed a vascular cause for the SAH in 91% of cases.

Treatment

The natural history of spontaneous SAH in pregnancy suggests that the appropriate management is dictated by the underlying source of the haemorrhage. Since rupture of an intracranial aneurysm in pregnancy leads to fatal recurrent bleeding, prompt diagnosis and surgical treatment should be carried out as for the non-pregnant patient. On the other hand, detection of an AVM does not require prompt surgical intervention unless there is a life-threatening haematoma, since recurrent haemorrhage during that pregnancy is rare. The well-being of the foetus requires to be constantly borne in mind during investigation and surgical treatment.

Neurosurgical Management

The patient should be admitted to a neurosurgical ward and the obstetric team should be consulted forthwith. Early investigation with angiography is necessary once the possibility of eclampsia or other rarer causes of SAH has been excluded. Further treatment will depend on the source of haemorrhage.

Intracranial Aneurysms

Since the incidence of recurrent haemorrhage is high, early surgical intervention is mandatory. It should, however, be remembered that induced hypotension (Cannell 1959; Robinson et al. 1972; Pool 1965) and osmotic diuretics (Wilson and Sedzimir 1959) may have a deleterious effect on the foetus. The planning of surgical treatment should aim for short uncomplicated surgery. Obliteration of the aneurysm from the circulation remains the, ideal goal. However, if this appears to be impossible in certain difficult aneurysms, such as those in the carotid–ophthalmic area, lesser surgical therapy, such as carotid ligation, may be advisable.

S. C., a 30-year-old housewife, experienced sudden onset of headache and vomiting on 9 June 1975. She was in the 38th week of her first pregnancy. She later developed neck stiffness and was admitted to the local hospital, where a lumbar puncture revealed uniformly blood-stained CSF. She was transferred to the maternity ward of the hospital. On examination, there were no focal neurological signs other than neck stiffness. Bilateral carotid angiography revealed an aneurysm on the anterior communicating artery and another on the proximal segment of the right middle cerebral artery near the origin of the lenticulostriate vessels. There was no evidence of spasm (Fig. 14.1). The patient was put on ε-aminocaproic acid (Epsikapron) 3 g at 3-hourly

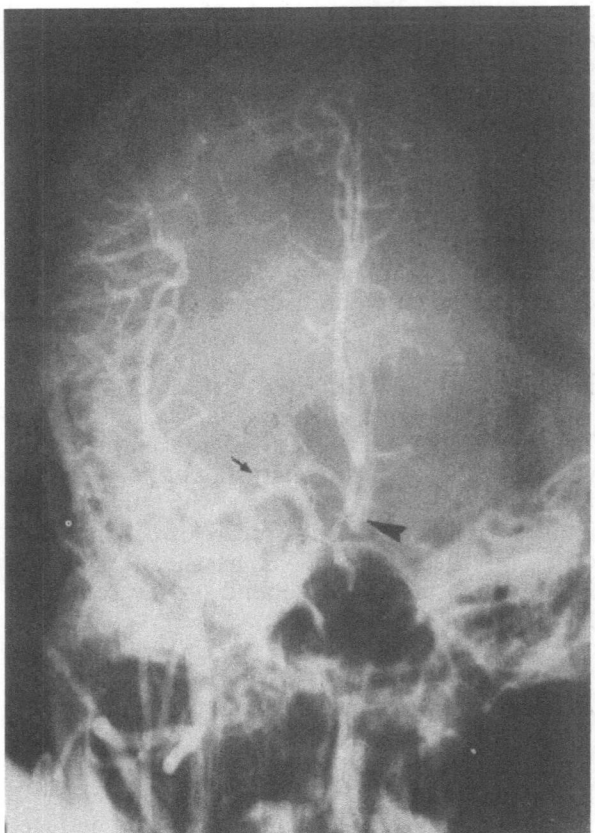

Fig. 14.1. Right carotid angiogram showing anterior communicating artery aneurysm (*arrowhead*) and a small aneurysm (*arrow*) arising from the M_1 segment of the right middle cerebral artery, near the lenticulostriate vessels.

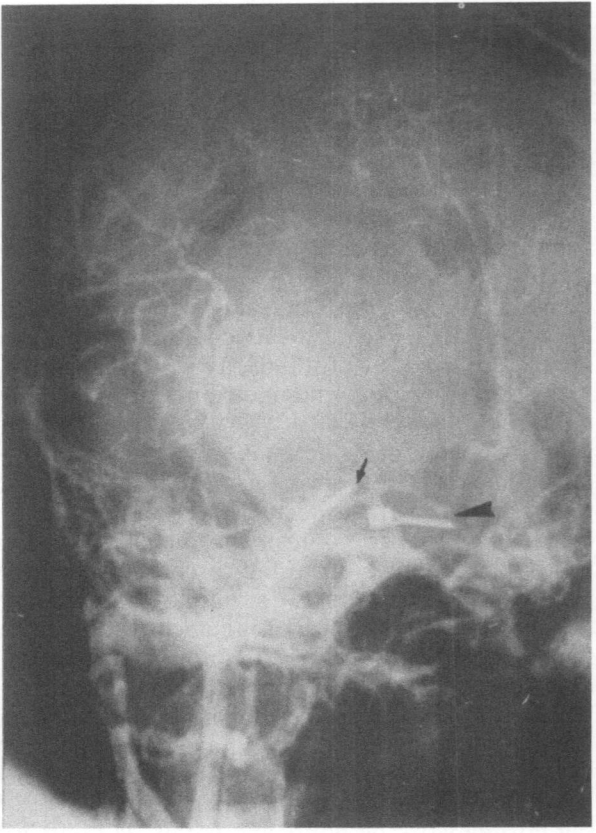

Fig. 14.2. Postoperative right carotid angiogram shows that the anterior cerebral artery and the middle cerebral artery aneurysms have been successfully clipped.

Arteriovenous Malformations

If an AVM appears to be the source of SAH, there is no indication for immediate surgery until the pregnancy is completed at full term. A large haematoma associated with an AVM should, however, be removed and the AVM excised.

When no source of SAH is revealed by complete angiographic investigation, the patient is treated with routine medical care.

S. R., an 18-year-old student, collapsed at a party on the night of 30 December 1980. She felt as if she was "about to have a brain haemorrhage", and walked into the toilet but did not return. She had to be helped out by her boyfriend and was not able to talk or walk unaided. The right side of the body felt weak, and there was asymmetry of the right side of the face. When seen at a nearby hospital she was conscious with no neck stiffness. There was a persistent right visual field defect and fluctuating right hemiparesis. She had no history of previous headache

intervals, and elective Caesarean section was carried out on 13 June 1975. A healthy boy was delivered. The patient was transferred to the neurosurgical ward on 18 June, where, on examination, she had no focal neurosurgical sign and blood pressure was 130/90 mmHg. On 20 June 1975, a right frontotemporal craniotomy was performed, and both aneurysms were clipped successfully. The patient was well in the immediate postoperative period. Three days later she developed left hemiparesis and was put on isoprenaline and lignocaine infusion, after which there was gradual improvement in her neurological deficit and the hemiparesis completely resolved within 2 days. Repeat angiography a week later showed satisfactory clipping of both aneurysms (Fig. 14.2).

or migraine. The patient had been amenorrheal for 4 months, and had an abortion several months earlier. She was transferred to the neurosurgical unit for further management. On examination, the patient was conscious and cooperative. She had expressive dysphasia, right temporal hemianopia, right facial palsy, right hemiparesis, grade 0 in the arm and grade 1–2 in the leg, and right sensory loss. There was no neck stiffness and fundi were normal. All reflexes on the right side were brisk. The right plantar was extensor. Blood pressure was 120/80 mmHg. Cardiovascular and respiratory systems were normal. CT scan showed a left temporal haematoma (Fig. 14.3) and angiography revealed a small AVM, with its main supply from the left middle cerebral branches and a mass effect (Fig. 14.4). On 2 January 1981, a left frontotemporal craniotomy with excision of the AVM and evacuation of the haematoma was performed. Postoperatively, the right hemiparesis and dysphasia improved with intensive physiotherapy and speech therapy. She was seen in consultation with an obstetrician, and it was decided to continue with the pregnancy. By May 1981 there was marked improvement in her speech and grade 4 power in the right upper and lower limbs. There was impairment of position

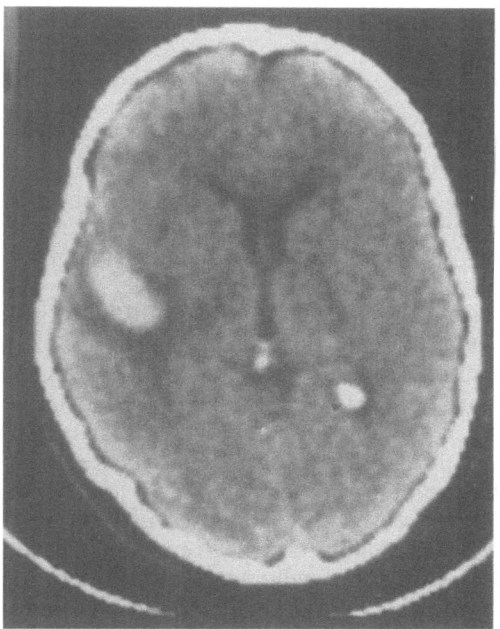

Fig. 14.3. CT scan showing left temporal haematoma.

sense in the right upper limb. She has been on phenytoin 100 mg three times daily prophylactically. She was delivered of a healthy male at full-term spontaneously.

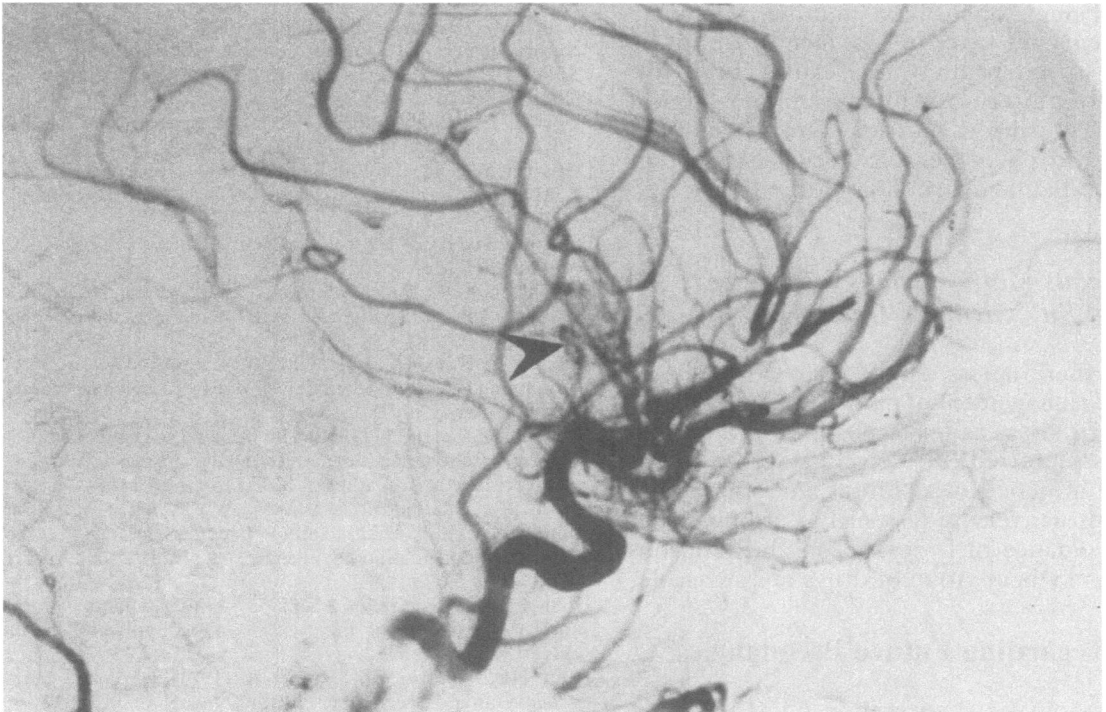

Fig. 14.4. Left carotid angiogram showing a small left temporal AVM (*arrowhead*) with the main feeding vessels from the middle cerebral artery.

Obstetric Management

Obstetric management largely depends on the time of SAH and the effectiveness of surgical management. Though Caesarean section offers no special advantage, and haemorrhage can occur even during this procedure, 6 of the 11 patients described in this report underwent Caesarean section before the haemorrhage was treated.

Hansen and Ueland (1966) found a steady increase in cardiac output as labour progressed in patients receiving only narcotic and local anaesthetics for delivery. In patients with caudal analgesics, no significant change in cardiac output was noted until post-partum, when it was 60% above the prelabour value.

Ergotamine elevates blood pressure and is a serious threat in patients with pre-eclampsia and in patients with SAH who have not undergone operation. Syntocinon is preferable for the management of the third stage in such cases. Blood pressure should be monitored and controlled with suitable doses of chlorpromazine.

Intracranial Aneurysms

If an aneurysm is treated successfully, the obstetric management should be as routine. If rupture of an aneurysm takes place near term, it is advisable to carry out Caesarean section, followed shortly afterwards by appropriate surgical treatment of the aneurysm. If a ruptured aneurysm proved inoperable during early pregnancy, therapeutic abortion is justified.

Arteriovenous Malformations and Other Sources of Subarachnoid Haemorrhage

Although there is less risk of recurrent haemorrhage, the management of delivery should aim for reduction of stress as far as possible. If a vaginal delivery is preferred, the second stage of labour should be modified by epidural anaesthesia and low forceps delivery to lessen the cardiovascular stress. Avoidance of hypertension and judicious use of the oxytocin group of drugs are advisable.

Advice Regarding Future Pregnancies

If the symptomatic aneurysm or AVM has been removed from the circulation, additional pregnancies pose no risk of SAH. If, however, a

ruptured aneurysm proved inoperable, another pregnancy should be avoided. The incidence of rebleed from an AVM is also significant as three of the AVMs which were not operated on for different reasons bled again—one after 2 years (patient died), one after 4 years and one after 6 years—though not in relation to pregnancy. A further patient had a rebleed during the same pregnancy. Obstetricians should be informed of the patient's neurological history so that appropriate care can be taken to avoid physical and psychological stress during labour. The patient and her practitioner are informed directly of the precise implications for the patient of a subsequent pregnancy. Decisions regarding sterilisation should be considered on obstetric rather than neurosurgical grounds (Amias 1970), or when an inoperable aneurysm is present (Pool 1965).

References

Amias AG (1970) Cerebral vascular disease in pregnancy. 1. Haemorrhage. J Obstet Gynaecol Br Comm 77:100–120
Barno A, Freeman SW (1976) Maternal deaths due to spontaneous subarachnoid haemorrhage. Am J Obstet Gynecol 125:384–392
Cannell MB, Botterell EH (1956) Subarachnoid haemorrhage in pregnancy. Am J Obstet Gynaecol 72:844–855
Cannell DE (1959) Subarachnoid haemorrhage in pregnancy. Proc R Soc Med 52:950–954
Copelan EL, Mabon RF (1962) Spontaneous intracranial bleeding in pregnancy. Obstet Gynecol 20:373–378
Department of Health and Social Security Report on Health and Social Subjects, No. 26. (1982) H.M.S.O. London, p 122
Dimsdale H (1962) Neurological emergencies in pregnancy. Proc R Soc Med 55:571–575
Donaldson JO (1978) Neurology in pregnancy. Cerebrovascular disease, Chap. 7. W.B. Saunders, Philadephia London Toronto
Garcia CA, Dulcey S, Dulcey J (1979) Ruptured aneurysm of the spinal artery of Adamkiewicz during pregnancy. Neurology 29:394–398
Hansen JM, Ueland K (1966) The influence of caudal analgesia on cardiovascular dynamics during normal labour and delivery. Acta Anaesthesiol Scand [Suppl] 23:449–452
Heron JR, Hutchinson EC, Boyd WN, Aber GM (1974) Pregnancy and subarachnoid haemorrhage and intravascular coagulation syndrome. J Neurol Neurosurg Psychiatry 37:521–525
Hirsh J, Cade JF, Gallus AS (1972) Anticoagulants in pregnancy—a review of indications and complications. Am Heart J 83:301–305
Hunt HB, Schifrin BS, Suzuki K (1974) Ruptured berry aneurysm and pregnancy. Obstet Gynecol 43:827–837
Kerr MG (1968) Cardiovascular dynamics in pregnancy and labour. Br Med Bull 24:19–24
Kirby JC, Jaindyl (1984) Cerebral CT findings in toxaemia of

pregnancy. Radiology 151:114

Lombardo L, Mateos JH, Barroeta FF (1968) Subarachnoid haemorrhage due to endometriosis of the spinal canal. Neurology 18:423–428

Minielly R, Yuzpe AA, Drake CG (1979) Subarachnoid haemorrhage secondary to ruptured cerebral aneurysm in pregnancy. Obstet Gynecol 53:64–70

Newman MJD (1958) Spinal angioma with symptoms in pregnancy. J Neurol Neurosurg Psychiatry 21:38–41

Pedowitz P, Perell A (1957) Aneurysms complicated by pregnancy. Part II. Aneurysms of the cerebral blood vessels. Am J Obstet Gynecol 73:736–749

Pool L (1965) Treatment of intracranial aneurysms during pregnancy. JAMA 192:209–214

Robinson JL, Hall CJ, Sedzimir CB (1972) Subarachnoid haemorrhage in pregnancy. J Neurosurg 36:27–33

Robinson JL, Hall CS, Sedzimir CB (1974) Arterio-venous malformations, aneurysms and pregnancy. J Neurosurg 41:63–70

Walton JN (1953) Subarachnoid haemorrhage in pregnancy. Br Med J I:869–871

Weigle EH (1955) Pregnancy complicated by subarachnoid haemorrhage following anticoagulant therapy of subacute bacterial endocarditis. Am J Obstet Gynecol 69:888–891

Wilson F, Sedzimir CB (1959) Hypothermia and hypotension during craniotomy in a pregnant woman. Lancet II:947–949

15 Subarachnoid Haemorrhage in Infancy, Childhood and Adolescence

Introduction

Hare, in 1849, first reported an adolescent with SAH due to a ruptured posterior communicating artery aneurysm (McDonald and Korb 1939). In 1871 Eppinger described a 15-year-old boy who collapsed at gymnastics and died 3 days later. At autopsy a ruptured anterior cerebral artery aneurysm was found, associated with coarctation of the aorta. Subarachnoid haemorrhage is an uncommon but well documented disease in childhood and adolescence: Only 2.7% of all cases of SAH occur in patients under 20 years of age (Locksley 1966)

The aetiology of SAH in childhood and adolescence is similar to that in the adult population, but a separate study in this age group is justified for several reasons. Firstly, there is a different incidence of specific pathologies producing SAH. In children, one-third of cases will be due to a bleeding arteriovenous malformation, one-third to a ruptured aneurysm, and in one-third no cause will be found (Laitinen 1964; Locksley 1966; Sedzimir and Robinson 1973).

Secondly, childhood aneurysms differ in several important respects from those in the adult population. Aneurysms in childhood are usually symptomatic, and few, if any, are discovered at routine angiography (Thompson et al. 1973) or autopsy (Housepian and Pool 1958; McCormick 1971). In addition, aneurysms often show unusual features, e.g. a different location on the circle of Willis compared with those in adults, a tendency to be larger and more peripherally located, and a reduced tendency to be multiple. These differences may reflect a different pathogenesis and encourage a new look at the pathogenesis of aneurysm formation. In a large proportion of children no cause for the SAH may be found. Cryptic malformations are more commonly seen at autopsy in children than in adults. This would suggest that they may play an important role in producing intracranial or subarachnoid haemorrhage in this age group.

Finally, since the surgical mortality and morbidity in this age group tends to be low (Richardson 1979), prompt diagnosis and treatment is vitally important.

Material

We have included in the childhood and adolescent age group, patients who are 20 years of age or less. In the period 1960–1983 there were 167

Some material from this chapter was used in Hourihan, Gates and McAllister (1984) J Neurosurg 60:1163–1166 cases of proven SAH. This does not include SAH in the neonatal period, which will be discussed separately at the end of this chapter.

Cause

The aetiology of SAH in this series is outlined in Table 15.1 and compared with that in other series in Table 15.2.

Subarachnoid haemorrhage was due to an aneurysm in approximately 52.1% and an AVM in 26.3% of cases. In 19.2% of cases no cause for the bleed was found on four vessel angiography. This contrasts strikingly with our experience in the adult population, where an aneurysm was demonstrated in 73.4% of cases, and an AVM in only 6.4% of cases (see Chap. 5).

Comparison of this series with earlier studies shows an increase in the number of cases due to an aneurysm and a decrease in the number of cases in which no lesion is found. Recent improvements in angiographic technique and their more widespread utilisation in children probably account for the greater incidence of vascular lesions in recent series.

Aneurysms

Aetiology

The aetiology of saccular aneurysms is discussed in Chap. 3. For a condition thought to be congenital in origin, it is rather surprising that it is rare for aneurysms either to rupture or to be found as an incidental finding at cerebral angiography or autopsy in childhood. Stehbens (1975) argues for a purely degenerative pathogenesis for cerebral aneurysms, but this would hardly apply in aneurysms of infancy and childhood, where it is rare to find histological evidence of either inflammation or atheroma. Bremer (1943) and Padget (1948) have postulated that saccular aneurysms arise from enlarged stumps of vestigeal vessels of the foetal cerebrovascular network.

Lipper et al. (1979) have suggested a possible difference in the pathogenesis between childhood aneurysms and those in adults. An unusually large, congenital, medial defect may be the initiating factor in children, whereas degenerative and haemodynamic factors, with or without an underlying medial defect, may be the basis for the increasing frequency of aneurysms with age. In addition, in the under 5 year age group, aneurysms, as mentioned previously, showed some unusual features compared with the adult population. This perhaps suggests that a different pathogenesis underlies aneurysms in the paediatric age group.

Presentation

Aneurysms in infancy and childhood usually present with an intracerebral haemorrhage. A review of the literature reveals only one aneurysm discovered before rupture, a case presenting with diabetes insipidus (Shucart and Wolpert 1972). In the period 1960–1983 we found only one case of an aneurysm presenting clinically but without an SAH. This was a female patient of 18 years who

Table 15.1 Subarachnoid haemorrhage—1960-1983 (167 cases)

	No.	%
Aneurysm	87	52.1
Arteriovenous malformation	44	26.3
No cause	32	19.2
Other causes	4	2.4
Tumour	2	
Hypertension in association with coarctation	1	
Moya Moya disease	1	

Table 15.2. Aetiology of SAH (0–20 years) (%)

		No.	Aneurysm	AVM	No lesion
Laitinen	(1964)	59	35.5	20.3	44
Locksley	(1966)	128	32	31.2	36.7
Sedzimir and Robinson	(1973)	124	40.4	26.6	25.8
Unpublished Newcastle series	(1983)	167	52.1	26.3	19.2

had a left posterior communicating artery aneurysm that presented with a third nerve palsy, although there was no evidence of SAH at surgery. Subsequent to this survey we have seen two further cases: (1) A 15-year-old male presented with epilepsy while watching television. Plain skull X-rays showed curvilinear calcification in the right temporal region. Angiography showed a middle cerebral artery aneurysm. At operation there was no evidence of haemorrhage. The aneurysm was successfully clipped and the epilepsy has been controlled. (2) A 15-year-old female with a giant right parasellar aneurysm presented with headaches and progressive swelling of the right eye. On examination there was a right sixth nerve palsy, a partial right third nerve palsy, absent right corneal reflex and absent fine touch and pin prick in the right fifth nerve first and second distribution. CT showed a right parasellar ring enhancing lesion suggesting an aneurysm. A right carotid angiogram showed a 2 cm right internal carotid ophthalmic aneurysm (largely thrombosed) with mass effect displacing the internal carotid artery medially. An EC/IC anastomosis followed by right carotid ligation was carried out with good results.

The most frequent presentation of SAH in childhood and adolescence, like in adults, is a sudden onset of severe headache with nausea and vomiting, which may or may not be associated with an impairment of conscious state. In infants, coma and hemiparesis are more common presenting features (Becker et al. 1978). In children a history of head injury can confuse the clinical picture and lead to a delay in diagnosis. Differentiation from head injury or meningitis may be aided by the use of CT scanning.

Age at Rupture

Aneurysms most commonly ruptured during the second decade. Review of the literature shows that in the first decade the peak incidence of presentation is in the under 2 year age group. In this series, only three cases presented in the first decade, the youngest patient being 6 years of age. The age distribution at presentation of 87 aneurysm cases is shown in Fig. 15.1.

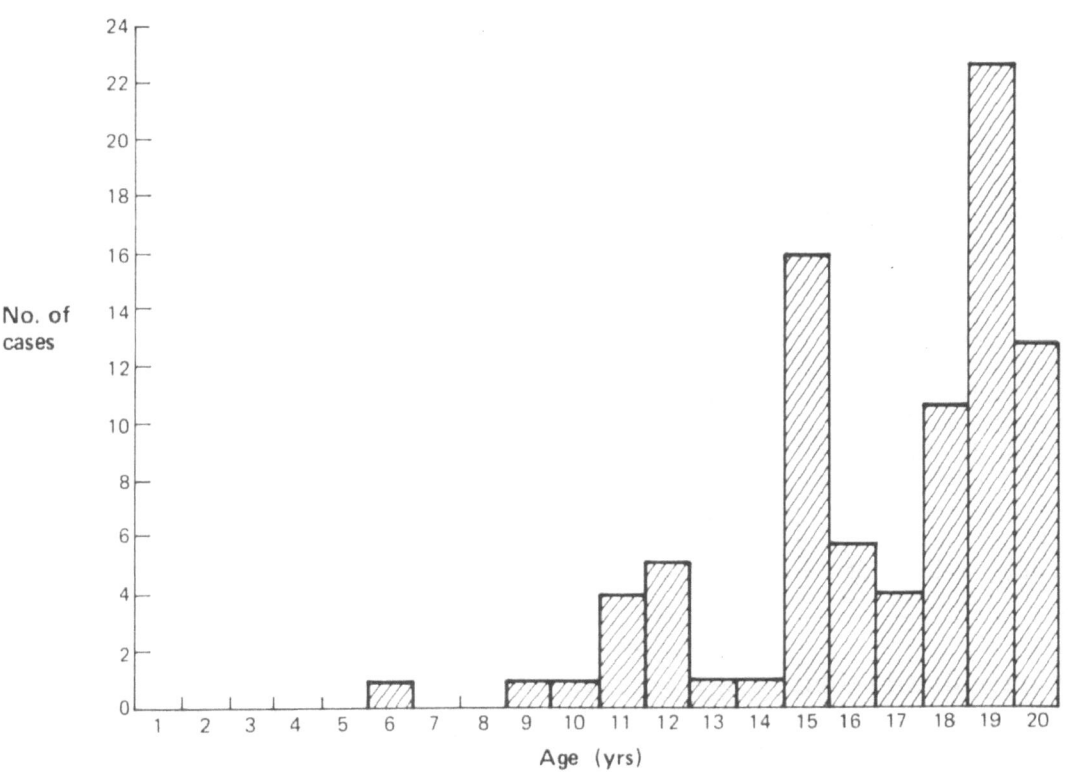

Fig. 15.1. Age of presentation in SAH due to ruptured aneurysms (87 cases).

Location

The location of aneurysms is shown in Table 15.3. In the second decade one finds a striking tendency for them to be located at the internal carotid artery bifurcation (Fig. 15.2). Such aneurysms occurred in 29.5% of cases, compared with the 4.5% reported in adults (Locksley 1966). A similar high incidence at this location was reported by Sedzimir and Robinson (1973) and Patel and Richardson (1971). There was a low incidence of middle cerebral artery and posterior circulation aneurysms.

Orozco et al. (1978) reviewed 27 cases of aneurysm in the under 5 year age group reported in the literature. They showed several interesting features. There is a predominance of males, and the majority of cases present in the first 2 years of life. The most common sites for aneurysms are the middle cerebral artery and posterior circulation, which shows a strikingly different distribution from those in the second decade of life. There is a tendency for aneurysms to be peripheral in location (Fig. 15.3) and they are often large (Fig. 15.4). Large aneurysms acting as pseudotumours have been reported by Lemmen and Schneider (1953), Jane (1961), Lapras et al. (1966), Pickering et al. (1970) and Arai et al. (1972).

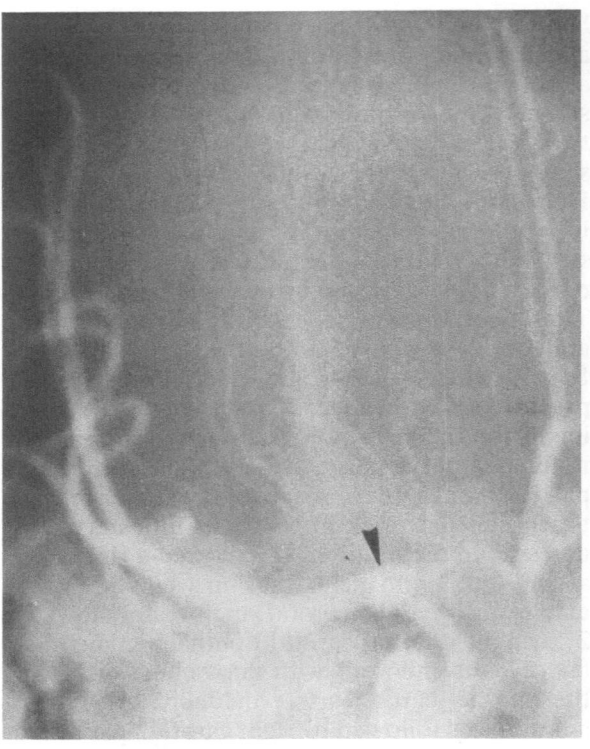

Fig. 15.2. Carotid angiogram, showing an internal carotid bifurcation aneurysm (*arrowhead*). Bifurcation aneurysms, when small, may be superimposed on the internal carotid and middle cerebral arteries and therefore could be missed.

Sex Incidence

There is a preponderance of males in our own series, the male–female ratio being 1.7:1. This contrasts strikingly with the adult population, where there is a female preponderance of 3 to 2.

Multiple Aneurysms

The incidence of multiple aneurysms in childhood and adolescence is low. A 6%–8% incidence of multiple aneurysms has been reported (Patel and Richardson 1971: Sedzimir and Robinson 1973). Multiple aneurysms were present in only eight patients (9.2%) in this series. This contrasts with a 29% incidence in adults in this unit (see Chap. 5).

Associated Congenital Lesions

Co-existence of cerebral aneurysms with a variety of congenital lesions has been reported, but this association is not significant, except with polycys-

Table 15.3. Location of aneurysms (79 cases of single aneurysms and eight cases of multiple (two) aneurysms

Site	Single aneurysm	Multiple aneurysms	Total no.	%
Anterior cerebral	2	1	3	3.1
Anterior communicating	21	4	25	26.3
Pericallosal	1	0	1	
Middle cerebral	11	5	16	16.8
Peripheral middle cerebral	1	0	1	
Internal carotid				
Bifurcation	26	2	28	29.5
Posterior communicating	10	2	12	12.6
Ophthalmic	3	0	3	3.1
Vertebrobasilar junction	1	0	1	
PICA	2	1	3	3.1
Basilar tip	1	0	1	
Posterior cerebral	0	1	1	
Total	79	16	95	

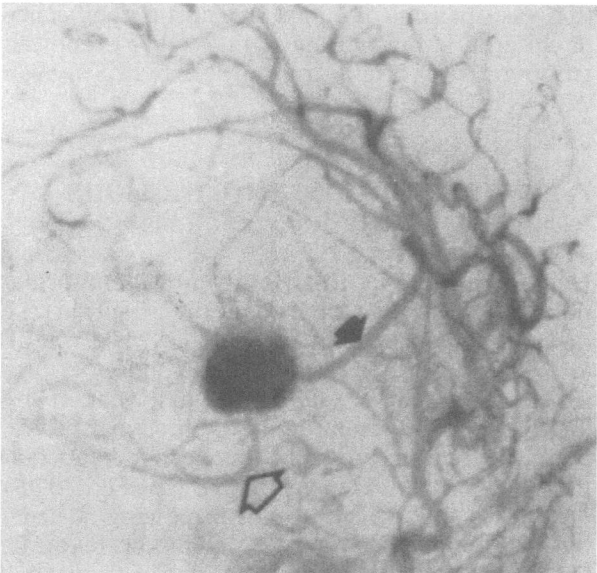 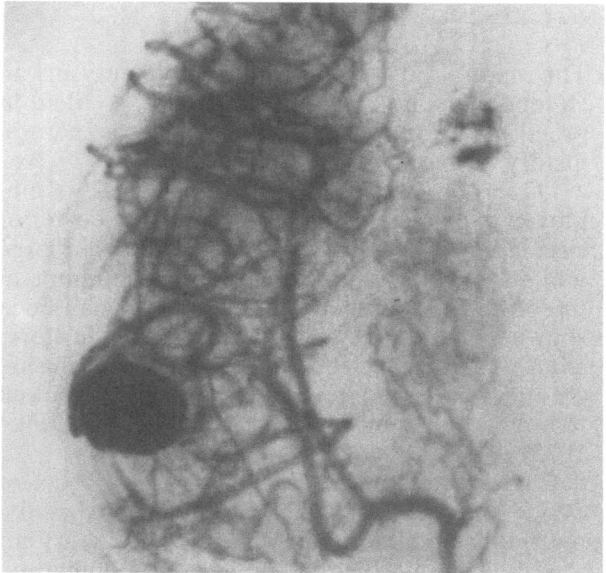

Fig. 15.3. Large peripherally located middle cerebral artery aneurysms in a neonate. (Courtesy of Dr. D. Hungerford)

tic kidney disease and coarctation of the aorta. The authors have reviewed 245 reported cases of childhood aneurysm in the literature and found 13 cases of coarctation of the aorta (5.3%) and three cases of polycystic kidney (1.2%). Additional congenital lesions that have been reported include a case of primitive trigeminal artery (Oroz-

co et al. 1978), a case of agenesis of the corpus callosum (Garcia-Chavez and Moosy 1965) and a case of fibromuscular hyperplasia (Bolander et al. 1978). Ferry et al. (1974) described a case of generalised vascular dysplasia with multiple aneurysmal dilatations of the carotid, basilar, vertebral and iliac arteries.

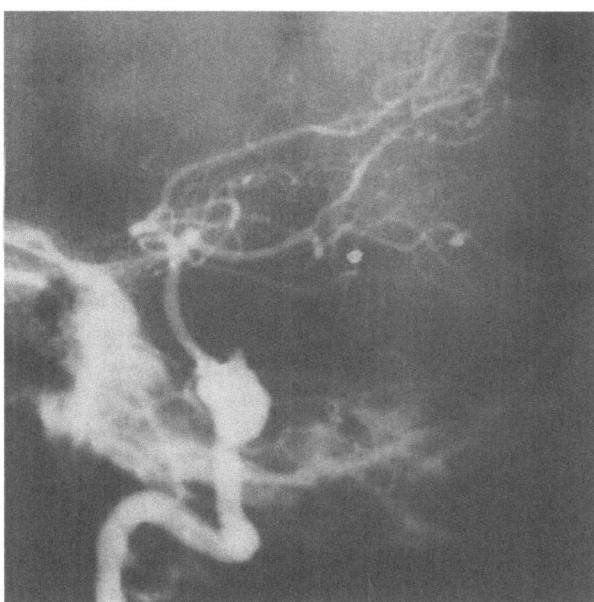

Fig. 15.4. Vertebral angiogram in a 15-year-old female with SAH showing a large vertebrobasilar junction aneurysm.

Angiographic Technique

Children with proven SAH, like adults, require the same early and complete four vessel angiography. Clinical features and CT scan findings obviously will help determine the extent and pattern of angiography. Direct puncture or selective percutaneous femoral catheter cerebral angiography can be employed. The latter is preferred since one can obtain multiple selective vessel studies from a single puncture. Children do have an increased tendency to thrombo-embolic complications associated with the femoral catheterisation; Jacobson et al. (1980) reported a 4% incidence in the under 5 year age group. Thrombus formation can be minimised by the use of thin walled heparinised catheters, thus reducing the surface area for formation of the thrombus. We have also found it useful to infuse dextran 40 during the catheter procedure to reduce the tendency to thrombosis. We use the paediatric femoral cerebral catheters manufactured by William Cook (Europe) Limited.

Treatment

The natural history of ruptured aneurysms in childhood is not well documented, so that in practice our approach is based on the natural history in the adult population.

Direct clipping of the aneurysm neck is employed whenever possible in our Unit. Posterior circulation aneurysms in childhood may be large and fusiform and in these cases an attempt at direct clipping may be hazardous. It has been shown that some of these large fusiform aneurysms are best treated by gradual occlusion of one vertebral artery. This procedure is well tolerated by young patients (Amacher and Drake 1975).

Children are more resilient to the effects of SAH, and there is general agreement that the morbidity and mortality of ruptured aneurysms are more favourable than in the adult population. Vasospasm is less of a problem, children appearing to be less affected by it. Certainly at autopsy, brain infarction is rarely seen in cases in which the pre-morbid angiogram has shown severe spasm (Richardson 1979). This compares strikingly with a high necropsy incidence (75%) of cerebral infarction in adults with ruptured intracranial aneurysms (Crompton 1964). Ostergaard and Voldby (1983) reported a 53% incidence of vasospasm in their childhood series, but none of the patients were in grade 4 or 5, and they suggest

that vasospasm is of minor prognostic significance in children. Amacher and Drake (1975) reported an operative mortality rate of less than 5% even with very large lesions.

Arteriovenous Malformations

Haemorrhage due to arteriovenous malformations (AVMs) has not been described in the new-born and is rare in early infancy. Kelly et al. (1978) point out the difference in mode of presentation of AVMs seen in the first year of life and those seen thereafter. In the first year of life, massive shunting producing congestive heart failure (e.g. vein of Galen aneurysms, see Fig. 13.19) or strategically placed lesions producing obstructive hydrocephalus are the common features. Auscultation of the skull in this group frequently reveals a bruit which is related to the large size of the lesion. In older children SAH and seizures are the more frequent presenting features.

Perret and Nishioka (1966) recorded that less than 20% of cases of SAH due to AVMs were in the under 20 year age group. In this series of 167 cases of SAH in the under 20 age group, 44 were due to an AVM (26.3% of cases). The age at the time of initial SAH is summarised in Fig. 15.5. The youngest patient was 6 years of age. There were 25 females and 19 males.

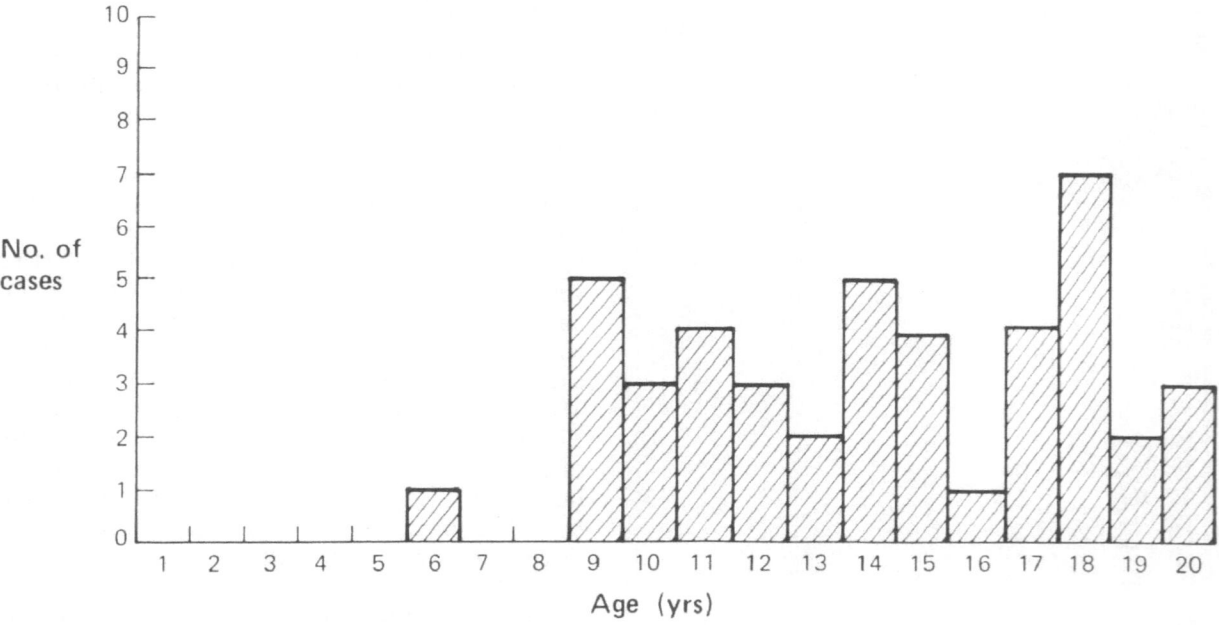

Fig. 15.5. Age of presentation in SAH due to AVMs (44 cases).

Site

In 40 cases (91%) the AVM was supratentorial in location. Right and left sides were about equally affected. Four cases (9%) were infratentorial in location. The most commonly affected areas were the parietal lobe (37.5%) and the temporal lobe (20.5%) (Table 15.4). Our findings are in agreement with those of other authors (Ingraham and Matson 1969; Moyes 1969; So 1978), in that parietal lesions in the distribution of the middle cerebral artery predominate.

Table 15.4. Site of AVMs

Supratentorial	
Parietal	15
Deep	9
Superficial	5
Temporal	9
Temporoparietal	3
Temporal (deep extension into basal ganglia)	2
Occipital	3
Frontal	4
Basal ganglia	3
Tentorial hiatus	1
Infratentorial	4
	44

Clinical Features

Locksley (1966) reported in a group of AVMs in all age groups a 13% incidence of seizures and a 43% history of headache before the first SAH. In our group of 44 patients, however, nine had a history of seizures preceding the SAH and only five had periodic headache prior to the onset of the haemorrhage.

In our series 17 patients (39%) did not have any focal neurological signs. This is in contrast to the previous report of 20% by Milhorat (1978). The SAH was associated with hemiplegia or hemiparesis in 15 patients, monoparesis in two and hemianopia in three. The common finding of hemiparesis associated wth a bleeding AVM is not surprising since the majority are located within the territory of the middle cerebral artery. Two patients suffered a grand mal seizure at the time of SAH, but other presentations include coma (one case), headache leading to coma and respiratory arrest (one case), and meningitis-like illness with fever and neck stiffness (one case). The CT scans in such instances should prevent errors in diagnosis.

Diagnosis

Plain Skull X-rays

Plain skull X-rays occasionally demonstrate increased vascular markings and calcification associated with an AVM. In our experience, however, they provide relatively little information: Intracranial calcification occurred in only two cases and a prominent vascular groove associated with the malformation in only one case. In a further case there was evidence of raised intracranial pressure. A shift of the calcified pineal gland may indicate the presence of an intracerebral haematoma. Pineal calcification is unusual before the age of 10 years and in this series, pineal shift indicating a haematoma was not recorded. Kelly et al. (1978) reported abnormal plain skull X-ray findings in only 5 out of 29 patients presenting with an SAH or epilepsy. In three cases there was evidence of calcification of the AVM. One case had marked unilateral increase in venous channels on the skull X-ray and one had evidence of macrocephalus.

CT Scanning

CT scan findings in AVMs have been discussed in Chap. 6. CT was carried out in 13 cases, all of which showed an abnormality. CT proved valuable in:

1. Confirming a diagnosis of SAH, especially where the differential diagnosis lay between meningitis and SAH.
2. Demonstrating the site of a haematoma and revealing if there is any extension into the ventricular system. This is also helpful in preparing for precise angiography.
3. Confirming the presence of an AVM by demonstration of typical serpiginous contrast enhancement. This occurred in five out of the ten cases in which contrast-enhanced scans were carried out.
4. Pinpointing the diagnosis of a posterior fossa haematoma.
5. Diagnosing cryptic or largely thrombosed AVMs which may not be detectable at angiography (Figs. 15.6, 15.7).

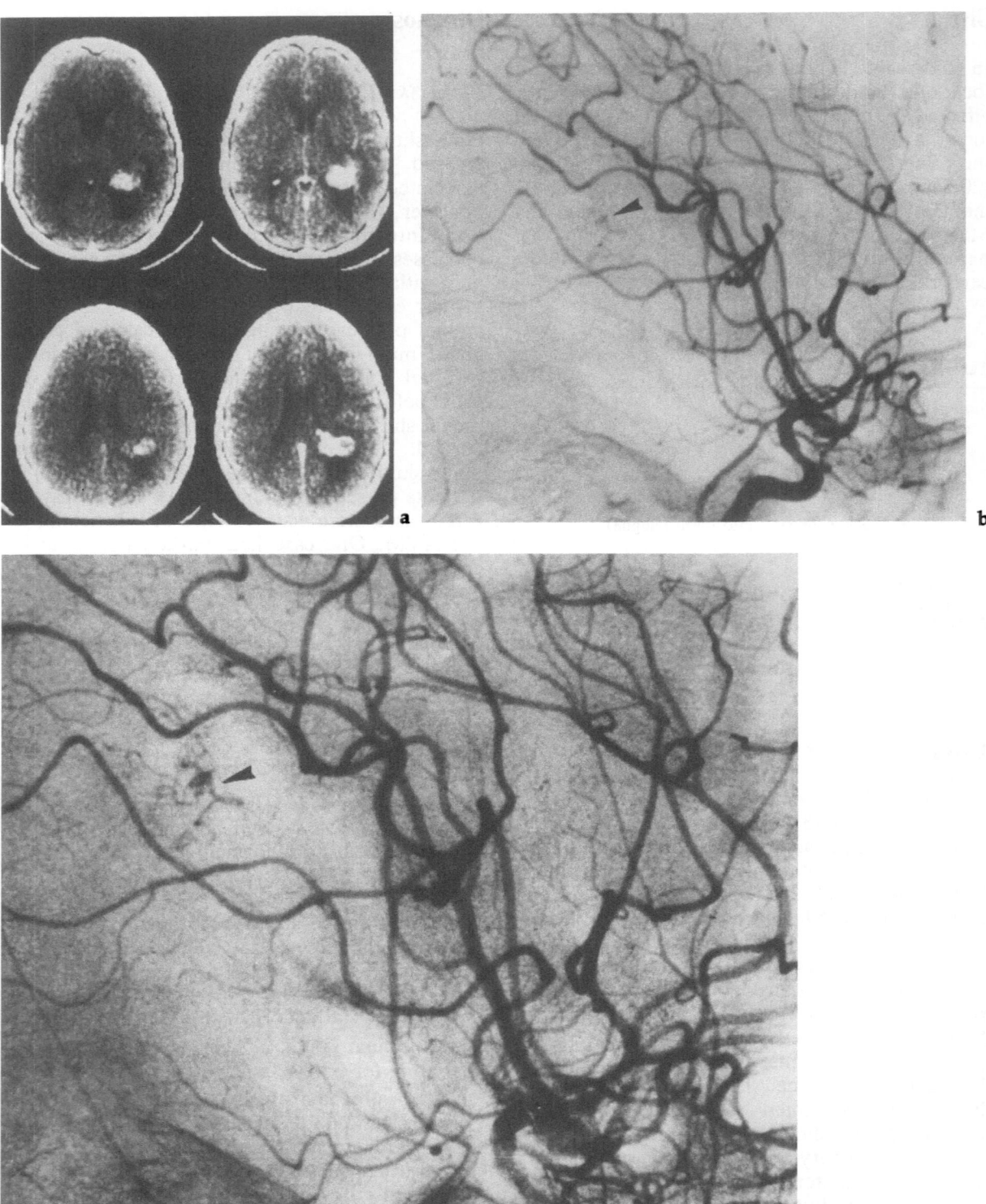

Fig. 15.6. a CT scan shows a high density lesion in the region of the trigone of the left lateral ventricle. After i.v. injection of contrast there is definite enhancement within and around this lesion, which shows minimal space-occupying effect and no surrounding oedema. **b** Right carotid angiogram showed a small suspicious area of abnormal vascularity (*arrowhead*) which was confirmed on **c** a magnification study (*arrowhead*). At operation an angioma was found with surrounding haemorrhage.

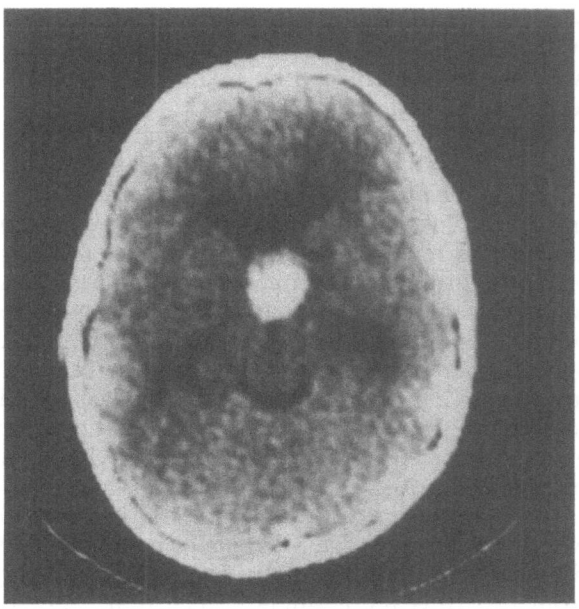

Fig. 15.7. CT scan in an 11-year-old child with a high density lesion consistent with a haematoma in the third ventricle, with no evidence of contrast enhancement. Four vessel angiography was normal. At surgery a haematoma was removed from the third ventricle and a small vascular malformation was seen, which was confirmed on histological examination.

Angiography

Angiography provides the definitive diagnosis of intracranial AVMs.

The size of AVMs varied widely from very small to very extensive, involving the larger part of the cerebral hemisphere. The majority of AVMs in this series (86.4%) were medium or small: in 24 cases (54.5%) the AVM was less than 2 cm in diameter and only six (13.6%) were classified as large. In Perret and Nishioka's series of AVMs in all age groups, only 8% were smaller than 2 cm (1966).

There is a relationship between the size of an AVM and its mode of presentation. Small AVMs are often deep and hemispheric in location and commonly remain silent until they rupture, when they frequently produce a massive haemorrhage. Large AVMs, however, are characterised by seizure or progressive motor deficit. Haemorrhage, if it occurs, is often less severe but may be recurrent.

Arteriovenous malformations could be divided into three types according to the angiographic pattern, as discussed in Chap. 7.

1. A typical AVM with large feeding arteries and draining veins (23 cases)
2. A small leash of vessels (capillary type AVM) with no evidence of draining veins (12 cases)
3. A small leash of vessels with a single draining vein (eight cases)

In one case angiography was not carried out, but an AVM was found at surgery.

The AVMs were supplied principally by the middle cerebral artery (55%), the posterior cerebral artery (29%) and the anterior cerebral artery (8.5%). In three cases the main supply was from the internal carotid artery, anterior choroidal artery and superior cerebellar artery respectively.

Treatment

In children, the initial mortality from rupture of an AVM is about 5%–10%, whilst with subsequent haemorrhages the mortality is in the order of 10%–20% (Milhorat 1978). The exact incidence of rebleeding in patients treated conservatively is unknown. Kelly et al. (1978) reported a mortality of 28% and morbidity of 22% in the patients with SAH treated conservatively. Of 14 children so treated, after the first SAH six (43%) died within 5 years (So 1978). One should remember that the majority of AVMs in children are small and these are more prone to recurrent bleed. Moreover, children have a long life expectancy. All cerebral AVMs in children should be treated surgically whenever possible.

The main aims of surgical treatment are (a) to evacuate the life-threatening intracerebral haematoma, and (b) total excision of the malformation. Surgical excision of an AVM in the presence of haematoma is often easily accomplished with little additional morbidity.

Very large AVMs and those deeply situated within the basal ganglia or thalamus are not usually amenable to surgical excision. More recently, embolisation techniques to augment the surgical treatment of AVMs have been introduced. Alternative types of treatment include radiotherapy, including conventional and proton beam therapy and stereotactic radiotherapy. These techniques have been described in Chap. 10.

Idiopathic (No Cause) Group

The idiopathic group will include children who have had a definite SAH but in whom aetiological factors, such as aneurysm, AVM or a haematological disorder, have been definitely excluded. Patients were included in this group only if they had a negative four vessel angiographic study. The idiopathic group accounted for 19.2% of cases, a somewhat lower incidence than the 35.7% reported by Locksley (1966) and 25.7% reported by Sedzimar and Robinson (1973).

Some haemorrhages may be due to small AVMs or AVMs which have been destroyed or largely thrombosed during the bleed, and therefore not shown at angiography. Cryptic malformations are more commonly seen at autopsy in children than in adults. Improved angiographic technique with magnification and subtraction will no doubt reveal smaller AVMs than was possible previously, and CT has proved useful (Leblanc and Ethier 1981) in demonstrating small (cryptic) and largely thrombosed AVMs not detected at angiography. They have suggested that an underlying AVM should be suspected even when the vascular nature is not demonstrated at angiography, if there is vascular enhancement of a high density lesion with no mass effect or surrounding oedema. The value of CT is clearly shown in the case illustrated in Fig. 15.6. A 14-year-old boy presented with a history of recurrent attacks of SAH. CT scan showed a small high density lesion consistent with a haematoma in the region of the trigone of the right lateral ventricle and after intravenous contrast there was definite evidence of some surrounding contrast enhancement (Fig. 15.6a). Conventional angiography was unremarkable, but in view of the CT findings, magnification studies with subtraction were performed, and showed a small vascular malformation (Fig. 15.6b). At surgery, an encapsulated, largely thrombosed cavernous angioma was found. In the pre-CT era this lesion could well have been missed, and therefore classified in the no lesion or idiopathic group. Another case of cryptic AVM is shown in Fig. 15.7. Even with CT many cryptic AVMs will still escape detection on account of their small size, destruction by haemorrhage, or difficulties in interpretation of various types of contrast enhancement found in association with a haematoma.

One of our patients who had an SAH at the age of 10 years with negative four vessel angiography had a repeat SAH 5 years later, and on this occasion angiography showed a small frontal AVM. It seems likely that the initial haemorrhage was due to a small cryptic malformation undetected at angiography.

Sedzimir and Robinson (1973) reported on the follow-up of 28 patients in whom no cause for the SAH could be found. The follow-up period varied from 1 to 17 years. In 26 cases (93%) there was no evidence of recurrent haemorrhage. Two patients had a recurrent bleed: one (14 years later) was found at angiography to have an aneurysm of the bifurcation of the right internal carotid artery, and another patient, who at the age of 11 years had negative three vessel angiography, was found to have a small AVM 5 years later. Focal or generalised fits subsequently occurred in eight patients (28.6%).

Our experience with 26 of the 32 patients in whom no cause for the SAH could be found, and who we were able to follow for periods ranging from 2 to 10 years, is similar. Recurrent haemorrhage (5–10 years later) occurred in four patients (15.4%) In these patients angiography demonstrated an AVM in two patients and an internal carotid bifurcation aneurysm in one; in the other patient no abnormality was seen on four vessel angiography at follow-up.

The current evidence available in this "no lesion group" suggests that the long-term prognosis is generally good, but one should be cautious since 10%–15% of these children are likely to have another SAH.

Rare Causes

The variety of potential rare causes of SAH in childhood and adolescence is greater than in adults.

Mycotic Aneurysms

Aneurysms due to bacterial endocarditis are extremely rare in childhood and will usually be accompanied by other stigmata of the disease, such as fever, cardiac signs and symptoms and embolic phenomena. These aneurysms are discussed in further detail in Chaps. 3 and 7.

Coarctation of the Aorta

Severe hypertension, which accompanies coarctation of the aorta, favours the development of aneurysms with subsequent SAH. Intracranial haemorrhage may also occur without an associated aneurysm (Baker and Shelden 1936).

Bleeding Disorders

Bleeding rarely occurs in the neonate but usually appears during the first year of life. Cerebral haemorrhage is the commonest cause of death in haemophiliacs. It is often initiated by trivial trauma and is usually followed by continuous oozing of blood which gradually results in an extensive intracranial haemorrhage. Visconti and Hilgartner (1983) reported 18 central nervous system bleeding episodes in eight patients with haemophilia A or B or von Willebrand's disease. SAH was the presenting feature of the disease in only one case—a 9-month-old infant. Haemorrhage was subarachnoid in 13 cases, subarachnoid and intracerebral in two cases, subdural in two cases, and in one case there was a spinal epidural haematoma.

The importance of blood tests to detect the rare case of hypofibrinogenaemia producing SAH has been emphasised by Wieczorek et al. (1970).

Thrombocytopenia, either idiopathic or in association with other disease, e.g. leukaemia, is the commonest cause of intracerebral haemorrhage. In leukaemia, intracerebral and subdural haemorrhage can be the presenting or one of the earliest clinical features (Hyland 1961). It occurs more frequently with acute rather than chronic and with myeloid rather than lymphatic types of leukaemia (Phair et al. 1964). There is evidence of abnormal bleeding elsewhere in the body by the time cerebral haemorrhage occurs.

Moya Moya Disease

Moya Moya disease, with its characteristic angiographic blush of tiny vessels at the base of the brain resembling "a puff of smoke", can lead to cerebral infarction, cerebral haemorrhage and subarachnoid haemorrhage. Subarachnoid haemorrhage, however, is an unusual feature under the age of 15 years. We have seen only one case in this age group (Fig. 15.8).

Cerebral Tumours

Cerebral tumours may rarely give rise to SAH. Figure 15.9 is the CT scan of a 16-year-old girl

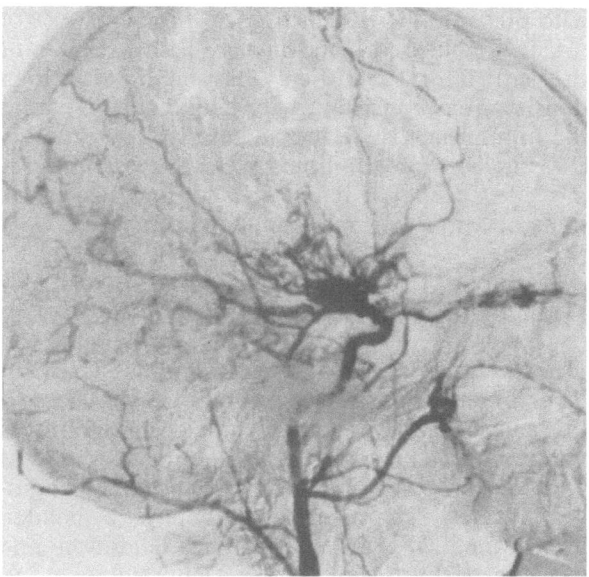

Fig. 15.8. A 10-year-old female patient who had a previous history of migrainous type headaches, and presented with an SAH. Cerebral angiography shows the typical angiographic features of Moya Moya disease.

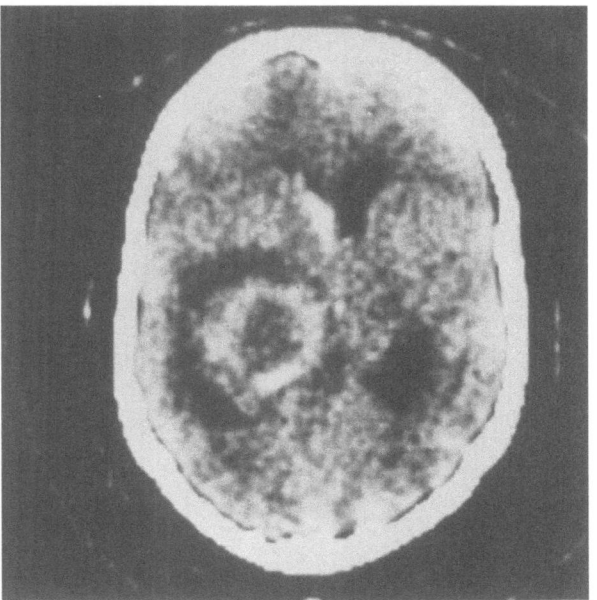

Fig. 15.9. A 17-year-old female with three previous episodes of SAH. Bilateral carotid angiography at the referring hospital had been reported as normal. CT scans taken at the time of the last SAH show a large mass in the region of the trigone of the left lateral ventricle. The ventricular system in the vicinity of the mass shows considerable dilatation. There are scattered areas of high density in the mass and in the frontal horn, consistent with haematoma. At surgery, a choroid plexus papilloma was found and successfully removed.

who presented with a history of three episodes of SAH. CT shows a mass in the dilated trigone of the left lateral ventricle associated with high density areas consistent with haemorrhage within the tumour and the left frontal horn. At surgery a choroid plexus papilloma was successfully removed. Cerebellar haemorrhage may also occur in association with malignant tumours.

Drug Abuse

One should remember that drug abuse (particularly amphetamine) may produce cerebral vasculitis causing SAH in young adults. Angiography is very valuable to exclude an aneurysm or AVM and to confirm a diagnosis of vasculitis. Angiography may characteristically show a beaded appearance with alternating vasodilatation and vasoconstriction (Fig. 15.10) (Rumbaugh et al. 1971). Repeat angiography may show return to

normality when the drug is stopped (Margolis and Newton 1971; Chynn 1975). Whether the vasculitis is due to an antigen antibody hypersensitivity response or impurities following self-administration is unknown.

Spinal Arteriovenous Malformations

Riche et al. (1982) reviewed 38 cases of AVM of the spinal cord in children. In 19 cases the presentation was of sudden impairment of motor functions, often related to physical effort. There was evidence of associated SAH in eight cases. Symptoms resembling those of SAH occurred in ten cases, and in many of these cases back pain focused attention on the spinal cord as the source of the haemorrhage. In three cases the symptoms were those of a simple SAH, but it was due to the paucity of cerebral involvement that myelography

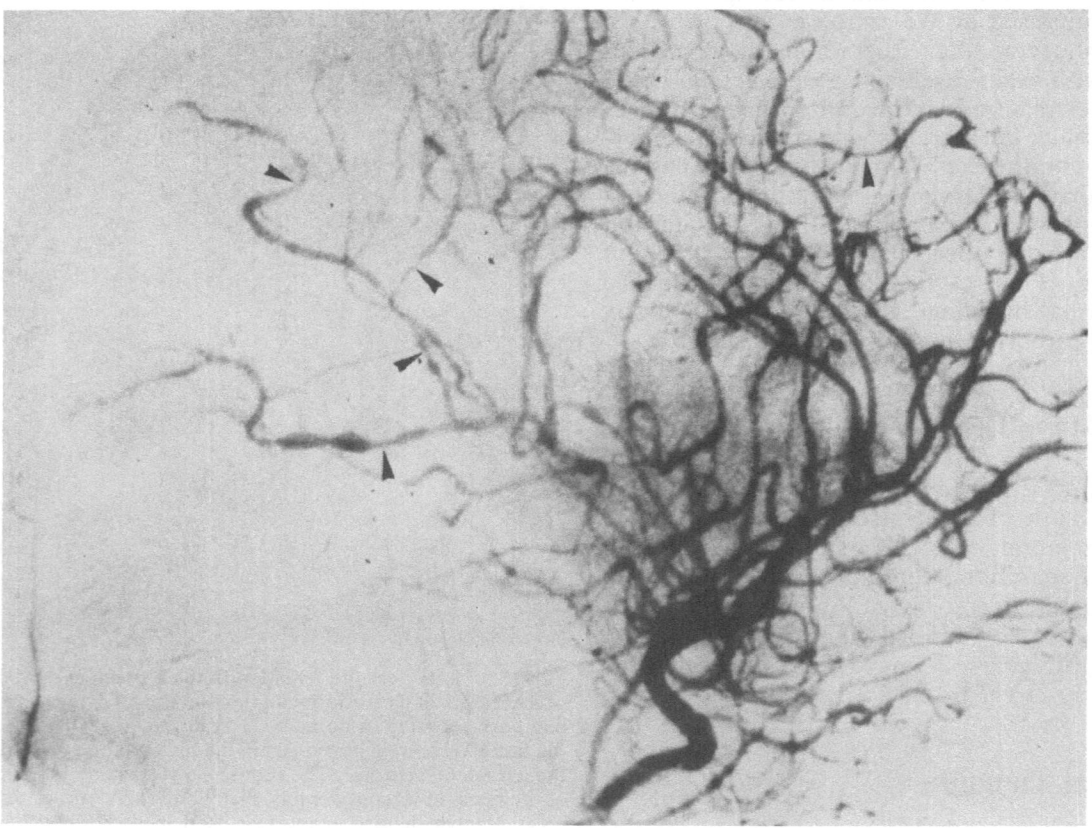

Fig. 15.10. Carotid angiogram showing multiple areas of arterial constriction (*arrowheads*) and dilatation typical of an arteritis.

was carried out and the source of the haemorrhage found. The location of the AVMs was cervical in 28% of cases, thoracic in 21% and thoracolumbar in 51%. The malformations had an intramedullary or mixed location in 82% of cases.

Bony changes occurred in 12 cases; mostly they consisted in widening of the spinal canal, but there was also scolloping of the vertebral body, erosion of pedicles or kyphoscoliosis. There was one case of vertebral body angioma (Cobb's syndrome). There was a frequent association with deep or cutaneous angiodysplasias (13 cases) (34%), including port-wine stained angiomas, Weber-Rendu-Osler disease, Klippel-Trenaunay disease and Cobb's syndrome.

Riche et al. emphasise that the short-term natural evolution of these angiomas is catastrophic. Early treatment is advised and the advantages of preliminary embolisation or simultaneous embolisation and operation is stressed. Embolisation alone proved effective in three cases.

Neonatal Intracranial Haemorrhage

Three main types of intracranial haemorrhage can occur in neonates.

1. Subdural haemorrhage
2. Periventricular, intracerebral or intraventricular haemorrhage
3. Subarachnoid haemorrhage

More rarely, intracerebellar haemorrhage in small preterm infants has also recently been described (Volpe 1977).

Subdural Haemorrhage

Subdural haemorrhage occurs when a traumatic delivery causes either a rupture at the junction of the vein of Galen and the immobile straight sinus, tearing of the superficial cerebral veins as they enter the sagittal sinus, or falx laceration with rupture of the inferior sagittal sinus. The majority of these patients die, particularly those who have a laceration at the level of the tentorium or the falx.

Periventricular, Intracerebral (Intraventricular) Haemorrhage

The proven associations with periventricular haemorrhage are low gestation, respiratory disease requiring ventilation and, particularly, pneumothorax. The overall incidence in babies under 1500 g is 45%–50%, and in babies under 1000 g, nearer 90%. There is no proven association with serious hypoxic events at birth. Bleeding arises classically from the subependymal, germinal matrix at the level of the foramen of Munro, producing a periventricular haematoma, frequently with an intraventricular extension.

Subarachnoid Haemorrhage

Subarachnoid haemorrhage is the most common variety of neonatal intracranial haemorrhage. It is commonly seen in prematurity and neonatal asphyxia. The source of the bleeding is usually venous, and the prognosis is generally good.

Clinical Features

Volpe (1977) describes three major syndromes. Firstly, minor haemorrhage with no signs or symptoms; this occurs particularly in premature infants, and accounts for 75% of all cases of SAH in babies. Secondly, presentation with seizures, especially in full-term infants. Seizures often characteristically have their onset on approximately the second day of life. In the interictal period, these babies often appear remarkably well, so that the description of "well baby with seizures, is appropriate. There may be recurrent apnoeic spells. A third syndrome, which is rare, is massive SAH with a rapidly fatal course. These infants have usually sustained a severe hypoxic injury with an element of trauma at birth.

Diagnosis

Cerebrospinal fluid is nearly always blood-stained and shows xanthochromia. CT and real time ultrasound have proved very useful diagnostic tools in the diagnosis, management and follow-up of neonatal intracranial haemorrhage.

CT can confirm the presence of SAH (Fig. 15.11). It will also demonstrate germinal matrix or subependymal haematomas and clearly show the extent of any intraventricular blood

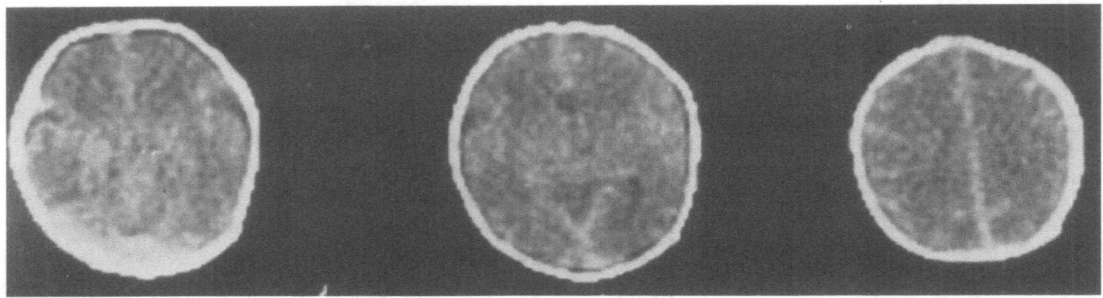

Fig. 15.11. CT scan in a neonate showing blood in the subarachnoid space.

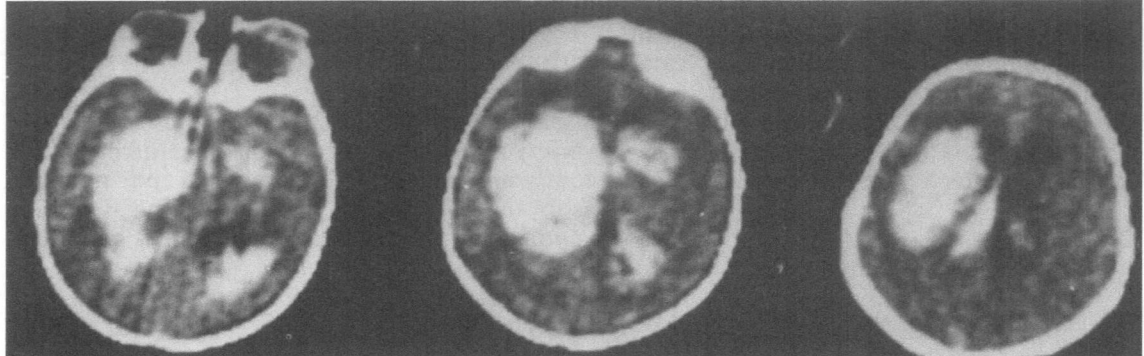

Fig. 15.12. CT scan in a neonate showing extensive intracerebral and intraventricular blood.

clots (Fig. 15.12). Demonstration of acute enlargement of the ventricular system may allow immediate institution of life-saving ventricular drainage and shunting. Progressive hydrocephalus is a common sequela following SAH in those cases surviving intraventricular bleeding, and this is clearly demonstrated on follow-up CT examination.

Real time ultrasound can provide detailed images of the neonatal brain in the axial, coronal and sagittal planes. The echogenicity of an intracranial structure depends on its abrupt interface with neighbouring structures. The cerebral fissures and cisterns, choroid plexus, lateral ventricular walls, falx and tentorium have abrupt interfaces, and are clearly shown as strongly echogenic structures that provide reliable anatomical landmarks (Fig. 15.13). High resolution real time ultrasound equipment can be easily transported to the neonatal intensive care unit. The infant can be scanned in the incubator without sedation and without disturbing life-support equipment. Rapid identification of intracranial anatomy is easily possible, making use of specially designed hand-held transducers and the real time display. Real time ultrasound compares favourably with CT in that it is not only less expensive but involves no ionising radiation and is, therefore, an ideal method of monitoring response to therapy. The technique and normal anatomy of real time ultrasound of the neonatal cranium have been described by Schuman et al. (1981).

Real time ultrasound can easily distinguish the typical small germinal matrix haemorrhage which is usually self-limiting and carries a good prognosis (Fig. 15.14) from the more serious cerebral and intraventricular haemorrhages (Fig. 15.15), which may lead to porencephaly and/or hydrocephalus (Fig. 15.16)). Real time ultrasound, however, is not as effective as CT in detecting primary SAH.

Prognosis

In general, the prognosis for infants with primary SAH without serious traumatic or hypoxic injury is good (Volpe 1977). If we look at the three major syndromes previously described, those in-

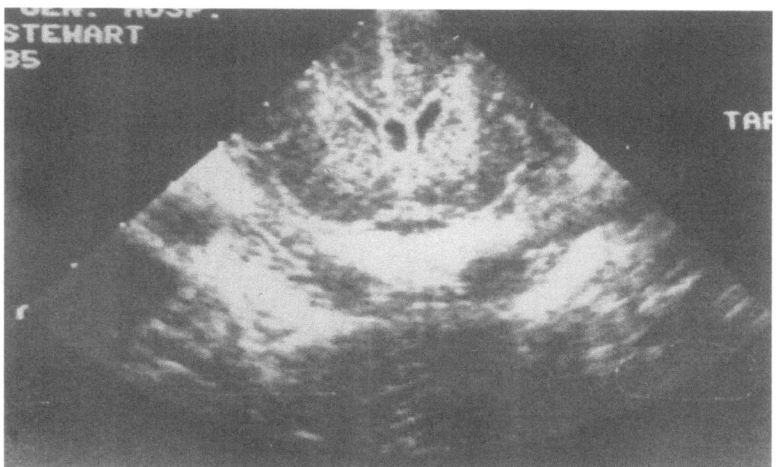

Fig. 15.13. Real time ultrasound. Coronal section showing normal sized ventricles. Note the cavum septum pellucidum. (By kind permission of Dr. David Milligan)

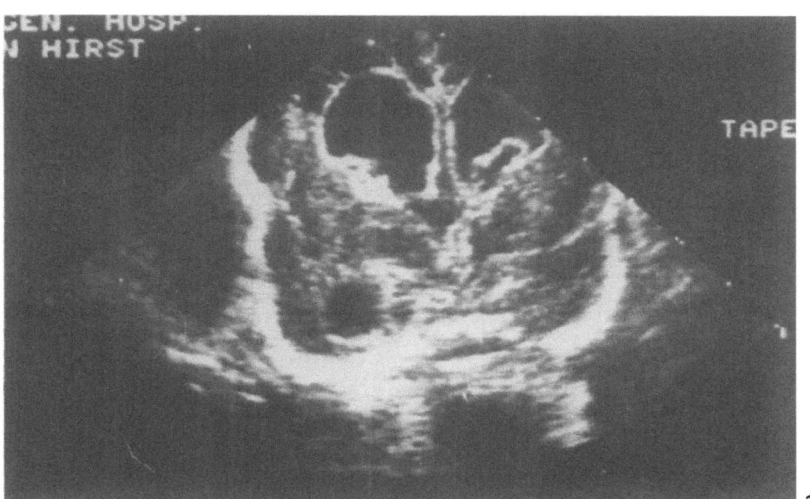

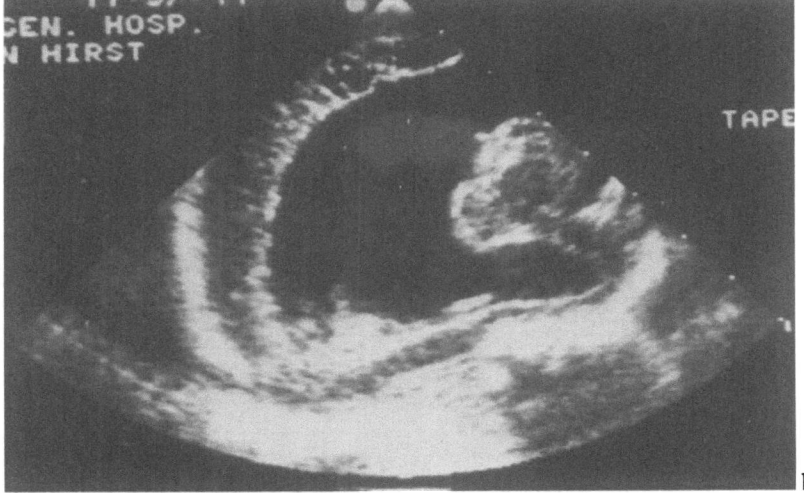

Fig. 15.14a, b. Real time ultrasound **a** Coronal section showing bilateral germinal matrix haemorrhage. The haemorrhage on the left side shows a central translucency due to liquefaction. There is hydrocephalus with periventricular lucencies. **b** Sagittal section again showing germinal matrix haemorrhage, hydrocephalus and periventricular lucencies. (By kind permission of Dr. David Milligan)

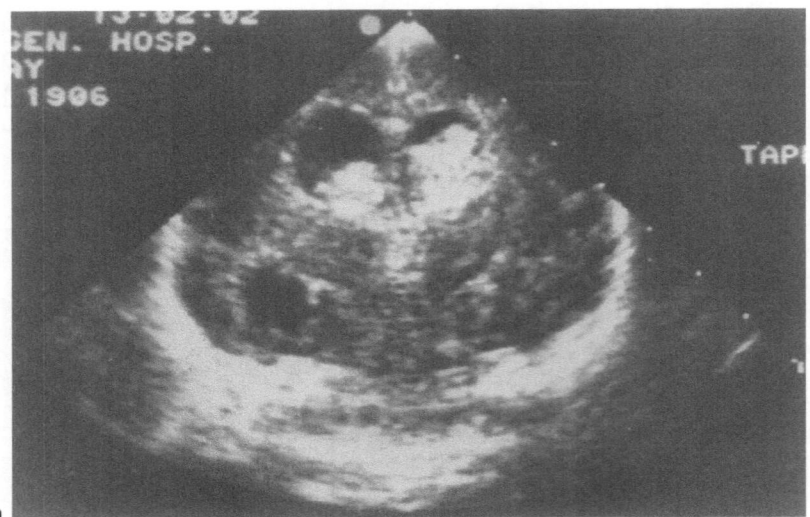

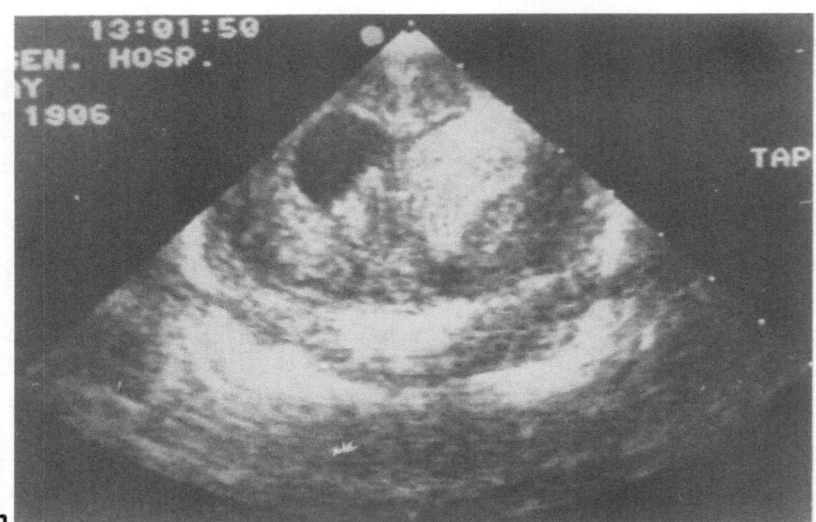

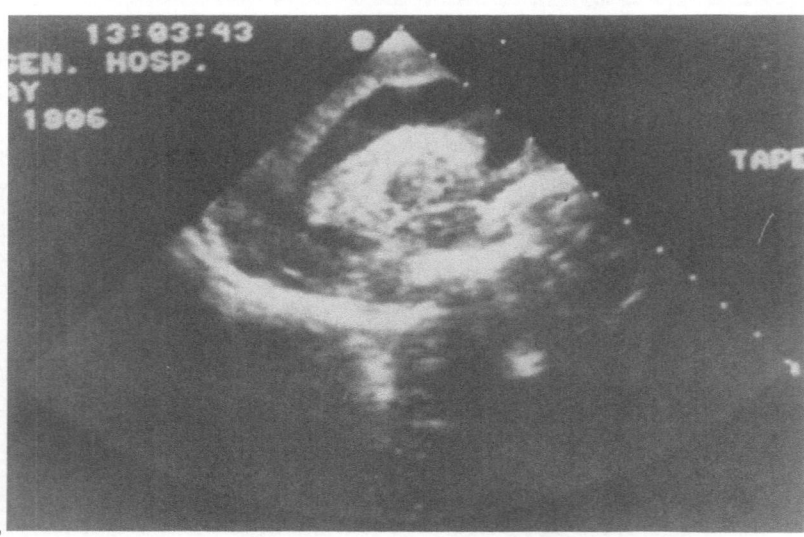

Fig. 15.15a–c. Real time ultrasound. **a, b** Coronal and **c** sagittal sections showing bilateral extensive intraventricular haemorrhages. (By kind permission of Dr. David Milligan)

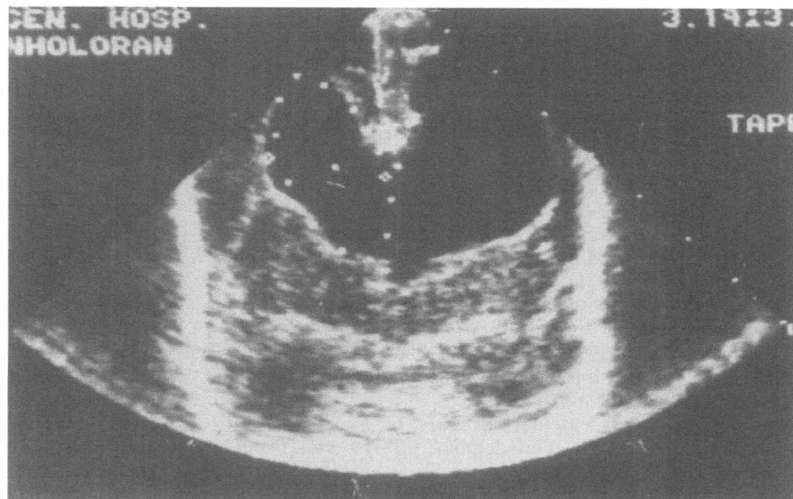

Fig. 15.16. Real time ultrasound. hydrocephalus. (By kind permission of Dr. David Milligan)

fants with minor haemorrhage and minimal signs uniformly do well. Infants presenting with seizures are normal at follow-up in approximately 90% of cases. Those presenting with massive SAH either die or are left with a serious neurological deficit.

The major complication following intracranial haemorrhage is the development of hydrocephalus, and the importance of CT scanning or real time ultrasound in detecting this complication has been stressed. The incidence of hydrocephalus (i.e. progressive ventricular dilatation requiring surgical interference) in pre-term babies who survive haemorrhage which ruptures into the ventricle is only now being adequately documented; it is probably of the order of 50% in those babies who develop significant ventricular dilatation associated with the bleed, but very much lower in those whose bleed is less severe.

References

Amacher AL, Drake CG (1975) Cerebral artery aneurysms in infancy, childhood and adolescence. Childs Brain 1:72–80

Arai H, Sugiyama Y, Kawakami S, Miyazawa N (1972) Multiple intracranial aneurysms and vascular malformations in an infant. Case report. J Neurosurg 37:357–360

Baker TW, Shelden WD (1936) Coarctation of the aorta with intermittent leakage of a congenital cerebral aneurysm. Am J Med Sci 191:626–633

Becker DH, Silvenberg GD, Nelson DH, Hambeny JW (1978) Saccular aneurysm of infancy and early childhood. Neurosurgery 2:1–5

Bolander H, Hassler O, Liliequist B, West KA (1978) Cerebral aneurysm in an infant with fibromuscular hyperplasia of the renal arteries. Case report. J Neurosurg 49:756–759

Bremer JL (1943) Congenital aneurysms of the cerebral arteries. An embryologic study. Arch Pathol 35:819–831

Chynn KY (1975) Acute subarachnoid haemorrhage. JAMA 233:55–56

Crompton MR (1964) Cerebral infarction following rupture of cerebral berry aneurysm. Brain 87:263–280

Eppinger H (1871) Stenosis aortae congenita. Seu isthmus persistens. Vjechr Praktheilk 112:31–67

Ferry PC, Kerber C, Peterson D, Gallo AA (1974) Arteriectasis, subarachnoid haemorrhage in a three months old infant. Neurology 24:494–500

Garcia-Chavez C, Moosy J (1965) Cerebral artery aneurysm in infancy. Association with agenesis of the corpus callosum. J Neuropathol Exp Neurol 24:492–501

Housepian EM, Pool JL (1958) A systematic analysis of intracranial aneurysms from the autopsy file of the Presbyterian Hospital 1914–1956. J Neuropathol Exp Neurol 17:409–423

Hyland HH (1961) Non-aneurysmal intracranial haemorrhage. Neurology 11:165–168

Ingraham FD, Matson DD (1969) Neurosurgery of infancy and childhood, 2nd edn. Thomas, Springfield Ill., pp 749–766

Jacobson B, Curtin H, Rubenson A, Sörensen SE (1980) Complications of angiography in children and means of prevention. Acta Radiol [Diagn] 21:257–261

Jane TA (1961) A large aneurysm of the posterior inferior cerebellar artery in a one year old child. J Neurosurg 18:245–247

Kelly JJ, Mellinger JF, Sundt TM (1978) Intracranial arteriovenous malformations in children. Ann Neurol 3:338–343

Laitinen L (1964) Arteriella aneurysm and subarachnoid alblodning hos barn. Nord Med 71:329–333

Lapras C, Goutelle A, Brunat M, Duchaume JP (1966) Les aneurysmes intracraniens chez l'enfant. A propos de quatra observations. Neurochirurgie, 14:891–900

Leblanc R, Ethier R (1981) Computerised tomographic patterns of angiographically occult arteriovenous malformations of the brain. Can J Neurol Sci 8:7–13

Lemmen LJ, Scheider RC (1953) Aneurysm in the third ventricle. Neurology 3:474–476

Lipper S, Morgan D, Krigman MR (1979) Congenital saccular aneurysm in a 19 days old neonate. Case report and review of the literature. Surg Neurol 10:161–165

Locksley HB (1966) Natural history of subarachnoid haemorrhage, intracranial aneurysms and arteriovenous malformations. Based on 6,368 cases in the co-operative study. J Neurosurg 25:219–239

Margolis MT, Newton TH (1971) Methamphetamine (speed) arteritis. Neuroradiology 2:179–192

McCormick WF (1971) Problems and pathogenesis of intracranial arterial aneurysms. In: Moosy J, Janeway R (eds) Cerebral vascular diseases. Grune and Stratton, New York London pp 219–231

McDonald CA, Korb M (1939) Intracranial aneurysms. Arch Neurol Psychiatry 42:298–328

Milhorat TH (1978) Vascular disorders. In: Paediatric neurosurgery. F.A. Davis, Philadelphia, pp 311–345 (Contemporary Neurology Series)

Moyes PD (1969) Intracranial intraspinal vascular anomalies in children. J Neurosurg 31:271–278

Orozco M, Trigueros F, Quintana F, Dierssen G (1978) Intracranial aneurysms in early childhood. Surg Neurol 9:247–252

Ostergaard JR, Voldby B (1983) Intracranial arterial aneurysms in children and adolescents. J Neurosurg 58:832–837

Padget DH (1948) The development of the cranial arteries in the human embryo. Contrib Embryol, Carnegie Inst Washington, Pub 212, pp 205–262

Patel AN, Richardson HE (1971) Ruptured intracranial aneurysms in the first two decades of life. A study of 58 patients. J Neurosurg 35:571–576

Perret GE, Nishioka H (1966) Arteriovenous malformations. An analysis of 545 cases of cranio-cerebral arterio-venous malformations and fistulae reported to the co-operative study. J Neurosurg 25:467–490

Phair JP, Anderson RE, Namiki H (1964) The central nervous system in leukaemia. Ann Intern Med 61:863–875

Pickering LK, Hogan GR, Gilbert EF (1970) Aneurysms of the posterior inferior cerebellar artery: rupture in a new born. Am J Dis Child 119:155–158

Richardson AE (1979) Aneurysm in childhood. In: Pia A, Langmaid C, Zierski J (eds) Cerebral aneurysm. Advances in diagnosis and therapy. Springer, Berlin, Heidelberg, New York, pp 376–378

Riche MC, Modenesi-Freitas J, Djindjian M, Merland JJ (1982) Arterio-venous malformation (AVM) of the spinal cord in children. A review of 38 cases. Neuroradiology 22:171–180

Rumbaugh CL, Bergeron RT, Fang HCH, McCormick R (1971) Cerebral angiographic change in the drug abuse patient. Radiology 101:335–344

Sedzimir CB, Robinson J (1973) Intracranial haemorrhage in children and adolescents. J Neurosurg 38:269–281

Schuman WP, Rogers JV, Mack LA, Alvord EC Jr, Christie DP (1981) Real time sonographic sector scanning of the neonatal cranium—technique and normal anatomy. Am J Neuroradiol 2:349–356

Shucart WA, Wolpert SM (1972) An aneurysm in infancy presenting with diabetes insipidus. J Neurosurg 37:368–370

So Sing Cho (1978) Cerebral arterio-venous malformations in children. Childs Brain 4:242–250

Stehbens WE (1975) Ultrastructure of aneurysms. Arch Neurol 32:798–807

Thompson JR, Harwood-Nash DC, Fitz CR (1973) Cerebral aneurysms in childhood. Am J Roentgenol 118:163–175

Visconti EB, Hilgartner MW (1983) Recognition and management of CNS haemorrhage in haemophilia. Paediatrician 9:127–137

Volpe JJ (1977) Neonatal intracranial haemorrhage. Pathophysiology, neuropathology and clinical features. Clin Perinatol 4:77–102

Wieczorek V, Brodkorb W, Remde W (1970) Subarachnoidal Blutung bei verstärkter Fibrinolyse. Münch Med Wochenschr 112:366–369

16 Spinal Subarachnoid Haemorrhage

Introduction

Spinal SAH is rare and often misdiagnosed because of its variable clinical presentation and the frequent paucity of signs referable to the spinal cord and cauda equina. The earliest observations of this condition were those by Duverney (1733) and Morgagni (1761).

In 1928 Michon described the sudden and agonising pain in the back, "coup de poignard" (or the stab of a dagger), as being classically associated with spinal SAH. The majority of cases of spinal SAH are due to arteriovenous malformations of the spinal cord, but there have been several reports of haemorrhage associated with spinal neoplasms since the original description by Andrew-Thomas in 1930.

Reviews on the subject have been published by Walton (1953, 1956), Henson and Croft (1956), Heidrich (1965), Prieto and Cantu (1967), Aminoff (1976) and Djindjian M. (1978).

Aetiology

A large number of conditions have been reported in the literature as causing spontaneous spinal SAH.

Arteriovenous Malformations

Arteriovenous malformations (AVMs) are the most frequent cause of bleeding into the spinal subarachnoid space. About 10%–26% of spinal AVMs present as acute SAH (Aminoff 1976; Djindjian M. 1978). Djindjian M. (1978) reported that 55% of the SAHs were in patients below the age of 15 years. In the majority of cases SAH occurs from angiomas with a shunt of large volume.

The risk of haemorrhage appears to be greater in females and in patients with cervical angiomas. Aminoff (1976), in a recent analysis of 59 cases of spinal AVM which had presented with SAH, showed that 42% occurred in the cervical region. In the majority of cases SAH occurs in AVMs which are partly or completely intramedullary (Djindjian M. 1978). Coexistent intracranial and spinal AVMs have been reported (Hash et al. 1975), and Parkinson and West (1977) have reported spontaneous SAH, first from an intracranial and then from a spinal AVM.

Tumours

Spinal tumours may occasionally be the cause of an SAH (Fig. 16.1). The majority of reported cases have been due to tumours of the conus medullaris or cauda equina, the most frequent histological types being ependymoma (Abbott

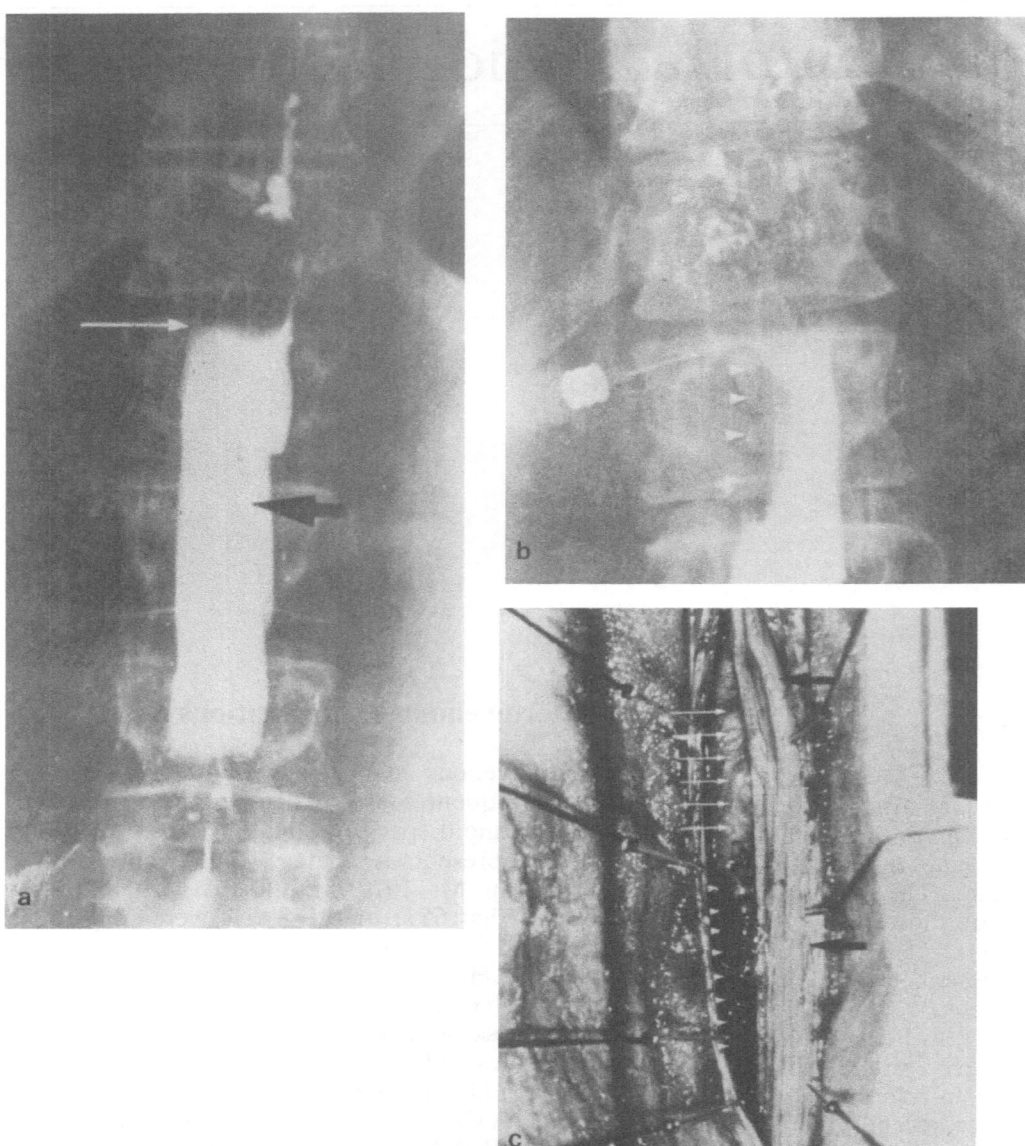

Fig. 16.1a–c. Patient with a T12/L1 neurofibroma, who had a spinal SAH during myelography. **a** Myelogram showing intradural extramedullary lesion at T12/L1. **b** Rescreen myelogram 10 days later now shows an irregular filling defect at L1 below the tumour site (*arrowheads*). **c** At operation a typical neurofibroma (*white arrows*) was seen, and immediately below the tumour is a blood clot (*arrowheads*) corresponding to the irregular filling defect shown in *b*. (Reproduced by courtesy of the Journal of Neurosurgery)

1939; Fincher 1951; Mendelsohn and Mora 1958; Odom 1961; Nassar and Correll 1968; Gibberd et al. 1972; Buge et al. 1974; Nijensohn et al. (1974), and neurofibroma (Krayenbuhl 1947; Fincher 1951; Halpern et al. 1958; Prieto and Cantu 1967; Gautier Smith 1967; Gnollmus 1975; Rice et al.

1978). Abbott (1939) described a very interesting case of spinal SAH in a 16-year-old boy who developed severe backache and bilateral leg pain following attempts at a high jump. This was followed by headache, weakness and flexor spasms of the left leg, nuchal rigidity and a positive Kernig's sign. Diagnostic lumbar puncture showed a uniformly blood-stained CSF. The patient recovered satisfactorily, but over the ensuing 14 months had 25 similar attacks. Myelography was eventually carried out and showed a block at L1, and at surgery a large encapsulated ependymoma attached to the filum terminale, associated with extensive amounts of blood clot, was found.

Other reports of tumours associated with spinal SAH include meningioma (Nassar and Correll 1968), meningioblastoma (Roger et al. 1949), meningeal sarcoma (in a 3.5-month-old child; Tarlov and Keener 1953), capillary angioblastoma (Henson and Croft 1956), spongioblastoma (Rodger et al. 1949), melanoblastoma (Heidrich 1970), cervical astrocytoma (Bhandari 1969), spinal haemangioblastoma (Kormos et al. 1980) and spinal cavernous haemangioma (Heimberger et al. 1982). Lombardo et al. (1968) reported a very unusual case of spinal endometriosis with repeated spinal SAH related to the patient's menstrual periods.

It has been postulated that friable vessels within the tumour or bridging veins from the tumour capsule to surrounding membranes rupture as a result of differential movement of the spinal contents relative to the spinal canal (Nassar and Correll 1968).

Spinal SAH following myelography is rare, but has been described by Rice et al. (1978) in a patient with a conus neurofibroma (Fig. 16.1).

Djindjian M. et al. (1978) in an analysis of 50 cases of spinal SAH due to tumour found that ependymoma was the cause in 64% of cases and neurofibroma in 18%. The remaining 18% were due to meningioma (two cases), astrocytoma (five cases), haemangioblastoma (one case) and meningeal sarcoma (one case).

Spinal Arterial Aneurysms

Spinal arterial aneurysms are rare and are often associated with an AVM (Herdt et al. 1971). The incidence of an AVM associated with an aneurysm in the spinal cord is about 6%–7%; the same as in the brain (Miyamoto et al. 1983).

Spinal aneurysms may present as cord compression (Hopkins et al. 1966; Leech et al. 1976) or SAH (Henson and Croft 1956; Garcia et al. 1979; Moore et al. 1982). The incidence of spinal SAH increases when an AVM is associated with an aneurysm (Miyamoto et al. 1983). In such a situation, the source of haemorrhage is often the

aneurysm (Herdt et al. 1971). The haemodynamic disturbance associated with AVM is an important factor in the development of spinal aneurysm (Miyamoto et al. 1983). In a case of spinal SAH, if an AVM is observed on investigation, a coexistent saccular aneurysm should be excluded (Herdt et al. 1971). Caroscio et al. (1980) reviewed the literature, and found only 14 cases of spinal AVMs associated with aneurysms, to which they added one case of their own.

In 1981, Vincent successfully clipped the first spinal aneurysm.

Trauma

Spinal SAH resulting from trauma is exceedingly rare. Minor trauma or strenuous physical activity has been implicated as a precipitating factor in some cases of SAH arising from an AVM or tumour. Norell (1965) described a case in which migration of a threaded Steinmann pin from an acromioclavicular joint into the spinal canal produced SAH. Spinal SAH following lumbar puncture has been described by King and Glas (1980) and Rengachary and Murphy (1974).

Blood Dyscrasias

Blood dyscrasias can give rise to spinal SAH (Walton 1953; Wilson 1955) and it has been reported in association with anticoagulant therapy (Yohl 1955; Middleston 1965; Bouzarth and Gutterman 1968).

Other Causes

Henson and Croft (1956) reported a case of spinal SAH in a 24-day-old child with spina bifida and meningocele due to rupture of a mycotic aneurysm on a lumbar artery.

Other reported causes of spontaneous spinal SAH include coarctation of the aorta (Wyburn Mason 1943; Watson 1967), polyarteritis nodosa (Henson and Croft 1956), systemic lupus erythematosus (Fody et al. 1980) and pseudoxanthoma elasticum (Kito et al. 1983). Alexander et al. (1982) have described a patient with primary Sjögren's syndrome in which spinal SAH occurred as a result of necrotising anterior spinal arteritis. The cause of a spinal SAH may remain undiagnosed even after extensive investigation (Swann et al. 1984).

Clinical Features

The classical history is of a sudden onset of back pain, initially at the site of the lesion and later spreading to the rest of the back, followed by radicular pain and meningism. The diagnosis will be obvious when SAH is accompanied by paraplegia or quadriplegia. The diagnosis is ultimately confirmed at lumbar puncture, which will show a uniformly blood-stained CSF. However, the distinction between spinal and cranial SAH may be difficult and will be described later.

Henson and Croft (1956) divided the clinical features of spinal SAH into three groups:

1. Those produced by blood in the spinal subarachnoid space. This gives rise to the sudden and often severe back pain at the site of the lesion which usually then spreads to the abdomen or down the leg in a sciatic distribution. A past history of recurrent episodes of back pain suggestive of intermittent spinal SAH is common (Coroscio et al. 1980; Henson and Croft 1956; Prieto and Cantu 1967). There may be signs of spinal meningeal irritation, e.g. rigidity of the spine, opisthotonus, and marked hyperaesthesia in the distribution of the affected nerve roots. Kernig's sign is always positive. If, however, the spinal haemorrhage results in a focal haematoma, there may be spinal cord compression and only local meningeal signs (Ruff 1978).

2. Intracranial extension of the haemorrhage. This may give rise to headache, vomiting, photophobia, disturbance of conscious level and other signs of raised intracranial pressure which typically may be delayed for some hours after the onset of back pain. Loss of consciousness was reported in 12% of patients with spinal SAH (Caroscio et al. 1980), but Prieto and Cantu (1967) state that it is rare. These features occur more frequently if the bleeding occurs in the cervical region and occasionally its onset is so dramatic and severe that confusion with an intracranial source of haemorrhage may occur. In such a situation the negative results of four vessel angiography may be misleadingly reassuring.

3. Damage to the spinal cord and nerve roots. Neurological evidence of spinal cord dysfunction in the acute period is often absent but may result from either haematomyelia or from compression of the cord by blood clot. Djindjian R. (1978) states, however, that neurological signs associated with spinal SAH result from the phenomenon of cord softening, which very likely follows early spasm of the arterial feeders to the AVM.

Organisation of the blood clot may be responsible for continued compression of the cord long after the haemorrhage, or this may arise from the development of arachnoid adhesions. Hydrocephalus which requires a shunt is also a rare complication.

Differential Diagnosis

The differential diagnosis of sudden onset of back pain followed by radicular pain and meningism would include consideration of acute disc prolapse, epidural abscess, poliomyelitis and spinal vascular accident. A diagnostic lumbar puncture will confirm the presence of an SAH and help differentiate it from these other conditions. Differentiation between SAH of intracranial and spinal origin is extremely important since it may save the patient needless cerebral angiographic investigation. Pia (1978) has emphasised the difficulty in making the diagnosis. In ten out of 25 cases an intracranial SAH due to aneurysm was assumed and cerebral angiography carried out. In seven of these cases, subsequent recurrent haemorrhage occurred. In nine cases a spinal SAH was not entertained, of which five cases were misdiagnosed as other spinal lesions, e.g. tumour (two cases), myelitis (one case), anterior spinal syndrome (one case) and trauma (one case). Aminoff (1976), in his analysis of spinal SAH cases, states that the majority of the patients were initially investigated by carotid and vertebral angiography to visualise an intracranial source of the bleed. This is not surprising considering that the majority of haemorrhages occur from cervical AVMs.

The following features may help suggest a spinal rather than an intracranial origin of an SAH

1. Lumbar and radicular pain more severe than backache
2. A normal level of consciousness
3. Rapidly clearing cerebral symptoms while lower cord symptoms remain severe or grow worse
4. Neurological signs of cord or root dysfunction
5. A previous history of acute back pain or sciatica in the absence of trauma

6. A bruit audible over the spine
7. The presence of subhyaloid haemorrhages would be suggestive of an intracranial origin since this has not been described in association with spinal SAH

Investigations

Apart from diagnostic lumbar puncture the following investigations are usually carried out:

Plain X-Rays

Plain X-rays of the spine will be normal in the majority of cases. Particularly in children, large AVMs can produce an enlargement of the spinal canal with pedicular erosion (Fig. 16.9). Similar changes may also be produced by ependymomas and neurofibromas in the region of the conus, which are the most common tumours to give rise to a spinal SAH. More specific plain X-ray changes indicating the possibility of an underlying AVM (e.g. segmental vertebral haemangioma, calcification in the AVM) are exceedingly rare. The plain X-ray changes in 150 cases of AVM of the spinal cord reported by Djindjian R. (1978) are shown in Table 16.1. He pointed out that in one-third of cases plain X-rays were helpful in determining the anatomical site of the malformation.

Table 16.1. Plain X-rays of the spine: 150 cases of spinal angioma (Djindjian R., 1978)

Evidence of expanding intraspinal lesion:	
Enlargement of the spinal canal	15 cases
Erosion of pedicle	11 cases
Erosion of posterior aspect of the vertebral body	4 cases
Localised scoliosis or kyphoscoliosis	15 cases
Localised signs:	
Segmental vertebral angioma	5 cases
Spina bifida	5 cases
Calcification in AVM	1 case

Myelography

Myelography in the presence of an AVM shows the typical multiple serpiginous filling defects or "bag of worms" appearance due to hypertrophied arteries and veins (Figs. 16.2, 16.3). A similar appearance, however, may be produced by prominent vessels in association with a tumour causing obstruction, by highly vascular tumours (e.g. haemangioblastomas) and by the redundant nerve root syndrome and lumbar canal stenosis (Fig. 16.4). In the presence of adhesive arachnoiditis secondary to recurrent SAHs, the myelographic appearances may be atypical. In the series reported by Djindjian R. (1978) myelography was abnormal in 93% of cases: in 62% there was the specific appearance of an angioma and in 31% there was evidence of a block or delay on screening without a typical appearance. In 7% of cases the myelogram was normal. Small AVMs not demonstrated at myelography may, however, be subsequently shown by selective spinal angiography (Djindjian R. 1978). Filling defects due to blood clot may be demonstrated if myelography is carried out in the early stages of the disease (Fig. 16.5). Emergency myelography in the presence of spinal cord compression may demonstrate evidence of extramedullary compression by haematoma or the presence of a haematomyelia (Fig. 16.6). Myelography is preferably carried out using the non-ionic water-soluble contrast media, since Myodil may react with blood and its breakdown products in the subarachnoid space, thus increasing the risk of developing arachnoiditis. In addition, one will also avoid the problem of retained Myodil obscuring vascular detail on subsequent spinal angiography.

Spinal Computerised Tomography

CT may show evidence of abnormal contrast enhancement in the region of abnormal vessels of an AVM (Di Chiro et al. 1977). Enlarged arteries or veins on the surface of the spinal cord may be demonstrated as abnormally enhancing structures on contrast-enhanced studies, or as filling defects in a metrizamide-enhanced subarachnoid space (Haughton and Williams 1982). CT will also demonstrate evidence of blood clot in the subarachnoid space or within the spinal cord (haematomyelia). Abnormal enhancement of a vascular malformation and a tumour may be indistinguishable at CT. The pattern and time course of the enhancement on dynamic CT studies, however, may help differentiate the two (Haughton and Williams 1982). CT scanning with i.v. contrast enhancement may prove a useful screening test prior to definitive spinal angiography. Dramatic demonstration of spinal AVMs at CT following intra-arterial injection of contrast has also been described (Nagashima et al. 1981). It remains

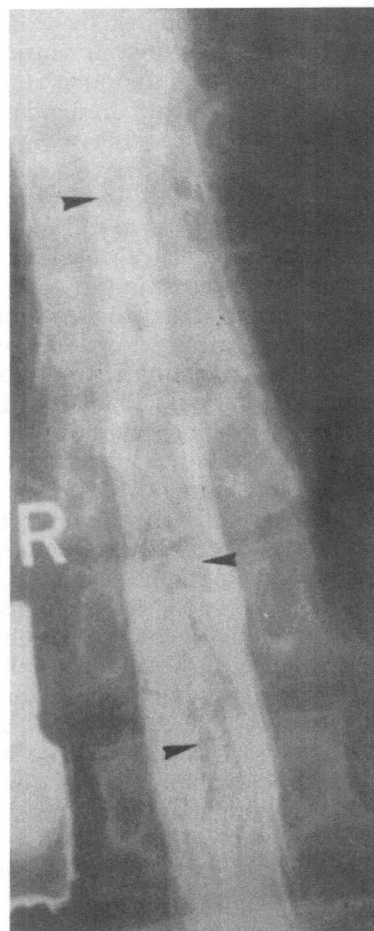

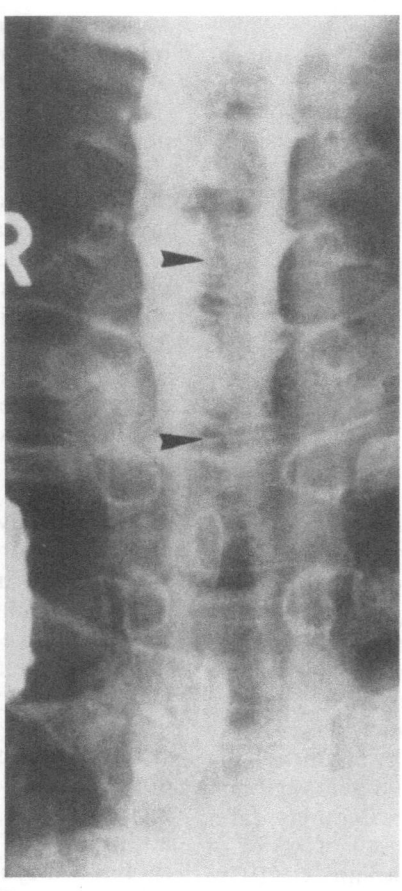

Fig. 16.2a, b. Iopamidol myelogram showing an extensive AVM (*arrowheads*) in the region of the conus and in the dorsal and cervical region.

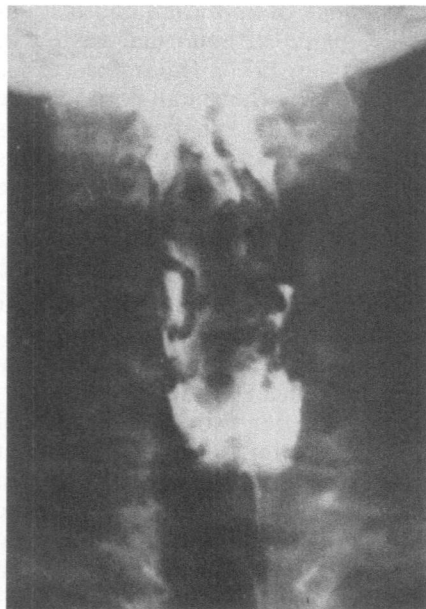

Fig. 16.3. Myodil myelogram showing multiple serpiginous filling defects or "bag of worms" appearance characteristic of an AVM.

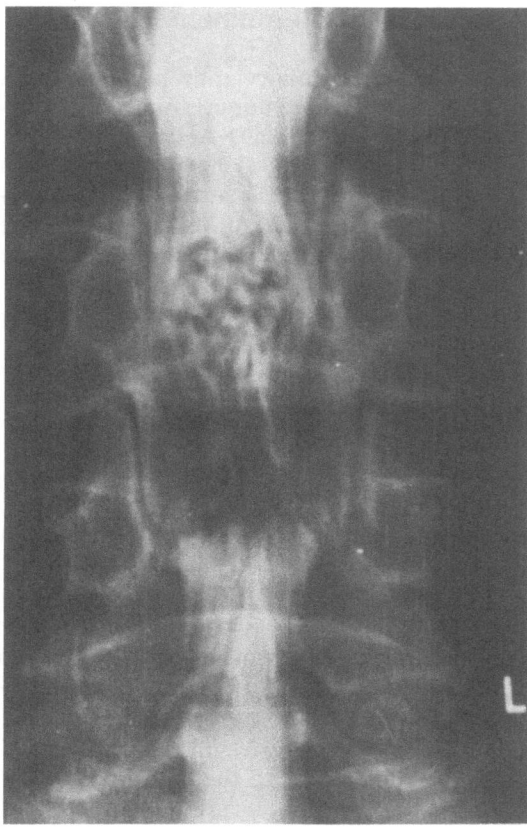

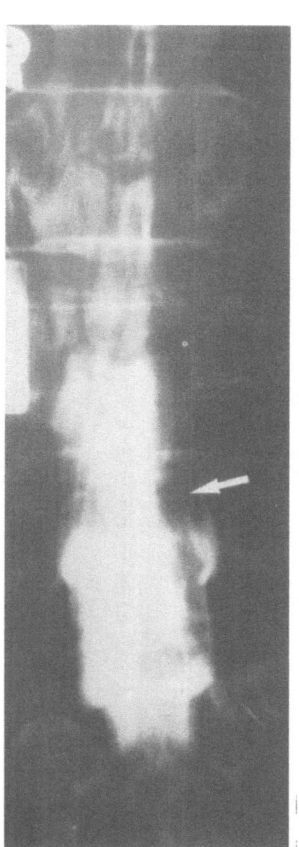

Fig. 16.4. A patient with lumbar canal stenosis with a large L4/5 disc protrusion. There are prominent serpiginous intradural filling defects which may be due to redundant nerve roots or prominent veins.

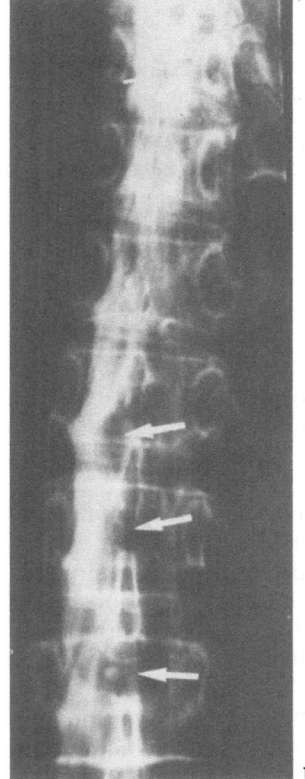

Fig. 16.5a, b. Female of 45 years with sudden onset of back pain followed by neck stiffness and a positive Kernig's sign. L.P. was uniformly blood-stained, and myelography showed multiple defects due to blood clot in the subarachnoid space (*arrows*) in the lumbar and dorsal regions. A repeat myelogram 2 months later showed disappearance of the clot but no AVM could be seen.

Nuclear Magnetic Resonance

Nuclear magnetic resonance may prove to be a valuable non-invasive technique for demonstrating spinal AVMs and spinal SAH and its cause. Modic and Weinstein (1984) have reported two cases of spinal AVM (one central and one thoracic) in which NMR scans using SE_1 technique clearly differentiated the soft tissue mass of the AVM from the CSF and spinal cord.

Selective Spinal Angiography

If an AVM has been demonstrated at myelography, and surgical treatment is contemplated, selective spinal angiography should be carried out to:

1. Demonstrate arterial feeders
2. Demonstrate the relationship of the AVM to the cord, e.g. dural vs intradural and intramedullary vs posterior
3. Define the artery of Adamkiewicz and see whether it contributes to the AVM

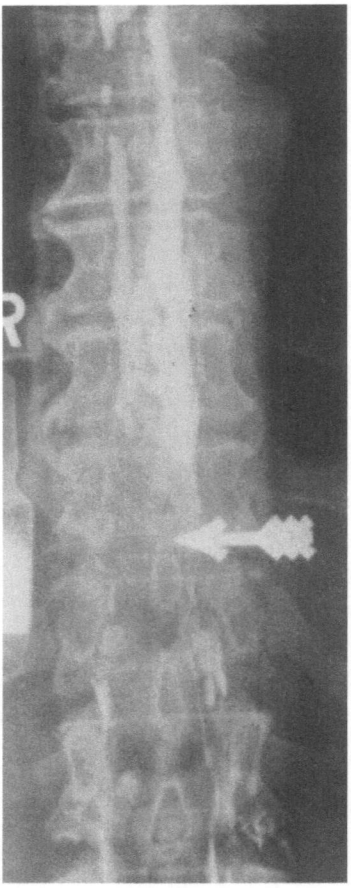

Fig. 16.6. A 60-year-old female presenting with sudden onset of interscapular pain followed by fluctuating weakness of the legs and bladder retention. On examination there was neck stiffness and a positive Kernig's sign. Cisternal puncture revealed uniformly blood stained CSF and myelography showed an almost complete block at D11 (*arrow*). At operation, an extensive subdural haematoma was found and evacuated. In addition there was evidence of a spinal cord AVM.

difficult, however, to decide at CT whether an AVM is superficial to or lying within the spinal cord, and this, of course, is crucial to the question of operability.

Guinto et al. (1984) have suggested a combined technique of intrathecal metrizamide and arterial injection of contrast medium during dynamic CT to demonstrate clearly the exact relationship of the AVM to the spinal cord, where this relationship cannot be resolved at myelography and angiography.

CT may be a useful follow-up examination after surgical or embolisation attempts to assess the effectiveness of treatment.

Anatomy of Spinal Vessels

The spinal cord is supplied by a single anterior spinal and paired posterior spinal arteries, which in turn are fed by the radiculo-medullary arteries. A detailed description of the blood supply of the spinal cord is provided by Lazorthes (1978). The spinal cord can be divided into three distinct vascular territories according to their unequal blood supply (Lazorthes 1978) (Fig. 16.7).

a) *The Cervicothoracic Region (C1–D2).* The first four cervical segments (C1–C4) are supplied by the anterior spinal artery, which originates from the convergence of two branches arising from the vertebral arteries. The last four cervical segments and first two thoracic segments (C5–D2) constitute the cervical enlargement and have an independent blood supply from two to four large radicular arteries originating from the vertebral arteries and the ascending and deep cervical arteries. The lowest radicular artery, which follows the course of the seventh and/or eighth cervical root, is the most important and has been designated the artery of the cervical enlargement.

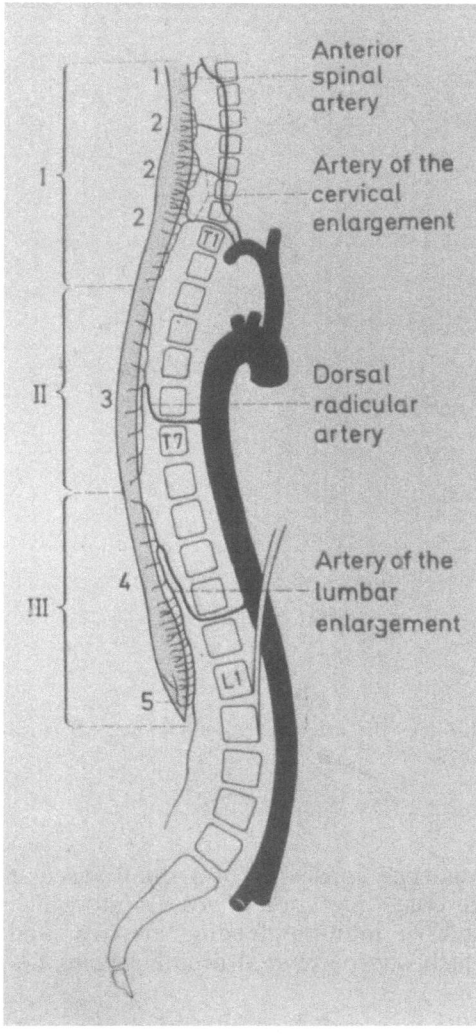

Fig. 16.7. The three vascular territories of the spinal cord (Lazorthes 1978).

b) *The Midthoracic Region (D3–D7).* The midthoracic region has a poorer blood supply and is, therefore, more prone to ischaemia. The anterior spinal artery is usually supplied by a single radiculo-medullary artery, most frequently the right or left fourth intercostal.

c) *The Thoracolumbar Region (D8 to Conus).* The anterior spinal artery is supplied by one large artery—the radiculo-medullary magna (artery of the lumbar enlargement, artery of Adamkiewicz). The origin of this vessel is very variable, but the most common site of origin is from the left intercostal or lumbar arteries between D9 and L2.

Technique

The patient is examined under general anaesthetic, since injection of ionic contrast into the intercostal arteries under local anaesthesia produces considerable discomfort to the patient.

The use of non-ionic contrast media (iopamidol, iohexol) enables one to carry out pain-free spinal angiography under local anaesthesia. In addition, Kendall (1979) has shown that the complication rate of selective spinal angiography with non-ionic contrast media is significantly less.

The patient is catheterised from the femoral route, using a femoral-visceral catheter (No. 3 for adults). The arteries supplying the suspected area of interest are first catheterised under fluoroscopic control, until the vessels supplying the AVM are located. In the cervical region, this may mean catheterisation of the vertebral arteries and the costocervical, thyrocervical and deep cervical arteries. Examination of the dorsolumbar region may in fact require selective catheterisation of up to ten pairs of intercostal arteries and five pairs of lumbar arteries. Once the site of the AVM is established, however, the examination can safely be limited to selective catheterisation of three pairs of vessels above and below the lesion.

Type of Arteriovenous Malformation

It is possible to distinguish two main types of AVM (Djindjian R. 1978):

1. Those with a posterior blood supply, which are called extramedullary or retromedullary, and which constitute approximately 40% of cases. This type never has an intramedullary component and only very rarely produces an SAH.
2. Those with an anterior or mixed (anterior or posterior) blood supply, which constitute 60% of cases. The majority of spinal SAHs occur with this type of AVM.

In Djindjian's series, 93% of the AVM were partly or completely intramedullary, and only 7% extramedullary. At angiography the AVM consists of:

1. Arterial feeding vessels
2. An angiomatous mass of variable size and appearance
3. Draining veins (Fig. 16.8)

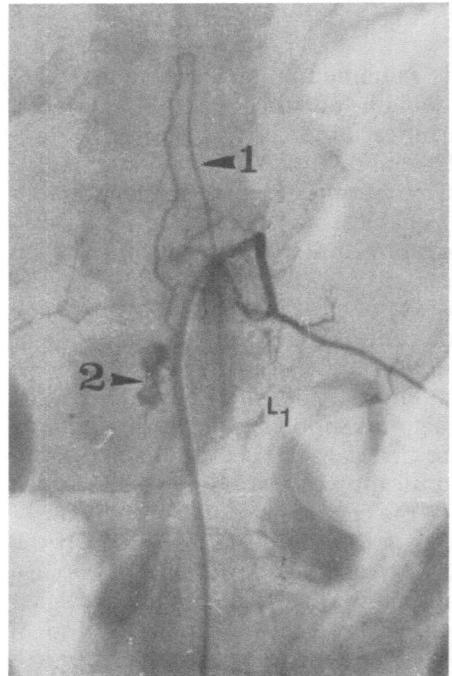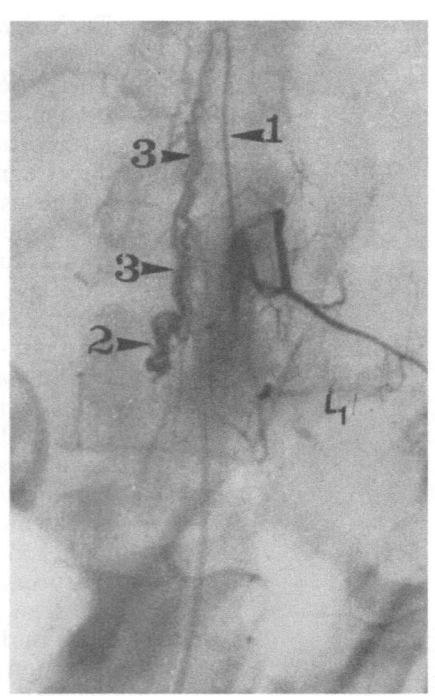

Fig. 16.8a, b. Typical AVM consisting of (*1*) arterial feeding vessel, in this case the artery of Adamkiewicz, (*2*) small angiomatous mass and (*3*) ascending draining veins.

Feeding Vessels

Arterial feeding vessels are likely to be multiple in about 70% of cases. In the cervical region they are usually multiple and come from the vertebral arteries, the thyrocervical trunk, the costocervical trunk and the deep cervical arteries (Fig. 16.9).

In the dorsal region, the feeding artery is the anterior superior radiculo-medullary artery; it may arise on the right or left from the third, fourth or fifth intercostal artery, or, as is very often the case, from a common trunk ascending from the fourth or fifth intercostal artery.

In the thoracolumbar region the feeding artery is the artery of Adamkiewicz (Fig. 16.8).

Angiomatous Mass

Three patterns can be distinguished (Ommaya et al. 1969; Di Chiro et al. 1971; Di Chiro and Wener 1973):

1. A simple arteriovenous fistula in which no angiomatous mass is seen, and the recognition of the change from arterial to venous is difficult, even on histological examination.

2. A glomus type consisting of a small vascular plexus or conglomeration of vessels into which run single or multiple feeding arteries, and from which one or several draining veins depart (Fig. 16.8).

3. A juvenile type, in which multiple large feeding vessels supply a very large vascular mass which fills the spinal canal and usually penetrates the spinal cord (Fig. 16.9).

Venous Drainage

The venous drainage of intramedullary AVMs is into the anterior spinal vein which runs on the anterior aspect of the cord behind the anterior spinal artery.

Digital Subtraction Angiography

Intravenous digital subtraction angiography (DSA) can demonstrate larger AVMs but is not adequate to define the feeding vessels. In addition, small AVMs will be missed (Doppman et al. 1983).

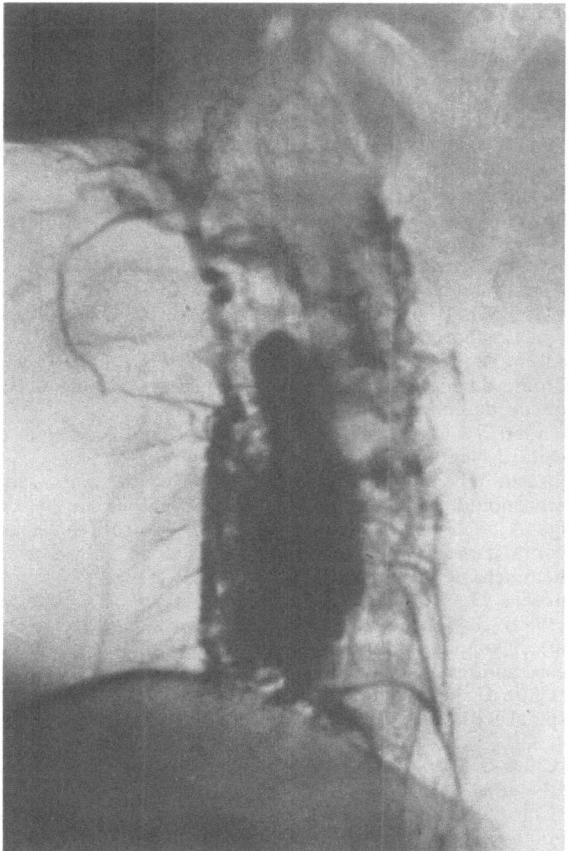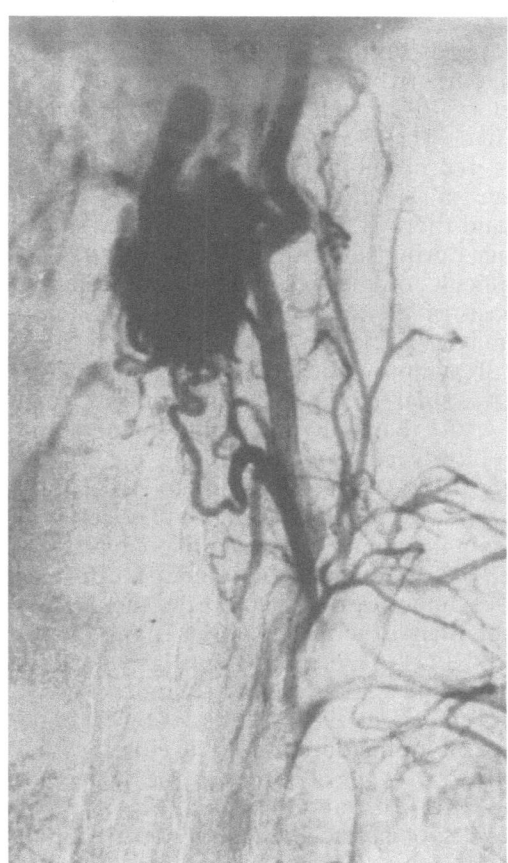

Fig. 16.9. Selective subclavian angiogram (**a** lateral and **b** AP projections) showing large juvenile type AVM of the cervical region with multiple feeding vessels from the vertebral artery, costocervical trunk and deep cervical trunk.

Selective intra-arterial DSA provides excellent diagnostic studies with significantly lower doses of contrast media and, therefore, decreased risk of spinal cord damage.

Natural History and Outcome

Aminoff (1976) has made a very detailed study of 63 cases of spinal AVM presenting with SAH. A patient who has had a spinal SAH has just over a 50% chance of developing a subsequent bleed, and in about 40% of these it will occur within 1 year. The overall mortality from spinal SAH was 15%.

Management of Spinal Arteriovenous Malformations

In evaluating the surgical treatment of spinal AVMs, the natural course of untreated cases should be borne in mind. Spinal vascular malformations remain asymptomatic for many years. However, once the patients begin to have symptoms, either slow progression or repeated episodes of increasing deficit will ensue. In 19% of cases the disease progresses rapidly, and patients become severely disabled within 1–2 months if not treated. In another 31% the disease has a subacute course. The remaining 50% have a very slow progressive course (Aminoff and Logue 1974).

The ideal method of treatment for an AVM is surgical excision based on pre-operative selective angiography. Successful surgical treatment of AVMs depends on their position and type. Posterior angiomas which are fed by the posterior lateral arteries are usually extramedullary and are comparatively easy to excise. Anteriorly placed angiomas, fed by the anterior spinal arterial system, have a significant intramedullary component, and there is a considerable risk of spinal cord injury during surgical excision.

It is difficult to assess operability of the lesion on the basis of the angiogram alone, and sometimes it may even be misleading (Post and Stein 1982). All symptomatic AVMs should be explored. A spinal cord AVM, in contrast to a cerebral AVM, has only one or two feeders and angiographically controlled selective ligation of the feeding arteries has been found to give a good result (Ommaya et al. 1969). Unlike cerebral AVMs, spinal angiomas are supplied by "nonessential" vessels, such as the intercostal or lumbar arteries, and they do not exert the sump effect because of their slow flow phenomenon (Doppman et al. 1971). Decompressive laminectomy alone makes the patient worse (Ommaya et al. 1969; Post and Stein 1982). If the lesion is found to be inoperable, the dura should be closed with a patch graft to prevent adhesion to the surface of the spinal cord (Post and Stein 1982).

The results of surgical excision depend upon the pre-operative condition of the patients (Krayenbuhl et al. 1969; Aminoff and Logue 1974; Post and Stein 1982). In about 80%–90% of patients, surgery will help in arresting or improving the neurological deficit (Post and Stein 1982). There were only three patients with poor results in Krayenbuhl et al.'s 1969 series of 17 patients.

Radiation therapy was found not to be beneficial in the treatment of spinal vascular malformations (Post and Stein 1982).

Embolisation of the AVM, using various substances, has also been practised in recent years (Doppman et al. 1971; Hilal et al. 1978). The technique is not feasible when the feeding arteries originate from the vertebral artery or when the posterior lateral feeding arteries arise from a common trunk, which also contributes to the anterior spinal artery system. The embolisation of spinal AVM is also limited because of the flow pattern of the feeding arteries (Doppman et al. 1971). With the advent of superselective catheterisation techniques, and the use of polymerizing agents (Kerber 1975), embolisation of spinal AVM may result in total obliteration of the lesion.

References

Abbott KH (1939) SAH from an ependymoma arising in the filum terminale. Bull Los Angeles Neurol Soc 4:127–132

Alexander EL, Craft C, Dorsch C, Moser RL, Provost TT, Alexander GE (1982) Necrotizing arteritis and spinal subarachnoid haemorrhage in Sjögren's syndrome. Ann Neurol 11:632–635

Aminoff MJ, Logue V (1974) The prognosis of patients with spinal vascular malformation. Brain 97:211–218

Aminoff MJ (1976) Spinal angiomas. Blackwell, Oxford London Edinburgh Melbourne

Andrew-Thomas F, Schaeffer H, De Marte LT (1930) Syndrome d'hémorrhagie mée réalisee par une tumeur de la queue de cheval. Paris Med 77:292–296

Bhandari YS (1969) SAH due to cervical cord tumour in a child. J Neurosurg 30:749–751

Bouzarth WF, Gutterman P (1968) Delayed traumatic subarachnoid haemorrhage. JAMA 205:880–881

Buge A, Phillipon J, Poisson M (1974) Hydrocéphalie au cours d'une épendymome de la queue de cheval avec hémorrhagie menargée. Nouv Pres Méd 2:1083–1086

Caroscio JT, Brannan T, Budah M, Huang YP, Yahr M (1980) Subarachnoid haemorrhage secondary to spinal arteriovenous malformation and aneurysm—report of a case and review of the literature. Arch Neurol 37:101–103

Di Chiro G, Doppman JL, Ommaya AK (1971) Radiology of spinal cord arterio-venous malformations. Prog Neurol Surg 4:329–354

Di Chiro G, Wener RL (1973) Angiography of the spinal cord. J Neurosurg 39:1–20

Di Chiro G, Doppman JL, Wener L (1977) Computed tomography of spinal cord arteriovenous malformations. Radiology 123:351–354

Djindjian M (1978) Clinical symptomatology and natural history of AVMs of the spinal cord.—A study of the clinical aspects and prognosis based on 150 cases. In Pia HW, Djindjian R (eds). Spinal angiomas. Advances in diagnosis and therapy. Springer, Berlin New York Heidelberg, pp 75–83

Djindjian R (1978) Angiographs in angiomas of the spinal cord. In: Pia HW, Djindjian R (eds) Spinal angiomas. Advances in diagnosis and therapy. Springer, Berlin New York Heidelberg, pp 98–136

Doppman JL, Di Chiro G, Ommaya AK (1971) Percutaneous embolisation of spinal cord arteriovenous malformation. J Neurosurg 34:48–55

Doppman JL, Kandy HG, Miller DL, Oldfield E, Di Chiro G (1983) Intraarterial digital subtraction angiography of spinal arteriovenous malformations. Am J Neuroradiol 4:1081–1085

Duverney GJ (1682) Histoire de l'Academie Royale des Sciences (1733) Tome II, p 28

Fincher EF (1951) Spontaneous SAH in intradural tumours of the lumbar sac—a clinical syndrome. J Neurosurg 8:576–584

Fody EP, Netsky MG, Mrak RE (1980) Subarachnoid spinal hemorrhage in a case of systemic lupus erythematosus. Arch Neurol 37:173–174

Garcia CA, Dulcey S, Dulcey J (1979) Ruptured aneurysm of the spinal artery of Adamkiewicz during pregnancy. Neurology 29:394–398

Gautier Smith PC (1967) Clinical aspects of spinal neurofibromas. Brain 90:359–394

Gibberd FB, Ngan G, Swan GF (1972) Hydrocephalus, subarachnoid haemorrhage and ependymomas of the cauda equina. Clin Radiol 23:422–426

Gnollmus J (1975) Spinal subarachnoid haemorrhage with Schwannoma. Acta Neurochir 31:253–256

Guinto FC, Nauta HJW, Haslim H, Pislarodi APM (1984) Dynamic computed tomography scanning with combined metrizamide and arterial bolus injection in arteriovenous malformation of the spinal cord. Surg Neurol 22:181–185

Halpern L, Foldman S, Peyser E (1958) SAH with papilloedema due to spinal neurofibroma. Arch Neurol Psychiatry 79:138–141

Hash CH, Grossman CB, Shenkin HA (1975) Concurrent intracranial and spinal cord arteriovenous malformations. Case report. J Neurosurg 43:104–107

Haughton VM, Williams AL (1982) Computed tomography of the spine. Mosby, St. Louis Toronto London, pp 42–45

Heidrich R (1965) Spinale subarachnoid Blutung. Munch Med Wochenschr 107:2011

Heimberger K, Schnaberth G, Koo W, Pendl G, Auff E (1982) Spinal cavernous haemangioma (intradural extramedullary) underlying repeated subarachnoid haemorrhage. J Neurol 226:289–293

Henson RA, Croft PB (1956) Spontaneous spinal subarachnoid haemorrhage. Q J Med 25:53–66

Herdt JR, Di Chiro G, Doppman JL (1971) Combined arterial and arteriovenous aneurysm of the spinal cord. Radiology 99:589–593

Hilal SK, Sane P, Michelson WJ et al. (1978) The embolisation of vascular malformations of the spinal cord with low viscosity silicone rubber. Neuroradiology 16:430–433

Hopkins CA, Wilkie FL, Vons D (1966) Extramedullary aneurysm of the spinal cord. J Neurosurg 24:1021–1023

Kendall BE (1979) Spinal angiography with metrizamide. In: Grainger RG, Lamb JT (eds) Myelographic techniques with metrizamide. Nyegaard U.K. Ltd., pp 147–152

Kerber CA (1975) Intracranial cyanoacrylate. A new catheter therapy for AVM. Invest Radiol 10:536

King OJ, Glas WW (1960) Spinal subarachnoid haemorrhage following lumbar puncture. Arch Surg 80:574–577

Kito K, Kobayashi N, Mori H et al. (1983) Ruptured aneurysm of the anterior spinal artery associated with pseudoxanthoma elasticum. Case report. J Neurosurg 58:126–128

Kormos RL, Tucker WS, Bilbao JM, Gladstone RM, Bass AG (1980) Subarachnoid haemorrhage due to spinal cord haemangioblastoma. Case report. Neurosurgery 6:657–660

Krayenbuhl H (1947) Spontane spinale Subarachnoidalblutung und akute Rückenmarkskompression bei intraduralem, spinalem Neurinom. Schweiz Med Wochenschr 77:692

Krayenbuhl H, Yasargil MG, McClintock HG (1969) Treatment of spinal cord vascular malformation by surgical excision. J Neurosurg 30:427–435

Lazorthes G (1978) Blood supply and vascular pathology of the spinal cord. In: Pia HW, Djindjian R (eds) Spinal angiomas. Advances in diagnosis and therapy. Springer, Berlin Heidelberg New York, pp 1–17

Leech PJ, Strokes BAR, Apsimon T, Harper C (1976) Unruptured aneurysm of the ambient spinal artery presenting as paraparesis. J Neurosurg 45:331–333

Lombardo L, Mateos JM, Barroeta FF (1968) Subarachnoid haemorrhage due to endometriosis of the spinal canal. Neurology 18:423–426

Mendelsohn RA, Mora F (1958) Spontaneous SAH caused by ependymoma of the filum terminale. J Neurosurg 15:450–463

Michon PL (1928) Coup de poignard rachidien. Presse Med 36:964

Middleston GD (1965) A case of spinal SAH complicating anticoagulant therapy. Br J Clin Pract 19:414–415

Miyamoto S, Kikuchi H, Karasawa J, Ikota T, Nagata I (1983) Spinal cord arteriovenous malformations associated with spinal aneurysms. Neurology 13:577–580

Modic MT, Weinstein MA (1984) Nuclear magnetic resonance of the spine. Br Med Bull 40:183–186

Moore DW, Hunt WE, Zimmerman JE (1982) Ruptured anterior spinal artery aneurysm repair via a posterior approach. Neurosurgery 10:626–630

Morgagni JB (1761) De sedibus et acausis morborum. Venetiis

Nagashima C, Yamaguchi T, Tsuji R (1981) Arteriovenous malformation of the spinal cord: Computed tomography with intra-arterial enhancement. J Comput Assist Tomogr 5:586–587

Nasser SI, Correll JW (1968) SAH due to spinal cord tumours. Neurology 18:87–94

Nijensohn DE, Laventman J, Miller RH, Gomez MR (1974) Repeated occult spinal subarachnoid haemorrhage and spinal cord ependymoma, Minn Med 57:687–699

Norell H Jr (1965) Migration of a threaded Steinmann pin from an acromio-clavicular joint into the spinal canal. J Bone Joint Surg [Am] 47:1024–1026

Odom GL (1961) Vascular lesions of the spinal cord: malformations, spinal subarachnoid and extradural haemorrhage. Clin Neurosurg 8:196–236

Ommaya AK, Di Chiro G, Doppman JL (1969) Ligation of arterial supply in the treatment of spinal cord AVM. J Neurosurg 30:679–692

Parkinson D, West M (1977) Spontaneous subarachnoid haemorrhage first from an intracranial then from a spinal arteriovenous malformation. Case report. J Neurosurg 47:965–968

Pia HW (1978) Symptomatology of spinal angiomas. In: Spinal angiomas—advances in diagnosis and therapy. In: Pia HW, Djindjian R (eds) Spinal angiomas. Advances in diagnosis and therapy. Springer, Berlin Heidelberg New York, pp 48–74

Post KD, Stein BM (1982) Surgical management of spinal cord tumours and AVMs. In: Schmidek HH, Sweet WH (eds) Operative neurosurgical techniques. Grune and Stratton, New York London, pp 1445–1475

Prieto A Jr, Cantu RC (1967) Spinal subarachnoid haemorrhage associated with neurofibroma of the cauda equina. J Neurosurg 27:63–69

Rengachary SS, Murphy D (1974) Subarachnoid haemorrhage following lumbar puncture causing compression of the cauda equina. J Neurosurg 41:252–254

Rice JF, Shields CB, Morris CF, Neely BD (1978) Spinal SAH during myelography. J Neurosurg 48:645–648

Roger H, Paillas JE, Duplay J (1949) Hémorragie méningée spinocérébrale révélatrice d'une tumuer de la queue de chaval chez 2 jeunes sujets. Bul Med Soc Med Hop 64:37–40

Ruff RL (1978) Cord compression from spinal SAH (letter). Arch Neurol 37:467

Swann KW, Ropper AH, New PFJ, Poletti CE (1984) Spontaneous spinal subarachnoid hemorrhage and subdural haematoma. Report of two cases. J Neurosurg 61:975–980

Tarlov IM, Keener EP (1958) SAH and tumour implants from spinal sarcoma in an infant. Neurology 3:384–390

Vincent FM (1981) Anterior spinal artery aneurysm presenting as a SAH. Stroke 12:230–232

Walton JN (1953) Subarachnoid haemorrhage of unusual aetiology. Neurology 3:517

Walton JN (1956) Subarachnoid haemorrhage. Livingstone, Edinburgh

Watson AB (1967) Spinal subarachnoid haemorrhage in a patient with coarctation of aorta. Br Med J IV:278

Wilson SAK (1955) Neurology, 2nd edn, vol 3. Butterworth, London

Wyburn-Mason R (1943) The vascular abnormalities and tumours of the spinal cord and its membranes. Kimpton, London

Yohl ET (1955) Spontaneous intraspinal haemorrhage and paraplegia complicating bishydroxycoumarol therapy. Arch Neurol Psychiatry 73:570–572

17 Future Developments

Introduction

Subarachnoid haemorrhage is a potentially lethal and yet eminently curable disease. Based on the incidence of SAH, which is 10.3 per 100 000 of the population according to Garaway et al. (1979), about 6 000 persons in the United Kingdom will suffer an SAH due to an aneurysmal rupture annually. Kassell and Drake (1983) have quoted an incidence of 12 per 100 000 for the United States, with an annual incidence of 28 000 patients with aneurysmal SAH. The surgical treatment of ruptured aneurysm has undoubtedly improved, with neurosurgeons like Yasargil and Fox (1975) reporting a remarkably low operative mortality of 1.9%. However, it has been estimated that only 30% of patients habouring a ruptured aneurysm survive without major disability (Kassell and Drake 1983).

Figure 17.1 shows Kassell and Drake's analysis of the various outcomes in this group of 28 000 patients, which will form the basis of the discussion in this chapter. Clearly, the factors which may result in a better outcome include improvement in diagnosis, earlier referral to specialist centres, prevention of rebleeding, and a better understanding and treatment of vasospasm and its ischaemic complications.

In addition, in this chapter we will evaluate the potential value of the new imaging techniques (e.g. computerised tomography, position emission tomography, digital vascular angiography and magnetic resonance imaging) in the management of patients with SAH.

Prevention of Subarachnoid Haemorrhage

It can be seen from Fig. 17.1 that a little over 10% of patients will die of SAH without warning. Ideally, one would like to be able to detect the presence of an aneurysm or AVM so that it could be surgically treated before fatal bleeding occurs. What we need is an accurate, non-invasive test, so that patients at risk, e.g. those with a family history of SAH, patients with polycystic kidneys or coarctation of the aorta, hypertensive patients, and particularly those with suspected warning leaks, can be screened. The potential role of the less invasive neuroradiological techniques, such as digital subtraction angiography (DSA) and computerised axial tomography scanning (CT scan) will be discussed later in the chapter. Once having identified patients harbouring an underlying asymptomatic aneurysm or AVM, we need to establish more accurate criteria for predicting the risk of a subsequent SAH. Dell (1982) suggested that the risk of rupture of an asymptomatic aneurysm is of the order of approximately 15% in the 10- to 50-year-old age group, and slightly less

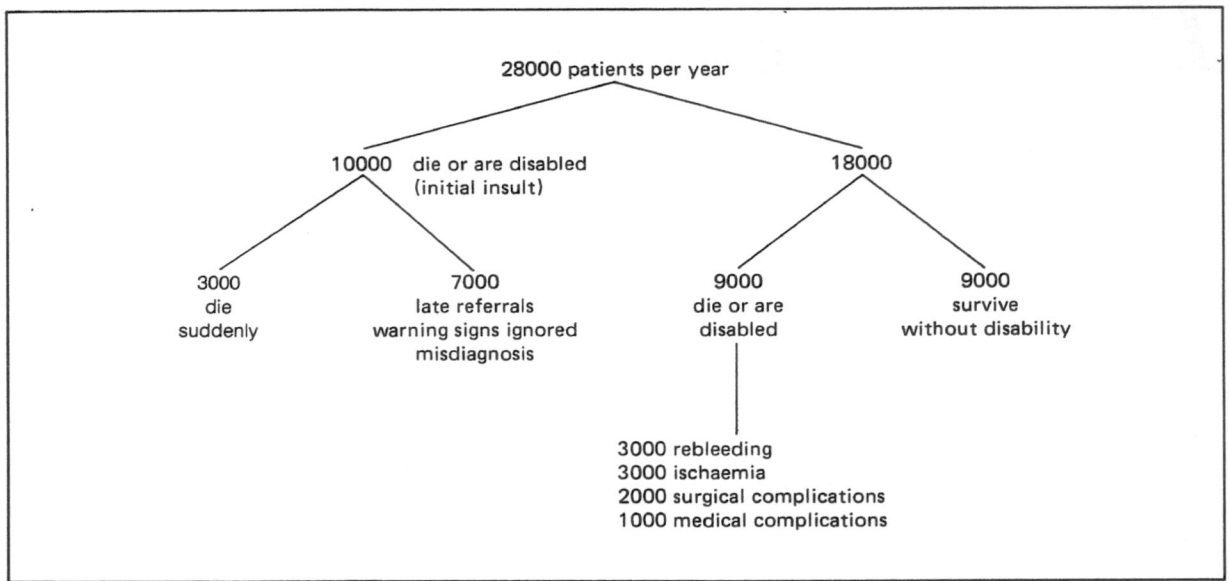

Fig. 17.1. Kassell and Drake's algorithm for patients with SAH in the United States.

Improved Diagnosis

It is surprising how frequently SAH is still misdiagnosed. The classic presentation is usually easy to recognise, but it may frequently present in a more subtle bizarre way, and the physician's index of suspicion must be high. The clinical manifestations of SAH, including some of the more atypical features, have been discussed in Chap. 4, and the differential diagnosis of more common presentations has been described in Chap. 5.

Twenty-five per cent of patients will die or be disabled prior to reaching a neurosurgeon, and it is in this group that perhaps the most immediate improvement in the prognosis of SAH can be made. This group consists of patients in whom the warning signs are ignored by either themselves or their attending physician. The diagnosis of SAH is not made at the time of the initial haemorrhage or it is only made retrospectively, and rather tragically, at the time of a second, usually more severe or even fatal haemorrhage.

Undoubtedly the most frequently ignored early warning sign is that of abrupt onset of severe headache. In such circumstances one must entertain the diagnosis, and once thought of, it is not difficult to confirm by lumbar puncture or by CT scanning, if it is available.

Treatment of the Complications of Subarachnoid Haemorrhage

If we turn our attention to the right-hand side of Fig. 17.1, one can see that of the 64% of patients who survive to reach a neurosurgical centre, approximately half of these will die or be severely disabled as a result of rebleeding, cerebral infarction and surgical or medical complications. The remainder of this group do well with current therapy.

Rebleeding

Drake (1968) has stated that "it is probably true that if we could learn how to keep a patient safe from re-bleeding for a week or longer, especially in the obtunded patient with cerebral symptoms, the problems of surgery of ruptured intracranial aneurysms would nearly be solved". The recent trends aimed at preventing rebleeding have included (a) early surgery and (b) the use of antifibrinolytic therapy. Although it has generally been accepted that the peak incidence of rebleeding is at the end of the first week following the initial rupture of an aneurysm, more recent evidence from the Co-operative Aneurysm Study would suggest that the peak incidence for rebleeding may be in the first 2 days (Kassell and Drake 1983). Thus, the rationale of early surgery is to clip the aneurysm before the peak incidence of rebleeding, and also prior to the onset of vasospasm. The role of early surgery for ruptured intracranial aneurysms, however, remains controversial. Recent reports of early surgery have been encouraging, with favourable outcomes in approximately 70% of cases (Suzuki et al. 1979; Weir and Aronyk 1981). Timing of aneurysm surgery has been the subject of a large multinational co-operative study organised by the University of Iowa in collaboration with 68 neurosurgical centres (including Newcastle) in 15 countries. Data were collected on 3521 cases, to hopefully resolve the dispute about early surgery. A preliminary report on this study has been published recently (Kassell and Torner 1984). The early surgery group (0–3 days) and late surgery group (7–14 days) compiled in this study were extraordinarily similar as regards key prognostic factors. After statistical adjustment for differing prognostic factors there was no statistically difference between the two planned intervals for mortality and good recovery (Kassel, Torner and Jane 1985, personal communication).

The overall management results determined at 6 months after SAH were disappointing considering the high percentage (80%) who were in good condition on admission. Only 58% were classified as having a good recovery according to the Glasgow Outcome Disability Scale and 27.0% had died. In 16% the patient had a vegetative survival or was moderately to severely disabled. It is interesting to note that the leading cause of mortality and morbidity was vasospasm, which had twice the importance of rebleeding in this regard.

There is evidence that antifibrinolytic therapy reduces the incidence of rebleeding (Sengupta et al. 1976). The effectiveness of these drugs has not been definitely proved, however, despite an abundance of literature. The multicentre randomised controlled double blind trial (Lindsay et al. 1983) demonstrated that antifibrinolytic therapy with tranexamic acid does not improve outcome in patients with SAH as assessed at 3 months. This is not due to failure in antifibrinolytic action as rebleeding was reduced from 24% in the control group to 9% in the treatment group, but

to a concurrent increase in the incidence of ischaemic complications. These authors suggest that by taking measures to reduce ischaemic complications, antifibrinolytic therapy may still have a role in the management of SAH. The current evidence suggests that although antifibrinolytics may decrease the incidence of rebleeding, the overall mortality is unaltered due to an increased incidence of cerebral infarction (Kassell et al. 1984).

Vasospasm

Vasospasm remains a challenging and, as yet, unsolved problem in the management of patients with SAH. Three aspects have received considerable attention in the recent medical literature: (a) prediction of vasospasm, (b) prevention of vasospasm and (c) treatment of vasospasm.

Prediction

It would be of considerable value to predict early those patients who are likely to develop vasospasm and its neurological ischaemic complications. The amount of blood demonstrated at CT in the subarachnoid cisterns may be very useful in predicting the incidence and severity of vasospasm (Kistler 1982). Tazawa et al. (1983) demonstrated a high correlation between prominent enhancement of the basal subarachnoid cisterns on the CT scan during the first 3 days after the onset of SAH and the subsequent development of symptomatic vasospasm. If these reports are confirmed, then it is possible that the CT scan may be useful in predicting those patients who are likely to experience vasospasm with its ischaemic complications.

Nornes and Aaslid (1983) have described a transcranial Doppler method of evaluating vasospasm and its time course following SAH by determination of the flow velocities in the middle cerebral arteries. A recent report (Aaslid et al. 1984) suggests that the technique may prove a useful bedside technique for assessment of vasospasm.

Prevention

In theory one should be able to prevent vasospasm by carrying out early surgery with removal of blood clots from the basal subarachnoid cisterns. Mizukami et al. (1982) have reported a low incidence of symptomatic vasospasm in those patients in whom the postoperative CT scan confirms that blood has been successfully removed. Recent experimental work has suggested that lavage of the subarachnoid cisterns with a fibrinolytic solution may be beneficial (Peterson et al. 1980).

Treatment

At present the underlying mechanism and thus the treatment of vasospasm has not been elucidated. There is no ideal animal model and the vasoconstrictor substances have not been identified. Numerous drugs which have been used for experimental and clinical studies to relieve vasospasm have been reviewed by Wilkins (1980). Recently, the calcium channel blocking agents, such as Nephedipine and Nimodipine, have been shown to be successful in preventing and reversing experimental vasospasm (Cohen and Allen 1979). A clinical report of the value of topically applied Nimodipine in the prevention of symptomatic vasospasm has recently been reported by Auer et al. (1982). Auer (1984) reports on 65 patients operated within 48–72 h of the SAH who were treated with Nimodipine locally and systematically. Only 6% of patients developed delayed ischaemic neurological deficit presumably related to vasospasm, and the deficit was permanent in only 3% of cases. This compares favourably with results from the International Cooperative Study on the timing of aneurysm surgery, in which the rate of delayed ischaemic neurological deficit was 30%, with permanent impairment in 15% (Kassell and Torner 1984). One could argue, however, that Auer's excellent results were as much due to early surgery as Nimodipine therapy. Grotenhuis et al. (1984) were unable to show any change in cerebral vessel calibre at angiography in patients with vasospasm after intracarotid slow bolus injection of Nimodipine. The importance of reduced cerebral perfusion in the production of ischaemia following SAH has already been discussed in a previous chapter, and we know that blood flow is directly proportional to the perfusion pressure. In a number of cases ischaemic deficit resulting from vasospasm can be reversed by increasing the intravascular volume and arterial pressure (preferably after clipping of the aneurysm). Naloxone has been shown to increase local cerebral blood flow (Faden et al. 1982) and prostacyclin is a very powerful vasodilator; both these drugs may have a future role to play in the management of vasospasm and cerebral ischaemia (Awad et al. 1983).

Merory et al. (1980) measured the cerebral blood flow by the non-invasive xenon clearance technique in patients having surgical treatment of a ruptured intracranial aneurysm. The groups of patients were defined by the presence or absence of a postoperative rise of cerebral blood flow. In 29 patients there was a rise in cerebral blood flow on the first postoperative day; of these, 24 were alert and only four were drowsy. In contrast, of the 16 patients with no rise in cerebral blood flow, only four were alert.

Improved Surgical Techniques

The two major advances in surgical technique in recent years have been the development of the torsion bar clip and the increased use of the operating microscope. Surgery of giant aneurysms, however, still remains a formidable task. The introduction of the technique of extracranial/intracranial by-pass procedure has helped in solving some of the problems of treating giant aneurysms. Balloon occlusion has been used successfully in the management of caroticocavernous fistulae (Serbinenko 1974), and although the treatment of aneurysms with detachable balloons has been reported (Debrun et al. 1981), the technique is more difficult since the arterial blood flow does not always carry the balloon to the aneurysmal pouch. There is a risk of rupture when the balloon is inflated. In some circumstances it is possible to retain the arterial blood flow, but in others the anatomical features of the aneurysm make occlusion of the parent vessel necessary.

Methods of surgical obliteration of aneurysms may be altered in future. Alksne and Smith (1980) reported stereotactic occlusion of 22 anterior communicating artery aneurysms, with promising results. The patients whose aneurysms could be treated trans-sphenoidally enjoyed the best outcome. With the help of computers, calculation of the precise location of the target may be possible in future, to make the stereotactic method a worthwhile advance.

Another future possibility of aneurysmal obliteration is the percutaneous introduction of a glue-like material, which may be injected through a small calibre catheter, which, under fluoroscopic control, has been placed at the origin of the aneurysm. With human capabilities, if it is possible to land on the moon with a group of scientists directing the machine from a control room, it is not inconceivable that a team of neurosurgeons, neuroradiologists and others may achieve obliteration of an aneurysm without craniotomy.

Technical advances in the treatment of arteriovenous malformations include embolisation techniques and stereotactic radiotherapy. These techniques are at present undergoing evaluation, and have been discussed in Chap. 13.

New Imaging Techniques

During the last decade significant new developments in diagnostic imaging technology have taken place, including computerised tomography, positron emission tomography, digital vascular imaging and nuclear magnetic reasonance. The clinician now has a variety of non-invasive and invasive diagnostic procedures with which to investigate patients with SAH. The exact role which these new developments will have in the diagnosis and management of SAH is yet to be evaluated. It seems appropriate, however, to review their potential applications.

Computerised Tomography

CT scanning, as outlined in Chap. 6, has already made revolutionary contributions to the diagnosis and management of patients with SAH. The technology of computerised tomography has continued to advance, with numerous computer software developments, including fast scanning times, which are especially valuable for the restless patient, multiplanar CT reconstruction and dynamic scanning facilites. New generation high resolution CT systems undoubtedly will be able to demonstrate small aneurysms with contrast-enhanced scans, which could be used for screening high-risk patients (Fig. 17.2). The value of CT in predicting the likely development of vasospasm has already been discussed. Dynamic CT scanning using a bolus intravenous contrast injection, making use of regional transit times of contrast, has been used to estimate cerebral blood flow, but it is limited by the fact that it cannot provide quantitative flow values. Dynamic CT scanning, using the rate of clearance of stable xenon, has been used to provide precise quantitative information about cerebral blood flow. Though safe, xenon has the disadvantage of being both expensive and an anaesthetic.

Positron Emission Tomography

Positron emission tomography (PET) is a technique for measuring radio-isotope tracer concentrations regionally within the body. The great attraction of positron emission tomography is that it can show us not only brain anatomy, but also function. At the Hammersmith Hospital in London, the ECAT positron camera and oxygen[15], a short-lived positron emitting isotope of oxygen, have been used for non-invasive tomography measurement of regional cerebral blood flow, oxygen extraction and oxygen utilisation quantitatively (Frackowiak and Wise 1983). The technique so far has mainly been applied to the study of normal cerebral physiology and to patients with stroke and dementia. There has been relatively little work done on patients with SAH, mainly because the currently installed PET scanners are not in neurosurgical centres. The technique will clearly demonstrate a brain infarct before CT changes are apparent, and it can distinguish between ischaemic and infarcted brain. It can demonstrate the change from ischaemia to infarction.

Serial studies of patients with SAH would therefore be of great value, both for research and for clinical management purposes. In addition, the results of existing and new therapeutic treatments, for example, in ischaemia due to vasospasm, could be evaluated. Follow-up studies may prove helpful in recognising patients who appear suitable for surgery on clinical grounds, but who will, nevertheless, subsequently develop neurological deterioration. Powers et al. (1985) studied regional cerebral blood flow (rCBF) and regional metabolic rate of oxygen (rCMRO$_2$) with PET in four patients with SAH and hemiparesis due to cerebral vasospasm. With resolution of vasospasm two patients recovered and two remained hemiparetic. Their findings suggest that accurate quantitative measurements of rCBF and rCMRO$_2$ may be useful in differentiating patients with reversible ischaemic neurological deficit from those with irreversible infarction. Positron emission tomography requires a cyclotron with a supply of short-lived isotopes, and since this is extremely expensive and requires an expensive team, the technique is likely to be limited to a relatively small number of medical centres.

Digital Subtraction Angiography

One of the most significant developments in diagnostic imaging recently has been the introduc-

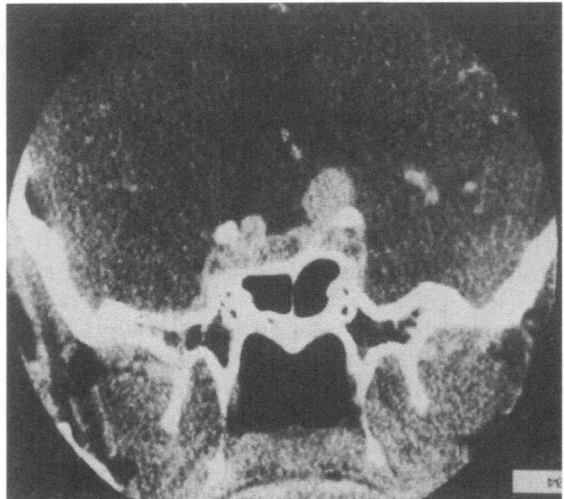

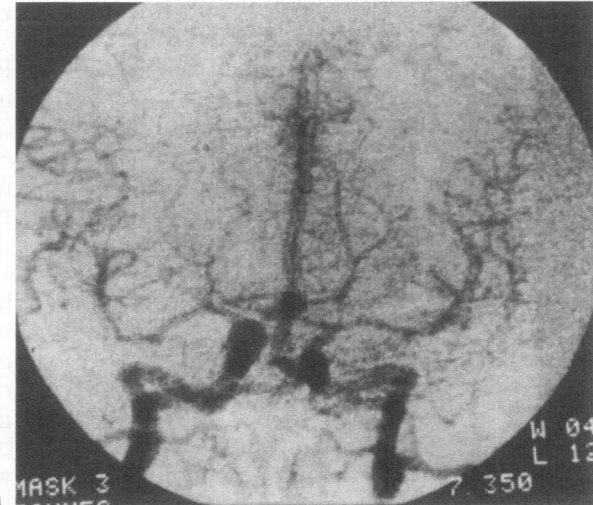

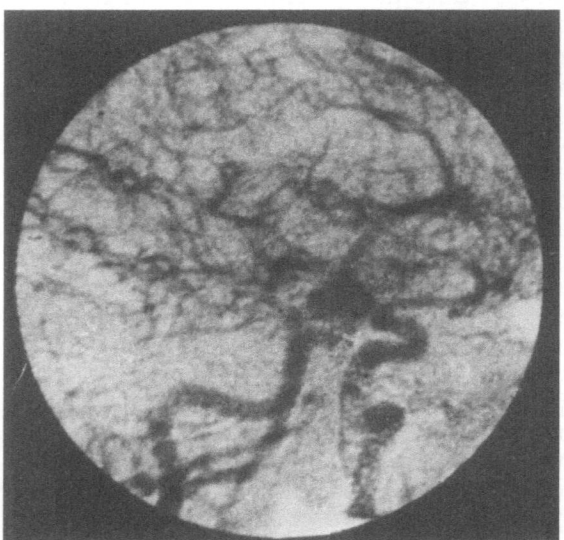

Fig. 17.2. a Contrast-enhanced direct coronal CT scan of the sella, showing an enhancing lesion consistent with an aneurysm arising from the internal carotid artery below its bifurcation. **b, c** IV-DSA: AP and oblique projections confirm the presence of a posterior communicating artery aneurysm.

tion of digital subtraction angiography (DSA), which makes it possible to visualise extracranial and, to some degree, intracranial arterial structures following intravenous injection of contrast media. This technique is made possible by real time digital processing of X-ray transmission data from image intensified video fluoroscopy systems. High-risk and asymptomatic patients can be screened by this technique with a significantly reduced risk. In addition there is likely to be a significant saving in X-ray film costs. The spatial resolution of intravenous DSA, however, is inferior to that obtained with conventional cut-film angiography.

Technique

The procedure consists of puncturing a peripheral arm vein in the antecubital fossa or the femoral vein, and inserting a catheter, which is screened under television control, into the superior vena cava. Usually 50 cc of contrast media, such as Urografin 370 mg, or non-ionic contrast media, such as iopamidol 370 or iohexol 370, are injected by pressure pump at the rate of 20 cc per second. Fluoroscopic images of the area of interest are taken and converted to digital data before the injection of contrast media, and will act as a masked image. The subsequent fluoroscopic im-

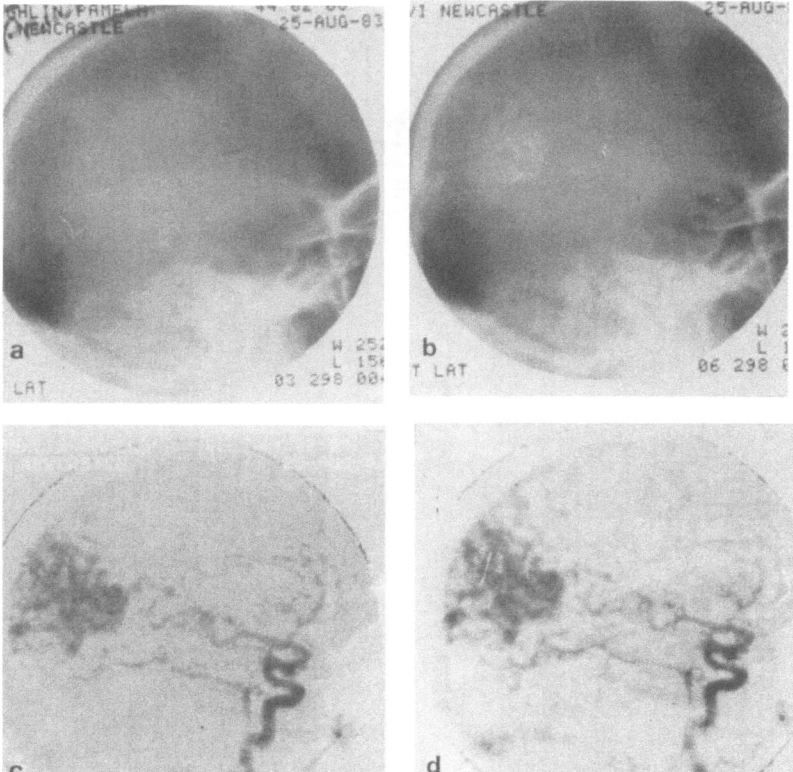

Fig. 17.3a–d. Intracranial AVM shown by IV-DSA. **a** Patient's head before i.v. injection of 50 cc of iopamidol 370. **b** Patient's head with contrast in AVM. **c** Image obtained by subtracting **a** from **b**. **d** Contrast enhancement of **c**.

ages during and after the arrival of contrast media in the arteries are also digitalised and have the masked image subtracted from them, and the resultant angiographic images are viewed in real time (Fig. 17.3). Contrast medium concentration as low as 2% within a vessel can be visualised with intravenous digital vascular imaging, whereas, without subtraction, contrast concentrations of 40%–50% would be required to provide images of equal diagnostic value.

The major limitations of the technique are related to spatial resolution, diagnostic difficulties due to overlapping of vessels and motion artefact resulting from swallowing or discomfort due to injection of the contrast medium. The use of non-ionic contrast media may reduce such motion artefacts. In some cases of patient motion, computer techniques of remasking the image or re-registration can be used to enhance the resolution of the vessels of interest.

It is convenient to distinguish between intravenous digital subtraction angiography (IV-DSA) and intra-arterial digital subtraction angiography (IA-DSA).

Intravenous Digital Subtraction Angiography

Intravenous DSA provides increased contrast resolution, but at the expense of spatial resolution of the intracranial vessels. This, together with the problems of overlapping of vessels, makes the demonstration of the intracranial arterial anatomy at the present time inferior to that achieved with conventional angiography. Intravenous DSA in the current state of the art will not replace conventional angiography, since it will not reliably demonstrate small aneurysms or clearly show the anatomy of an aneurysm's neck or its relationship to important surrounding vessels. Aneurysms larger than 1 cm can be demonstrated fairly reliably (Fig. 17.4) and large aneurysms will be clearly demonstrated (Fig. 17.5). Intravenous DSA has been used for postoperative assessment of the effectiveness of aneurysm clipping (Fig. 17.6).

Intravenous DSA may prove valuable in patients with a life-threatening haematoma to demonstrate or exclude a significant sized aneurysm or AVM prior to emergency surgical treatment.

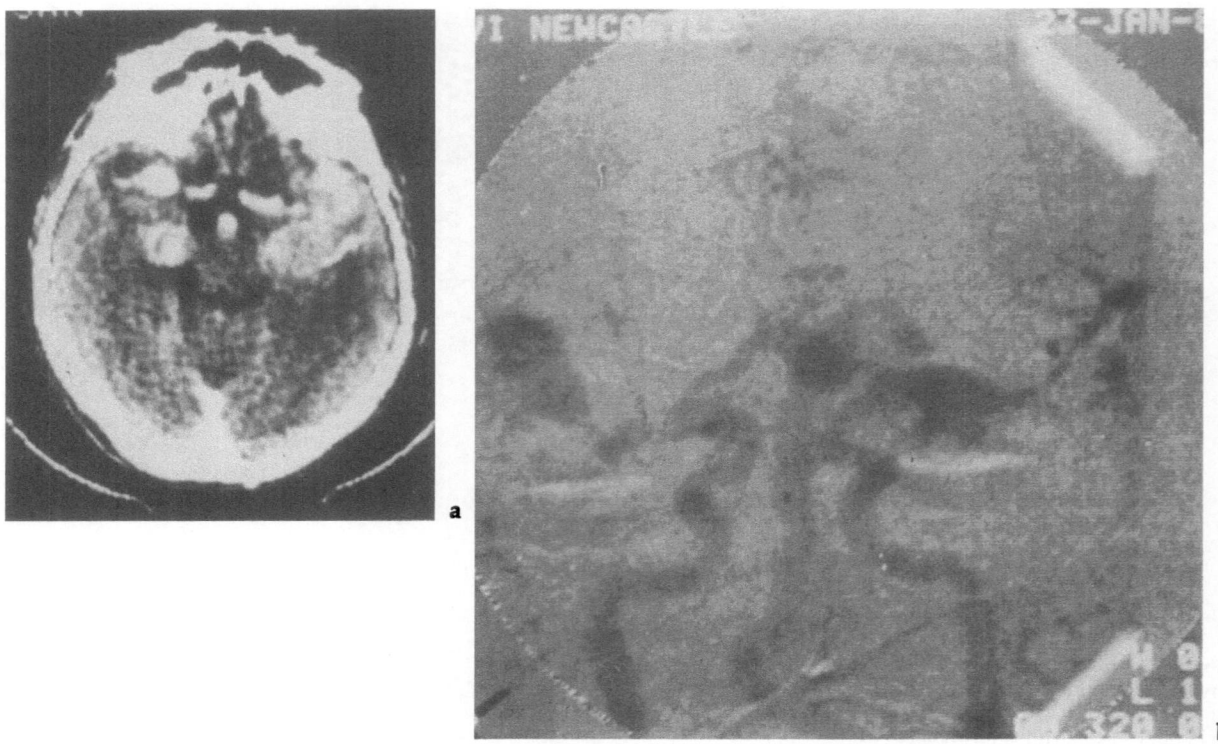

Fig. 17.4. a Contrast-enhanced CT scan showing bilateral enhancing lesions suggestive of multiple aneurysms. **b** IV-DSA confirms the presence of multiple large aneurysms.

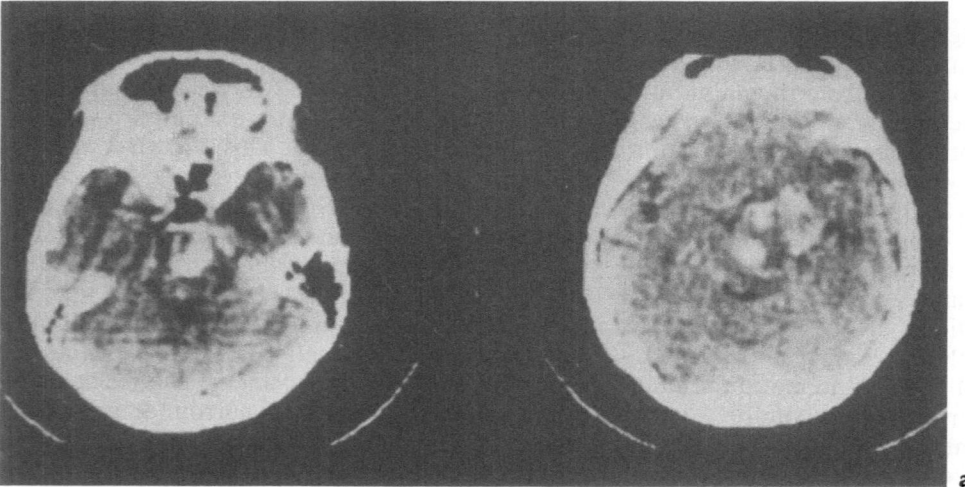

Fig. 17.5. a Contrast-enhanced CT scan showing an enhancing lesion in the right thalamic region. **b** IV-DSA showing a large partially thrombosed aneurysm. **c** Angiogram on the same case confirms that there is a large partly thrombosed aneurysm arising from the posterior cerebral artery itself.

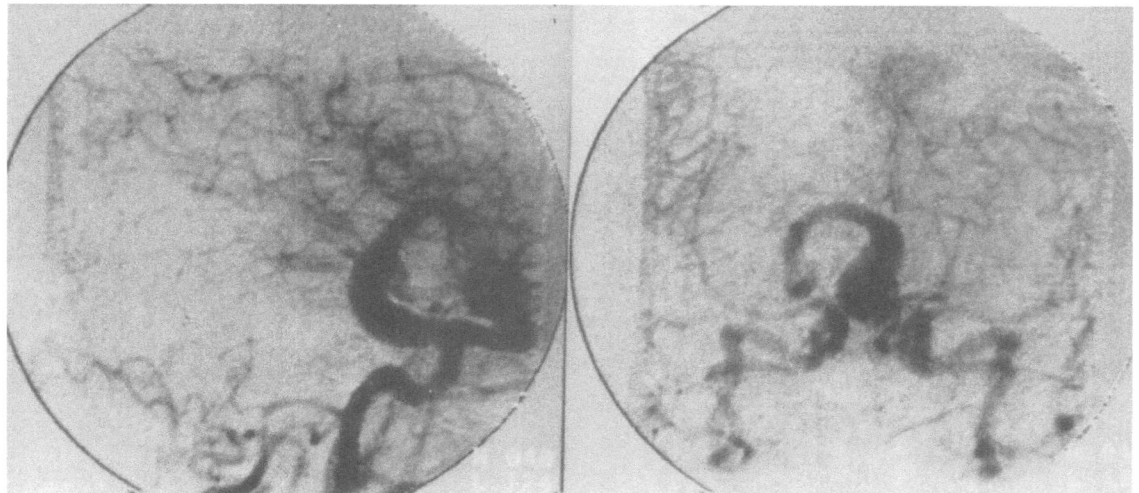

Fig. 17.5b

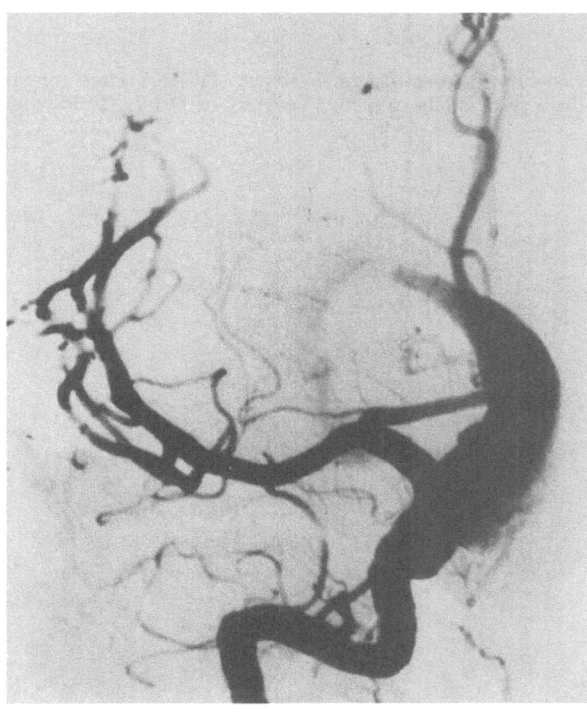

Fig. 17.5c

Because of excellent patient tolerance and low risk, it could be used to assess the natural history of incidental aneurysms or incompletely obliterated aneurysms following surgery. Intravenous DSA has proved reliable in demonstrating preoperative spasm. In the patient with aneurysm rupture who deteriorates and in whom CT scanning has excluded a rebleed, an IV-DSA study can provide documentation of arterial spasm required prior to the institution of medical therapy; in addition it can potentially assess the response to that therapy (Pinto et al. 1983).

Intravenous DSA will demonstrate medium and large intracranial arteriovenous malformations (Fig. 17.7), but again conventional angiography is required to show the precise anatomy of the feeding vessel and draining veins. Intravenous DSA is entirely satisfactory for checking postsurgical or postembolisation obliteration of an AVM.

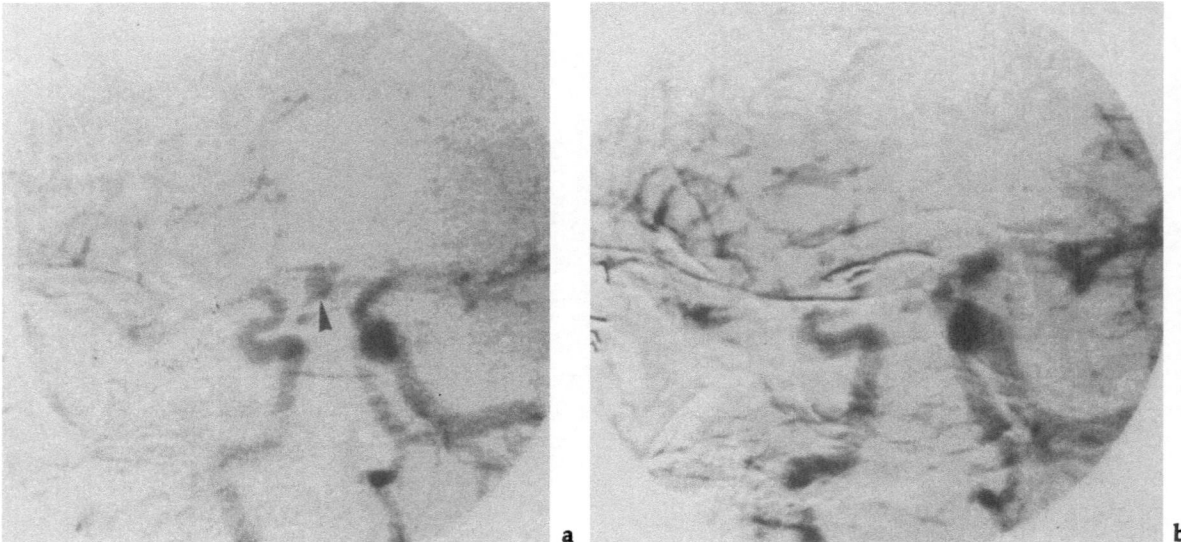

Fig. 17.6. a IV-DSA showing an anterior communicating artery aneurysm (*arrowhead*). **b** Repeat IV-DSA after surgery confirms that the anterior communicating artery aneurysm has been successfully clipped. (Courtesy of Dr. J. Occleshaw)

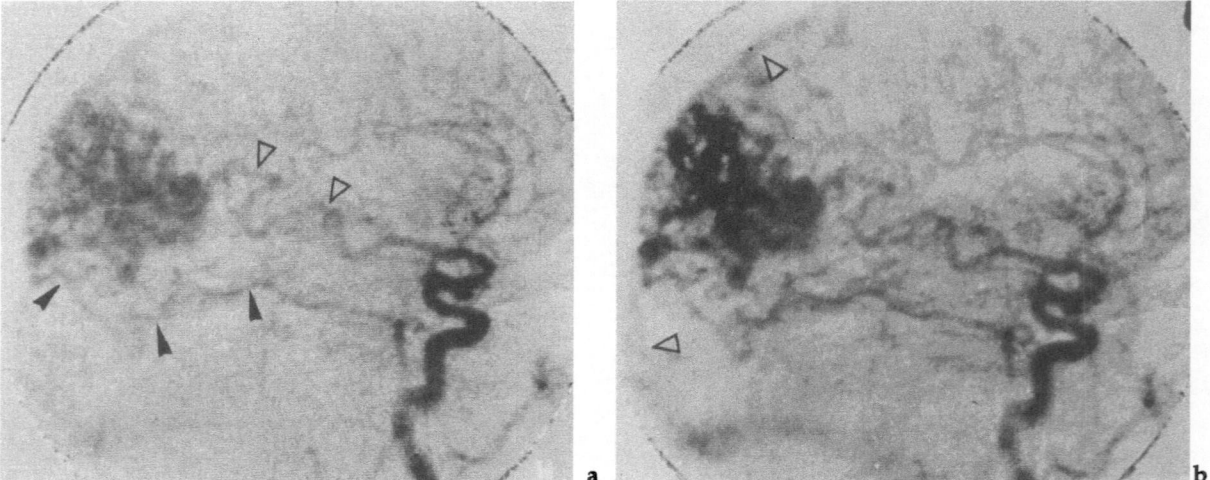

Fig. 17.7. a IV-DSA (50 cc iopamidol injected over 2 s) showing a parietal AVM with clearly demonstrated feeding vessels from the middle cerebral artery (*open arrowheads*) and posterior cerebral artery (*closed arrowheads*). **b** Slightly later phase shows early venous drainage into the sagittal sinus (*open arrowheads*).

Intra-arterial Digital Subtraction Angiography

Because of its inherent improved contrast sensitivity, IA-DSA requires less contrast media to produce a diagnostic study. The other advantage is that being real time, a subtracted image is immediately available, and one should certainly not forget the significant savings in the cost of X-rays film with this technique. An example of an IA-DSA examination, using a significantly lower contrast dosage, is demonstrated in (Fig. 17.8). In patients where selective catheterisation of the major vessels proves impossible, due to vessel tortuosity, injection of the major vessels arising from the aortic arch can provide a perfectly adequate diagnostic study. The lower dosage of

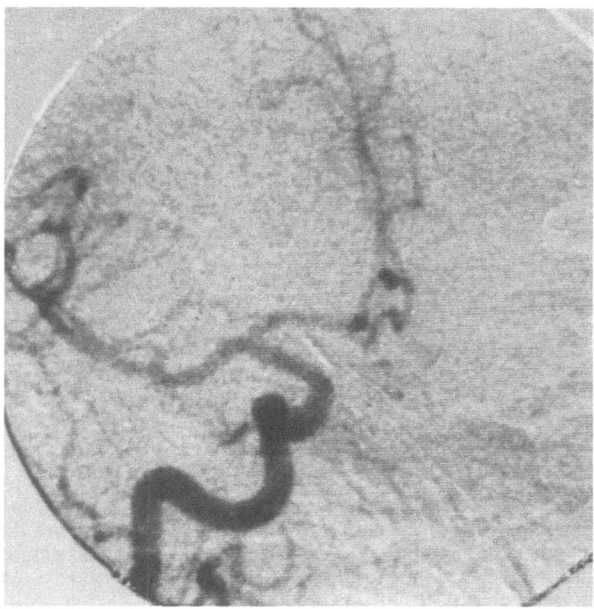

Fig. 17.8. IA-DSA showing that diagnostic studies can be obtained with small dosages of contrast media.

contrast media required and the immediate subtracted images provided make IA-DSA a very useful technique during embolisation procedures.

Functional DSA Imaging

Intravenous DSA does provide some insight into the distribution of cerebral blood flow and collateral blood flow patterns, since all vessels fill simultaneously with contrast and real time images are obtained. There does appear to be some promise that in the future it will be possible to use digital data obtained with this technique to provide quantitative information about blood flow.

Future Prospects for DSA

Intravenous DSA is likely to have limited applications in SAH, perhaps in the postoperative assessment of aneurysm or arteriovenous malformation surgery. The main role of DSA in SAH will be its intra-arterial applications. Intra-arterial DSA will probably result in shorter procedure times and the use of smaller amounts of contrast media. The concentration of contrast media can be reduced to a third and one can therefore use finer catheters (e.g. 3 or 4 F gauge) for the procedure. This should add to the safety of the procedure and significantly reduce film and non-ionic contrast

media costs. Future experience may show that the optimal system of angiographic investigation involves switching between digital and conventional angiographic techniques. Digital subtraction angiography could provide a suitable angiographic "road map" to pin-point the site (or sites) of the lesion in patients with SAH, followed by selective conventional angiography (including magnification studies) to provide more precise detail of vascular anatomy.

Magnetic Resonance Imaging[1]

Magnetic resonance imaging (MRI) is a new non-invasive method of interrogating the internal structure of the body which completely avoids the use of ionising radiation and does not appear to be associated with any significant hazard. It employs radiofrequency (RF) radiation in the presence of a carefully controlled magnetic field to produce cross-sectional maps of the body in every plane which portray the distribution density of hydrogen nuclei and parameters reflecting their motion in cellular water and lipids (the so-called T_1 and T_2 relaxation times). As with CT, there is excellent display of soft tissue detail, but with MRI there is the additional advantage of being able to manipulate the contrast between different tissues by altering the pattern of RF which is applied and this includes the ability to highlight blood vessels without the use of contrast media.

Where an aneurysm or arteriovenous malformation presents with a spontaneous SAH the purpose of any preliminary examination is to try and identify the site of bleeding so that selective angiography can be applied to identify the causal lesion. Where the clinical presentation of a large aneurysm is related to its mass effect or of an angioma to "steal" effects, the principal objective of investigation is to separate these lesions from other possible pathology. Where clinical presentation follows haemorrhage the size and position of the associated haematoma is readily assessed whether this be subarachnoid in situation or parenchymal (Fig. 17.9). Occasionally rupture occurs into the ventricular system and if the haematoma is large there may be a considerable mass effect. Acute haemorrhage is associated with a lengthening of both T_1 and T_2 relaxation times but early in the natural history of a resolv-

---

[1] The section "Magnetic Resonance Imaging" is provided by courtesy of Professor B. Worthington.

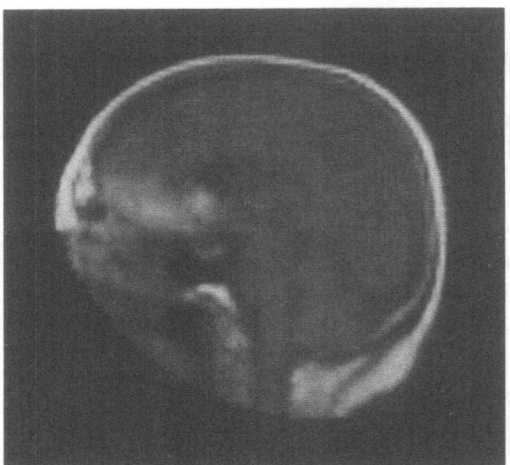

Fig. 17.9. Ruptured anterior communicating artery aneurysm showing subfrontal haematoma.

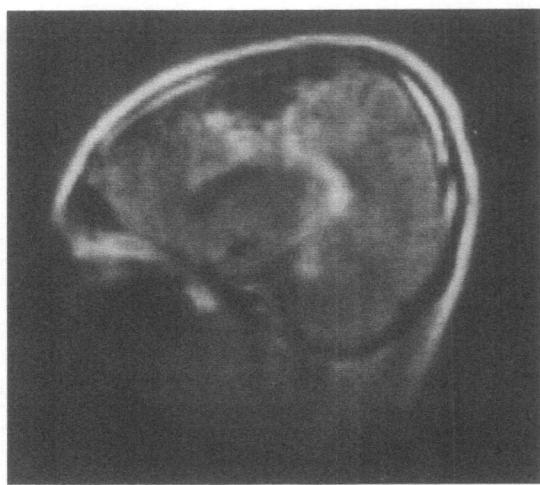

Fig. 17.11. Parasagittal NMR scan showing parasagittal angioma which has bled downwards into the hemisphere; the clot has ruptured into the ventricle. The blood in rapid motion within the angioma results in a zero signal and the vessels appear black.

ing haematoma it becomes associated with a considerably shortened T_1 time. The scan appearances parallel those seen at CT with the additional perspective of direct coronal and sagittal views. The area of liquefaction within resolving clots is readily appreciated on MRI scans and by the use of T_2 weighted scans the reaction in the brain surrounding the clot is well shown.

MRI scans are exquisitely sensitive in demonstrating infarction which gives areas of lengthened T_1 and T_2 relaxation times. As with CT, the

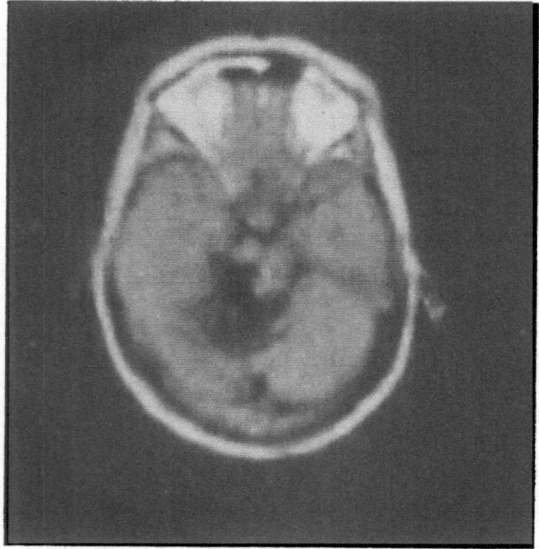

Fig. 17.10. Transverse axial NMR scan showing an angioma involving the brain stem and left cerebellar hemisphere.

development of a communicating hydrocephalus from obstructed basal cisterns is also readily shown.

Using spin sequences which highlight blood flow angiomas can be demonstrated without the need for contrast media (Figs. 17.10, 17.11). MRI only obviates the requirement for angiography where the size, position or condition of the patient precludes treatment. The technique offers a simple method for assessing the results of surgery or embolisation in achieving ablation. Flow-dependent sequences also allow a certain diagnosis of giant aneurysms where the patent lumen can be distinguished from any thrombus lining the wall, and the effects of treatment can also be assessed (Fig. 17.12). The dislodgement of a clip within the high magnetic field is a serious potential hazard for patients who may have to be examined after surgery. It is important, therefore, that non-ferromagnetic clips are employed (e.g. Kean et al. 1985). Bleeding into the subarachnoid space may also be a complication of a head injury (Fig. 17.13) or a primary intracerebral bleed in a hypertensive patient (Fig. 17.14).

Future Prospects for MRI

The authors have no direct experience with MRI as yet but can foresee several potentially valuable applications in SAH. MRI is a tremendously

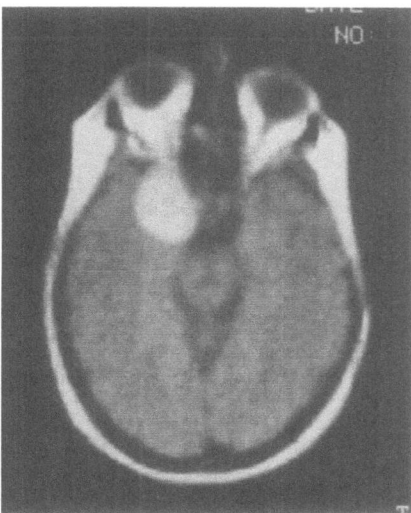

Fig. 17.12. Transverse axial NMR scan showing a large left parasellar aneurysm which has been treated by ligation. The blood within the lumen of the aneurysm has clotted, accounting for the high signal.

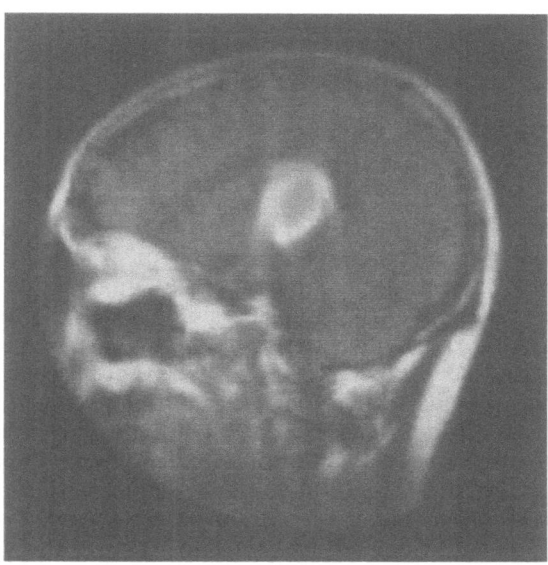

Fig. 17.14. Parasagittal NMR scan showing a haematoma in the basal ganglia. There is a central low density area which probably represents an area of liquefaction.

exciting technique since it potentially provides anatomical, physiological and biochemical information about the brain in a non-invasive manner. MRI and its clinical applications are described in detail in the British Medical Bulletin, vol. 40 (Steiner and Radda 1984).

The imaging of nuclei other than hydrogen—particularly phosphorus and sodium—is an exciting prospect. Sodium appears to be a very sensitive indicator of ischaemia and infarction and

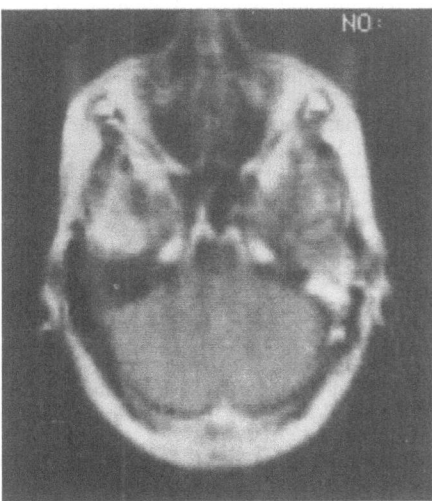

Fig. 17.13. Transverse axial NMR scan showing contusion in the anterior third of the left temporal lobe. There is a haematoma in the right middle ear cleft accounting for the patient's deafness.

preliminary results have been reported by Maudsley and Hilal (1984). It may prove possible with sodium imaging to detect reversible ischaemia prior to irreversible infarction. We are not aware, however, of any studies of sodium imaging carried out in patients with SAH.

MRI provides a non-invasive method of imaging blood flow. It seems highly likely that in the future MRI will provide quantitative measurements of cerebral blood flow. Early recognition by MRI of low cerebral blood flow may enable one to reverse any associated neurological progression by the early use of induced hypertensive therapy.

MRI systems are now developed which permit hydrogen (^{1}H) imaging of the head and localised natural abundance phosphorus (^{31}P) and carbon (^{13}C) MRI chemical shift spectroscopy (Bottomley et al. 1984). The system permits joint assessment of anatomy, metabolism and biochemistry in the head. MRI spectroscopy may find a major application in basic medical research into SAH. MRI has been shown to be an accurate method of measuring brain pH using MRI phosphorus spectroscopy (Cady et al. 1983; Petroff and Pritchard 1983). There is evidence that reduced cerebral blood flow from vasospasm leading to brain ischaemia is associated with raised lactate and a low pH measured serially in the CSF (Voldby and Enevoldsen 1982). MRI spectroscopy studies of brain pH may therefore provide an early indication of impending reduced cerebral blood flow and brain ischaemia.

Digital Tomosynthesis

Maravilla et al. (1983) have reported on this technique and its clinical applications. In digital tomosynthesis the X-ray tube and image intensifier are moved through a single tomographic sweep during which mulptiple video images are rapidly recorded. Each individual frame projects a two-dimensional picture of the anatomy from a slightly different angle. Its potential value is in providing a better definition of three-dimensional spatial relationship of complex vascular anatomy. It may prove extremely helpful where the neck of an aneurysm and its relationship to surrounding vessels is difficult or impossible to demonstrate on conventional angiography. In AVMs its ability to demonstrate three-dimensional anatomy may aid in the identification of feeding arteries and draining veins.

I-123 Iodoamphetamine Brain Scans

A recently developed isotope is I-123, used in chemical combination with amphetamine. It is lyophilic, which enables it to pass from the bloodstream across the blood–brain barrier and enter the brain. Brain scanning with I-123 may prove a sensitive technique for determining regional ischaemia following subarachnoid haemorrhage.

Conclusion

The management of patients with SAH remains difficult, crucial and controversial. Subarachnoid haemorrhage is now a potentially curable disease, but identification of patients in the early stages is only possible by continuing education on the subject for all concerned. Successful management requires early referral to a co-ordinated team of neurologists, neurosurgeons, neuroradiologists and neuro-anaesthesiologists experienced in the condition. The latest imaging techniques outlined in this chapter will almost certainly have a major impact on the diagnosis and management of patients with SAH. Modern techniques of intravascular surgery, such as repair of the arterial wall to seal the neck of an aneurysm or obliteration of

the AVM with a catheter technique, offer new hope. Various research activities to understand the genesis of cerebral ischaemia and its therapy promise a brighter future.

References

Aaslid R, Huber P, Nornes H (1984) Evaluation of cerebrovascular spasm with transcranial Doppler ultrasound. J Neurosurg 60:37–41

Alksne JF, Smith RW (1980) Stereotaxic occlusion of 22 consecutive anterior communicating artery aneurysms. J Neurosurg 52:790–793

Auer LM (1984) Acute operation and preventive nimodepine improve outcome in patients with ruptured cerebral aneurysms. Neurosurg 15:57–66

Auer LM, Ito Z, Suzuki A, Ohta H (1982) Prevention of symptomatic vasospasm by topically applied nimodipine. In: Auer LM, Heppner F, Symon L (eds) Aneurysm surgery in the acute stage. Springer, New York, pp 297–302

Awad I, Little JR, Lucas F, Skrinska V. Slugg R, Lesser RP (1983) Treatment of acute focal cerebral ischaemia with prostacyclin. Stroke 14:203–209

Bottomley PA, Hart HR Jr, Edelstein WA, Schenck JF, Smith LS, Leue WM, Mueller OM, Redington RW (1984) Anatomy and metabolism of the normal human brain studied by magnetic resonance at 1.5 Tesla. Radiology 150:441–446

Cady EB, Costello AM, Dawson MJ, Delpy DT, Hope PL, Reynolds EO, Tofts PS, Wilkie DR (1983) Non-invasive investigation of cerebral metabolism in newborn infants by phosphorus nuclear magnetic resonance spectroscopy. Lancet I:1059–1062

Cohen R, Allen GS (1979) Cerebral arterial spasm. The role of calcium in in vitro and in vivo analysis of treatment with nifedipine and nimodipine. In: Wilkins RH (ed) Cerebral arterial spasm. Williams and Wilkins, Baltimore, pp 527–532

Debrun G, Fox A, Drake C et al. (1981) Giant unclippable aneurysms treated with detachable balloons. Am J Neuroradiol 2:167–173

Dell S (1982) Asymptomatic cerebral aneurysms—assessment of the risk of rupture. Neurosurgery 10:162–166

Drake CG (1968) Discussion of Hunt, L.E., Hess, R.M., risk related to time of surgery in intracranial aneurysms. J Neurosurg 28:19–20

Faden AI, Hallen Beck JM, Brown CQ (1982) Treatment of experimental stroke, comparison of naloxone and thyrotropin releasing hormone. Neurology 32:1083–1087

Frackowiak RSJ, Wise RJS (1983) Positron tomography in ischaemic cerebrovascular disease. Neurological clinics 1 (1):183–200. W.B. Saunders, Philadelphia

Garaway WM, Whishnant JP, Furlan AJ, Phillips LH II, Kurland LT, O'Fallon WM (1979) The declining incidence of stroke. N Engl J Med 300:449–452

Grotenhuis JA, Bettag W, Othmar Fiebach BJ, Dabir K (1984) Intracarotid slow bolus injection of nimedipine during angiography for treatment of cerebral vasospasm after SAH. A preliminary report. J Neurosurg 61:231–240

Kassell NF, Drake CG (1983) Review of the management of saccular aneurysms. Neurological clinics 1 (1):73–86. W.B. Saunders, Philadelphia

Kassell NF, Torner JC (1984) Research in progress. The international cooperative study on timing of aneurysm surgery—An update. Stroke 15:566–570

Kassell NF, Torner JC, Adams HP (1984) Antifibrinolytic therapy in the acute period following aneurysmal subarachnoid hemorrhage. J Neurosurg 61:225–230

Kean DM, Worthington BS, Firth JL, Hawkes RC (1985) The effects of magnetic resonance imaging on different types of microsurgical clips. J Neurol Neurosurg Psychiatry 48:286–287

Kistler JP (1982) Predicting symptomatic vasospasm in patients with subarachnoid haemorrhage from a ruptured saccular aneurysm. Advances in Neurosurgery, 1–5. Harvard Medical School, Dept. of Continuous Medical Education, 25 Shattuck Street, Boston, MA

Lindsay KW, Vermeulen R, Murray G, Cheah F, Hijdra A, Muizelaar JP, Schannong M, Teasdale GM, Van Crevel H, Van Gijin J (1983) A multicentre double blind controlled trial of tranexamic acid in SAH. Society of British Neurological Surgeons Handbook, Liverpool

Maravilla KR, Murray RC, Deck M, Horner S (1983) Clinical application of tomosynthesis: A preliminary report. AJNR 4:277–280

Maudsley AA, Hilal SK (1984) Biological aspects of sodium-23 imaging. Br Med Bull 40:165–166

Merory J, Thomas DJ, Humphrey PRO, du Boulay GH, Marshall J, Ross-Russel RW, Symon L, Silkha E (1980) Cerebral blood-flow after surgery for recent subarachnoid haemorrhage. J Neurol Neurosurg Psychiatry 32:214–221

Mizukami M, Kawase T, Usami T, Tazawa T (1982) Prevention of vasospasm by early operation with removal of subarachnoid blood. Neurosurgery 10:301–307

Nornes H, Aaslid R (1983) Transcranial Doppler evaluation of cerebrovascular spasms and their time course following subarachnoid haemorrhage. Abstracts of seventh European congress of neurosurgery, Brussels, p 3

Peterson EW, Choo SH, Lewis AJ (1980) Lysis of blood clot and experimental treatment of subarachnoid haemorrhage.

In: Wilkins RH (ed) Cerebral arterial spasm. Williams and Wilkins, Baltimore, pp 625–627

Petroff OA, Pritchard JW (1983) Cerebral PH by NMR (letter). Lancet II:105–106

Pinto RS, Kricheff II, De Filipp G, Flamm ES, Lin JP (1983) Vasospasm secondary to ruptured aneurysm assessment by digital intravenous angiography. Am J Neuroradiol 4:283–285

Powers WJ, Grubb RL, Baker RP, Mintun MA, Raichle ME (1985) Regional cerebral blood flow and metabolism in reversible ischaemia due to vasospasm. J Neurosurg 62:539–546

Sengupta RP, So SC, Villarejo-Ortega FJ (1976) Use of epsilon aminocaproic acid (EACA) in the pre-operative management of ruptured intracranial aneurysms. J Neurosurg 44:479–484

Serbinenko FA (1974) Balloon catheterisation and occlusion of major cerebral vessels. J Neurosurg 41:125–145

Steiner RE, Radda GK (1984) Nuclear magnetic resonance and its clinical applications. Br Med Bull 40:113–204

Suzuki J, Onuma T, Yoshimoto T (1979) Results of early operation on cerebral aneurysms. Surg Neurol 11:407–412

Tazawa T, Mizukami M, Kawase T, Usami T, Togashi O, Hyodo A, Eguchi T (1983) Relationship between contrast enhancement on computed tomography and cerebral vasospasm in patients with subarachnoid haemorrhage. Neurosurgery 12:643–648

Volby B, Enevoldsen EM (1982) Intracranial pressure changes following aneurysm rupture. Part 2: Associated cerebrospinal fluid lactacidosis. J Neurosurg 56:197–204

Weir B, Aronyk K (1981) Management mortality and the timing of surgery for supratentorial aneurysm. J Neurosurg 54:146–150

Wilkins RH (1980) Attempted prevention or treatment of intracranial arterial spasm. A survey. Neurosurgery 6:198–210

Yasargil MG, Fox JL (1975) The microsurgical approach to intracranial aneurysms. Surg Neurol 3:7–14

Subject Index